Volume 6

Pelvic Ring and Hip

EUROPEAN FEDERATION OF NATIONAL ASSOCIATIONS
OF ORTHOPAEDICS AND TRAUMATOLOGY

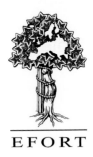

EFORT

SURGICAL TECHNIQUES
in
Orthopaedics and Traumatology

Coordinated by Professor Jacques Duparc
Honorary Chairman, Orthopaedic Department, Hôpital Bichat, Paris, France

Volume 6

Pelvic Ring and Hip

Associate Editors

Pär Slätis - Erwin Morscher
André Kaelin - Roberto Giacometti Ceroni

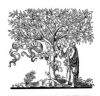

ELSEVIER

Paris, Amsterdam, New York, Oxford, Shannon, Tokyo

SURGICAL TECHNIQUES
in
Orthopaedics and Traumatology

Coordinated by Professor Jacques Duparc

In this collection:

1. General Knowledge   ISBN 2-84299-414-0

2. Spine   ISBN 2-84299-415-9

3. Shoulder   ISBN 2-84299-416-7

4. Arm, Forearm and Elbow   ISBN 2-84299-417-5

5. Wrist and Hand   ISBN 2-84299-439-6

6. Pelvic Ring and Hip   ISBN 2-84299-440-X

7. Femur and Knee   ISBN 2-84299-441-8

8. Lower Leg, Ankle and Foot   ISBN 2-84299-442-6

8 volume collection (full set)   ISBN 2-84299-443-4

Also available: the prestigious 4 volume Hardbound Package. Attractive loose-leaf binders allow continual updating. Includes quarterly updates and Internet access to the full text articles. For further information, please contact Editions Scientifiques et Médicales Elsevier or see: www.surgical-techniques-efort.com or www.elsevier.fr.

© 2003 Éditions scientifiques et médicales Elsevier SAS. Tous droits réservés. All rights reserved
23, rue Linois, 75724 Paris cedex 15, France
http://www.elsevier.fr – http://www.surgical-techniques-efort.com

Printed by SGIM, 10, rue du Parc, Parc Industriel Euronord, 31150 Bruguières, France

Bookbinding by Atenor, 11, rue de Lutèce, 78500 Sartrouville, France

Imprimé par SGIM, 10, rue du Parc, Parc Industriel Euronord, 31150 Bruguières, France

Façonnage par Atenor, 11, rue de Lutèce, 78500 Sartrouville, France

Dépôt légal N° : 03-558 - Janvier 2003   ISBN : 2-84299-440-X

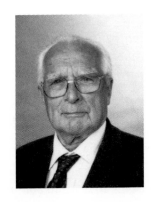

Preface

First and above all, this collection dedicated to surgical techniques in orthopaedics and traumatology is truly European.

It is published under the auspices of the European Federation of National Associations of Orthopaedics and Traumatology (EFORT), which at present groups 35 national associations. The creation of EFORT in 1992 resulted from the wish to form a European orthopaedic community. This has been made all the more important by the need to organise and standardise the training and qualifications of all European orthopaedists, according to the requirements and advice of the orthopaedic section of the European Union of Medical Specialists (UEMS).

Over the past 30 years, Europe has reclaimed its position among the leaders in the development of orthopaedics and traumatology. There has been a great deal of creativity. Among the many new contributions, we can mention the progress in osteosynthesis techniques due to the intramedullary nailing developed by Küntscher and the methods of internal fixation for fractures invented and developed mainly in Switzerland. The development of total joint replacement in the United Kingdom has revolutionised our field. Mention must also be made of the original ideas of Ilizarov, which were introduced and developed by the Italian School. We should add the Swedish National Survey of Hip and Knee Arthroplasties, initiated by the late Goran Bauer and continued by Peter Herberts, and the contributions to treatment of spinal pathology by R. Roy Camille and J. Dubousset of France. The above list is far from complete and will grow as new advances are made.

There is no doubt that Europe has an important role to play in the future of orthopaedics and traumatology.

This extraordinary growth and the development of increasingly sophisticated techniques in our field has made teaching and training more arduous. It has been suggested that the knowledge required by a general orthopaedic surgeon has increased 40 times over the past 40 years.

For all these reasons, EFORT decided to publish a collection covering the surgical techniques for all aspects of locomotor pathology in adults and children, without excluding non-operative treatment.

Thanks to the Editorial Board of EFORT, I have the honour - and also the very heavy responsibility - to be Editor of this work. For such a task, a large team was necessary, the members of which are listed at the end of this preface.

The collection is divided into eight sections, each under the responsibility of one or more Associate Editors. They have played an important part in selecting and contacting the contributing authors, in reviewing and coordinating the manuscripts. I must warmly thank these Associate Editors, who have accepted to undertake this additional work along with their surgical practice. They have played an essential role in its creation and publication.

The first section, "General Knowledge", is devoted to the general problems encountered in the practice of orthopaedic surgery: anaesthesia, prevention of deep venous thrombosis and infection, bone grafts, etc. The seven sections that follow concern the anatomical sites: the spine; shoulder; arm, elbow and forearm; hand and wrist; hip and pelvis; femur and knee; lower leg, ankle and foot.

It must be emphasised that this collection does not represent the work of a single group, school or institution, but rather results from the contributions of specialists and leaders in their fields throughout Europe. This explains its diversity. This collection is naturally written in English, which, as John Goodfellow put it, is the "new Esperanto" permitting scientific communication.

Each article must be considered as a separate entity and can be read without referring to the others. This has lead to some unavoidable overlapping, which we have tried to reduce to a minimum.

Most of the articles are devoted mainly to the surgical techniques themselves, which are described step by step and copiously illustrated. Variations of the techniques are discussed, as well as complications and clinical results. Some articles devote more discussion to the indications when this is necessary for the choice of treatment.

In general, the articles largely cover current orthopaedic practices. Most of these have already been widely tested by the orthopaedic community. Nevertheless, some articles discuss newer techniques, such as meniscal allograft transplantation, computerised pedicular screw fixation, video-assisted anterior approach to the spine, etc. It seems appropriate to include these new techniques which are already known to a large public but which have not yet been tested by time.

There are now two presentations of this collection. The first is the prestigious 4-volume, loose-leaf Hardbound Package which includes quarterly updates and access to the articles on Internet. The second, this edition, is divided into eight paperback volumes which may be purchased separately, allowing the specialised orthopaedic surgeon to select those parts of the collection devoted to his daily activities.

Many thanks to the editorial team at Elsevier - Sylvie Vercken, Agnès Brunel, Evelyne Lambert and Annabel Courage. I cannot too deeply express my appreciation to Gregg Colin for her assistance in the preparation of the manuscripts. Without her help, this publication would not have been possible.

Most of all, I would like to thank the authors and the Associate Editors who have contributed their time and their expertise to create this publication.

Jacques Duparc
Editor

The aim of EFORT, the European Federation of National Associations of Orthopaedics and Traumatology, is to promote science and education in the field of orthopaedics and traumatology.

The EFORT collection "Surgical Techniques in Orthopaedics and Traumatology", first published in 2000, was therefore a major step forward in demonstrating the great variety of European orthopaedic techniques.

Thanks to the unstinting work of Professor J. Duparc and the entire editorial board, in the short time since this collection has been launched it has attained a place in all the major European libraries. The next important step is the introduction of the new paperback edition. This will allow our orthopaedic colleagues who have specialised in a specific field to focus on one or several topics in which they are particularly interested.

On behalf of EFORT, I also want to thank the publisher, Elsevier, who accepted to join us in this editorial adventure to enhance orthopaedic operative techniques in Europe.

Nikolaus Böhler
President
European Federation of National Associations
of Orthopaedics and Traumatology (EFORT)

Patronage Committee

EFORT   Jacques Duparc, Michael A R Freeman, Erwin Morscher, Otto Sneppen, Paolo Gallinaro, Nikolaus Böhler

UEMS   Rafael Esteve de Miguel, Marc Speeckaert

Scientific Committee

Jacques Duparc, George Bentley, Henri Dorfmann, John Kenwright, Roger Lemaire, Frantisek Makai, Antonio Navarro, Panayotis N Soucacos, Nikolaus Böhler, Joachem Eulert, Frantz Langlais, Lars Lidgren, Pier Giorgio Marchetti, Wolfhart Puhl, Tibor Vízkelety

Editor

Jacques Duparc, MD, Professor
Honorary Chairman of Orthopaedic Department
Hôpital Bichat
Paris, France

Associate Editors

1. General Knowledge

Roger Lemaire, MD
Professor and Chairman
Department of Orthopaedic and Trauma Surgery
University Hospital
Liège, Belgium

2. Spine

Claus Carstens, MD
Head of Department
Paediatric Orthopaedics
Orthopaedic Hospital, University of Heidelberg
Heidelberg, Germany

Alain Deburge, MD
Professor, Department of Orthopaedics and Traumatology
Hôpital Beaujon
Clichy, France

3. Shoulder

Mario Randelli, MD
Professor
Istituto Clinico Humanitas
Milan, Italy

Jens-Ole Søjbjerg, MD, Professor
Department of Orthopaedics
University Hospital of Aarhus
Aarhus, Denmark

Jón Karlsson, MD, PhD
Department of Orthopaedics
Sahlgrenska University Hospital/Östra
Göteborg, Sweden

4. Arm, Forearm and Elbow

Norbert Gschwend, Prof Dr med
Orthopaedic Department
Schulthess Klinik
Zurich, Switzerland

Piet M. Rozing, MD
Department of Orthopaedic Surgery
Leiden University Medical Center
Leiden, The Netherlands

5. Wrist and Hand

Jean-Yves Alnot, MD, Professor
Chief of Orthopaedic Department
Upper Limb and Nerve Surgery Unit
Hôpital Bichat
Paris, France

Panayotis Soucacos, MD, FACS
Professor and Chairman
Department of Orthopaedic Surgery
University of Ioannina School of Medecine
Ioannina, Greece

6. Pelvic Ring and Hip

André Kaelin, MD
Paediatric Orthopaedic Unit
Hôpital des Enfants
Geneva, Switzerland

Erwin Morscher, MD, Professor
Felix Platter Hospital
Basel, Switzerland

Pär Slätis, MD, Professor
Orthopaedic Hospital of the Invalid Foundation – Helsinki
Grankulla, Finland

Roberto Giacometti Ceroni, MD
Istituto Galcazzi
Milan, Italy

7. Femur and Knee

Paul Aichroth, MD, MS FRCS
Emeritus Consultant Orthopaedic Surgeon
Knee Surgery Unit, The Wellington Hospital
London, United Kingdom

John Fixsen, MA, M.Chir, FRCS
Department of Orthopaedic Surgery
Great Ormond Street Hospital for Chidren
London, United Kingdom

René Verdonk, MD, PhD
Department of Orthopaedic Surgery
Ghent University Hospital,
Ghent, Belgium

Ate Wymenga, MD
Knee Reconstruction Unit
Sint Maartenskliniek
Nijmegen, The Netherlands

8. Lower Leg, Ankle and Foot

Tomás Epeldegui Torre, MD, PhD
Hospital Nino Jesus
Madrid, Spain

Nikolaus Wülker, MD, Professor
Orthopaedic Department
Orthopädische Klinik und Poliklinik
Tubigen, Germany

Table of Contents
Volume 6 - Pelvic Ring and Hip
Surgical Techniques in Orthopaedics and Traumatology

Preface

Table of Contents - Volume 6

Participating authors

Approaches to the hip and acetabulum (P Koch, R Ganz, JW Mast, M Beck, H Nötzli, S Nazarian, DL Fernandez, KA Siebenrock, B Isler, M Weber, F Hefti) 55-400-A-10

Hip dislocation and femoral head fractures (M Bircher) 55-400-B-10

Fractures of the femoral neck (A Alho) 55-400-C-10

Intertrochanteric osteotomy for nonunion of the femoral neck (RK Marti, EL Raaymakers) 55-400-D-10

Trochanteric and subtrochanteric fractures (I Kempf) 55-400-E-10

Acetabular fractures (G Zinghi, A Moroni) 55-400-F-10

Fractures and dislocations of the pelvic ring (T Pohlemann, A Gänsslen, H Tscherne) 55-410-A-10

Proximal femoral and pelvic fracture in children (A Kaelin, D Ceroni) 55-410-B-10

Dysplasia dislocation of the hip: conservative treatment and open reduction (A Dimeglio, D Moukoko) 55-410-D-10

Pelvic osteotomies in the treatment of congenital dislocation and subluxation of the hip (developmental dysplasia of the hip: DDH) (TL Vízkelety, G Szőke, JA Fixsen) 55-410-E-10

Acetabuloplasties and shelf operations (G Bollini, M Jacquemier, JL Jouve) 55-420-A-10

Chiari osteotomy of the hip (W Schwägerl, P Zenz) 55-420-B-10

The Bernese periacetabular osteotomy (M Weber, R Ganz) . . . 55-420-C-10

Legg-Calve-Perthes disease (A Catterall) 55-420-D-10

Slipped capital femoral epiphysis (H Carlioz, P Mary) 55-420-E-10

Hip deformity in cerebral palsy (JU Baumann, R Brunner) . . . 55-430-A-10

Congenital proximal femoral deficiency (JA Fixsen, FP Monsell) 55-430-B-10

Femoral neck lengthening osteotomy (FNLO) (EW Morscher, F Hefti, CC Hasler) 55-430-C-10

Classification of total hip arthroplasties (THA) (J Witvoet) . . . 55-430-D-10

The Exeter cementing technique for the femur (M Fagan, G Gie, G Heyse-Moore, A Lee, R Ling, A Timperley) 55-430-D-20

Tribology of hip joint replacement (L Sedel) 55-430-E-10

Dislocations of total hip prostheses (D Huten, J Vidil, J Duparc) 55-440-A-10

Cement removal from the femoral cavity (B Bradnock) 55-440-C-10

The cementless total hip arthroplasty (G Scheller, L Jani) 55-440-D-10

Total hip replacement in congenital hip disease (G Hartofilakidis, T Karachalios) 55-440-E-10

Total hip arthroplasty for ankylosed hips (M Kerboull, L Kerboull, M Hamadouche) 55-450-A-10

Classification and treatment methods of acetabular deficiencies (EW Morscher, R Elke, B Berli) 55-450-B-10

Acetabular reconstruction with impacted bone grafting and cement (TJJH Slooff, BW Schreurs, JWM Gardeniers, P Buma) 55-450-D-10

Acetabular revision with armature, allografts and cemented prosthesis (M Kerboull, L Kerboull) 55-450-E-10

Femoral revision with impaction cancellous allografting (G Gie, RSM Ling, J Timperley) 55-460-A-10

Revision total hip replacement: transfemoral approach and noncemented implantation (H Wagner, M Wagner) . . . 55-460-B-10

Revision of failed femoral prostheses: transfemoral approach and cementless distally-locked stem (C Picault, P Vives) . . . 55-460-B-20

The infected hip prosthesis (A Lortat-Jacob) 55-460-C-10

Hip joint resection (A Lortat-Jacob) 55-460-D-10

Arthrodesis of the hip (A Lortat-Jacob) 55-460-E-10

Osteotomies of the upper femur: varisation, valgisation, derotation (ME Müller) 55-470-A-10

Osteonecrosis of the femoral head (P Gallinaro, A Massè) 55-470-B-10

Resection of periacetabular tumours (Segment II) and reconstruction (R Kotz, R Windhager) 55-470-C-10

Resection of ischiopubic tumors (pelvic region 3) (N Fabbri, M Mercuri, M Campanacci) 55-470-D-10

Hip rotationplasty (W Winkelmann) 55-470-E-10

Hip disarticulation (R Baumgartner) 55-480-A-10

Hemipelvectomy (hindquarter amputation) (W Winkelmann) . . . 55-480-B-10

Resection and reconstruction in proximal femoral malignancies (F Langlais) 55-480-C-10

Hip arthroscopy (RN Villar, A Arora) 55-480-D-10

Soft tissue coverage of trochanteric and sacral sores (C Oberlin, C Touam, N Ameur, P Greant, A Bhatia) 55-480-E-10

Index - Volume 6

Participating Authors
Volume 6 - Pelvic Ring and Hip
Surgical Techniques in Orthopaedics and Traumatology

Alho A 55-400-C-10

Ameur N 55-480-E-10

Arora A 55-480-D-10

Baumann JU 55-430-A-10

Baumgartner R 55-480-A-10

Beck M 55-400-A-10

Berli B 55-450-B-10

Bhatia A 55-480-E-10

Bircher M.................. 55-400-B-10

Bollini G 55-420-A-10

Bradnock B 55-440-C-10

Brunner R 55-430-A-10

Buma P 55-450-D-10

BW Schreurs 55-450-D-10

Campanacci M 55-470-D-10

Carlioz H 55-420-E-10

Catterall A................. 55-420-D-10

Ceroni D 55-410-B-10

Dimeglio A................ 55-410-D-10

Duparc J 55-440-A-10

Elke R 55-450-B-10

Fabbri N 55-470-D-10

Fagan M 55-430-D-20

Fernandez DL 55-400-A-10

Fixsen JA 55-410-E-10
55-430-B-10

Gallinaro P 55-470-A-10

Gänsslen A 55-410-A-10

Ganz R 55-400-A-10
55-420-C-10

Gardeniers JWM 55-450-D-10

Gie G 55-430-D-20
55-460-A-10

Greant P 55-480-E-10

Hamadouche M............ 55-450-A-10

Hartofilakidis G............ 55-440-E-10

Hasler CC 55-430-C-10

Hefti F...................... 55-400-A-10

Hefti F...................... 55-430-C-10

Heyse-Moore G 55-430-D-20

Huten D 55-440-A-10

Isler B 55-400-A-10

Jacquemier M.............. 55-420-A-10

Jani L....................... 55-440-D-10

Jouve JL..................... 55-420-A-10

Kaelin A 55-410-B-10

Karachalios T.............. 55-440-E-10

Kempf I..................... 55-400-E-10

Kerboull L................... 55-450-A-10
55-450-E-10

Kerboull M.................. 55-450-A-10
55-450-E-10

Koch P 55-400-A-10

Kotz R...................... 55-470-C-10

Langlais F 55-480-C-10

Lee AJC..................... 55-430-D-20

Ling RSM................... 55-430-D-20
55-460-A-10

Lortat-Jacob A.............. 55-460-C-10
55-460-D-10
55-460-E-10

Marti RK.................... 55-400-D-10

Mary P...................... 55-420-E-10

Massè A 55-470-A-10

Mast JW 55-400-A-10

Mercuri M.................. 55-470-D-10

Monsell FP 55-430-B-10

Moroni A.................... 55-400-F-10

Morscher EW............... 55-430-C-10
55-450-B-10

Moukoko D................. 55-410-D-10

Müller ME 55-470-A-10

Nazarian S 55-400-A-10

Nötzli H 55-400-A-10

Oberlin C.................... 55-480-E-10

Picault C..................... 55-460-B-20

Pohlemann T 55-410-A-10

Raaymakers EL 55-400-D-10

Scheller G 55-440-D-10

Schwägerl W 55-420-B-10

Sedel L...................... 55-430-E-10

Siebenrock KA 55-400-A-10

Slooff TJJH 55-450-D-10

Szôke G..................... 55-410-E-10

Timperley J 55-430-D-20
55-460-A-10

Touam C 55-480-E-10

Tscherne H.................. 55-410-A-10

Vidil J....................... 55-440-A-10

Villar RN 55-480-D-10

Vives P...................... 55-460-B-20

Vízkelety TL................ 55-410-E-10

Wagner H................... 55-460-B-10

Wagner M................... 55-460-B-10

Weber M 55-400-A-10
55-420-C-10

Windhager R 55-470-C-10

Winkelmann W 55-470-E-10
55-480-B-10

Witvoet J 55-430-D-10

Zenz P 55-420-B-10

Zinghi G..................... 55-400-F-10

Surgical Techniques in Orthopaedics and Traumatology 55-400-A-10

Approaches to the hip and acetabulum

P Koch
R Ganz
JW Mast
M Beck
H Nötzli
S Nazarian
DL Fernandez
KA Siebenrock
B Isler
M Weber
F Hefti

Abstract. – Nine surgical approaches to the hip and the acetabulum which have proved to be valuable are described. The features of each approach – its specific indications, advantages and disadvantages, limitations and risks – are pointed out. This chapter provides an overview of a selection of approaches favoured by the authors. At the beginning of each section is provided a list of recommended reference literature for the study of more detailed practical information. It is emphasised that a thorough knowledge of the surgical anatomy of the hip is of fundamental importance for a safe and optimal execution of the different approaches.

Keywords: hip, acetabulum, surgical approaches, ilioinguinal approach, anterior approach (Smith-Petersen), anterolateral approach (Watson-Jones), transgluteal approach, transtrochanteric approach, trochanteric flip approach, posterior approach (Kocher-Langenbeck), transfermoral approach to the femur, inferior approach (Ludloff).

Introduction [1, 11, 14, 16]

Surgical approaches to the hip provide the necessary exposure to accomplish the desired surgical plan. No single approach is useful for all hip pathology and combined simultaneous approaches are only required for complex problems. Each approach has specific indications, advantages and disadvantages, limitations and risks.

We provide an overview of the various approaches to the hip and the acetabulum which have been proven to be valuable and

P Koch, M.D., Maurice E. Müller Foundation for Continuing Education, Research and Documentation in Orthopaedic Surgery, Murtenstrasse 35, CH-3001 Bern; Orthopädische Abteilung, Lindenhofspital, CH-3012, Bern, Switzerland.
R Ganz, M.D., Professor, Klinik für Orthopädische Chirurgie, Universität Bern, Inselpital, CH-3010 Bern, Switzerland.
JW Mast, M.D., Professor, Department of Orthopaedic Surgery, Wayne State University, Hutzel Hospital, Detroit, USA.
M Beck, M.D., Klinik für Orthopädische Chirurgie, Universität Bern, Inselpital, CH-3010 Bern, Switzerland.
H Nötzli, M.D., Orthopädische Universitätsklinik, Balgrist, CH-8008 Zürich, Switzerland.
S Nazarian, M.D., Professor, Service d'orthopédie traumatologique et chirurgie vertébrale, Centre hospitalier régional et universitaire de Marseille, Hôpital de la Conception, F-13385 Marseille, France.
DL Fernandez, M.D. P.D., Associate Professor of Orthopaedic Surgery, Orthopädische Abteilung, Lindenhofspital, CH-3012 Bern, Switzerland.
KA Siebenrock, M.D., Klinik für Orthopädische Chirurgie, Universität Bern, Inselpital, CH-3010 Bern, Switzerland.
B Isler, M.D., Orthopädische Chirurgie, Kantonsspital, CH-8401 Winterthur, Switzerland.
M Weber, M.D., Klinik für Orthopädische Chirurgie, Universität Bern, Inselpital, CH-3010 Bern, Switzerland.
F Hefti, M.D., Professor, Kinderorthopädische Universitätsklinik, Kinderspital, CH-4005 Basel, Switzerland.

point out their special features. For more detailed practical information, it is necessary to study the reference literature given at the beginning of each section. We emphasise that a thorough knowledge of the surgical anatomy of the hip is of fundamental importance for a safe and optimal execution of the different approaches.

Ilioinguinal approach[(1)]

[7, 14]

FEATURE

This surgical approach develops intermuscular intervals allowing direct access to the anterior column of the acetabulum through three anatomic windows and indirect access to the posterior column through the second window.

INDICATIONS

– Fractures of the anterior wall or column.

– Certain fractures that associate dominant anterior column with posterior column patterns.

ADVANTAGES

An extensile anterior approach, it allows good access to fractures of the pelvic ring

[(1)] JW Mast

from the sacroiliac joint posteriorly to the pubic symphysis. Combination is possible with the iliofemoral approach. Recuperation from the operation is rapid and complete, as postoperatively the intervals close naturally, and the investing fascia layers may be closed anatomically and securely.

DISADVANTAGE

A propensity for myositis ossificans, but this is rare and, when present, remote from the articular surface.

RISKS

Postoperative impairment of the lateral femoral cutaneous nerve of the thigh is a common occurrence. Less commonly, imprecise closure of the floor of the inguinal canal may allow an inguinal hernia to occur. Rarely, intimal or direct injuries to the iliac or femoral vessels may occur as a result of a direct injury by dissecting instruments, or more commonly indirectly, through retraction. The most common vascular complication is that of an insidious thrombosis of the femoral artery which must be avoided by extreme care when operating through the second window of the wound.

TECHNIQUE

The patient is in the supine position.

The skin incision curves from the anterior superior iliac spine concavely upward and

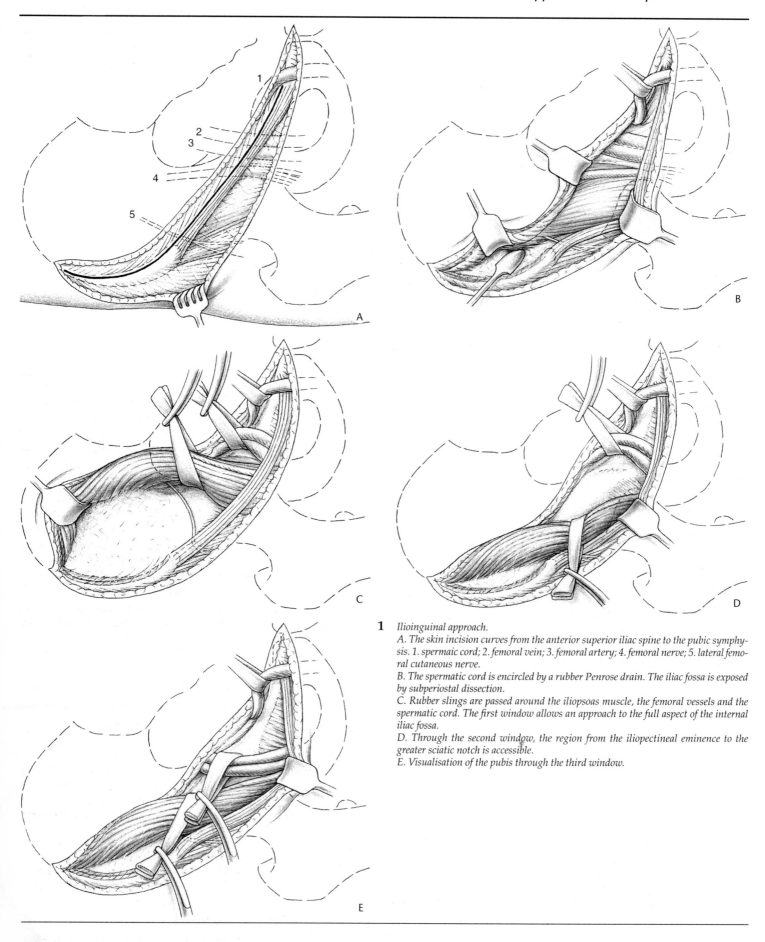

1 *Ilioinguinal approach.*
A. The skin incision curves from the anterior superior iliac spine to the pubic symphysis. 1. spermaic cord; 2. femoral vein; 3. femoral artery; 4. femoral nerve; 5. lateral femoral cutaneous nerve.
B. The spermatic cord is encircled by a rubber Penrose drain. The iliac fossa is exposed by subperiostal dissection.
C. Rubber slings are passed around the iliopsoas muscle, the femoral vessels and the spermatic cord. The first window allows an approach to the full aspect of the internal iliac fossa.
D. Through the second window, the region from the iliopectineal eminence to the greater sciatic notch is accessible.
E. Visualisation of the pubis through the third window.

medially to reach the midline just proximal to the pubic symphysis (*fig 1A*). The incision is deepened until the fascia overlying the iliac crest and the aponeurosis of the external oblique is encountered. The round ligament/spermatic cord is found emerging from the external inguinal ring and is encircled by a rubber Penrose drain.

The conjoint insertion and origins of the abdominal muscles and hip abductor muscles are incised along the iliac crest. The internal iliac fossa is exposed by subperiostal dissection of the iliacus muscle with a periosteal elevator *(fig 1B)*. The external oblique is incised 1 cm proximal to the external ring including the decussation of its fibres with the anterior sheath of the rectus abdominus. The distal leaf of the aponeurosis of the external oblique is retracted distally along with the distal leaf of the anterior sheath of the rectus abdominus muscle. The junction of the origins of the conjoint tendon of the internal oblique and the transversus abdominus from the inguinal ligament is identified. The Penrose drain is replaced around the spermatic cord/round ligament internal to the external inguinal ring so that retracting it upward exposes the floor of the inguinal canal *(fig 1B)*.

An incision is then made through the common origins of the internal oblique and transversus abdominus at the edge of the inguinal ligament, leaving 2-3 mm of fascial margin to facilitate wound closure. The dissection opens the anterior aspect of the psoas sheath exposing the iliopsoas muscle and the femoral nerve. After retracting the spermatic cord/round ligament upward, the incision is continued medially through the transversalis fascia overlying the vascular sheath of the common femoral vessels. The exposure is continued through the floor of the inguinal canal by incising the conjoint tendon and insertion of the rectus abdominus on the body of the pubis.

Between the medial border of the iliopsoas muscle and the common femoral artery, the iliopecineal fascia is prepared and incised to the iliopectineal eminence, and then along the pelvic brim as far posterior as the region of the sacroiliac joint. The periosteum is elevated from the pelvic brim and down the quadrilateral plate to the edge of the greater sciatic notch inferiorly. A periosteal elevator is used to strip the periosteum and pectineus muscle from the superomedial surface of the pubic ramus. Occasionally, the obturator artery, vein, or both may have an anomalous origin and have a direct communication from the obturator canal to the common femoral vessels. This relatively rare configuration was referred to historically as the "corona mortis". If encountered, it should be isolated, tied and cut to allow full mobilisation of the soft tissues in the region of the "windows".

Large rubber slings are then passed around the iliopsoas muscle and the femoral vessels *(fig 1C)*. Dissection at the base of the pubic ramus exposes the obturator nerve and vessels, and by medial retraction of these structures and the spermatic cord, the anterior border of the obturator canal in the region of the cotyloid notch along the anterior aspect of the quadrilateral plate *(fig 1D)*.

The exposure as developed gives a full visualisation through the first wound interval of the entire inner aspect of the internal iliac fossa, including the sacroiliac joint and lateral 1 cm of the sacrum, the pelvic brim, and inferiorly, the sciatic buttress anterior to the angle of the greater sciatic notch and inferiorly to the ischial spine *(fig 1C)*. Through the second window, the iliopectineal eminence and anterior margin of the obturator foramina along with the quadrilateral plate posteriorly to the greater sciatic notch are accessible *(fig 1D)*. Through the third window, access is possible to the root of the pubic ramus including, inferiorly, the obturator canal, the pubic ramus, tubercule, body and pubic symphysis *(fig 1E)*.

Anterior approach (Smith-Petersen) – iliofemoral extension[2]

[9, 11, 19]

FEATURE

This is an anterior approach to the hip joint and the upper part of the pelvis exploiting the internervous plane between the sartorius and rectus muscles with the femoral nerve, and the tensor and gluteus medius and minimus muscles with the superior gluteal nerve *(fig 2A)*.

INDICATIONS

– Open reduction of congenital dislocation of the hip, pelvic osteotomies (Salter, Pemberton, Chiari, periacetabular, shelf arthroplasty).

– Hip fusion.

– ORIF (Open reduction with internal fixation) of certain acetabular fractures (anterior column lateral to the iliopectineal eminence, transverse fractures, certain T-shaped fractures).

– ORIF of femoral head fractures.

– Hip joint revision (acetabular labrum, intraosseous ganglion, intra-articular tumor).

ADVANTAGES

– A straightforward approach in a true internervous plane.

– Excellent exposure to the anterior and lateral parts of the hip joint.

Possible extension:

– posteriorly along the iliac crest externally and/or internally (with osteotomy of the anterior superior iliac spine).

– distally (along the anterolateral aspect of the thigh in the lateral interval between vastus lateralis and rectus).

---

(2) M Beck

DISADVANTAGES

– Long lasting abductor weakness, when extended to the external iliac wing.

– Broad scar in the distal part of the incision, if extended to the external side.

RISKS

– Damage to the lateral femoral cutaneous nerve with consecutive paraesthesia of the lateral aspect of the thigh.

– Ectopic ossifications anterior and lateral of the hip joint capsule.

– Abductor morbidity and weakness.

TECHNIQUE

The patient is in the supine position.

The skin incision follows the anterior half of the iliac crest to the anterior superior iliac spine, from there curving distally and laterally *(fig 2B)*.

Careful dissection through the subcutaneous fat to avoid cutting the lateral femoral cutaneous nerve. Incision of the fascia on the medial aspect of the tensor *(fig 2C)*.

Detachment of the tensor and partial detachment of the gluteus medius from the iliac crest and wing, retraction of the tensor laterally and the sartorius medially *(fig 2D)*.

Detachment of the direct and reflected head of the rectus femoris, retraction of the rectus medially.

Incision of the deep (innominate) fascia underneath the rectus and ligation of the ascending branch of the lateral femoral circumflex artery.

Exposure of the joint by careful release of the iliopsoas (iliaco-capsular muscle), partly attached to the anteroinferior aspect of the joint capsule *(fig 2E)*.

■ *Extension*

Further detachment of the gluteus medius and minimus from the iliac wing to expose the outer aspect of the innominate bone *(fig 2E)*.

Osteotomy of the anterior superior iliac spine with detachment of the origin of the sartorius muscle and the inguinal ligament *(fig 2F)*. Detachment of the external oblique, internal oblique and iliacus to expose the internal iliac fossa and the iliopectineal eminence, as well as the joint capsule *(fig 2G)*. Anterior capsulotomy and surgical hip dislocation by external rotation *(fig 2H)*.

■ *Closure*

Refixation of the osteotomy of the iliac spine by means of a screw and transosseous reattachment of the musculature to the iliac crest.

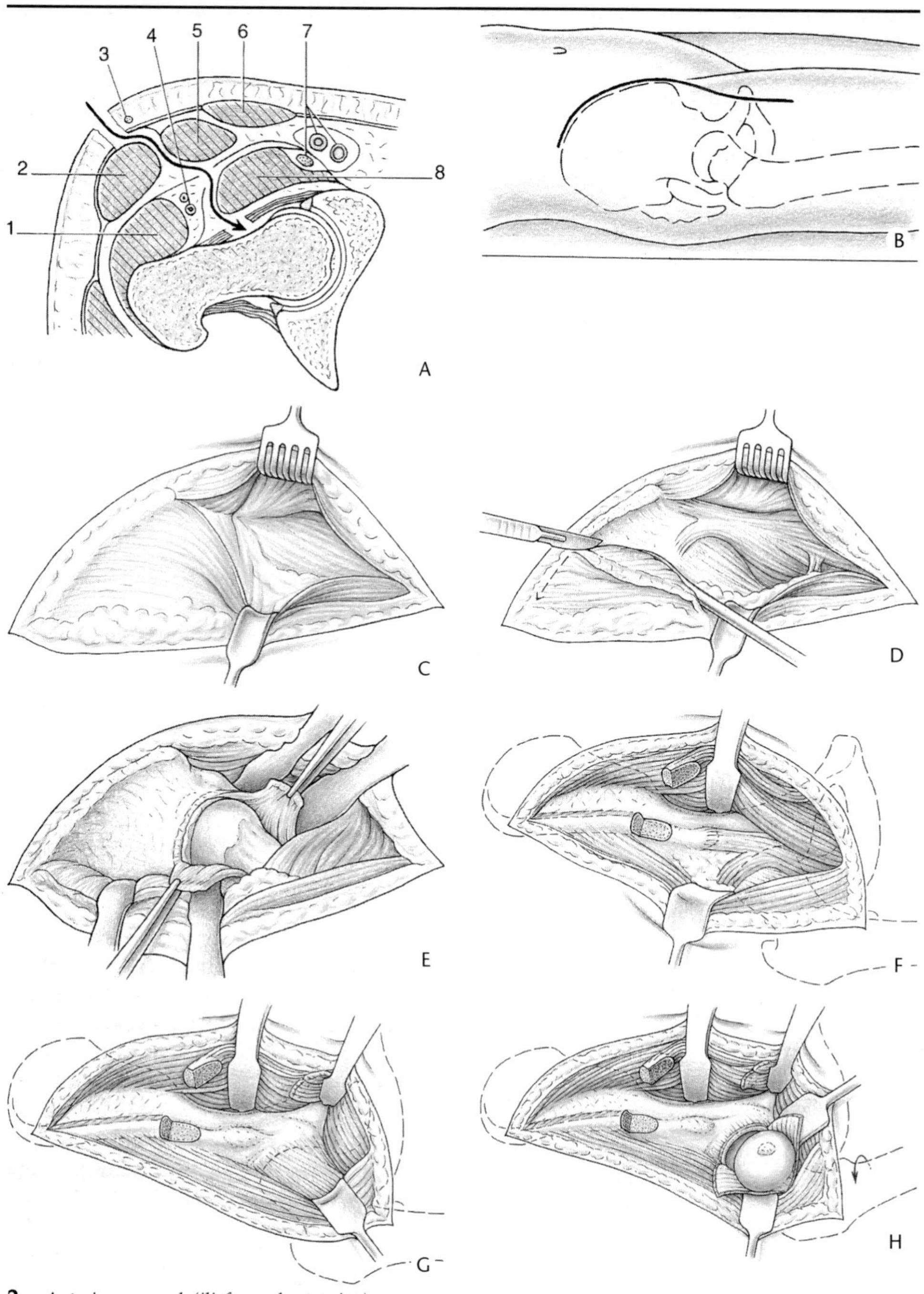

2 *Anterior approach (iliofemoral extension).*
A. Anterior approach to the hip joint. 1. gluteus medius muscle; 2. tensor fasciae latae muscle; 3. lateral femoral cutaneous nerve; 4. lateral circumflex femoral artery; 5. rectus femoris muscle; 6. sartorius muscle; 7. femoral nerve, artery, vein; 8. iliopsoas.
B. Patient in supine position. The skin incision follows the anterior half of the iliac crest, curving distally and laterally.
C. Incision of the fascia on the medial aspect of the tensor muscle.
D. Detachment of the tensor fasciae latae muscle and partially of the gluteus medius muscle from the iliac crest.
E. Exposure of the outer aspect of the innominate bone. Anterior joint capsule widely incised.
F. Detachment of the sartorius muscle and the inguinal ligament by osteotomising the anterior superior iliac spine.
G. Exposure of the internal iliac fossa and the joint capsule.
H. Surgical dislocation of the hip by external rotation.

Anterolateral approach (Watson-Jones)(3) [1, 22]

FEATURE

An approach using the anatomical interval between the gluteus medius and tensor

(3) H Nötzli

fasciae latae to reach the anterior hip capsule.

INDICATIONS

– Femoral neck fractures.

– Hemiarthroplasty and primary THA (with additional partial desinsertion of the gluteus medius and minimus on the anterior aspect of the trochanter).

ADVANTAGES

Approach follows anatomical structures.

DISADVANTAGES

Limited exposure of the proximal femur due to endangering the branches of the superior gluteal nerve crossing from underneath the gluteus medius to the tensor fasciae latae.

RISKS

– Damage to the superior gluteal nerve and denervation of the tensor fasciae latae.

– Abductor weakness due to partial desinsertion of the gluteus medius and minimus.

TECHNIQUE

The patient is in supine position with the greater trochanter overhanging the edge of the operating table.

Lateral skin incision following the femoral axis, centred over the greater trochanter and usually curved anteriorly in its proximal third toward the anterosuperior iliac spine. Equal thirds of length of the incision lie proximal to, over and distal to the greater trochanter (fig 3A).

The subcutaneous and the fascia incision follow the skin incision. In the proximal third, the fascia split is placed between the visible belly of the tensor muscle and the anterior border of the gluteus maximus. The interval between gluteus medius and tensor fascia latae is developed. Branches of the lateral circumflex vessels are ligated or coagulated. Care has to be taken not to advance far above the acetabular rim in order to avoid injury to the end branches of the superior gluteal nerve feeding the tensor muscle. By retracting the latter anteriorly and the gluteus medius muscle posteriorly, the anterior hip joint capsule is brought into view and the capsule can be progressively freed (fig 3B). The plane between the straight muscle of the thigh and the anterior acetabular rim is developed. Then, the layer between the joint capsule and the ileopsoas muscle and the ileocapsularis, respectively, is dissected. For osteosynthesis of the proximal femur, the vastus lateralis is mobilised from the capsule and the tendinous insertion at the tuberculum innominatum is incised in a L-shaped fashion. For hip arthroplasty, the tendinous insertions of the gluteus medius and minimus at the anterior aspect of the greater trochanter are incised until the underlying bursa becomes visible (fig 3C). In order not to harm the musculature during insertion of a prosthesis, a partial detachment of these muscles, preferably with an osteotome for easy reattachment, may be advisable. A T-shaped opening of the capsule can then be performed (fig 3D).

In THA, the femoral neck is osteotomised in situ or after dislocation of the femoral head

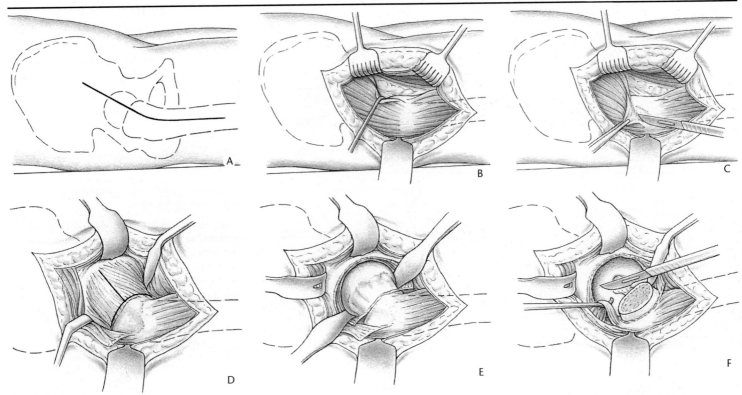

3 *Anterolateral approach.*
A. Curved anterolateral skin incision, centred over the greater trochanter.
B. Exposure of the anterior hip joint capsule.
C. Incision of the anterior part of the tendinous insertion of the gluteus medius and minimus muscle.
D. T-shaped capsulotomy.
E. Anterior capsulectomy. Femoral neck osteotomy using retractors with rounded beak for soft tissue protection.
F. Posterior capsulotomy or capsulectomy with additional cutting of the piriformis tendon.

(fig 3E). A partial or complete resection, especially of the posterior capsule, and cutting of the tendon of the piriformis muscle provide adequate mobility of the proximal femur *(fig 3F)*.

■ ***Closure***

The careful reinsertion of the detached portions of the gluteus medius and minimus muscles is mandatory, as well as the reinsertion of the vastus lateralis if detached. Fascia, subcutaneous tissue and skin are usually sutured over one subfascial drain.

Transgluteal approach[(4)]

[2, 6, 15]

FEATURE

A lateral direct approach to the hip through a longitudinal division of the gluteus medius and vastus lateralis in the direction of their musculotendinous fibres allowing to maintain the anatomical continuity of these muscles and their function.

INDICATIONS

Hemiarthroplasty, primary and revision THA.

---

(4) S Nazarian

ADVANTAGES

– Patient in supine or lateral decubitus.

– Spares the musculotendinous longitudinal continuity between the glutei and vastus lateralis muscles, and therefore facilitates the postoperative rehabilitation.

– Spares the gluteal nerves and vessels.

– Optimal exposure of the acetabulum and proximal femur.

DISADVANTAGES

– Transitory weakness of abductor muscles.

– Limitation in revision surgery in case of extended bone loss.

RISKS

– Ectopic ossification in glutei muscles on greater trochanter.

– Loss of the continuity of the musculotendinous fibres by careless detachment of the tendinous junction of the three muscles.

– Damage of the neurovascular pedicle between the gluteus medius and minimus, if its position is not recognised.

TECHNIQUE

The patient is in the supine or lateral decubitus position.

The skin incision is straight and centred over the middle of the projection of the greater trochanter *(fig 4A)*. Its length depends on the thickness of the subcutaneous tissue (usually 15 to 20 cm, of which 1/3 above and 2/3 below the tip of the greater trochanter).

The incision of the gluteal fascia is straight and in the axis of the fibres, centred at the projection of the greater trochanter. Its supratrochanteric segment passes between the sheath of the tensor fasciae latae in front and the gluteus maximus behind.

The transgluteal incision is a longitudinal division of the gluteus medius and vastus lateralis muscles in the direction of their fibres. The line of division is centred at the middle of the greater trochanter, equidistant between its anterior and posterior borders. The neurovascular bundle is located at 3 to 5 cm above the tip of the greater trochanter. So the supratrochanteric part of the incision should not extend beyond 3 cm above this tip; it is carried out by introducing the scissors through the lower fibres of the gluteus medius and opening them in the direction of these fibres. The aim of this approach is to reach directly the anterior and cranial aspects of the joint, getting behind the anterior musculotendinous strap resulting from the incision, of which the continuity must be preserved. This anterior musculotendinous strap can be schematised as a digastric muscle complex including a cranial belly, an intermediate tendon and a

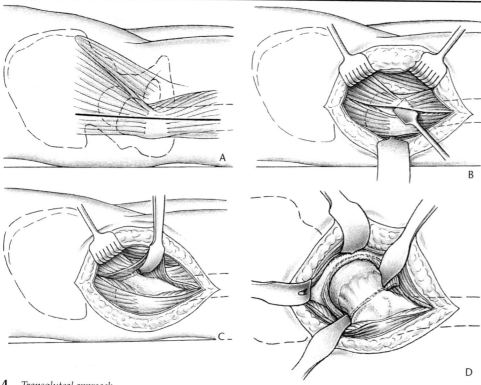

4 *Transgluteal approach.*
A. Straight lateral skin incision over the greater trochanter.
B. Disinsertion of the intermediate tendon from the anterior part of greater trochanter.
C. Visualisation of the capsule.
D. Exposure for femoral neck osteotomy.

caudal belly. The cranial belly includes the anterior fibres of the gluteus medius and the gluteus minimus. The caudal belly is formed by the anterior fibres of the vastus lateralis. The intermediate tendon results from the fusion of the tendinous fibres of the three muscles and is inserted on both the lateral and anterior aspects of the greater trochanter.

Once the anterior part of the vastus lateralis is detached from the femur and maintained anteriorly by a retractor, the intermediate tendon is very meticulously disinserted from the anterior part of the lateral aspect of greater trochanter and then from its anterior aspect (*fig 4B*). The disinsertion of the fibrotendinous junction is the cardinal step in this approach, as the preservation of its integrity is the condition of the effective use of this approach. This continuity may be maintained by various technical procedures imposed by the presence of Sharpey's fibres. Once the inner part of the tendon is detached from the anterior aspect of the greater trochanter, the gluteus minimus can be stripped off the capsule, and this cleavage can be performed from below upwards by means of a sharp rasp which breaks up the tendinous expansions to the capsule (*fig 4C*). However, anteriorly the gluteus minimus is not the only precapsular structure. To reach the anterior margin of the acetabulum and insert an angled retractor on it, it is still necessary to detach the rectus femoris from the capsule and especially to strip off the most lateral fibres of the iliacus muscle (the so-called iliocapsularis), which are inserted

directly onto the anterior aspect of the capsule, just in front of the femoral head. This procedure frees the capsule as far as the cranial aspect of the acetabular rim. After T-shaped opening of the anterior capsule, the femoral neck osteotomy is performed, protecting the underlying structures by retractors having a long and rounded peak (*fig 4D*). A posterior acetabular retractor can easily be placed once the head and the neck are removed. A perfect exposure is then allowed, using 3 or 4 retractors.

The closure of the incision is simple, the two margins of gluteus medius and vastus lateralis coming in contact with each other. Transosseous reattachment of the fibrotendinous junction at its anatomical site of insertion reinforces the interrupted suture of the two margins of the incision.

Transtrochanteric approach[5] [3, 4, 23]

FEATURE

Trochanteric osteotomy provides a wide exposure of the acetabulum, posterior column, posterolateral iliac wing and proximal femur, since it allows easy and atraumatic separation of the abductors and external rotator muscles proximally.

_____
[5] DL Fernandez

INDICATIONS

The transtrochanteric approach is rarely used, since other approaches are equally adequate for most reconstructive hip procedures. However, it is still clearly indicated in:

– Primary hip arthroplasty with important varus deformity after a previous intertrochanteric osteotomy for which a rebalance of the abductor muscles is mandatory.

– Primary total hip arthroplasty in CDH with high dislocation.

– Revision hip arthroplasty (revision of the acetabular component without removal of the femoral head, extensive scarring due to several previous operations, ectopic periacetabular ossification or recurrent total hip dislocation).

– Intertrochanteric osteotomies when a substantial correction of the neck angle and/or flexion-extension is planned.

– Fractures of the posterior column with posterior or lateral wall comminution in which a trochanteric slide approach would give slightly less exposure to the anterolateral iliac wing due to the maintenance of the continuity of the anterior gluteus medius and vastus lateralis.

ADVANTAGES

– Wide exposure of the posterior column, hip joint, and posterolateral iliac wing.

– The trochanteric osteotomy allows improvement of the abductor lever arm by trochanteric repositioning (lateral and/or distal displacement).

– Prevention of trochanteric avulsion in osteoporotic bone during surgery.

DISADVANTAGES

The transtrochanteric approach implies additional surgery for osteotomy and refixation of the greater trochanter (time, blood loss).

RISKS

Potential nonunion with a significant proximal migration of the greater trochanter and metal-induced trochanteric bursitis are known complications.

TECHNIQUE

The patient is in the supine or lateral position.

The skin incision is lateral, straight or slightly curved posteriorly.

After longitudinal incision of the fascias, the anterior and posterior borders of the gluteus medius and minimus are visualised. The tip

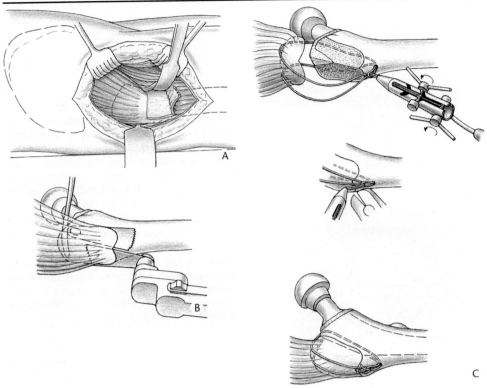

5   *Transtrochanteric approach.*
A. L-shaped detachment of the vastus lateralis at the greater trochanter.
B. A chevron biplanar osteotomy is performed using an inserted saw plate for orientation.
C. Refixation of the gluteal muscle with a simple tension band wire tightened by turning the cranks. The cerclage is fixed by simply bending the wire under tension.

of the greater trochanter is found in the anterior aspect of the gluteus medius muscle with a blunt tip elevator. An L-shaped detachment of the vastus lateralis at the greater trochanter is carried out (*fig 5A*). An anterior cut of a chevron biplanar osteotomy is made by externally rotating the leg, followed by the second cut in internal rotation. A free saw blade is inserted in the anterior cut to facilitate completion of the posterior cut at a convex angle of approximately 120° (*fig 5B*). The muscles are then reflected superiorly from the hip capsule and lateral ilium. Superior exposure is limited by the superior gluteal pedicle and by the superior gluteal nerve branch to the tensor anteriorly. The short external rotators are usually detached with this approach, but this is not obligatory, unless exposure of the ischium is necessary. Detachment with the piriformis insertion is, however, indicated if preoperative limitation of internal rotation is present. The capsulotomy may be performed posteriorly, superiorly or anteriorly. The hip can be dislocated anteriorly or posteriorly.

The chevron type of trochanteric osteotomy optimises healing due to its larger contact surface, and provides good rotation stability, therefore allowing refixation with a simple tension band wire (*fig 5C*). If the trochanter fragment splits longitudinally during the procedure, an additional transverse compression wire is recommended.

Trochanteric flip approach(6) [12, 18]

FEATURE

This approach maintains the anatomical continuity of gluteus medius and minimus and vastus lateralis muscles together with the osteotomised greater trochanter.

INDICATIONS

– Joint preserving surgery for various hip pathologies.

– Acetabular fractures, especially with posterosuperior involvement.

– Difficult primary total hip arthroplasty requiring a wide exposure.

– Revision total hip arthroplasty.

ADVANTAGES

The trochanteric flip approach provides a wide exposure to the hip joint. There is less risk of cranial migration of the reattached greater trochanter than after performing a classical trochanteric osteotomy. There is also a low nonunion rate of the greater trochanter.

DISADVANTAGE

Limited weight-bearing is necessary until the greater trochanter has healed.

(6) KA Siebenrock

RISKS

A trochanteric osteotomy performed too medially endangers the blood supply to the femoral head (the ascending branch of the medial femoral circumflex artery).

TECHNIQUE

The patient is in the lateral decubitus position.

Skin incision: straight lateral (*fig 6A*).

Proximally, the interval between the gluteus medius and tensor fascia lata muscle is split. Distally, the fascia lata is incised longitudinally. The posterior border of the gluteus medius muscle and the vastus lateralis muscle is identified with the leg in internal rotation (*fig 6B*). The vastus lateralis is incised and elevated at its posterior border. A plane osteotomy is performed with an oscillating saw. To prevent the osteotomy from being too medial and thereby risking damage to the medial femoral circumflex artery, a small part of the most posterior portion of the gluteus medius tendon has to remain initially attached to the proximal femur (*fig 6C*). After the osteotomy, these fibres are eventually cut sharply, allowing the trochanteric fragment to be flipped anteriorly. The osteotomy runs lateral to the insertion of the short external rotators, which remain attached to the proximal femur (*fig 6D*). The ascending branch of the medial femoral circumflex artery crosses posterior to the obturator externus tendon and runs cranially, anterior to the remaining external rotators. The trochanteric fragment is further mobilised anteriorly by releasing the gluteus minimus and vastus lateralis muscles from the underlying capsule and bone. This is facilitated by putting the leg in progressive external rotation and flexion. Wide exposure of the hip capsule is provided. A Z-shaped capsulotomy is performed with the proximal limb adjacent to the acetabulum and the distal limb adjacent to the femur (*fig 6E*). With the leg brought into external rotation, adduction and flexion, the femoral head will subluxate or dislocate completely anteriorly. Complete dislocation will provide exposure to the femoral head and the entire acetabulum (*fig 6F*).

Exposure of the pelvic bone posterior and superior to the hip joint will be obtained with the leg in internal rotation and extension, and gentle retraction of the external rotator muscles.

■ *Closure*

Reattachment of the greater trochanter can be done with cerclage wires or non-absorbable sutures in osteoporotic bone, or with cortical screws in good bone.

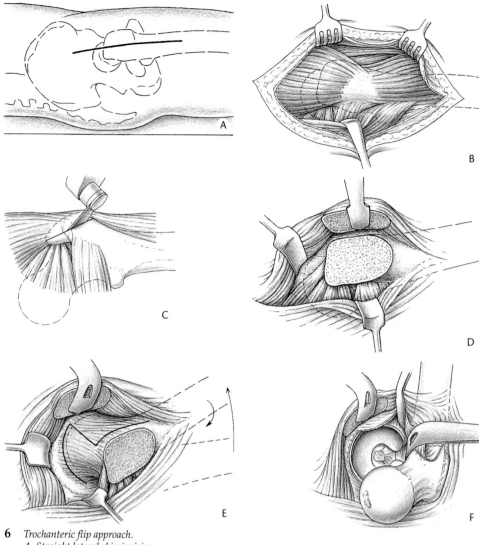

6 *Trochanteric flip approach.*
A. Straight lateral skin incision.
B. The posterior border of the gluteus medius muscle is identified.
C. A mid-trochanteric plane osteotomy is performed.
D. The short external rotators remain attached to the proximal femur.
E. A Z-shaped capsulotomy is carried out with the distal limb adjacent to the femur anteriorly.
F. Exposure of the femoral head and the entire acetabulum.

The fascia lata is split in the iliotibial tract along its fibres and continued proximally into the fibres of the gluteus maximus muscle in the direction of, and to within 8 cm from, the posterior superior iliac spine. The osseous insertion of the gluteus maximus is visualised and can be divided if necessary.

After development of the subgluteal space, the following structures can be identified: the greater trochanter, the posterior border of the gluteus medius, the piriformis, the triceps coxae (obturator internus and gemelli), the quadratus femoris, the sciatic nerve and the vastus lateralis (*fig 7B*).

For the deep dissection, the piriformis tendon is divided and the piriformis muscle is reflected, thus exposing the greater sciatic notch (*fig 7C*). The interval between triceps and quadratus is identified and the triceps coxae is divided at a short distance from the posterior border of the greater trochanter. Within the divided triceps, the obturator internus tendon is identified and followed to the lesser sciatic notch. A blunt retractor can be placed into the lesser sciatic notch in front of the triceps muscle. The interposed muscle protects the sciatic nerve against the retractor. In this way, both the greater and the lesser sciatic notches, the retroacetabular surface and the posterior aspect of the hip joint capsule are exposed. The posterior borders of the gluteus medius and minimus can only be mobilised to a very limited extent without damage to the musculature. If more exposure is needed in the supra-acetabular region, the trochanter-flip extension can provide it without injury to the hip abductors.

The hip joint capsule can be incised along the acetabular rim in its posterior circumference. The joint can be distracted, inspected or even dislocated, if necessary.

Closure is simple by suturing the capsule, suturing the piriformis and obturator internus tendons, suturing the osseous insertion of the gluteus maximus if it was divided, and by reapproximating the fascia lata and the split gluteus maximus.

Posterior approach (Kocher-Langenbeck)[7]
[8, 13]

FEATURE

A posterior approach to the hip joint with the possibility to expose the outer aspect of the entire posterior column. Abductors are in continuity with the femur.

INDICATIONS

– Hemiarthroplasty, THR, Revision-THR.

– ORIF of certain acetabular fractures.

– Hip joint revision after posterior dislocation.

ADVANTAGES

No detachment of hip abductors. Approach common and widely known.

DISADVANTAGE

Propensity for heterotopic ossifications.

RISKS

Femoral head circulation, insufficient refixation of the short rotators.

TECHNIQUE

The position of the patient is either prone or lateral decubitus. The hip should remain extended and the knee flexed whenever possible to avoid undue tension on the sciatic nerve.

The skin incision is angled with the angle at the tip of the greater trochanter (*fig 7A*). The superior limb is directed posteriorly toward the posterior superior spine; the inferior limb is directed along the femoral shaft.

Transfemoral approach to the femur[8] [10, 17, 21]

FEATURE

The transfemoral approach allows a wide exposure of the femoral canal and the hip joint. It elevates the anterolateral femur, preserving its blood supply and the soft tissue continuity.

INDICATIONS

– Stem loosening in a deficient proximal femur (i.e. safe anchorage of a conventional stem is impossible).

[7] B Isler

[8] M Weber

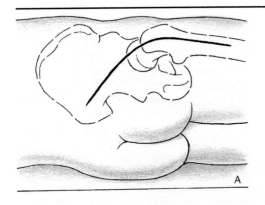

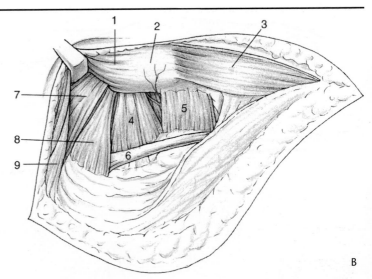

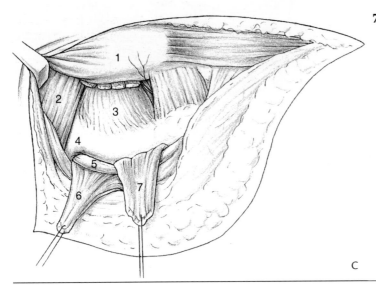

7 *Posterior approach.*
A. Curved posterolateral skin incision angled at the tip of the greater trochanter.
B. View of the posterior border of the greater trochanter and the gluteus medius muscle. The sciatic nerve has to be identified. 1. gluteus medius; 2. greater trochanter; 3. vastus lateralis; 4. triceps coxae; 5. quadratus femoris; 6. sciatic nerve; 7. gluteus minimus; 8. piriformis; 9. gluteus maximus.
C. Exposure of the posterior capsule. The piriformis and triceps coxae muscles are detached and reflected. 1. greater trochanter; 2. gluteus minimus; 3. capsule; 4. greater sciatic notch; 5. sciatic nerve; 6. piriformis; 7. triceps coxae.

– Removal of femoral components that cannot be extracted by any other means.

ADVANTAGES

Safe and rapid exposure of the medullary canal for component retrieval and debridement.

DISADVANTAGES

Reserved for revision operations where the proximal femur is destroyed, since the approach otherwise compromises the load-bearing capacity of the upper femur.

RISKS

– Technical errors result in uncontrolled propagation of fractures.

– Stripping the muscles devascularises the fragments (nonunion).

– Loss of soft tissue continuity weakens abductors.

TECHNIQUE

The patient is in the lateral decubitus position.

The skin incision is straight lateral (*fig 8A*).

The vastus lateralis is elevated from the intermuscular septum, but not off the linea aspera. According to the preoperative planning, the level of the transverse osteotomy is marked at the end of the lytic zone (*fig 8B*). With drill holes connected with a chisel, the semicircular osteotomy is performed (*fig 8C*). Using broad chisels, the osteotomy then passes along the linea aspera to proximal (*fig 8D*). At the level of the greater trochanter, the latter can either be split in half longitudinally, creating a transgluteal approach proximally, or it can be left intact and be elevated with the anterolateral femur (comparable to the trochanter flip approach). The anterior counter-osteotomy is performed at 150-180° opposite to the posterior osteotomy. A narrow chisel is inserted through the muscle and several cuts are made to create an incomplete anterior osteotomy (*fig 8E*). Alternatively, the anterior osteotomy can be performed inside-out. If the lateral fragment is very thin and somewhat elastic, it can be elevated through the posterior osteotomy, and a chisel can be passed at the side of the prosthesis to cut the anterior cortex. Proximally, the gluteus medius and minimus need to be mobilised. The osteomuscular

flap is then elevated by inserting lamina spreaders in the posterior osteotomy until the anterior osteotomy is completed and the fragment becomes mobile. Careful external rotation and adduction of the leg will further facilitate the exposure.

Closure of the approach is achieved by suture or wire cerclage. Only if the soft tissue continuity of the abductors to the femur has been lost is there a need for proximal-to-distal fixation.

Inferior approach (Ludloff)[9] [5, 10]

FEATURE

This is a simple approach to the infantile hip joint and also to the sciatic bone, requiring minimal dissection. Blood loss is minimal and it provides the most direct approach to the obstacles that prevent concentric reduction of the hip, i.e. the iliopsoas tendon, transverse acetabular ligament, and contracted inferoanterior capsule of the hip joint. It also allows a fairly

[9] F Hefti

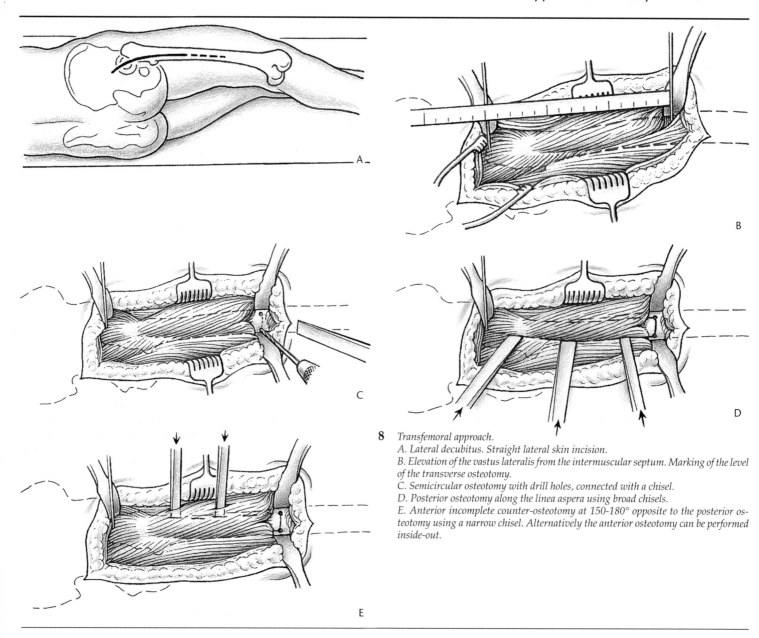

8 *Transfemoral approach.*
A. Lateral decubitus. Straight lateral skin incision.
B. Elevation of the vastus lateralis from the intermuscular septum. Marking of the level of the transverse osteotomy.
C. Semicircular osteotomy with drill holes, connected with a chisel.
D. Posterior osteotomy along the linea aspera using broad chisels.
E. Anterior incomplete counter-osteotomy at 150-180° opposite to the posterior osteotomy using a narrow chisel. Alternatively the anterior osteotomy can be performed inside-out.

good approach to the anterior (intra-acetabular) sciatic bone.

INDICATIONS

Open reduction of the hip (not in teratologic dislocation and not after walking age).

Steel-type triple osteotomy.

ADVANTAGES

Simple, good cosmetics, minimal blood loss, good approach to the iliopsoas tendon, the transverse ligament, the inferoanterior capsule of the hip joint and the anterior aspect of the sciatic bone.

DISADVANTAGES

It does not allow thorough exploration and visualisation of the hip and the joint capsule. A slightly higher risk of avascular necrosis is reported (compared to the anterior approach). Therefore, plication of the lax capsule to prevent redislocation is not feasible.

TECHNIQUE

The patient is placed in the supine position, and the ipsilateral hip, hemipelvis, and entire lower limb are prepared and draped, allowing free mobility of the limb during surgery.

Skin incision: There are two alternative skin incisions, longitudinal and transverse. We prefer the longitudinal incision because of its better cosmesis (*fig 9A*).

The iliopsoas tendon and hip joint capsule may be reached by an approach posterior to the adductor brevis, anterior to the adductor brevis and posterior to the pectineus, or anterior to the pectineus (*fig 9B*).

With the hip flexed about 60°, slightly abducted, and externally rotated, the adductor longus muscle is palpated, and a straight longitudinal incision is made immediately behind the adductor longus muscle for a distance of 8 to 8 cm (*fig 9A*). It begins at the adductor tubercle and extends distally along the course of the muscle.

The subcutaneous tissue is divided in line with the incision. The deep fascia is divided.

The anterior and posterior margins of the adductor longus muscle are delineated, and the muscle is sectioned over a blunt elevator at its origin and retracted distally. The adductor brevis muscle is retracted anteriorly, and the anterior branches of the obturator nerve and vessels are visualised but not disturbed. By blunt digital dissection, the interval posterior to the adductor brevis is developed; the lesser trochanter is easily palpated in the intermuscular interval. The iliopsoas tendon is exposed, and the fatty tissue and the bursa over the tendon are elevated. The tendon is divided by a transverse incision and allowed to retract proximally.

The pectineus muscle is retracted medially and inferiorly, and the femoral vessels and nerve are retracted laterally. Two curved retractors are placed around the femoral neck and capsule, one superolaterally and the other inferomedially to expose the capsule of the hip joint (*fig 9C*). Next, the capsule is divided by a T-shaped incision with the longitudinal limb along the long

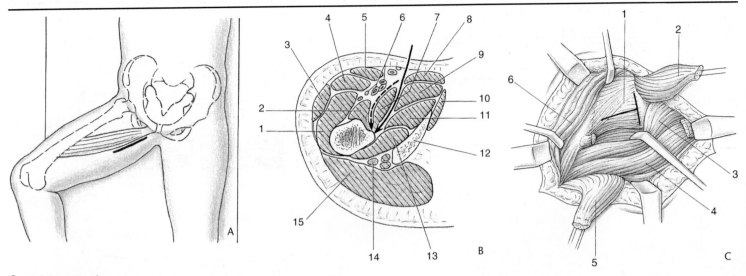

9 *Inferior approach.*
A. Straight longitudinal skin incision beginning at the adductor tubercle with the hip flexed, slightly abducted and externally rotated.
B. The medial inferior hip joint capsule may be reached by an approach posterior or anterior to the pectineus muscle. 1. vastus medialis; 2. iliopsoas; 3. tensor fasciae latae; 4. rectus femoris; 5. sartorius; 6. femoral nerve, artery, vein; 7. pectineus; 8. adductor longus; 9. adductor brevis; 10. gracilis; 11. adductor magnus; 12. ischium; 13. quadratus femoris; 14. sciatic nerve; 15. gluteus maximus.
C. Exposure of the inferior medial joint capsule, retracting the divided iliopsoas and adductor longus tendon. 1. capsule; 2. iliopsoas; 3. pectineus; 4. adductor brevis; 5. adductor longus; 6. femoral vein, artery, nerve.

axis of the femoral neck and the transverse limb along the margin of the acetabulum.

An alternative surgical approach is through a transverse oblique skin incision about 5 to 7 cm long centred over the anterior margin of the adductor longus about 1 cm distal and parallel to the inguinal crease. The deep fascia is divided. One should take care not to injure the saphenous vein, but if necessary it may be ligated and sectioned. The adductor longus muscle is sectioned at its origin and reflected distally. At the anterior margin of the adductor longus, the fibres of the pectineus muscle are identified.

One can approach the lesser trochanter by a route medial to the pectineus muscle to release the iliopsoas tendon. The pectineus muscle is retracted laterally, protecting the femoral vessels and nerve, and the adductor brevis muscle is retracted medially, bringing the iliopsoas tendon into view at its insertion to the lesser trochanter. A clamp is passed under the iliopsoas tendon and opened slightly. The tendon is then sectioned.

References

[1] Bauer R, Kerschbaumer F, Poisel S. Operative approaches in orthopedic surgery and traumatology. Stuttgart : Georg Thieme Verlag, 1987

[2] Bauer R, Kerschbaumer F, Poisel S, Oberthaler W. The transgluteal approach to the hip joint. *Arch Orthop Trauma Surg* 1979 ; 95 : 47-49

[3] Berry DJ, Müller ME. Chevron osteotomy and single wire attachment of the greater trochanter in primary and revision total hip arthroplasty. *Clin Orthop* 1993 ; 294 : 155-161

[4] Debeyre J, Duliveux P. Les arthroplasties de la hanche : Étude critique à propos de 200 cas opérés. Paris : Flammarion, 1954 : 1-91

[5] Etienne E, Lapeyrie M, Campo A. La voie d'accès interne de l'articulation de la hanche. *J Chir* 1946 ; 62 : 115-121

[6] Hardinge K. The direct lateral approach to the hip. *J Bone Joint Surg Br* 1982 ; 64 : 17-19

[7] Letournel E. Acetabulum fractures: classification and management. *Clin Orthop* 1980 ; 151 : 81

[8] Letournel E, Judet R. Fractures of the acetabulum. New York : Springer-Verlag, 1981 : 1-232

[9] Letournel E, Judet R. Fractures of the acetabulum. Berlin : Springer-Verlag, 1993

[10] Ludloff K. Zur blutigen Einrenkung der angeborenen Hüftluxation. *Z Orthop Chir* 1908 ; 22 : 272

[11] Masquelet AC, McCullough CJ, Tubiana R. Voies d'abord chirurgicales du membre inférieur. Paris : Masson, 1994

[12] Mercati E, Guary A, Myquel C, Bourgeon A. Une voie d'abord postéro-externe de la hanche. Intérêt de la réalisation d'un "muscle digastrique". *J Chir* 1972 ; 103 : 499-504

[13] Moore AT. The self locking metal hip prosthesis. *J Bone Joint Surg* 1957 ; 39 : 811-827

[14] Nazarian S, Müller ME. Voie d'abord de la hanche. *Encycl Méd Chir* (Éditions Scientifiques et Médicales Elsevier SAS, Paris), Techniques Chirurgicales - Orthopédie-Traumatologie, 44-600, 1998

[15] Nazarian S, Tisserand P, Brunet C, Müller ME. Anatomic basis of the transgluteal approach to the hip. *Surg Radiol Anat* 1987 ; 9 : 27-35

[16] Pellegrini VD, Evarts CM. Surgical approaches to the hip joint. In : Evarts CM ed. Surgery of the musculoskeletal system. New York : Churchill Livingstone, 1990 : 2735-2756

[17] Picault C. Voie d'abord transfémorale pour ablation d'implant et remplacement par la prothèse à verrouillage distal temporaire. Monographie Impact. Charnoz: Les Hortensias, 1993

[18] Schneeberger AG, Murphy SB, Ganz R. Die digastrische Trochanterosteotomie. *Oper Orthop Traumatol* 1997 ; 9 : 1-15

[19] Smith-Petersen MN. Approach to and exposure of the hip joint for mold arthroplasty. *J Bone Joint Surg Am* 1949 ; 31 : 40

[20] Wagner H. Revisionsprothese für das Hüftgelenk bei schwerem Knochenverlust. *Orthopäde* 1987 ; 16 : 295-299

[21] Wagner M, Wagner H. Der transfemorale Zugang zur Revision von Hüftendoprothesen. *Oper Orthop Traumatol* 1999 ; 11 : 278-295

[22] Watson-Jones R. Fracture of the neck of the femur. *Br J Surg* 1953 ; 36 : 787-808

[23] Weber BG. Zur Osteotomie des Trochanter major bei der Totalprothese des Hüftgelenkes. *Orthopäde* 1989 ; 18 : 540-544

Hip dislocation and femoral head fractures

M Bircher

Abstract. — Isolated hip dislocation is discussed and the early management outlined. The importance of early reduction and postoperative CT scanning is emphasised with particular reference to the need for the removal of entrapped fragments. Complications are discussed, including failed closed reduction, sciatic nerve palsy, retained bone fragments, hip instability, heterotopic ossification, avascular necrosis and osteoarthritis. The Pipkin classification of the femoral head fractures is described and the fact that it deals only with posterior dislocations is emphasised. The patho-anatomy and early management is described with special reference to the complex decision-making required to decide the surgical approach. Femoral head fractures in association with other injuries of the proximal femur are discussed, as well as the poor outcome with Pipkin Type III and type IV injuries.

Keywords: hip, dislocation, femoral head fracture, Pipkin classification.

Hip dislocation

INTRODUCTION

High energy is required to dislocate the normally stable and deeply-seated hip joint. Associated soft tissue and skeletal injuries are common. The delay before reduction strongly influences the outcome and relocation needs to be performed as an emergency [14].

POSTERIOR DISLOCATION

■ Assessment and closed reduction

Clinically, a posterior dislocation is obvious except in the grossly obese. The hip is flexed and internally rotated with shortening of the affected limb. Injury to the sciatic nerve must be assessed. An AP pelvis view will demonstrate the dislocation. Associated fractures are common. In a good quality non-rotated AP X-ray film of the pelvis, the femoral head will appear smaller on the affected side, indicating the direction of the dislocation (fig 1).

After general assessment and resuscitation, emergency arrangements should be made to relocate the hip. A general anaesthetic with

Martin Bircher, MBBS FRCS(Edin) FRCS(Eng), Consultant Trauma and Orthopaedic Surgeon. The Pelvic Unit Department of Orthopaedics, St. George's Hospital NHS Trust, Blackshaw Road, London SW17 OQT, England.

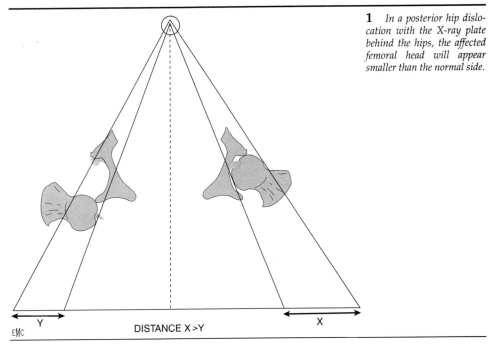

1 *In a posterior hip dislocation with the X-ray plate behind the hips, the affected femoral head will appear smaller than the normal side.*

DISTANCE X > Y

good relaxation is advised to reduce the risk of iatrogenic femoral neck fracture. Preparations must also be made to allow the surgeon to proceed to an open reduction if necessary. The reduction manoeuvre is best carried out on a radiolucent operating table under image intensification [1]. The pelvis is stabilised by downward pressure on both iliac crests.

Longitudinal traction is then applied to the affected limb in the direction the femur is held. Under progressive traction, the hip is then gently further flexed and internally rotated. In thin patients, the femoral head can be palpated in the buttock and gentle direct pressure can be applied to assist reduction. The hip should relocate with a palpable "clunk", after which the limb is carefully extended and externally rotated. Hip stability is then assessed. This is done both clinically and radiographically. In a pure dislocation, the hip will be stable in the

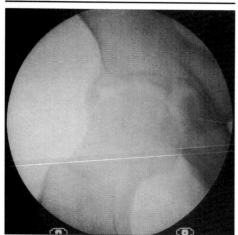

2 *Theatre image intensifier view. Entrapment of fragments. Hip standing off.*

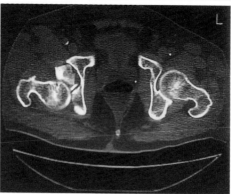

3 *CT scan of hips. Entrapment of fragments. The AP pelvis looked superficially normal, but the femoral head on the right was smaller.*

sagittal plane to 90 degrees. Incarcerated fragments and occult posterior wall injuries alter stability. Crepitus should alert the treating surgeon to the fact that associated local injuries are present *(fig 2)*. In the past, femoral or tibial skeletal traction was recommended for up to six weeks following reduction. After successful reduction, with no retained intra-articular fragments, there is no documented evidence that a period of traction alters the outcome. Light skin traction can be applied for patient comfort and the patient then mobilised within a few days as pain allows.

The period of non-weight-bearing is controversial and no firm data are available to support a prolonged weight-bearing regimen. Epstein [5] suggests weight-bearing when the pain and spasm subside.

A post operative CT scan is mandatory. Incarcerated fragments, occult posterior wall fractures with or without subluxation and impaction of the articular surfaces usually require further surgery. Plain AP X-rays at two and four weeks are sufficient to monitor stability. Patients must be followed up for between 2 to 4 years to assess femoral head viability. An MRI scan in the early postoperative period will delineate chondral bruising. The significance of these lesions is still generally unknown, and it may be possible in the future with such investigations to produce an accurate long-term prognosis. Follow-up MRI scans may alert the treating team to the development of avascular necrosis.

■ Failed closed reduction

This occurs in 2-7% of simple posterior dislocations of the hip and can be due to a torn acetabular labrum, interposition of disrupted external rotator muscles, or button holing of the femoral head through the posterior capsule. The patient can be placed on the operating room floor to allow better leverage, but an experienced surgeon should be able to recognise when closed reduction is not possible. The patient then needs to be placed either in the lateral or prone position on the operating table. A Kocher-Langenbeck incision is used. The femoral head will be obvious underneath the abductor mass. The sciatic nerve needs to be identified and protected. The hip is then washed out prior to relocation. Stability must be recorded and associated injuries dealt with as indicated.

■ Sciatic nerve palsy

A preoperative palsy is reported in approximately 8-19% of patients depending on the specific injury. The peroneal component is most commonly injured. Spontaneous recovery does occur and functional results are acceptable, although full recovery is rare. The severity of the palsy and the delay before reduction will clearly influence the outcome.

■ Retained bone fragments *(fig 3)*

These are usually associated with occult posterior wall injuries and/or femoral head fractures. They may not be recognised on ordinary X-rays. Plain films may demonstrate a loss of joint space congruence and opacities within the joint. Incarcerated bone debris requires prompt removal with copious joint lavage. The Kocher-Langenbeck approach is recommended. Chondral defects invisible on the CT scan will usually be found at surgery.

■ Posterior hip instability

Posterior instability is associated with posterior type acetabular fractures. Longitudinal tibial or femoral traction should be temporarily applied, oblique X-rays and CT scan arranged, and operative correction of the instability planned.

■ Hetertopic ossification

This can occur even after conservative treatment and appears to be more severe when associated with head injury.

■ Avascular necrosis and osteoarthritis

The quoted rate for avascular necrosis varies from 6% to 40%. It is important to distinguish between avascular phenomena and post-traumatic osteoarthritis. Severe chondral damage leads to osteoarthritis, whereas avascular necrosis is usually related to circulatory disturbances in association with simple dislocations. Simple dislocations have a higher rate of avascular necrosis than fracture dislocations [7]. It has been shown that a delayed reduction will strongly impair the outcome after dislocation of the hip. Although various times are quoted (for example 6, 12, 24 hours), common sense dictates that the hip should be relocated as soon as possible.

ANTERIOR DISLOCATION

■ Assessment and closed reduction

Isolated anterior dislocation is an unusual injury and is outnumbered by posterior dislocations in an average ratio of 1:10. This injury usually presents with extension, adduction and external rotation of the limb. In moderately sized patients, the femoral head will be palpable somewhere between the anterior superior iliac spine and the groin. In the extremely rare obturator dislocation, the femoral head will be palpable in the inner upper thigh. The lower limb in this situation is held in wide abduction. The anterior dislocation of the hip is obvious on an AP X-ray with the femoral head being larger than that on the other side. The usual preoperative work-up, as outlined for posterior dislocations, needs to be followed. A general anaesthetic is recommended and iatrogenic fracture of the femoral head and neck is a real danger. Specific reposition manoeuvres are the Allis or reverse Bigelow manoeuvre. They involve traction in line of the femur, gentle abduction and flexion, followed by internal rotation and extension. The hip will relocate with a clunk and stability is checked. Post operative X-rays and CT scans are arranged to exclude associated local injuries, and in particular intra-articular fragments. Skin traction is applied and the patient moblised, as pain allows. Regular clinical and radiological checks are made. A failed closed reduction, a progressive neurological lesion and circulatory disturbance to the lower limb, retained bone fragments and anterior instability all require further surgical investigation and treatment.

■ Complications

Early vascular compromise (femoral artery) is a concern and early exploration is

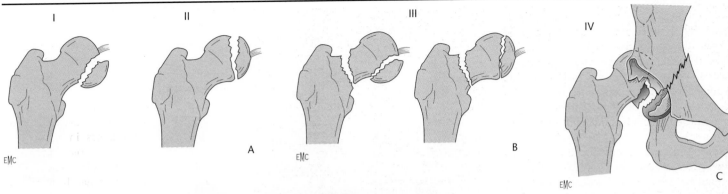

4 *The Pipkin classifiction for head fractures. Types I and II (A), III (B), and IV (C).*

required. Iatrogenic fracture of the femoral neck requires reduction and fixation. Avascular necrosis rates are lower following anterior dislocation as opposed to posterior dislocation [4, 10] due to asymmetrical femoral head circulatory anatomy. Chondral injuries predispose to the early development of osteoarthritis. The anterior Smith-Petersen surgical approach is advocated to treat irreducible dislocations. Chemical prophylaxis with indomethacin may be used in order to avoid heterotopic bone ossification.

Hip dislocation associated with femoral head fracture

INTRODUCTION

These are such unusual injuries that during an average orthopaedic surgical career only a few lesions will be encountered. Most large series are usually a combination of many surgeons' experience [11].

CLASSIFICATION

Thompson and Epstein in 1951 [12] produced a comprehensive classification of dislocation of the hip and described femoral head fractures as type V injuries. Within this type V group, Pipkin in 1957 [9] further subdivided femoral head injuries into four groups occurring in association with posterior dislocation (*fig 4*). The classification considers the femoral head fractures in relation to the fossa of the head. It should be observed, however, that the fracture also has a cleavage plane with reference to the anterior and posterior part of the femoral head (*fig 5*). Femoral head fractures do occur both in association with anterior dislocation and with more complex acetabular fractures. In rare cases, the femoral head can be fractured without actual dislocation.

SURGICAL TREATMENT

To understand the rationale for surgical treatment and, more importantly, to decide the best surgical approach, the direction of

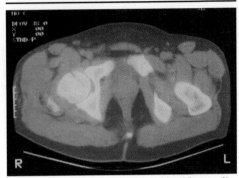

5 *Typical orientation of the femoral head fracture line following a posterior dislocation. Plain X-rays are usually very unclear.*

force, the capsular injury and the exact position of the femoral head fracture needs to be clearly understood. The advent of CT scanning has greatly improved the 3-dimensional interpretation of these injuries. By using Pipkin's classification, it is possible to assess the correct surgical approach for each of these rare and rather unique injuries. Brumback et al [2] go somewhat further in defining the injuries, but their classification has not provided more support for surgical decision-making than the Pipkin classification.

■ *Pipkin Type I injury: Posterior dislocation of the hip with fracture of the femoral head caudad to the fossa*

The femoral head injury is caudal to the fossa of the head of the femur. It is due to direct impingement of the femoral head against the acetabular rim during dislocation and relocation. Normal resuscitative measures must be adopted, the sciatic nerve assessed, and prompt arrangements made for relocation of the hip as for any isolated dislocation. An AP X-ray may not clearly show the head fragment lying within the acetabulum. Indeed, these injuries are often missed. Following successful relocation of the hip, an X-ray should be taken in theatre. This may demonstrate a concentric reduction or more rarely a blocked reduction. If the hip does not reduce, arrangements should be made for opening the joint. If the hip

reduces, gentle skin traction may be applied. A postoperative CT scan will allow accurate assessment of the fracture. If the postoperative CT scan demonstrates a small fragment off the weight-bearing surface, this fragment may well heal in a normal or slightly displaced position. However, comminution and occult chondral damage is accurately appreciated only at operation. Comminution and chondral damage may account for some of the poor results of conservative treatment of the type I injury. With reliable techniques and a better understanding of the injury, a more aggressive approach can be undertaken. Surgical procedures for type I injuries are either fragment excisions or fragment fixation. Additional benefit of surgical intervention is gained by lavage of the joint.

■ *Pipkin Type II Injury: Posterior dislocation of the hip with fracture of the femoral head cephalad to the fossa*

This is an avulsion fracture as the ligamentum teres is attached firmly to the fragment. The medial fragment attached to the ligamentum teres does not displace as in a Type I injury. Therefore, prompt relocation of the hip may result in an initial acceptable reduction. In the acute phase, rapid relocation should be performed in a standard manner. During reduction, the medial fragment may, however, turn on the ligamentum teres and block the reduction. Emergency arrangements need to be made to open the hip and relocate and fix the fragment. The proximal part of the fracture may involve a significant portion of the weight-bearing surface of the femoral head. If the fracture remains displaced, an accurate, stable anatomical fixation should be undertaken.

■ *Pipkin Type III Injury: Type I or Type II injury associated with fracture of the femoral neck*

The femoral neck injury is usually an intracapsular fracture. The blood supply to the femoral head is further jeopardised from this second insult. Although a rare injury, the prognosis for this type of fracture is poor. The Type III injury can be produced during the closed reduction of Type I and Type II fractures. A Type III injury requires operative treatment. In an elderly patient, hemiarthroplasty or total joint replacement is the treatment of choice. In the young, anatomical reduction and stabilisation of the femoral neck fracture needs to be undertaken as an emergency. If an accurate reduction of the femoral neck fracture cannot be achieved by closed methods, an open reduction of the lesion is done through an anterior approach, avoiding the posterior capsular structures. Once the femoral neck fracture is reduced and accurately fixed, attention can be turned to the femoral head fracture. In Type I injuries, excision of the fragment is advocated, and in Type II injuries, direct fixation through the chondral surface provides good stability. The time lapse from injury to surgical intervention strongly influences the outcome, and delayed treatment has a poor prognosis.

■ *Pipkin Type IV Injury: Type I or Type II injury associated with fracture of the acetabular rim*

Acetabular fracture associated with any femoral head fracture is considered a Type IV injury. The management is usually dictated by the acetabular injury. Major posterior column injuries should be approached through a Kocher-Langenbeck incision. Unlike Type I and Type II Pipkin injuries, the acetabular fracture allows better visualisation of the femoral head fracture line. Direct reduction and retrograde fixation can be more easily achieved. Small fragments of the femoral head should be excised, but large fragments should be retained and stabilised. The recent development of a Kocher-Langenbeck incision combined with a digastric slide offers an approach where the posterior column injury and the femoral head fracture can be fixed under direct vision.

COMMENTS ON THE SURGICAL APPROACHES

■ *Posterior dislocation of the hip with fracture of the femoral head*

In both Type I and Type II injuries, the fragment detached from the femoral head is anterior and medial. As one graduates from Type I or Type II injuries, the vertical component begins to encroach upon the superior weight-bearing surface of the femoral head. There are four considerations before deciding on the surgical approach:

– The state of the soft tissues.

– The direction of dislocation.

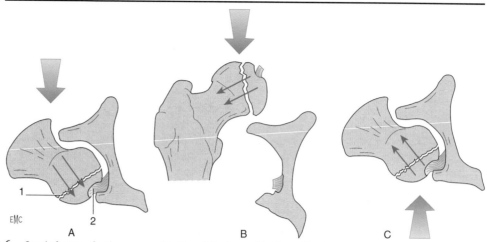

6 *Surgical approaches (open arrows) in Type II fractures of the femoral head.*
A. A posterior approach to the undislocated hip does not provide direct visualisation of the femoral head fracture. Fixation of the fragment has to be guided by an image intensifier.
B. Posterior approach with additional transection of the ligamentum teres. The fragment can be fixed (arrows) under direct visual control. Division of the ligamentum teres, however, devascularises the fragment.
C. Anterior approach. Direct visualisation and fixation of the fragment. The blood supply is retained.

– Medial fragment viability.

– The method and ease of fixation.

Epstein [6] stated that any surgical approach which impairs the blood supply to the femoral head was inadvisable. He suggested that, as the dislocation was posterior, a posterior approach should be used. His opinion, however, has not been corroborated by surgical experience. A posterior approach certainly causes less damage to the soft tissues. Yet, it is almost impossible from this approach to directly visualise fracture Type I injuries, and it can be unmanageable in Type II injuries. Further, in Type II injuries, the hip has to be dislocated in order to see the fracture of the head. This makes it impossible to relocate the medial fragment without cutting the ligamentum teres (*fig 6*). Cutting the ligamentum teres turns this into a free osteochondral graft. Although only a minor part of the blood supply to the adult femoral head comes through the ligamentum teres, it seems illogical to completely devascularise the medial fragment. For this reason, an anterior approach has been advocated. Trueta in 1957 [13] elegantly demonstrated that the blood supply provided to the femoral head via the anterior hip capsule is minimal. Type I and Type II injuries are easily approached through the anterior Smith-Petersen approach. In females, the scar can be unpleasant, and therefore a more horizontal incision can be used. The anterior hip capsule is easily identified underneath the reflected head of rectus femoris. The rectus femoris can be tagged and divided and a T-shaped capsuleotomy is performed. With gentle external rotation of the hip, the fracture will be visualised. A femoral distractor can be applied to further open the joint to facilitate visualisation. The fracture can be stabilised with Herbert type screws

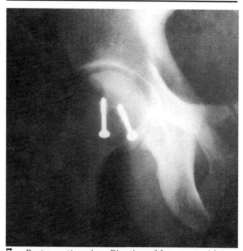

7 *Postoperative view. Fixation of fragment with two countersunk cancellous screws. Herbert screws or other small screws can be used.*

or buried with countersunk cancellous screws (*fig 7*). A small trap door can be made in the articular cartilage to allow placement of the screws in the bone. The trap door is closed after the screw head is buried. Biodegradeable rods are available, but probably do not afford enough stability. The joint should be thoroughly irrigated. There is little literature to strongly support either a posterior or an anterior approach. Swiontkowski et al in 1992 [11], in a series collected from a number of surgeons, compared 12 patients treated through a Kocher-Langenbeck approach with 12 patients treated through an anterior Smith-Peterson type approach. In the Kocher-Langenbeck group, 7 had Type II injuries and 7 had Type I fractures. Fractures of the Smith-Petersen group were equally split. Using a posterior approach, surgeons in three cases had to abandon fixation and resect the femoral head piecemeal. In another case, the posterior approach was

Hip dislocation and femoral head fractures

abandoned and an anterior approach was used to resect the fragment. Thus, in 4 out of 12 cases, the preoperative plan was altered. A further 3 cases were treated by resection. This leaves 5 cases out of the 12 where fixation was performed. In one of these 5 cases, the screws did not engage the medial femoral fragment. This demonstrates the difficulties associated with the posterior approach. There were no such technical problems encountered using an anterior approach. The operative time in the posterior approach group in the Swiontkowski series was 4.1 hours compared to 2.9 hours in the anterior approach dozen. The blood loss was also increased by 50% in the posterior group. Swiontkowski et al [11] did not report an increased incidence of avascular necrosis using the anterior approach. There was a significantly increased risk of heterotopic ossification. No prophylaxis was used, and he comments that the use of indomethacin and/or radiation may eliminate this complication. If this particular complication problem is removed from the results, then the anterior group results are significantly better than those of the posterior group. Marchetti et al in 1996 [8] studied 33 patients with femoral head fractures followed up for an average of 49 months. The results were good in 69%, fair in 18% and poor in 15%.

There were no excellent results. These figures were similar to that of the Swiontkowski series. Marchetti concluded that the Pipkin classification was a useful predictor of outcome, but could not demonstrate the advantages suggested by Brumback et al in 1987 [2]. With modern imaging techniques, the trend towards operative treatment of Type I and Type II injuries will increase. Treatment following accurate scanning and choice of the correct approach can produce good results. No significant follow-up studies, however, have so far revealed excellent results. It must therefore be concluded that a normal functional outcome after these injuries is improbable.

ANTERIOR DISLOCATION OF THE HIP WITH FRACTURE OF THE FEMORAL HEAD

Anterior dislocations are very unusual. Brumback et al [2] estimated that only 10% of femoral head fractures in the literature were associated with anterior dislocation. They are usually produced by a direct blow on an extended hip. The dislocating force may produce a deep impression or a shear fracture of the femoral head caused by impingement on the sharp anterior inferior rim of the acetabulum. De Lee et al [3] reported 12 indentation fractures in 22

anterior hip dislocations, of which 9 had adequate follow-ups. Six of these had significant evidence of post-traumatic osteoarthritis two years following injury. Thus, anterior dislocation is apt to cause severe chondral injury, and in this respect differ from the Pipkin type of fractures. The ligamentum teres is often torn, but not usually included in the fracture fragment as in Type II Pipkin injury. The damage is much more cephalad, approaching the weight-bearing portion of the femoral head. CT scanning following prompt reduction of the dislocation will delineate fracture lines and define whether or not reconstruction is possible. Removal of the debris seems logical, and if any fragments are large enough, fixation should be considered.

CENTRAL DISLOCATION OF THE HIP WITH FRACTURE OF THE FEMORAL HEAD

The central dislocation should be promptly reduced and held with tibial femoral traction. Trochanteric traction should not be used. Definitive work-up is then carried out if operative treatment is planned. The femoral head fracture can be either excised, or in very rare incidences, relocated and fixed with transchondral screws at the time of the acetabular reconstruction.

References

[1] Allis OH. The hip. Philadelphia : Dornan Printer, 1985

[2] Brumback RJ, Kenzora JE, Levitt LE, Burgess AR, Polk A. Fracture of the femoral head. In : Proceedings of the Hip Society, 1986. St Louis : CV Mosby, 1987 : 181-206

[3] Delee JC, Evans JA, Thomas J. Anterior dislocation of the hip and associated femoral head fracture. *J Bone Joint Surg Am* 1980 ; 62 : 960-964

[4] Epstein HC. Traumatic dislocation of the hip. *Clin Orthop* 1973 ; 92 : 116-142

[5] Epstein HC. Traumatic dislocation of the hip. Baltimore : Williams and Wilkins, 1980

[6] Epstein HC, Wiss DA, Cozen L. Posterior fracture dislocation of the hip with fractures of the femoral head. *Clin Orthop* 1985 ; 201 : 9-17

[7] Letournel E, Judet R. Fractures of the acetabulum. Berlin : Springer-Verlag, 1993

[8] Marchetti ME, Steinberg GG, Coumas JM. Intermediate term experience of Pipkin fracture dislocation of the hip. *J Orthop Trauma* 1996 ; 10 : 455-461

[9] Pipkin G. Treatment of grade IV fracture dislocation of the hip. *J Bone Joint Surg Am* 1957 ; 39 : 1027-1042

[10] Stewart MJ, Milford LW. Fracture dislocation of the hip. *J Bone Joint Surg Am* 1954 ; 36 : 315-342

[11] Swiontkowski MF, Thorpe M, Seiler JG, Hansen ST. Operative management of displaced femoral head fractures. *J Orthop Trauma* 1992 ; 6 : 437-442

[12] Thompson VP, Epstein HC. Traumatic dislocation of the hip. *J Bone Joint Surg Am* 1951 ; 33 : 7-46

[13] Trueta J. The normal vascular anatomy of the human femoral head during growth. *J Bone Joint Surg Br* 1957 ; 39 : 358-359

[14] Upadhyay SS, Moulton A. The long term results of traumatic posterior dislocation of the hip. *J Bone Joint Surg Br* 1981 ; 63 : 548-551

Fractures of the femoral neck

A Alho

Abstract. – Intracapsular, low-energy femoral neck fractures are best divided into nondisplaced fractures and displaced fractures with and without comminution. High-energy shearing fractures are more vertical. Preoperative radiographical findings are important for the decision about treatment.

In children and young adults, immediate internal fixation is the most effective way to guarantee the viability of the femoral head. In the elderly patient, the choice is between internal fixation and replacement with endoprosthesis.

Good reduction is more important than the choice of the fixation implant. The technique of multiple screw fixation is described here. The complications of internal fixation are wound infection, subtrochanteric fracture, early failure of fixation, nonunion, and avascular necrosis of the femoral head with late segmental collapse.

Comparative studies have been in favour of cemented, bipolar hemiendoprostheses. An active patient may benefit from total hip replacement rather than hemiarthroplasty. The technique of bipolar hemiarthroplasty is described here. Complications of endoprosthesis are femoral fractures, dislocation of the hip, component loosening, infection, heterotopic ossification and protrusion of the prosthesis head.

Because of increasing survival of the elderly, the longevity of the implant is a matter of increasing importance. The choice between internal fixation and endoprosthesis is not fully settled. The re-operation rates in long-term studies have generally varied from 15 to 40% after internal fixation, and from 7 to 17% after arthroplasty. The pertinent question is not whether to treat the displaced femoral neck fractures with internal fixation or with prosthesis replacement, but to define the criteria for choice between these two treatment modalities.

In ipsilateral fractures of the hip and femoral shaft, the treatment alternatives are locked intramedullary nailing with either separate neck screws or a cephalo-medullary nail.

© 2000, Editions Scientifiques et Médicales Elsevier SAS. All rights reserved.

Keywords: hip, fractures, femoral neck fractures, dynamic hip screw, internal fixation, hemiarthroplasty.

Introduction

Hip fracture remains a severe injury at all ages. In the elderly, the incidence is increasing in European countries. This type of fracture consumes a significant portion of health care time and resources. Efficient surgical treatment and rehabilitation are the best guarantees for restitution of function and return to the pre-injury physical and social state. In younger individuals, the injury is an even greater challenge, since retaining the femoral head is the only alternative to ensure a well-functioning joint. Most femoral neck fractures are intracapsular and subcapital, and the terms are almost synonymous.

Antti Alho, M.D., Ph.D., Professor, Chief Orthopaedic Surgeon. ORTON Orthopaedic Hospital, Invalid Foundation, Tenholante 10, 00280 Helsinki, Finland.

MORPHOLOGY

Considering the proximal shaft and neck as tubes, the neck tube is anterior to the shaft; therefore, the anatomical neck axis and anteversion line do not coincide *(fig 1)*. The line connecting the centre of the head and the centre of the proximal shaft is anteverted $15 \pm 8°$ (range 0 to 30°) in relation to the posterior femoral condylar plane. The caput-collum-diaphysis angle is $125 \pm 7°$ (110-140°).

BLOOD CIRCULATION

The collateral circulation from the anterior (lateral) and posterior (medial) circumflex arteries is rich *(fig 2)*. These arteries anastomose and send out a number of anterior and posterior retinacular branches. The posterior circumflex artery ends by penetrating into the head at the superior border of the femoral neck and head, providing intraosseous blood supply. Injury

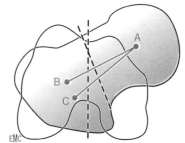

1 *Anteversion of the femoral neck. The real axis of the neck (AB) lies anterior to the centre of the proximal femoral shaft (C). Clinically, the axis is drawn from the head centre to the shaft centre (AC). The screw direction should be between the lines AB and AC.*

to this branch may be most critical for perfusion of the head. The artery of the ligamentum teres is derived from a branch of the obturator artery and participates in the perfusion of the head by 0-30% [19]. The safest way to open the capsule is by an

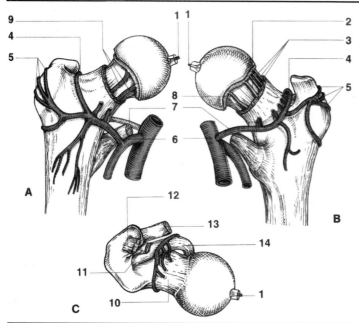

2 *Arterial circulation of the proximal femur. (Reprinted from Kempf I et al. Encyclopédie Médico-Chirurgicale. Appareil locomoteur, 14-076-A-10) 1. Artery of ligamentum teres; 2. cervical branch of posterior circumflex artery; 3. lateral epiphyseal arteries (main posterior superior branches); 4. anastomosis of the two circumflex arteries; 5. trochanteric branches; 6. anterior circumflex artery; 7. posterior circumflex artery; 8. retinacular artery; 9. retinacular artery; 10. joint capsule; 11. obturator internus; 12. gemelli; 13. piriformis; 14. obturator externus.*
  A. Anterior aspect.
  B. Posterior aspect.
  C. Superior aspect.

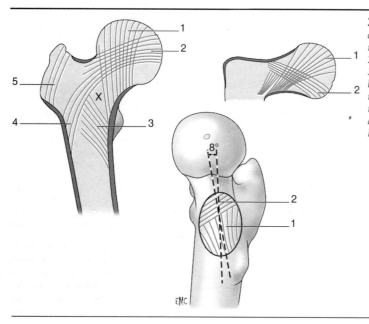

3 *The trabecular structure of the proximal femur. 1. Primary compressive trabeculae; 2. primary tensile trabeculae; 3. secondary compressive trabeculae; 4. secondary tensile trabeculae; 5. trochanteric trabeculae. X. Ward's triangle is the weakest cancellous bone region of the neck.*

anterior approach with a periacetabular extension.

In fracture of the femoral neck, the blood supply may be compromised for three reasons. The retinacular arteries are stretched and tethered; the branch entering the head may be disrupted and the head left only with blood supplied by the artery of the ligamentum teres. Secondly, bleeding inside an intact capsule increases the intracapsular pressure and hampers blood supply. Thirdly, if treatment is delayed, blood circulation is impaired and the risk of avascular necrosis of the head is increased [25]. Today, evaluation of a vascular compromise in a fresh fracture is not reliable, either with 99m technetium-MDP scintigraphy or with MRI.

OSSEOUS STRUCTURE AND MECHANICS

Several experimental models have been suggested to produce fractures of the femoral neck. Both bending and torsional forces act in the low-energy fractures. The most physiological model may be that of Hirsch and Frankel [17]. It mimics the compressive forces by the abductors and adductors acting in the direction of the femoral neck axis. High-energy fractures are more vertical and occur with a shearing mechanism.

The exact mechanism of fracture seems to be of limited importance for the mechanics of fracture fixation. The strongest structure of the neck, the calcar femorale, provides the most important single support for an implant. The strong subchondral cancellous bone of the head provides the best hold for the tip of a screw (fig 3). Calcar support for the distal screw(s) is important for fracture stability, since it provides a 3-point fixation. Parallel screws are superior to crossed screws [31].

The calculations by Pauwels [32] of hip joint stresses have been verified by in vivo measurements [7], which show that the load during symmetric two-legged stance is 0.7 times body weight and is increased in walking to 3.0 times body weight. The direction of the resultant force deviates about 16° from the vertical and about 30° from the axis of the femoral neck. The resultant force has a major component which compresses the fracture [17].

Although bone fragility is an important etiological factor of fractures in old age, the grade of osteoporosis is not essential for the choice of operative treatment. If implants are correctly positioned in internal fixation, they can obtain sufficient hold in fragile bone to bear the body weight and muscular forces, provided the conditions for uneventful healing of the fracture prevail. Osteoporosis does not affect the stability of a cemented femoral stem of an endoprosthesis.

Radiographic evaluation and classification of adult hip fractures

The fracture should be studied in good quality anteroposterior and lateral radiographs, paying attention to displacement, comminution and head fragment size. An anteroposterior view of the entire pelvis is preferable to a radiograph of only the hip.

Low-energy fractures are by far the most common. High-energy fractures, often sustained in traffic accidents, are regularly combined with other injuries [2]. The possibility of pathological and fatigue fracture should be kept in mind.

CLASSIFICATIONS

Pauwels [32] based his classification on the angle of the fracture line with the horizontal level (fig 4), postulating adverse healing conditions for the most vertical fractures.

The classification of Garden [14] is probably the most widely used (fig 5). Type 1 is an incomplete subcapital fracture. A minimal degree of lateral rotation creates the radiological illusion of impaction. Type 2 is a complete fracture without displacement. The inferior cortical buttress has been broken, but no tilting of the capital fragment takes place. Type 3 is a complete fracture with partial displacement. The two fragments retain their posterior retinacular attachment and crushing of the posterior cortex has not taken place. Lateral rotation of the distal fragment tilts the capital fragment into abduction and medial rotation. Type 4 is a complete fracture with full displacement.

In the AO classification [26], all proximal femoral fractures are grouped together (fig 6). The femoral neck fractures form group B. Type B1 fractures are subcapital, with slight displacement; type B2 fractures are transcervical; and type B3 fractures are

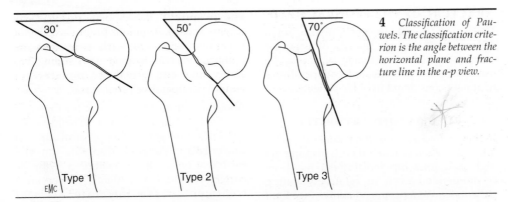

4 *Classification of Pauwels. The classification criterion is the angle between the horizontal plane and fracture line in the a-p view.*

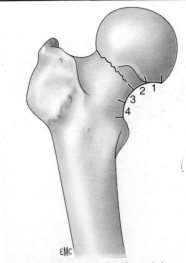

7 *Reconstruction of the calcar femorale by comparing the fractured side with the intact one.*

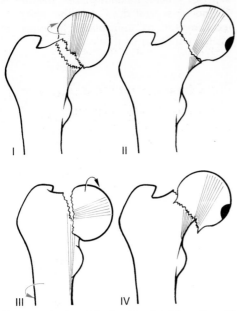

5 *Classification of Garden (Reprinted from Kempf I et al. Encyclopédie Médico-Chirurgicale. Appareil locomoteur, 14-076-A-10). 1. Impacted fracture; 2. nondisplaced fracture; 3. displaced fracture with varus tilting of the head; 4. fully displaced fracture.*

subcapital, nonimpacted and displaced. Each type is further divided in three subgroups.

Pauwels's classification, based on biomechanical calculations, does not predict healing of the common low-energy fractures fractures [4, 27]. Garden's classification has been widely used, but its value seems to be limited to a dichotomy between undisplaced and displaced fractures, partly due to the large interobserver variations [11, 13]. The same is true of the AO classification, which also seems to poorly predict the outcome of treatment [8].

Radiographic findings: To a great extent, the healing ability of a femoral neck fracture may be predicted from the preoperative radiological findings *(fig 7)* [4, 22, 27]. Indications of poor prognosis are 30° varus angulation of the head, cranial displacement by 20 mm *(fig 8)*, small head fragment (distance head-fracture line of 15 mm or less) *(fig 9)*, and comminution of the calcar *(fig 8, 10)*. When any of these signs were present [4], the fixation failed in 50% of the cases; if no adverse sign was present, the failure was 8%.

Intracapsular, low-energy femoral neck fractures may best be divided as follows:

– nondisplaced fractures;

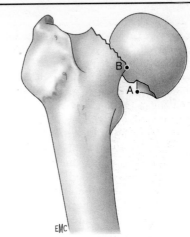

8 *Cranial displacement AB in the a-p view. Comminution of the calcar reduces effective calcar length and hampers reduction.*

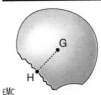

9 *The size of the head fragment is measured as the distance G-H between the centre of the femoral head and the fracture line.*

– displaced fractures;
– displaced fractures with comminution.

Principles of treatment in different age groups and conditions

PERSONS BELOW 60 YEARS OF AGE

Three percent of femoral neck fractures occur in patients aged 50 years or less [34]. In children and young adults, a united fracture with a well-vascularised femoral head guarantees the best long-term result. An immediate decompression of the intracapsular fracture haematoma by aspiration has been suggested to improve

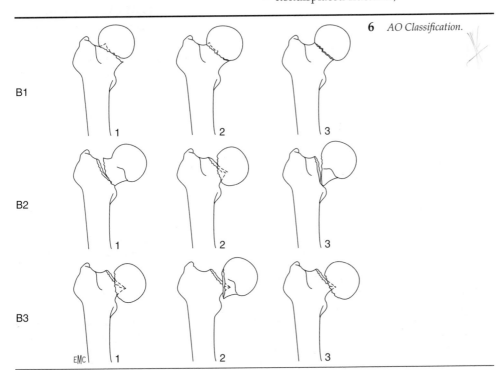

6 *AO Classification.*

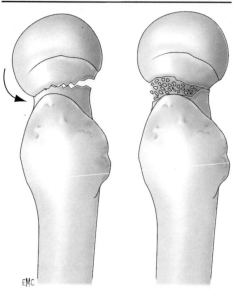

10 *Posterior comminution reduces fracture stability.*

blood supply. However, an early operation is the most effective way to guarantee the best possible blood perfusion [16]. It is advisable to aspirate the joint during the operation. Primary vascular bone grafting has been suggested in cases where jeopardy of blood circulation of the head is suspected. However, the effect has not been well documented. The same applies for primary valgus osteotomy, which may impair the already compromised blood supply of the femoral head. Between the ages of 40-60 years, endoprosthesis replacement may sometimes be warranted.

ELDERLY PATIENTS

Operative treatment presents many risks in the older patient, but these are outweighed by the higher risks and poor functional results of extended conservative treatment. Treatment of a displaced fracture in an elderly patient is controversial, the choice being between internal fixation and primary replacement with endoprosthesis. The choice has often depended more on tradition than on the comparative analyses of long-term outcome.

The risk of failure increases with the patient's age, and arthroplasty should be preferred in higher age groups. Elderly patients subject to epilepsy with seizures, parkinsonism, etc. are best treated with hemiendoprosthesis. A poorer than average physiological state may warrant endoprosthesis replacement at a younger age.

CONCURRENT HIP AND SHAFT FRACTURE

Concurrent hip and shaft fractures is most often a high-energy fracture combination encountered mainly under 40 years of age. Both fractures are best treated with internal fixation.

FRACTURE OF THE FEMORAL HEAD

This may occur in association with dislocation of the hip. The risk of avascular necrosis is high. Resorbable pins may be used in young patients and endoprosthesis treatment considered in older patients.

RHEUMATOID ARTHRITIS

In rheumatoid arthritis, the failure rates after internal fixation of femoral neck fractures are high, and total hip replacement has been recommended even in relatively young patients [37]. We recommend a lower age limit of 40 years.

PRE-EXISTING HIP DISEASE

Pre-existing hip disease makes total hip arthroplasty warranted. This is also the case concerning an old, undiagnosed fracture of the neck.

PATHOLOGICAL FRACTURE

Pathological fracture is usually caused by metastatic disease. A tumour work-up is made and the local tumour removed. Irradiation of the hip to treat malignancy increases the risk of hip fracture. Endoprosthetic replacement is usually the best choice.

FATIGUE FRACTURE

Stress fracture may occur in a young person in unusual strenuous activity. In an elderly patient, a metabolic disorder may be the cause. These fractures are best treated with multiple screw fixation.

Initial management

The choice of the treatment method depends on the type of fracture, time from fracture, radiological findings, and the age and physical and mental condition of the patient. Except for moribund patients, operative treatment should be preferred in all displaced fractures, since the risks of prolonged bed rest are higher than the risks of operation. If the choice is internal fixation, it is best to operate as soon as possible, in consideration of the vascularisation of the femoral head. Half of the elderly patients have a medical condition that should be treated preoperatively. The metabolic and cardiovascular condition of the patient can be improved by fluids and medication; in such cases, the operation should be postponed for those few hours this balancing requires. Since the risk of complications increases with increased waiting before surgery, reduction and internal fixation should be performed within 24 hours.

Preoperative care has two further goals: to prevent pressure sores and to reduce pain. The best pain relief may be obtained in semiflexion and outer rotation of the hip by placing the leg on a pillow.

The hospital's thrombosis prophylaxis scheme is used. Antibiotic prophylaxis is not necessary in cases with percutaneous pinning, whereas fixation with sliding hip screw and endoprosthetic replacement require perioperative prophylaxis.

About 5% of all femoral neck fractures are nondisplaced and impacted. Whether such patients are given the option of not undergoing surgery depends on the treatment policy of the institution. With the correct selection of patients, conservative treatment has a low rate of later displacement and an acceptable cost [30]. Conservative treatment is a natural choice in cases where a nondisplaced fracture is diagnosed several days after the injury. In most institutions, undisplaced fractures are treated with internal fixation.

Internal fixation with screws

PRINCIPLES OF SCREW FIXATION

The key factors are good fracture reduction and optimal placement of the screws, the most important screw position being inferoposterior *(fig 11)*. A multiple screw technique is described here.

POSITIONING OF THE PATIENT

The patient lies supine on an orthopaedic table *(fig 12)*. The leg is in neutral rotation and abduction in shoe traction. The knee is supported to prevent the hip from hanging. The correct position of the image intensifier is checked.

CLOSED REDUCTION

The quality of reduction has been shown to be far more important than the choice of implant. Reduction is usually achieved in traction and internal rotation of the leg *(fig 13)*. A push on the posterolateral aspect of the greater trochanter for impaction may be favourable *(fig 14)*. Poor reducibility is a poor prognostic sign [10].

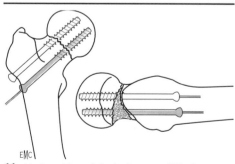

11 *Ideal position of the basic screw. Whether one or more screws are used, one should be positioned upon the calcar in the posterior lower quadrant of the neck. The thin outline depicts the position of the second screw.*

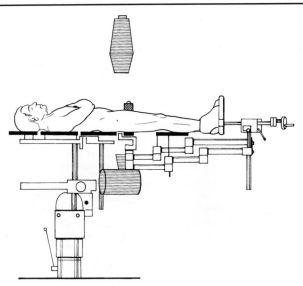

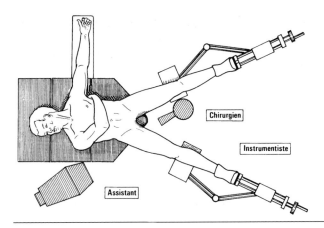

12 *Position of the patient on the traction table with the leg in extension and abduction with the knee supported. Note the position of the image intensifier. (Reprinted from Kempf I et al. Encyclopédie Medico-Chirurgicale, Techniques Chirurgicales, Orthopédie, 44-620).*

Chirurgien

Instrumentiste

Assistant

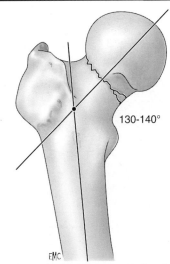

15 *The reduction should be anatomical, or in a 0-10° valgus position in the a-p view.*

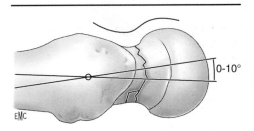

16 *In the lateral view, not more than 10° of deviation from the straight neck axis is allowed. The ventral contour of the neck should after reduction be anatomically formed as an 'S'. Loss of the normal contour is a sign of poor reduction, as seen when a posterior tilt distorts the line into a 'J'.*

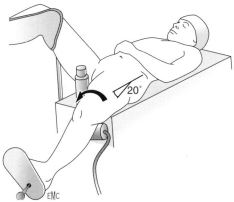

13 *The leg is adducted and rotated inwards.*

Criteria of reduction: After reduction, the head fragment should lie in direct, anatomical continuation of the femoral neck in the a-p and lateral views of the image intensifier *(fig 15, 16)*. No ad latus displacement and a maximum of 10° valgus of the head should be allowed. The anteversion, approximately 15°, is checked in relation to the posterior femoral condylar plane *(fig 1)* by using the image intensifier.

If the fracture of an elderly patient cannot be reduced satisfactorily, replacement with an endoprosthesis should be carried out. In a young patient, an open reduction should be performed.

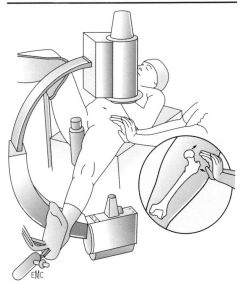

14 *A push posterolaterally may help in valgisation and impaction of the fracture.*

OPEN REDUCTION

After draping of the operative field, the hip is exposed through a Watson-Jones anterolateral approach and the joint capsule opened through a longitudinal anterior excision. The hip is flexed 20-30° to facilitate the exposure and fracture reduction. Once the fracture is reduced, guide pins are inserted for a provisional fixation and the

position controlled in the image intensifier. The screw fixation is performed as described below.

INTERNAL FIXATION

After preparation of the skin, the operative field is surrounded by a transparent adherent plastic drape that covers the entire side of the operation.

Several techniques (pin guides, cannulated screws, etc.) use the same principle of placing multiple screws in a parallel way in the femoral neck. The trabecular area below the greater trochanter, rather than the proximal lateral cortex, is the insertion site of the screws. This gives a course for the screw(s) more or less parallel to the axis of the femoral neck and prevents too high a location of the screw tips.

For preliminary orientation, a Kirschner wire is placed in front of the femoral neck parallel with its axis *(fig 17)*. A skin incision, 4 to 5 cm long, is made in alignment with the femoral shaft. Alternatively, stab incisions are used. A 4 mm Steinman pin is placed centrally in the neck and its position checked in the a-p and lateral views *(fig 18)*. The tip of the pin lies subchondrally 3 mm from the bone surface of the head. The length of the guide pin outside the bone is measured in order to obtain the screw length. The distal

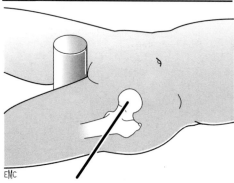

17 *Kirschner pin in front of the femoral neck for preliminary extraosseal orientation.*

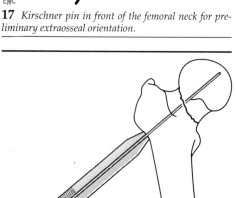

18 *Positioning of the intraosseal guide pin and measuring the length of screws.*

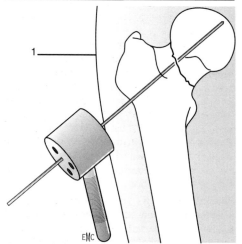

19 *Pin guide mounted on the guide pin. The pin guide may be used for percutaneous insertion of the screws, or placed on the fascia through an ample skin incision.*

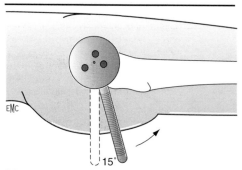

20 *Placement of the pin guide in the desired position between 0 and 15°.*

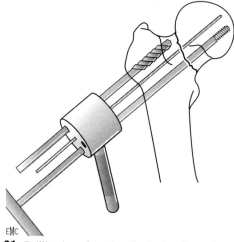

21 *Drilling is performed to the fracture line using a drill sleeve. When drilling a new hole the drill guide is kept in place by an already inserted screw. The screw should not perforate the subchondral bone.*

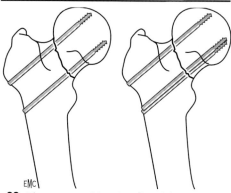

22 *The screws are driven into the subchondral bone.*

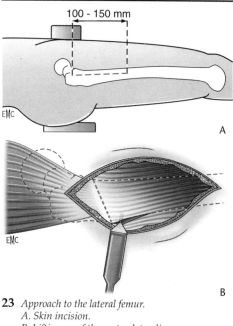

23 *Approach to the lateral femur.*
A. Skin incision.
B. Lifting up of the vastus lateralis.

POSTOPERATIVE CARE

The patient can usually be mobilised with a walker on the first postoperative day. In younger patients, partial weight-bearing is advisable for a period of 6 to 12 weeks. Weight-bearing as tolerated is allowed for an elderly patient who voluntarily limits loading of the injured limb [20].

Internal fixation with dynamic hip screw

PRINCIPLES OF SLIDING SCREW FIXATION

The screw gets extra support from the plate. The more lateral the fracture the more important the plate becomes. Positioning of the patient, closed reduction and open reduction are the same as described in the section on internal fixation with screws.

INTERNAL FIXATION

After preparation of the skin, the operative field is surrounded by a transparent adherent plastic drape that covers the entire side of the operation table. A Kirschner wire is placed in front of the femoral neck parallel with its axis *(fig 17)*. A skin incision, 10 to 15 cm long, is made in alignment with the femoral shaft *(fig 23)*. The fracture position is secured in a preliminary fashion with two Kirschner wires. The dynamic hip screw angle guide is placed against the femoral shaft so that the guide tube points to a line just proximal to the calcar femorale in the anteroposterior view and posterior to the centre of the femoral neck axis in the side view *(fig 24)*. The lateral cortex is opened with a 2-mm drill bit and a guide pin is inserted. The guide pin with its tip in the subchondral bone should remain in place

screw(s) should be 5 mm longer and the proximal screw 5 mm shorter than the length of the guide pin inside the bone.

A drill guide is introduced over the Steinman pin and put in the position chosen for insertion of the screws *(fig 19)*. We recommend positioning two screws in good contact with the calcar femorale. According to the surgeon's choice, 2 or 3 screws may be used *(fig 20)*. Protection sleeves are used around awls and drills.

When self-tapping screws are used, the holes are drilled to the fracture line *(fig 21)*. Tapping of the head fragment may be

necessary if the bone is hard. Perforation of the subchondral bone must be prevented to avoid later screw perforation. To retain the position of the fracture, it is important that a screw be fully attached before drilling, tapping and insertion of the next screw.

Careful choice of the site of screw insertion in the lateral cortex is of utmost importance to avoid stress sites due to unnecessary perforations of the bone. A suboptimal position of a screw may be preferable to an empty hole. The tips of the screws should lie at 3 to 5 mm from the cartilage *(fig 22)*.

After final checking of the screw positions, the protection sleeves, drill guide and Steinman pin are removed and the wound is closed.

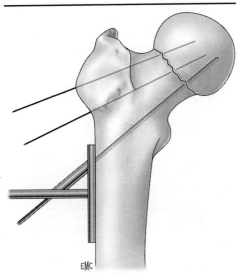

24 *Preliminary fixation with 2 Kirschner pins and insertion of the guide pin.*

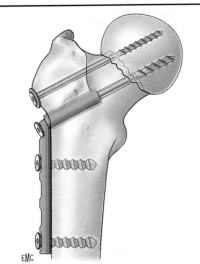

25 *Femoral neck fracture fixed with a dynamic hip screw and a cancellous screw.*

throughout the procedure. The threaded end helps to secure it in the bone. Slide the direct measuring device over the guide pin and read off directly the length of the pin within the bone.

The details of reaming are presented in the chapter on the treatment of trochanteric fractures. The drill hole should end 5 mm short of the subchondral bone plate. Set the reamer to the correct depth (e.g. 100 - 5 = 95 mm) and ream the hole. In hard cancellous bone, the thread should be pre-cut with a tap. Use the shorter of the two centring sleeves with the tap. The insertion of the screw is described in the treatment of trochanteric fractures. An additional cancellous screw proximal to the dynamic screw and parallel to it is advisable *(fig 25)*. After final checking of the screw positions, the protection sleeves, drill guide and Steinman pin are removed. The wound is closed.

POSTOPERATIVE CARE

The patient can usually be mobilised with a walker on the first postoperative day. In younger patients, partial weight-bearing is

Author	Implant	No. of patients	AVN*	Non-union	Reoper-ation	Follow-up
Frandsen et al 1979 [12]	Smith-P. nail	62	20 %	34 %	34 %	2 years
	Sliding nail plate	69	21 %	23 %	23 %	
Svenningsen et al 1984 [39]	McLaughlin nail	127	21 %	25 %	25 %	3 years
	Sliding hip screw	128	15 %	11 %	· 11 %	
Nordkild et al 1985 [28]	Sliding nail plate	19	21 %	26 %	32 %	2 years
	Sliding screw plate	30	10 %	14 %	23 %	

Table I. – Results of treatment of displaced femoral neck fractures with nails and screws

* Avascular necrosis of the femoral head

advisable for a period of 6 to 12 weeks. Weight-bearing as tolerated is allowed for an elderly patient who voluntarily limits loading of the injured limb.

Complications of internal fixation

WOUND INFECTION

Surgical debridement combined with antibiotics may allow saving the fixation. Alternatively, salvage with total hip replacement is indicated. A low-grade infection may result in gradual damage of the fixation and dislocation of the femoral head from the acetabulum.

SUBTROCHANTERIC FRACTURE

The insertion of solitary screws too obliquely, or multiple attempts at passing a guide wire or pin, may weaken the lateral cortex and result in subtrochanteric fracture. A sufficient trauma force may cause such a fracture after a technically adequate fixation. Fixation with a sliding hip screw and retaining any screw(s) that reliably connect the fragments of the original fracture are advised.

EARLY FAILURE OF FIXATION

The main causes of fixation failure are comminuted fracture, poor reduction and insufficient fixation. Most failures in elderly patients occur within the first 3 months. Small changes in the position of the fracture and implant(s) are common in control radiographs. Backing of screw(s) by 20 mm is ominous. A change of 5° or 10 mm in relation to the original position of the fracture or implant is suggestive of failure. All patients should be controlled 3 months after treatment, since most failures occur early and the decision to salvage a poorly-functioning, painful hip should not be postponed too long.

Salvage of failed internally fixed fracture. In a young patient, a new, more adequate osteosynthesis should be considered. Vascularised bone graft has been used as an adjunct, but controlled studies do not exist to show its effects. Bipolar cemented hemiendoprosthesis is a useful salvage operation in elderly persons 3 to 6 months

postoperatively. The alternative is total hip replacement which is considered in later failures, in cases with a damaged acetabulum and in pre-existing hip disease. Non-union is dealt with in another chapter.

Avascular necrosis of the femoral head (AVN) and late segmental collapse. AVN may occur even in a nondisplaced fracture. Whether the femoral head should be replaced by endoprosthesis depends on the symptoms and function.

Results of internal fixation

The results of internal fixation differ due to demographic factors, quality of surgery and type of osteosynthesis [23]. Good reduction is more important than the choice of the implant [1, 4].

Timing of the surgery is also important. Limited hospital resources may result in delays, but sufficient priority should be given to these fractures, since the vitality of the femoral head is inversely related to the length of the delay. The rate of late segmental collapse after avascular necrosis was halved in those patients treated within 6 hours after the injury, compared with patients treated later [25]. The re-operation rates in long-term studies have generally varied from 25 to 40%. A number of prospective studies with participation from one or a few institutions have yielded lower figures, around 15% [3, 38].

Many implants give satisfactory results, and controversies between studies may depend more on local variations in treatment policy than the type of implant. Three studies comparing a solitary nail, sliding nail with plate and sliding screw with plate speak in favour of the sliding screw plate *(table I)*. In a meta-analysis [29], screws were superior to pins, but their number could not be deduced from the results. A side-plate did not give any advantage.

Replacement by hemiendoprosthesis

PRINCIPLES OF HEMIPROSTHESIS REPLACEMENT

Replacement of the femoral head/neck by an implant eliminates the healing problems of fracture treatment. The technique of bipolar hemiarthroplasty is described here.

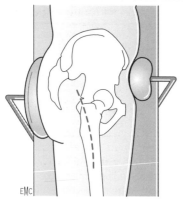

26 *Positioning of the patient with supports in front and behind. The dotted line indicates the skin incision.*

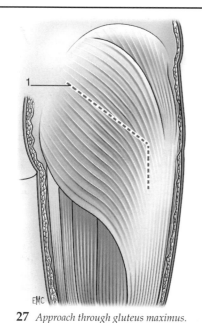

27 *Approach through gluteus maximus.*

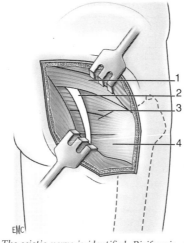

28 *The sciatic nerve is identified. Piriformis, gemelli and obturator internus are divided close to their insertion to femur. 1. Piriformis muscle; 2. sciatic nerve; 3. gemellus muscles; 4. quadratus femoris muscle.*

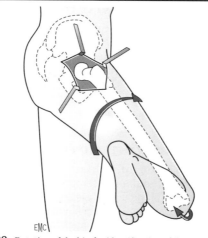

29 *Rotation of the hip for identification of the posterior capsule.*

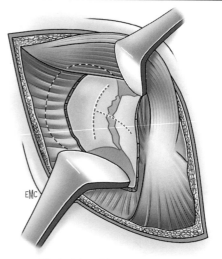

30 *Incision of the posterior capsule.*

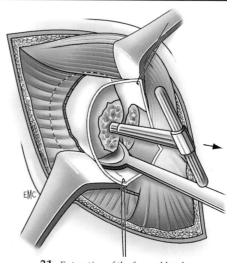

31 *Extraction of the femoral head.*

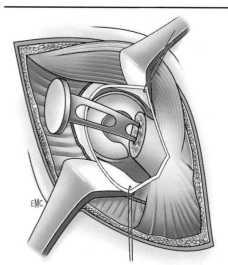

32 *Preparation of the femoral neck and medullary cavity.*

SURGICAL APPROACH

Anterior, anterolateral, transgluteal and posterior approaches all have their pros and cons. The surgeon's familiarity with a certain approach is most important. In this chapter, the posterior approach is presented.

The patient is placed in a lateral decubitus position lying on the unaffected side; the position is secured with supports *(fig 26)*. The skin is prepared down from the lower costal border to include the entire lower extremity. The leg is draped to permit free movement during the operation. The perineal region is carefully excluded from the operative field.

With the hip flexed, a curved incision is made extending from the posterior superior iliac spine over the greater trochanteric eminence and 10 cm distally along the posterolateral aspect of the thigh. The gluteus maximus is separated in line with its fibres to a level above the acetabulum without disturbing the femoral insertion *(fig 27)*. The incision is continued distally, opening the fascia lata, and the edges retracted. The sciatic nerve is visualised as it passes deep to the piriformis and superficial to the other external rotator muscles. A soft plastic tube may be placed about the nerve to facilitate its protection *(fig 28)*. The short extensors, the piriformis, obturator internus and externus and gemelli, and the upper part of the quadratus femoris are divided close to their attachments to the femur.

REPLACEMENT

The rotating manoeuvre of the leg *(fig 29)* helps in identifying the hip capsule, which is opened in a T-shape along the posterior border of the acetabulum and longitudinally along the neck *(fig 30)*. Internal rotation of the leg opens the fracture. The femoral head is extracted *(fig 31)* and its diameter measured for the correct size of the prosthesis head. Any excessive synovium and remnants of ligamentum teres are excised. A trial fit of the chosen prosthetic femoral head component is then performed. The insertion of the test implant should require considerable pressure, but total insertion should be possible. Removal should be difficult due to a suction effect which helps in preventing later dislocation. The ultimate resection of the femoral neck depends on the design of the implant. The anteversion, approximately 15°, is checked in relation to the posterior femoral condylar plane *(fig 1)*. The medullary cavity of the proximal femur is prepared with a rasp *(fig 32)*. A plug made of cancellous bone or plastic is inserted 2 cm distal to the tip of the prosthesis *(fig 33)*. The cavity is irrigated

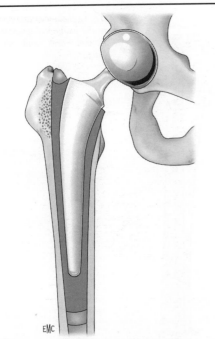

33 *Principles of cementing: distal plug and an even layer of cement around the prosthesis stem.*

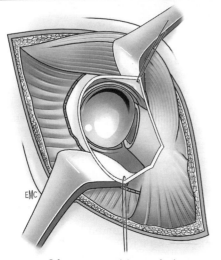

34 *Reduction of the prosthesis.*

and haemostasis secured with adrenaline or hydrogen peroxide swabs. High-viscosity polymethylmethacrylate cement is mixed in vacuum and inserted with a cement gun from distal to proximal. Pressure by thumbs or a flange is used to secure good cement filling of the trabecular bone. While the cement is plastic, the stem is inserted and its central position, correct depth and rotation checked. Excess cement is removed. After hardening of the cement, the head is inserted and the prosthesis reduced *(fig 34)*. Its stability in flexion and rotation is checked and the capsule closed. The operative field is irrigated to remove foreign materials and tissue debris. The wound is closed in layers over a closed suction drain.

POSTOPERATIVE CARE

The thrombosis prophylaxis regime is continued. A control radiograph is taken. Full weight-bearing, first with walking aids, is encouraged from the first postoperative day. The average time in hospital is 8 days. Hip flexion to 90° is allowed at 6 weeks.

Complications of endoprosthesis replacement

Complications related to the operation are peroperative fracture, dislocation of the hip due to improper sizing of the prosthesis head or malrotation of the stem, and component loosening because of imperfect cementing technique.

Infection of the implant is a serious complication. When it is detected at an early stage, surgical debridement and prolonged antibiotic treatment are required. Removal of a cemented stem from an osteoporotic femur may be difficult and result in splintering of the femur. It may be advisable to wait for signs of loosening under antibiotic coverage instead of immediately removing a stem which is still fixed. In a debilitated patient, removal of the implant only may be necessary. Otherwise, salvage by total hip replacement may be the choice.

Heterotopic ossification is a rare complication after bipolar hemiendoprosthesis replacement because of the limited raw bone surfaces.

Erosion of the cartilage and protrusion of the prosthesis head is a late complication and typically causes pain in the groin.

Results of endoprosthesis replacement

The problems of internal fixation are obviated by prosthetic replacement. The optimum lower age range for prosthesis replacement is not settled. Technical failure rates have been low, between 7% and 17%, after many types of primary prosthetic replacements.

An 80-year-old person having sustained a femoral neck fracture survives on average for 5 years. Therefore, the longevity of the therapeutic solution is a matter of increasing importance. Long-term results of the uncemented, unipolar Moore hemiendoprosthesis have been unfavourable with poor function and high cost of social care [18]. Studies comparing uncemented versus cemented hemiendoprostheses and unipolar versus bipolar implants have been in favour of cemented, bipolar hemiendoprostheses, and the differences in the quality of life are in favour of bipolar prostheses [21, 36]. Although the studies of motion in the two articulations of the bipolar cemented hemiendoprostheses, with a ball joint between the prosthesis head and shaft, are controversial, these designs have yielded improved functional results [24, 40]. Acetabular erosion in bipolar prostheses is halved compared with unipolar devices in long-term follow-up studies [21, 33, 40]. The survival

of bipolar hemiendoprosthesis, as a salvage operation several months after internal fixation in cases with an undamaged acetabulum, is similar to that of primary replacement [6].

Total hip replacement as the primary treatment for displaced femoral neck fracture has been controversial, and complication rates are higher than in replacement for coxarthrosis. A healthy, active patient may benefit from total hip replacement rather than hemiarthroplasty [15].

Comparison of internal fixation and endoprosthesis replacement

Lu-Yao et al [23] concluded that arthroplasty, particularly bipolar and total, is associated with fewer secondary operations than internal fixation. This is a major concern in elderly patients, since even minor operations in the elderly carry an increased risk of mortality. Percutaneous internal fixation of the femoral neck fracture is associated with a 5 to 10% perioperative mortality. The complication and mortality rates in prosthetic replacement and internal fixation are similar in many reports.

Today, the pertinent question is not whether to treat all displaced femoral neck fractures with internal fixation or prosthesis replacement, but to define the criteria for choice between these two treatment modalities.

A number of fractures carry a poor prognosis because of their character. Large displacement, comminution and small femoral head fragment and difficult fracture reduction make the fracture more suitable for endoprosthesis replacement in an elderly patient. Internally fixed fractures heal poorly in patients with rheumatoid arthritis.

Robinson et al [35] designed a physiological status score to decide the management of displaced fractures. They treated patients younger than 65 years of age with internal fixation and patients over 85 with hemoarthroplasty. Patients aged 65-85 years who were ambulant, medically fit, mentally alert and who had good bone stock were managed by reduction and internal fixation. The remainder were treated with hemiendoprosthesis. Alho et al [4] found that an 85-year-old patient has a doubled risk of failure after internal fixation compared with a patient 10 years younger.

The expense of surgery has been used as an argument in the choice of treatment. However, no reliable studies exist. The question of internal fixation or primary prosthesis replacement in displaced femoral neck fractures in the elderly is not fully settled.

Concurrent ipsilateral hip and shaft fractures

Ipsilateral fracture of the hip and femoral shaft is a typical fracture combination encountered in high-energy trauma and occurs in approximately 3% of femoral shaft fractures [5]. The cause is high-energy axial force in the direction of the long axis of the femur, dashboard injury being the best example. When the femur is compressed axially between the dashboard and the fixed pelvis in mid-position between abduction and adduction, it buckles and fractures. The same force shears the femoral neck; alternatively, a bending-type intertrochanteric fracture may occur by bending. Dissipation of the fracture energy at two sites may explain why the hip fracture is often undisplaced and noncomminuted. The fracture is cervical in 70% and trochanteric in 30% of the cases. A radiograph of the pelvis should be included in the emergency studies of all cases of high-energy trauma and/or femoral fracture to determine concurrent injuries.

Several combinations of internal fixation have been applied in the double fracture situation. Plate fixation of the shaft allows a free choice for the fixation of the hip fracture. However, plating necessitates an extensive exposure and the advantage is outweighed by problems of wound-healing, infection, delayed union and implant failure. The over-all results using the unlocked Küntscher nail have not been better. Nonunion and deep infection are rarer, but shortening and rotational malunion more common. Also, difficulties in positioning of hip screws with a nail in the medullary canal have resulted in re-operations. With a careful technique, screws may be driven into the femoral neck in front of or behind the nail.

After the introduction of locked intramedullary nailing, this technique has replaced most other treatment alternatives. It makes opening of the femoral fracture

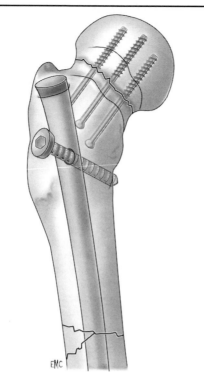

35 *Insertion of 2-3 screws to the femoral neck beside a locked intramedullary nail.*

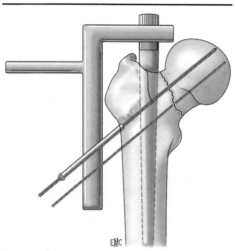

36 *Fixation of the fracture of the femoral neck by the proximal locking screws of a cephalo-medullary nail which also fixes the concurrent ipsilateral femoral shaft fracture.*

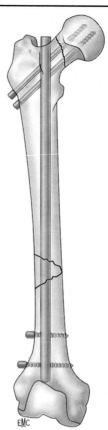

37 *Cephalo-medullary nail in the fixation of ipsilateral femoral neck and shaft fracture.*

unnecessary and efficiently controls the length and rotation of the shaft fracture. Separate screws are sufficient for the fixation of the neck fracture (*fig 35*). They may not control a trochanteric fracture adequately.

Cephalo-medullary nails with proximal screw(s) through the nail to the femoral neck (*fig 36*) and distal locking screws in the distal metaphysis (*fig 37*) have been designed to fix complex femoral fractures, comminuted subtrochanteric fractures and hip shaft fracture combinations [5, 9]. The results in recent reports are similar to the results of the first generation locked nails and separate hip screws. The complications of locked nailing have been fewer and the outcomes superior to plates and unlocked nails. The fixation of hip fracture with these implants requires special expertise.

References

[1] Alberts KA, Jervaeus J. Factors predisposing to healing complications after internal fixation of femoral neck fracture. *Clin Orthop* 1990 ; 257 : 129-133

[2] Alho A. Concurrent ipsilateral fractures of the hip and femoral shaft. A meta-analysis of 659 cases. *Acta Orthop Scand* 1996 ; 67 : 19-28

[3] Alho A, Austdal S, Benterud JG, Blikra G, Lerud P, Raugstad TS. Biases in a randomized comparison of three types of screw fixation in displaced femoral neck fractures. *Acta Orthop Scand* 1998 ; 69 : 463-468

[4] Alho A, Benterud JG, Rønningen H, Høiseth A. Prediction of disturbed healing in femoral neck fracture. *Acta Orthop Scand* 1992 ; 63 : 639-644

[5] Alho A, Ekeland A, Grøgaard B, Dokke JR. A locked hip screw-intramedullary nail (cephalo-medullary nail) for the treatment of fractures of the proximal part of the femur combined with fractures of the femoral shaft. *J Trauma* 1996 ; 40 : 10-16

[6] Benterud JG, Kok WL, Alho A. Primary and secondary Charnley-Hastings hemiarthroplasty in displaced femoral neck fractures and their sequelae. *Ann Chir Gynaecol* 1996 ; 85 : 72-76

[7] Bergmann G, Rohlmann A, Graichen F. In vivo Messung der Hüftgelenkbelastung. *Z Orthop* 1989 ; 127 : 672-679

[8] Blundell CM, Parker MJ, Pryor GA, Hopkins-Woolley J, Bhonsle SS. Assessment of the AO classification of intracapsular fractures of the proximal femur. *J Bone Joint Surg Br* 1998 ; 80 : 679-683

[9] Bose WJ, Corces A, Anderson LD. A preliminary experience with the Russel-Taylor reconstruction nail for complex femoral fractures. *J Trauma* 1992 ; 32 : 71-76

[10] Chua D, Jaglal SB, Schatzker J. Predictors of early failure of fixation in the treatment of displaced subcapital hip fractures. *J Orthop Trauma* 1998 ; 12 : 230-234

[11] Eliasson P, Hansson LI, Kärrholm J. Displacement in femoral neck fracture. *Acta Orthop Scand* 1988 ; 59 : 361-364

[12] Frandsen PA. Osteosynthesis of displaced fractures of the femoral neck. *Acta Orthop Scand* 1979 ; 50 : 443-449

[13] Frandsen PA, Andersen E, Madsen F, Skjødt T. Garden's classification of femoral neck fractures. An assessment of inter-observer variation. *J Bone Joint Surg Br* 1988 ; 70 : 588-590

[14] Garden RS. Low-angle fixation in fractures of the femoral neck. *J Bone Joint Surg Br* 1961 ; 43 : 647-663

[15] Gebhard JS, Amstutz HC, Zinar DM, Dorey FJ. A comparison of total hip arthroplasty and hemiarthroplasty for treatment of acute fractures of the femoral neck. *Clin Orthop* 1992 ; 282 : 123-131

[16] Gerber C, Strehle J, Ganz R. The treatment of fractures of the femoral neck. *Clin Orthop* 1993 ; 292 : 77-86

[17] Hirsch C, Frankel VH. Analysis of forces producing fractures of the proximal end of the femur. *J Bone Joint Surg Br* 1960 ; 42 : 633-640

[18] Jalovaara P, Virkkunen H. Quality of life after primary hemiarthroplasty for femoral neck fracture: six-year follow up of 185 patients. *Acta Orthop Scand* 1991 ; 62 : 208-217

[19] Judet J, Judet R, Legrange J, Dunoyer J. A study of the arterial vascularization of the femoral neck in the adult. *J Bone Joint Surg Am* 1955 ; 37 : 663-680

[20] Koval KJ, Sala DA, Kummer FJ, Zuckerman JD. Postoperative weight-bearing after a fracture of the femoral neck or an intertrochanteric fracture. *J Bone Joint Surg Am* 1998 ; 80 : 352-356

[21] Labelle LW, Colwill JC, Swanson AB. Bateman bipolar hip arthroplasty for femoral neck fractures. A five- to ten-year follow-up study. *Clin Orthop* 1990 ; 251 : 20-25

[22] Lamare JP. Fracture du col du fémur transcervicale. In : Conférence d'enseignement de la SOFCOT. Paris : Expansion Scientifique Française, 1979

[23] Lu-Yao GL, Keller RB, Littenberg B, Wennberg JE. Outcomes after displaced fractures of the femoral neck. A meta-analysis of one hundred and six published reports. *J Bone Joint Surg Am* 1994 ; 76 : 15-25

[24] Malhotra R, Arya R, Bhan S. Bipolar hemiarthroplasty in femoral neck fractures. *Arch Orthop Trauma Surg* 1995 ; 114 : 79-82

[25] Manninger J, Kazar G, Fekete G, Nagy FE, Zolczer L, Frenyo S. Avoidance of avascular necrosis of the femoral head, following fractures of the femoral neck, by early reduction and internal fixation. *Injury* 1985 ; 16 : 437-448

[26] Müller ME. The comprehensive classification of fractures of long bones. In : Müller ME, Allgöwer M, Schneider R, Willenegger H eds. Manual of internal fixation. Techniques recommended by the AO-ASIF group. Berlin : Springer-Verlag, 1991 : 118-150

[27] Nilsson LT, Johansson Å, Strömqvist B. Factors predicting healing complications in femoral neck fractures. *Acta Orthop Scand* 1993 ; 64 : 175-177

[28] Nordkild P, SonneHolm S, Jensen JS. Femoral neck fracture: sliding screw plate versus sliding nail plate: a randomized study. *Injury* 1985 ; 16 : 449-454

[29] Parker MJ, Blundell C. Choice of implant for internal fixation of femoral neck fractures. Meta-analysis of 25 randomised trials including 4, 925 patients. *Acta Orthop Scand* 1998 ; 69 : 138-143

[30] Parker MJ, Myles JW, Aand JK, Drewett R. Cost-benefit analysis of hip fracture treatment. *J Bone Joint Surg Br* 1992 ; 74 : 261-264

[31] Parker MJ, Porter KM, Eastwood DM, Schembi Wismayer M, Bernard AA. Intracapsular fractures of the neck of femur. Parallel or crossed Garden screws? *J Bone Joint Surg Br* 1991 ; 73 : 826-827

[32] Pauwels F. Der Schenkelhalsbruch, ein mechanisches Problem, Grundlagen des Heilungsvorganges, Prognose und kausale Therapie. *Z Orthop Chir* 1935 ; (suppl 63) : 1-138

[33] Reymond MA, Kohler O, Rothenbühler JP, Chevalley P, Regazzoni P. Prothèse céphalique pour fracture du col fémoral (702 cas) : résultats comparatifs des prothèses céphaliques simples et des prothèses intermédiaires. *Rev Chir Orthop* 1991 ; 77 : 419-424

[34] Robinson CM, Court-Brown CM, McQueen MM, Christie J. Hip fractures in adults younger than 50 years of age. *Clin Orthop* 1995 ; 312 : 238-246

[35] Robinson CM, Saran D, Annan IH. Intracapsular hip fractures. Results of management adopting a treatment protocol. *Clin Orthop* 1994 ; 302 : 83-91

[36] Schätzler A, Möllers M, Stedtfeld HW. Ergebnisse der Versorgung von Schenkelhalsfrakturen mit zementierten bipolaren Endoprothesen (Experience with bipolar hemiarthroplasty for fractures of the femoral neck.) *Zentralbl Chir* 1997 ; 122 : 1028-1032

[37] Strömqvist B, Kelly I, Lidgren L. Treatment of hip fractures in rheumatoid arthritis. *Clin Orthop* 1988 ; 228 : 75-78

[38] Strömqvist B, Nilsson LT, Thorngren KG. Femoral neck fracture fixation with hook-pins. *Acta Orthop Scand* 1992 ; 63 : 282-287

[39] Svenningsen S, Benum P, Nesse O, Furset OI. Internal fixation of femoral neck fractures. *Acta Orthop Scand* 1984 ; 55 : 423-429

[40] Wetherell RG, Hinves BL. The Hastings bipolar hemiarthroplasty for subcapital fractures of the femoral neck. *J Bone Joint Surg Br* 1990 ; 72 : 788-793

Intertrochanteric osteotomy for nonunion of the femoral neck

RK Marti
ELFB Raaymakers

Abstract. – *Nonunion and avascular necrosis of the femoral head or the combination of both are the main complications following fractures of the femoral neck. In spite of improved operative techniques, nonunion is still reported in 10 to 20% of cases. Nowadays, in cases of nonunion of the femoral neck, the surgeon is tempted to perform prosthetic replacement of the hip, an operation that is, in our view, reserved for elderly patients and those middle-aged patients with severely deformed femoral heads. In the others, a joint-saving procedure is indicated. We have gained extensive experience in the performance of a valgisation osteotomy as described by Pauwels in the 1930s. The essence of this operation is transformation of a nearly vertical fracture line into a nearly horizontal one, bringing the nonunion into almost a right angle to the forces acting on the hip joint. Even in the case of a severely collapsed femoral head, good results can be achieved by abduction osteotomies in young patients, postponing a total hip replacement or hip fusion for many years.*

© 2000, Editions Scientifiques et Médicales Elsevier SAS. All rights reserved.

Keywords: hip, femur, nonunion femoral neck, intertrochanteric osteotomy, valgisation osteotomy, Pauwels osteotomy, avascular necrosis of the femoral head, hip prosthesis.

Introduction

Nonunion or avascular necrosis of the femoral head or the combination of both are the main complications following fractures of the femoral neck. In spite of improved operative techniques, nonunion is still reported in 10 to 20% of cases. The reason for this high incidence is a combination of unfavourable biomechanical and vascular conditions caused by the fracture itself, poor reduction and inadequate internal fixation. Pauwels classified the femoral neck fractures based on their mechanical behaviour (*fig 1*). As a logical consequence of his theories, he designed for the treatment of nonunions an abduction osteotomy at the intertrochanteric level (*fig 2*), which converts shearing forces into compression [12]. Nowadays, in cases of nonunion of the femoral neck, the surgeon is tempted to perform a prosthetic replacement of the hip, the more so if there is also evidence of disturbed vascularisation of the head. This will provide rapid pain relief and mobilisation. However, long-term results of hip arthroplasties, especially in younger people and in the presence of bone atrophy, are not always as good as expected,

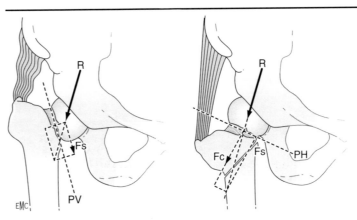

1 *Modified Pauwels classification of femoral neck fractures. In Type 1 fractures the cleavage plane is more horizontal because of impaction in valgus. The forces acting on the hip joint result in compression at the fracture site. These fractures are therefore relatively stable. The more vertical fractures of Type 2 and 3 cause the same forces to have a shearing and even distracting effect on the fracture. They are therefore unstable.*

Type 1   Type 2   Type 3

2 *Principles of the valgisation osteotomy designed by Pauwels. By taking out a lateral wedge, a steep fracture plane (PV) can be redirected into an almost horizontal one (PH). Mechanical analysis of the resultant force (R) acting on the nonunion shows how in the preoperative site shearing forces (Fs) dominate the fracture scene. After valgisation, R is almost parallel to the compression arm (Fc) of the parallelogram. R no longer displaces the fragments, but compresses them.*

René K Marti, M.D., PhD, Professor of Orthopaedics and Chief of the Department of Orthopaedic Surgery.
Ernst L.F.B Raaymakers, M.D., PhD, Associate Professor of Traumatology.
Academisch Medisch Centrum, Universiteit van Amsterdam, Postbus 22660, NL 1100 DD Amsterdam, The Netherlands.

and a less radical approach is worth considering. Avascularity of the femoral head has been found in up to 70% of displaced femoral neck fractures [4, 9, 10, 13, 15].

All references to this article must include: Marti RK and Raaymakers ELFB. Intertrochanteric osteotomy for nonunion of the femoral neck. Editions Scientifiques et Médicales Elsevier SAS (Paris). All rights reserved. Surgical Techniques in Orthopaedics and Traumatology, 55-400-D-10, 2000, 7 p.

The same authors have found that revascularisation, though slow and restricted, does occur, which explains the actual low percentage of deformities due to avascular necrosis (30%) after displaced fractures, as well as nonunions (50%). Furthermore, many patients with healed femoral neck fractures or nonunions, but having radiographic signs of avascular necrosis, present few clinical symptoms for many years.

The combination of femoral neck nonunion and suspected avascular necrosis of the femoral head is no contraindication to a valgisation osteotomy. Nonunion and osteotomy heal in these cases without any problem [9, 10]. Even in a partial collapse of the femoral head, good results can be achieved by abduction osteotomies in young patients, delaying a total hip replacement or hip fusion for many years. Total hip replacement as a salvage procedure after unstable internal fixation or nonunion of the femoral neck is reserved for elderly patients and patients with a severely deformed femoral head.

Our strategy

From 1973 until 1997, we treated 148 patients having a nonunion of the femoral neck after failed internal fixation or non-operative treatment. One patient got along with her handicap (shortening, limping) very well. The other 147 patients underwent surgery 4 weeks to 8 years after the femoral neck fracture. The following techniques were used.

HEMIPROSTHESIS - 30 PATIENTS

This method was chosen for the oldest group of patients. Their mean age was 78.9 years.

TOTAL HIP REPLACEMENT - 39 PATIENTS

These patients were younger (mean age 69.2 years). They were not considered for a valgisation osteotomy because of age over 70 years, severe osteoporosis or a total collapse of the femoral head.

VARIOUS INTERNAL FIXATIONS - 8 PATIENTS

Sometimes, delayed primary internal fixation, or even refixation with screws or an angled blade plate is possible without an osteotomy. This is especially a treatment option if leg length discrepancy is small or absent. This phenomenon is mainly seen after Pauwels type 2 fractures. Interposition of a corticocancellous bone graft in a recurrent nonunion of the femoral neck was performed in a young man with juvenile osteoporosis.

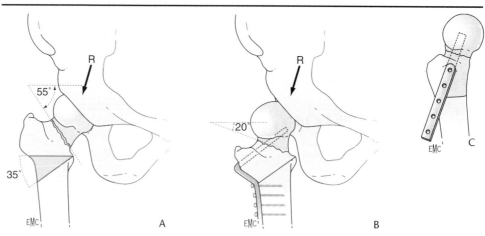

3 *A. Preoperative drawing of a femoral neck nonunion. The inclination of the nonunion is the angle between the perpendicular to the femoral shaft and the fracture line. In this example, the angle is 55°. The result (arrow) of the forces acting on the hip joint is a shearing force. In order to transform shearing into compression forces, the fracture line should be brought into a more horizontal position. Ideally, the new inclination angle should be 20°. Therefore, a lateral wedge of 35° must be taken out.*
B. Result of the preoperative planning. The inclination of the nonunion is now 20°. Mainly compressing forces are acting on the nonunion and will promote healing. The position of plate and screws is included in the drawing.
C. Retrotorsion of more than 15° should be corrected, and the position of the plate in the lateral view has to be included in the preoperative planning. Correction of these retrotorsions is mandatory in order to obtain an ideal position of the tip of the blade of the plate in the centre of the femoral head.

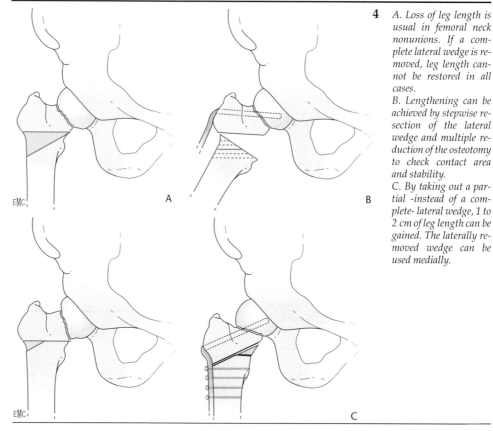

4 *A. Loss of leg length is usual in femoral neck nonunions. If a complete lateral wedge is removed, leg length cannot be restored in all cases.*
B. Lengthening can be achieved by stepwise resection of the lateral wedge and multiple reduction of the osteotomy to check contact area and stability.
C. By taking out a partial -instead of a complete- lateral wedge, 1 to 2 cm of leg length can be gained. The laterally removed wedge can be used medially.

VALGISATION OSTEOTOMY ACCORDING TO PAUWELS - 70 PATIENTS

These patients were 18 to 72 years old (mean age 49.5). Our strategy was to preserve the hip joint, certainly of our younger patients, but also in the active middle-aged group. Of course, the method has its limits. Severe incongruence of the femoral head leads to early osteoarthritis. Excavation of the head by moving hardware in unstable internal fixations offers too little chance for the nonunion to heal.

Surgical procedure

PREOPERATIVE PLANNING

The preoperative planning is performed by drawings from the plain X-rays. The amount of abduction is calculated on the AP view *(fig 3A, B, C)*. If the osteotomy cannot compensate for the loss of leg length, a partial wedge should be taken in order to gain leg length *(fig 4A, B, C)*. One of the reasons we prefer the intertrochanteric osteotomy to the subtrochanteric osteotomy

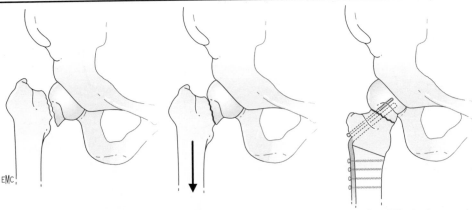

5   *Regaining of leg length by traction on the leg is sometimes possible, if there is enough mobility in the nonunion. Under maximal traction, a lag screw stabilises the new position before the valgisation osteotomy is performed.*

The intertrochanteric valgisation osteotomy is demonstrated in a typical case without significant angulation in the lateral view *(fig 3A)*. The patient is in the supine position on the operating table. A modified Watson-Jones anterolateral approach is advocated *(fig 6A)*. Sharp transverse dissection of the vastus lateralis at the intertrochanteric insertion is followed by careful release of the muscle out of the intermuscular septum to expose the lateral aspect of the femur. Ligation of the perforating vessels is obligatory. Arthrotomy of the hip joint by excision of the anterior capsula *(fig 6B)* is optional, depending on the mobility of the nonunion and the necessity for intraoperative reduction. In fibrous connected nonunions, a closed procedure is preferable. Two Kirschner wires are introduced in the sagittal plane for rotation control, one in the tip of the major trochanter and another distally from the future plate position. These wires should be inserted in a parallel way in the absence of a rotational deformity. Usually the leg is in external rotation. The corresponding angle between the K-wires marks the angle over which the future distal fragment must be internally rotated after the osteotomy. The K-wires should be parallel by then. A K-wire on the anterior side of the femoral neck marks the antetorsion of the neck *(fig 7A)*. Parallel to this guide wire in the frontal plane, a second K-wire is introduced respecting the calculated abduction correction and the antetorsion at the same time *(fig 7B)*. This guide wire can be replaced by a 6.5 mm cancellous bone screw in unstable nonunions, in order to avoid undue displacement of the nonunion during the introduction of the seating chisel. The bone

is the length of the osteotomy line in the former. The contact area is big enough, even after taking out a partial wedge. Theoretically, the ideal postoperative inclination angle to eliminate all shearing forces in the nonunion is approximatively 20°.

However, there is a limit to the degree of valgisation, given by the range of adduction, that can be reached in the hip joint. Exceeding the range of valgisation introduces an abduction contracture. Clinical assessment of the correction possibility can be documented by taking an AP X-ray in maximal adduction, but the real range of adduction is greater than clinical examination would suggest. Often the correction angle has to be evaluated during the operative procedure and falls between the optimal calculated angle and the maximal clinical adduction possibility. Severe flexion-extension-angulation deformity in the nonunion is rare. However, it must be corrected in the similar manner as for a slipped epiphysis *(fig 3C)*. Far more

frequent is the (external) rotational deformity, which has to be evaluated clinically. Femoral neck nonunions are usually atrophic. Although sometimes strong fibrous connection between femoral head and neck and almost no motion in the nonunion are observed, there is often enough mobility to allow lengthening and some correction of the varus deformity by traction on the leg as the first step *(fig 5)*. In this particular situation, the nonunion is partially reduced and fixed with one cancellous lag screw. The remaining inclination is then corrected by a valgisation osteotomy.

REQUIREMENTS

The ideal implant for the valgisation osteotomy is the AO 120° fixed angled blade plate. An alternative is the 95° condylar plate which can be bent to any desired angle, creating a similar shape as the 120° plate. Peroperatively, the use of an image identifier is recommended.

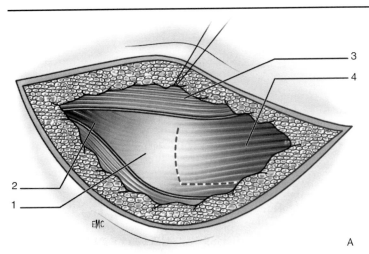

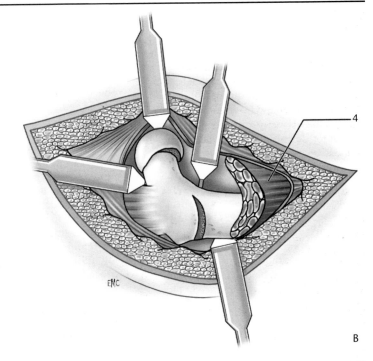

6   *A. Use a modified Watson-Jones anterolateral approach, where the major tro-chanter (1) is about in the middle. Split the fascia lata in line with the skin inci-sion. Develop the plane between gluteus medius and minimus (2) on one side and tensor fasciae latae (3) on the other. Expose the inter- and subtrochanteric region by making an L-shaped incision in the insertion of the vastus lateralis (4) and by reflecting the muscle ventrally.*
B. After excision of the ventral capsule, three Hohmann retractors are positioned. The first passes over the anterior rim of the acetabulum, the others over both sides of the femoral neck. 4. vastus lateralis.

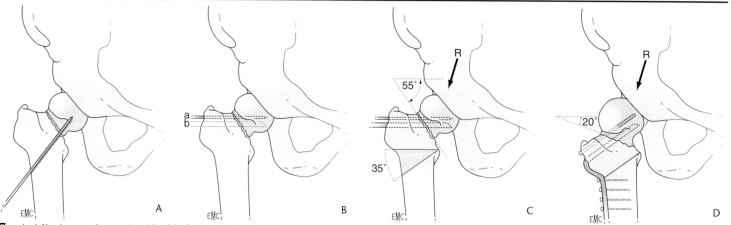

7 *A. A K-wire over the anterior side of the femoral neck marks the antetorsion of the neck.*
B. Parallel - in the lateral view - to the K-wire in fig 7A, a second K-wire (a) is introduced, respecting the calculated valgisation. Keep in mind that, if a 120°-angled blade plate is to be used, 30° of valgisation corresponds to a position of the blade perpendicular to the femur shaft. The K-wire must be introduced as high as possible in the neck and head, avoiding its interference with the future seating chisel (b).
C. The seating chisel is introduced exactly parallel to the second wire and as caudally in the femoral head as possible. Image intensifier control in both directions. Osteotomy parallel to the seating chisel and about 2 cm distal of it. After correction of rotational deformity, a second osteotomy will provide a complete or partial wedge.
D. Exchange the seating chisel for the blade of a 4-hole 120°-angled blade plate. Reduction of the osteotomy and fixation of the plate to the femur.

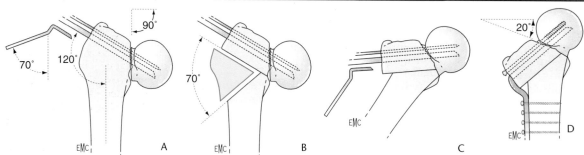

8 *The Y-shaped osteotomy allows a high valgisation degree and the medial displacement leads to direct support of the femoral head. Instead of this direct support, the laterally removed wedge can be used as a graft.*

of the femoral head is sometimes very hard.[1] The seating chisel is introduced parallel to the latter guide wire under image identifier control *(fig 7C)*. The lateral view is realised by bringing the hip joint into 90° flexion and slight abduction without changing the position of the tube. The proximal osteotomy is performed 2 cm distally and parallel to the seating chisel. A smaller amount of bone between the blade of the plate and the osteotomy increases the risk of break-out of the blade. In the presence of severe osteoporosis, the hold of the blade can be reinforced by a screw through the plate in the femoral head and by a tension-band wire around the abductor insertion at the major trochanter. In our example *(fig 3)*, a wedge of 35° is taken from the distal fragment.

There are different surgical techniques of wedge resection: complete, partial and step by step. The standard procedure is partial wedge resection in stages, allowing several osteotomy reductions using the seating chisel as a handle to check the clinical adduction possibility. After removal of the seating chisel, the blade of the chosen 120° angled blade plate is introduced. This is a

critical part of the procedure. In order to prevent a deviation of the blade, care must be taken that the exposure of the introduction point is excellent. The plate must be introduced by hand and not mounted on the device provided by the manufacturer. The blade is pushed forward parallel to the guide wire. The length of the blade must be at least 1 cm less than the distance over which the seating chisel has been driven in. The proximal fragment should have the possibility to glide over the blade towards the distal fragment.

The osteotomy is reduced by closing the wedge and applying the plate to the femoral shaft with a clamp. This action leads automatically to compression of the osteotomy. Whenever there is too much abduction in the hip joint at the end of the procedure, the position of the seating chisel should never be changed. There is only one chance for adequate grip of the chisel/blade. It is better to adapt the angle of the plate to the new situation. Fixation of the plate to the femur using the asymmetric DC-holes for additional compression concludes the procedure *(fig 7D)*. Finally, the residual range of adduction and the parallellity of the K-wires should be checked.

If the nonunion requires a valgisation of more than 50 degrees, the bony support can be increased by an alternative technique *(fig 8)*. A neutral position between abduction

and adduction should be aimed at. Even an abduction contracture of up to 10° can be accepted, but under these circumstances is it advisable to install traction-suspension for one or two weeks.

Complications and results

Valgisation osteotomy was performed in 70 patients. There was no hospital mortality. During the observation period, 19 (27%) of our patients died 4 months to 18 years (mean: 9.3 years) after the operation. Early complications were as follows. One postoperative haematoma was debrided and healed. Four times the angled blade plate had to be exchanged because the blade penetrated into the hip joint. A recurrent nonunion was encountered in 9 patients. One patient continued walking on a nonunion and felt well. His Harris Hip Score (HHS) was 84. Seven total hip replacements and 1 hemiarthroplasty were performed in the remaining 8 patients. Healing of the nonunion and osteotomy was achieved in 61 patients (87%). Twenty-six of them (43%) did not develop avascular necrosis or osteoarthritis. Their follow-up period was 0.5 - 16 years (mean 8 years). These patients had a mean HHS of 89 (67 - 100). Thirty-five patients (57%) with a healed nonunion

---

[1] Note: What is important for the healing of the nonunion is the abduction osteotomy and not the compression screw or the plate.

Table I. – Six patients with segmental collapse of the femoral head at the time of osteotomy.

Sex	Age at time of osteotomy	Reoperation or HHS-score	Interval between osteotomy and reoperation or length of FU
M	51 yrs	fusion	int: 1 y
F	31 yrs	THR	int: 14 y
F39	51 yrs	THR	int: 5 y
M	44 yrs	THR	int: 3 y
M	23 yrs	HHS 86	FU: 17 y
M	43 yrs	HHS 75	FU: 15 y

showed mild or serious signs and symptoms of segmental necrosis. In 6 of them, the deformity of the femoral head was already visible at the operation (*table I*). Interestingly, undisturbed healing of the nonunion was observed in each of these 6 cases. In 20 out of this group of 35 patients, a total hip replacement was performed, 0.5 - 18 years (mean 8.4 years) after the osteotomy. Fifteen others did not need any further (operative) treatment. Their follow-up period varied from 1 to 20 years (mean 12 years). The mean HHS is remarkably high: 79 (46-97). In total, 41 (26 + 15) patients out of 70 (59%) had no further operative treatment after a valgisation osteotomy.

Technical aspects, pitfalls and results of treatment

Healing of the femoral neck nonunion and the valgisation osteotomy is unproblematic in the presence of a vital femoral head. Osteoarthritis may develop as a consequence of the valgisation, but is rare. Of special interest are patients showing vascular disturbance of the femoral head with and without deformities at the moment of the intervention.

EXTREME VALGISATION

It is obvious that hip biomechanics are changed by the valgisation. Extreme valgisation may lead to a subluxation of the femoral head, especially in dysplastic hips. Therefore, younger patients have to be checked in regular intervals. If the hip becomes symptomatic, a secondary varisation might be indicated.

OSTEOTOMY IN THE PRESENCE OF VASCULAR DISTURBANCE WITHOUT DEFORMITY OF THE FEMORAL HEAD

A complete revascularisation is possible, but the final result is not predictable and can often be a well-tolerated collapse, a partial deformity, but also a normal head configuration (*fig 9*).

OSTEOTOMY IN THE PRESENCE OF AVASCULAR NECROSIS AND CONSECUTIVE DEFORMITY OF THE FEMORAL HEAD

In the presence of femoral head resorption and excavation of the necrotic femoral head, healing of the nonunion is compromised. The valgisation osteotomy is reserved for younger patients in which later arthrodesis might be indicated (*fig 10*).

TOTAL HIP REPLACEMENT AFTER VALGISATION OSTEOTOMY

In spite of the osteotomy, osteoarthritis may evolve, leading to a later indication for total hip replacement. In general, the technique is simple, but may be complicated by the anatomical alterations resulting from the valgisation osteotomy.

Discussion

Usually nonunions of the femoral neck are grossly displaced by shortening and rotation. If not, a simple (re)fixation of the initial fracture without complementary osteotomy can be successful. Hou [5] reports a small series of neglected fractures with shortening up to 5 cm. He was able to cure these nonunions with a pedicled autologous bone graft and to restore leg length in 4 of his 5 patients. The use of these grafts was popularised by Meyers in 1980 [11]. The initially reported success has not been reproduced in large series, and the procedure has been considered unreliable [1].

A surgical alternative for nonunions, characterised by little shortening and varisation, is slight valgisation combined with medialisation, creating a bony support

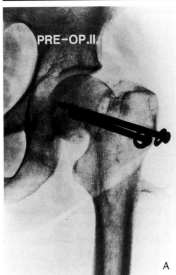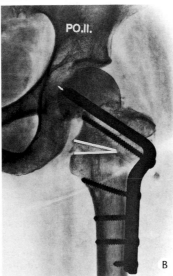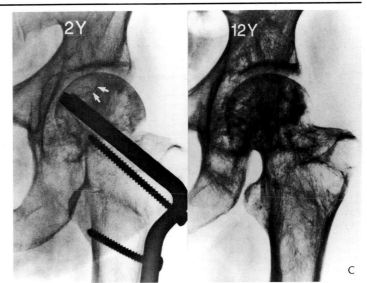

9   *A. Secondary displacement of a Pauwels type 3 fracture in a 43-year old female.*
B. Open-wedged 55° closed valgisation osteotomy. The further sliding of the plate is prepared by the seating chisel (arrow). Additional stability of the 120° plate is created by the proximal screw. The regular high density of the femoral head in comparison with the pertrochanteric area is typical for avascularity.
C. During the long follow-up, the regular density of the femoral head disappears, the competition between rebuilding and collapse ends in favour of a restructuring of the femoral head. Twelve years postoperatively the patient is free of pain, the walking distance is only slightly limited, the hip mobility is equal to that of the right side and the HHS is 91.

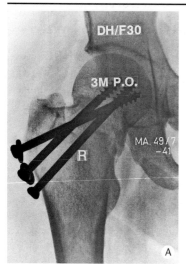
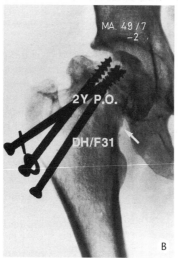
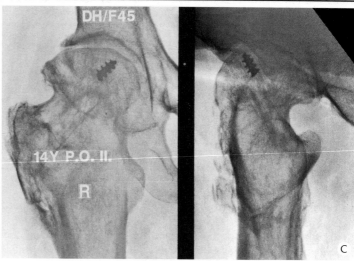

10 *This case of a young patient demonstrates that even in severe necrosis, secondary revascularisation is possible, leading to a significant delay of total joint replacement.*
A. Open reduction, impaction and screw fixation of a femoral neck fracture in a 30-year old woman.
B. Femoral head necrosis and secondary pathological fracture proximal to the healed femoral neck fracture (arrow). This phenomenon could be compared with an epiphyseal separation.
C. A still reasonable result after 14 years; HHS at that moment 83. 16 years after the primary fracture the now 46-year old patient received a total hip replacement.

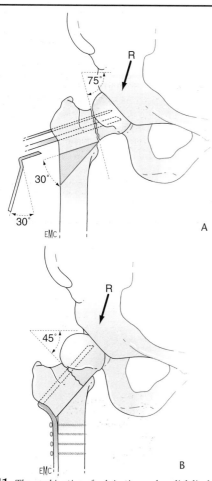

11 *The combination of valgisation and medial displacement osteotomy. In nonunions with minimal shortening, varisation and a rather long femoral head-neck fragment, a full wedge valgisation osteotomy can be performed. The medially displaced calcar creates direct support to the femoral head. Cancellous bone of the removed wedge is used as a graft.*

Table II. – Pauwels osteotomy for femoral neck nonunion. Review of the largest series.

Author	Year of publication	Number	Healed nonunion	Age limits
Weber and Cech [18]	1973	36	100 % (?)	"younger"
Lies and Scheuer [7]	1983	17	88 %	< 60 years
Walcher and Wiesinger [17]	1983	13	100 % (?)	< 40 years
Wentzensen and Weller [19]	1983	7	100 %	< 60 years
Ballmer et al [2]	1990	17	88 %	< 60 years
Anglen [1]	1999	13	100 %	?

to the femoral head (*fig 11*). The valgisation osteotomy designed by Pauwels represents a masterly mechanical concept. Not only can healing of the nonunion and osteotomy be achieved, but leg length discrepancy, rotational and angular deformity can be corrected at the same time. Osteotomies at the subtrochanteric level [6, 20] are less capable of correcting the inclination of the fracture line adequately. In addition, it is not possible to restore leg length and secondary total hip replacement becomes more difficult. Finally, the cancellous bone of the intertrochanteric region offers better healing qualities than the cortical bone at the subtrochanteric level [2]. We do not consider that preoperative traction [6, 16] is necessary. Restoration of leg length can be achieved by valgisation and varying the wedge taken from the distal fragment. We have never taken out a wedge of more than 55°. A 120°-plate as a standard implant is totally satisfactory in the case of a 50-60° correction. The question of whether a valgisation osteotomy interferes with the vascularity of the femoral head should be addressed. The findings of Calandruccio and Anderson [3] are important; they concluded that the vascular damage at the time of the fracture determines whether or not necrosis will develop. This conclusion is supported by the –not yet published– results of internal fixation of fresh femoral neck fractures in our institution. In a series of 228 patients who could be followed for 3-19 years, the frequency of avascular necrosis was the highest (57%) in the group of patients whose fractures did heal after internal fixation, but in a position other than the postoperative position. Temporary instability apparently has a greater impact on the vascularity than an osteotomy and the introduction of an angled blade plate (45% avascular necrosis).

We consider therefore, as did Pauwels, that femoral neck nonunion is above all a mechanical problem and that the addition of pedicled or unpedicled autologous bone graft [6, 14] is superfluous. Several authors who use the same technique as we have described have reported good early results [1, 2, 7, 17-19]. Together, these authors reported on 103 cases, which means that our series of patients is by far the largest ever published (*table II*). Walcher [17] considered radiographic signs of avascular necrosis in patients over 30 years of age as a contraindication for osteotomy. Our results show that it is worthwhile trying to save the joint of young patients, even in case of a segmental collapse (*table I*). A total hip replacement is considerably postponed and better conditions for hip replacement can be achieved. The results of the valgisation osteotomy related to age are listed in table III. It is obvious that patients in their sixties should not be excluded from having a joint-saving operation. In four of our patients, the proximal femoral fragment was

Table III. – Results of valgisation osteotomy related to age.

Age group/mean age/number of patients			Nonunion	Necrosis/arthrosis (preexistent excluded)	Total hip replacement/interval osteotomy-reoperation	Mean FU (no reoperation)	Mean HHS (no reoperation)
< 40 y/	28 yr/	13	0 %	54 %	23 % / 12 y	11 y	88
40-49 y/	42 yr/	17	25 %	54 %	15 % / 7 y	9 y	79
50-59 y/	55 yr/	27	4 %	54 %	44 % / 9 y	11 y	93
> 60 y/	65 yr/	13	33 %	25 %	25 % / 2 y	5 y	89

brought into too much valgus. The postoperative AP Garden Index was 180 degrees. This mechanically unfavourable situation caused a late osteoarthritis in three older patients, followed by total hip replacement. A younger patient had an intertrochanteric varus osteotomy 9 years after the Pauwels osteotomy.

Literature on the treatment of femoral neck nonunion is scarce. Reports on (total) hip replacement for nonunion are completely lacking.

It is our strategy to treat fresh femoral neck fractures with a hemiarthroplasty in patients over the biological age of 70 years. Logically, the same choice will be made for patients with a nonunion. Whether a hemiarthroplasty or a total hip replacement should be performed remains open. Approximately 8000 femoral neck fractures per year occur in The Netherlands. About 25% of these patients are under 70 years of age and should therefore be treated with internal fixation. According to the findings of Lu-Yao [8], at least 300 nonunions are produced in one year. We are afraid that the majority of these 300 nonunions in our country will be treated with an arthroplasty instead of a Pauwels osteotomy. Some missionary work still remains to be done!

References

[1] Anglen JO. Intertrochanteric osteotomy for failed internal fixation of femoral neck fracture. *Clin Orthop* 1997 ; 341 : 175-182

[2] Ballmer FT, Ballmer PM, Baumgartel F, Ganz R, Mast JW. Pauwels osteotomy for non-unions of the femoral neck. *Orthop Clin North Am* 1990 ; 21 : 759-767

[3] Calandruccio RA, Anderson WE. Post-fracture avascular necrosis of the femoral head: correlation of experimental and clinical studies. *Clin Orthop* 1980 ; 152 : 49-84

[4] Catto M. A histological study of avascular necrosis of the femoral head after transcervical fracture. *J Bone Joint Surg Br* 1965 ; 47 : 749-776

[5] Hou SM, Hang YS, Liu TK. Ununited femoral neck fractures by open reduction and vascularized iliac bone graft. *Clin Orthop* 1993 ; 294 : 176-180

[6] Huang CH. Treatment of neglected femoral neck fractures in young adults. *Clin Orthop* 1986 ; 206 : 117-126

[7] Lies A, Scheuer I. Schenkelhalspseudarthrosen bei Erwachsenen: Pathogenese, Therapie und Ergebnisse. *Unfallheilunde* 1983 ; 86 : 116-121

[8] Lu-Yao GL, Keller RB, Littenberg B, Wennberg JE. Outcomes after displaced fractures of the femoral neck. *J Bone Joint Surg Am* 1994 ; 76 : 15-23

[9] Marti RK, Raaymakers EL, Nolte P, Besselaar PP. Pseudarthrosen am proximalen Femur. *Orthopäde* 1996 ; 25 : 454-462

[10] Marti RK, Schüller HM, Raaymakers EL. Intertrochanteric osteotomy for nonunion of the femoral neck. *J Bone Joint Surg Br* 1989 ; 71 : 782-787

[11] Meyers MH. The role of posterior bone grafts (muscle pedicle) in femoral neck fracture. *Clin Orthop* 1980 ; 152 : 143-146

[12] Pauwels F. Der Schenkelhalsbruch ein mechanisches Problem Beilageheft zur Zeitschr f Orthop Chir, Band 63. Stuttgart : Enke, 1935 : 1-139

[13] Phemister DB. Repair of bone in the presence of aseptic necrosis resulting from fractures, transplantation and vascular obstruction. *J Bone Joint Surg Am* 1956 ; 38 : 769-787

[14] Schwetlick G, Weber U, Klingmuller V. Die Schenkelhalspseudarthrose nach medialer Schenkelhalsfraktur. Eine Indikation für das gefässgestielte Beckenkammtransplantat. *Unfallchirurg* 1989 ; 92 : 73-78

[15] Sevitt S. Avascular necrosis and revascularization of the femoral head after intracapsular fractures. *J Bone Joint Surg Br* 1964 ; 46 : 270-296

[16] Stewart MJ, Wells RE. Osteotomy and osteotomy combined with bone grafting for non-union following fracture of the femoral neck. *J Bone Joint Surg Am* 1956 ; 38 : 33-49

[17] Walcher K, Wiesinger H. Aufrichtungsosteotomie nach Pauwels oder Alloplastik bei der Schenkelhalspseudarthrose? *Aktuel Traumatol* 1983 ; 13 : 34-41

[18] Weber BG, Cech O. Schenkelhals-pseudarthrose. In : Weber BG, Cech Oeds. Pseudarthrosen: Pathophysiologie, Biomechanik, Therapie, Ergebnisse. Bern : Verlag Hans Huber, 1973 : 141-179

[19] Wentzensen A, Weller S. Die Pseudarthrose als Komplikation der Schenkelhalsfraktur. *Aktuel Traumatol* 1983 ; 13 : 72-76

[20] Zinghi GF, Specchia L, Ruggieri N, Galli G. The role of osteotomy in the treatment of pseudarthrosis of the neck of the femur in younger patients. *Ital J Orthop Traumatol* 1985 ; 11 : 341-348

Trochanteric and subtrochanteric fractures

I Kempf

Abstract. – Fractures of the trochanteric or subtrochanteric region represent a major health problem related to ageing of the population. Prevention will be a major challenge in coming decades. Stable osteosynthesis, which allows immediate mobilisation and, if possible, early weight-bearing, is the treatment of choice. There is a very limited place for prosthetic replacement.

About 60 to 70% of these fractures are unstable. The classifications are numerous and several point out the problem of stability, which is provided mainly by an intact inner cortical buttress, but also by the posteromedial part of the trochanteric massif.

Open surgical procedures are based on the use of sliding compression hip screws such as the AO Dynamic Hip Screw (DHS). The 130°- or 95°-angled blade-plates are of limited use. With the use of Dynamic Hip Screws, a stable osteosynthesis allowing immediate mobilisation is achieved. Full early weight-bearing is only possible in stable fractures. Technically easy to perform in simple cases, the operation is much more aggressive in displaced fractures and requires additional fixation.

Closed intramedullary procedures are mechanically more efficient because of the shorter lever arm of the implant. The Gamma Nails in their three versions – standard, trochanteric or long gamma – represent the latest advances in the treatment of trochanteric and subtrochanteric fractures. The technique is demanding: installation and reduction on a fracture table and permanent peroperative image intensifier control are mandatory. Applicable in all types of fractures, these procedures permit immediate weight-bearing, even in very unstable cases.

Prosthetic replacement is rarely indicated in trochanteric fractures. Severe coxarthrosis, tumour problems and local metabolic bone disorders may warrant endoprosthetic replacement.

Keywords: hip, fractures, trochanteric fractures, subtrochanteric fractures, classification, dynamic hip screws, Ender nailing, Gamma nails, prosthetic replacement.

Introduction

Trochanteric fractures located in well-vasularised cancellous bone are characterised by a very low nonunion and head necrosis rate, as opposed to transcervical fractures, and a good local prognosis. However, like neck fractures, which occur mostly in the elderly, the outcome may be extremely poor if there is prolonged bed-rest.

The imperative goals of treatment are early walking and immediate, full weight-bearing by means of a stable fixation.

The mean age of persons with fractures is very high – 74 years old – and females are predominant in the ratio of 2:1. The growing frequency of these fractures correlates with the combined role of age and ageing of the population. In developed countries, the incidence of such fractures has doubled between 1980 and 2000. Therefore, trochanteric fractures, like all other types of hip fractures, represent a growing social issue with serious economic, social and human consequences.

Prevention of fractures will be a very important challenge in forthcoming decades. It has been proven that in elderly people, a balanced phosphocalcic diet, the administration of calcium and vitamin D, and in females long-term treatment with oestrogen, as well as gentle physical activity, significantly reduce the incidence of hip fractures.

Anatomy – architecture – classification

ANATOMY – ARCHITECTURE – BIOMECHANICAL PROPERTIES

Of interest to the surgeon are the architecture and the biomechanical properties of the upper extremity of the femur – head, neck, and the greater and lesser trochanter – which can be compared to a crane or a street lamp. The frontal section *(fig 1)* shows both cortices in the trochanteric area:

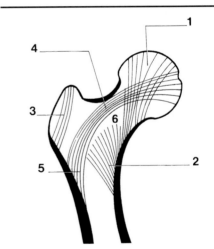

1 *Architecture of the proximal femur. 1. Principal compressive group; 2. secondary compressive group; 3. greater trochanter group; 4. principal tension group; 5. secondary tension group; 6. Ward's triangle.*

Ivan Kempf, *Professor, Emeritus Professor, Faculty of Medicine, Orthopaedic and Traumatology Surgeon, Laboratoire de Biomécanique, Institut d'Anatomie Normale, 4, rue Kirschleger, 67085 Strasbourg cedex, France.*

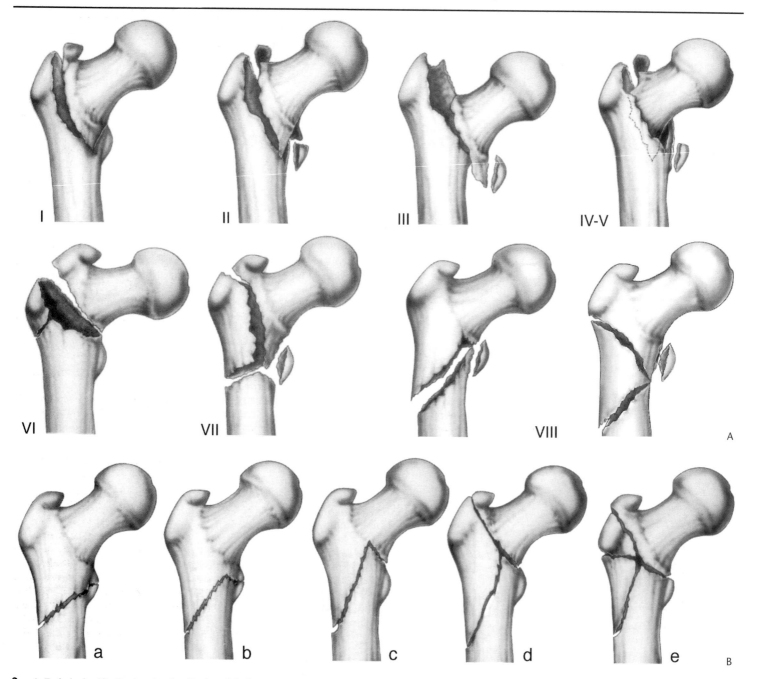

2 *A. Ender's classification based on localisation of the fracture.*
B. Subtrochanteric fractures. Classification according to Boyd and Evans. a. Evans reversed fracture; b. like a Basque roof; c. like a church tower; d. with trochanteric line; e. with trochanteric comminution.

— the medial cortex, or Adam's arch, is thicker than the lateral cortex; it plays a fundamental role in the load transfer from the pelvis through the head and neck to the femoral diaphysis. The precise reduction of this "arch" provides the stability of the fracture.

— the lateral cortex ends at the level of the insertion of the vastus lateralis at the root of the greater trochanter. Fixation devices must be inserted below this landmark into solid, cortical bone.

The spongy bone of the trochanteric region, which becomes more porotic in older patients, is a very well-vascularised one, so consolidation of fractures is the rule and non-unions are very rare. The trabeculae are disposed approximately along the line of the greatest compression and stress *(fig 1).*

Table I. – Correspondence between nomenclatures.

Pertrochanteric simple	Ender-Type 1
Pertrochanteric complex	Ender-Type 2 in external rotation
	Ender-Type 4, 5 in internal rotation with penetration
	(These differenciations are helpful for the reduction.)
Pertrochanteric with coxa valga	Ender-Type 3
Intertrochanteric	Ender-Type 6 displaced in coxa vara
Subtrochanteric	Ender-Type 7 divided into subgroups
Trochantero-diaphyseal	Ender-Type 8

CLASSIFICATION

A great number of classifications exist. In French-speaking countries, the classification always used is that of Decoulx and Lavarde [4] and Ramadier and Teinturier [16], based on anatomic criteria, whose types can easily be combined with the Ender classification [5], more-frequently used in the German-speaking world *(fig 2A).* The correspondence between both nomenclatures is provided in *table I.*

While the AO classification creates a universal common language for all traumatologists, it lacks a good description of subtrochanteric fractures, which represent an important group, being the most unstable

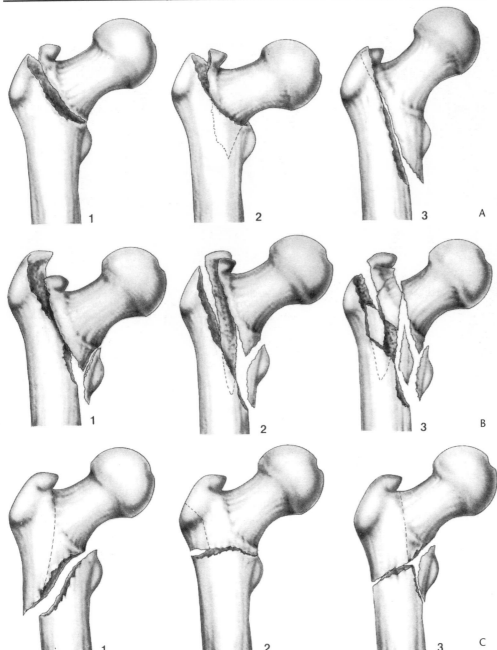

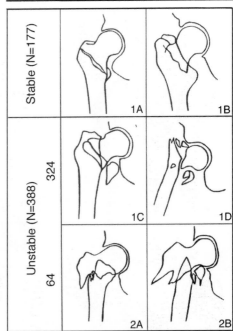

4 *Pertrochanteric fractures. Evans and Jensen classification based on the stability. (N=565).*

3 *AO classification. It is codified in 3 groups:*
A. Group A1: trochanteric, A1.1 along the trochanteric line, A1.2 pertrochanteric, A1.3 trochantero-diaphyseal below the lesser trochanter;
B. Group A2: pertrochanteric multifragmentary with 3 subgroups, A2.1 one intermediate fragment, A2.2 two intermediate fragments, A2.3 three and more intermediate fragments;
C. Group A3: intertrochanteric fractures, A3.1 oblique, simple, A3.2 transverse simple, A3.3 with medial wedge. In all three groups additional fractures can extend to the greater trochanter.

and difficult to treat. Well-described by Boyd and Evans [2, 6] *(fig 2B)*, they involve the lesser and/or the greater trochanter, and must be differentiated from the proximal diaphyseal femur fractures in which the trochanteric block is intact.

The AO classification *(fig 3)*, proposed and developed by M.E. Müller, S. Nazarian and P. Koch [15], represents a universal system that is more and more widely applied.

In the English-speaking world, the classification of Evans and Jensen [6, 7] *(fig 4)* is based mostly on the problem of stability. Stability is provided not only by an intact inner cortical buttress, but also by the

posteromedial and the posterior part of the trochanteric massif involving the lesser trochanter and the posterior crests. This stability is multidirectional, but only the single pertrochanteric fractures, Ender type 1, Evans type 1A and 1B, and AO type A1.1, are stable. All other types are unstable.

Operative treatment

The goal of the treatment is early walking and, if possible, with full weight-bearing. Conservative treatment with prolonged bed-rest is rarely indicated. Stable osteosynthesis

is the rule, performed either by open or closed methods, or by prosthetic replacement.

OPEN FIXATION: NAILS, PLATES, SCREW PLATES

In the early days of surgical treatment, trochanteric fractures were fixed with different types of articulated nail plates, which provided a large number of mechanical complications at the junction between the nail and the plate; these have now been completely abandoned and replaced by "monoblock" angled plates. Previously, the most frequently used plates were the AO-ASIF 130°-angled blade-plate, which is no longer recommended, and the AO-ASIF 95°-condylar plate, which is still in use [14].

■ *Surgical approach*

The patient is supine, either on a fracture table with closed reduction and the help of the image intensifier (one or preferably two apparatus), or on a conventional table with open reduction. Using a lateral approach, split the fascia lata in line with the skin incision to expose the trochantero-subtrochanteric region by making an L-shaped incision close to the insertion of the vastus lateralis and by reflecting the muscle forwards. This approach is identical for all types of fixation material in open procedures. For subtrochanteric fractures, the approach must be extended more or less distally.

■ *The 130°-angled AO blade-plate* *(fig 5)*

The operative technique is well-known and easy to perform in a simple undisplaced, or

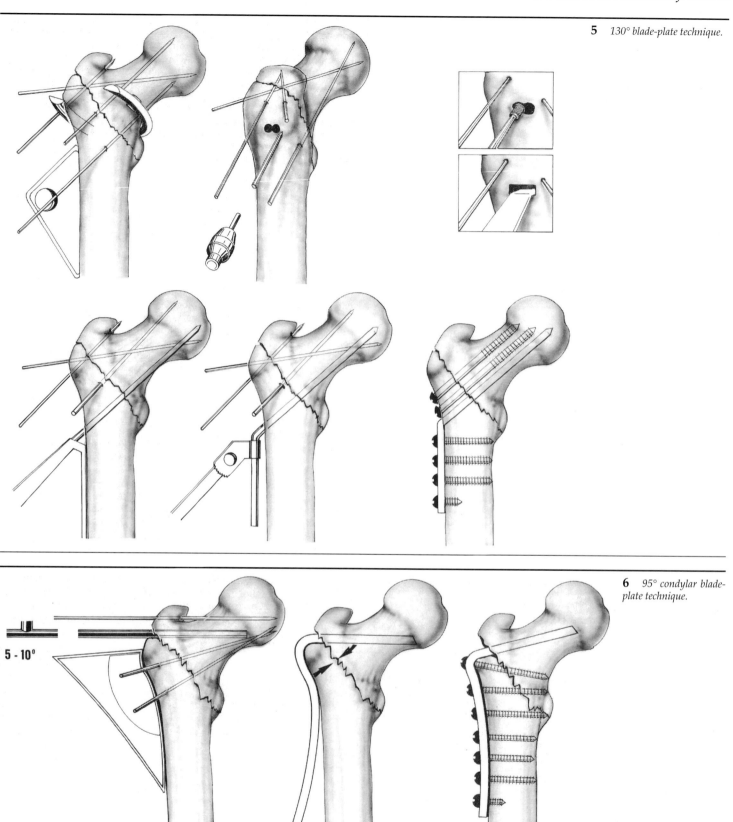

5 *130° blade-plate technique.*

6 *95° condylar blade-plate technique.*

slightly displaced, stable type Ender 1, AO A1.1 fracture, which represents a possible residual indication.

■ **The 95° condylar plate** *(fig 6)*

This material is more stable due to two possibilities of compression of the fracture line with one or two transverse screws and the preloaded plate. The plate requires a solid inner cortical buttress, and some surgeons favour these plates. However, there are some disadvantages.

In this procedure, adjunctions are necessary to improve stability in complex cases, such as additional, cancellous bone grafts when there is a bone defect, additional screw or wires, or when bone cement is no longer advisable as it blocks callus formation.

Modified procedures, such as immediate valgisation (Sarmiento) and medial translation (Dimon), are interesting concepts, but in practice, they have a very restricted field of application.

The main disadvantage of blade-plates is the lack of a sliding capacity, which can be responsible for mechanical complications, such as penetration into the joint space,

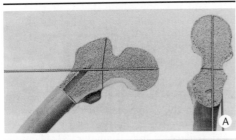

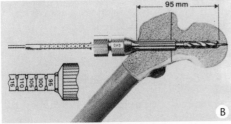

95 mm

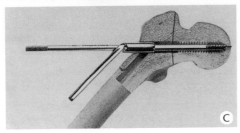

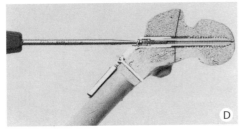

7 *DHS (Dynamic Hip Screw) technique.*
A. Positioning of the guide wire in the centre of the neck.
B. Drilling the hole with a long screw drill.
C. Introduction of the screw and positioning of the plate.
D. Compression of the fracture site.

loosening or breaking of the device itself. For these different reasons, the above devices have been largely abandoned.

■ *Compression screw plates*

At the moment, compression screw plates are the most widely used devices in the open treatment of trochanteric fractures. They are manufactured in two parts and improved technology has removed problems at the junction of screw and plate. The most frequently used screw plates are the AO Dynamic Hip Screw (DHS) [17] and other contemporary models, such as the THS or Howmedica Vitalium Compression Screw. They are the modern versions of older, well-proved devices, such as the Putti Hip Screw or the Pohl'sche Lasche.

Insertion technique with AO-ASIF Dynamic Hip Screw (DHS) *(fig 7)*

The screw exists in 11 lengths ranging from 65 to 115 mm. The CCD angles are basically 135° and 150°, with the possibility of

ordering special types, such as 140° and 145°. The most frequently used plates have four, five or six holes (on special request, 2 to 16 holes). More recently, an extension of the DHS using a trochanter stabilising plate has been developed for unstable intertrochanteric fractures [1].

Through a lateral approach, the fracture site is exposed and an open reduction is performed when operating on a normal table. The fracture is stabilised by driving a 2.5-mm-thick Kirschner wire into the head, very precisely placed in the centre of neck and head in both anteroposterior and axial views, which serves also as a guide-wire for the insertion of the screw. The hole for the screw is prepared with the 3-mm diameter drill-bit. After measurement of the length, the appropriate screw is placed, and then the plate is fixed with 4.5-mm cortical screws. The fracture site is compressed by using the special compression screw.

Like blade-plates, DHS and other types of compression hip screws permit good fixation for stable fractures, but additional grafts, screws or wires are required for complex fractures.

In general, open techniques are known to allow an anatomical reduction of the fracture, but in most cases, closed reductions are of good quality. In both techniques, a secondary collapse occurs, thus stabilising the fracture. The sliding capacity of most hip compression screws is a decisive advantage in comparison to "monoblock" blade-plates. However, open procedures increase the risk of devascularisation of the fragments, bleeding and infection. Last, but not least, the length of the lever arm of blade- and screw-plates does not allow immediate and full weight-bearing in unstable fractures.

CLOSED PROCEDURES

Closed procedures are less aggressive for periosteal vessels and achieve improved mechanical behaviour with a shorter lever arm.

Two methods can be qualified as closed intramedullary cephalo-cervico-diaphyseal nailing methods – Ender Nailing and Gamma Nailing – both derived from devices designed by G. Küntscher [12]. The Trochanteric Nail is used for the first method and the Y-Nail for the second method. Both have sliding possibilities.

■ *Ender Nailing*

In the original technique, the multiple rod, elastic nailing by Ender [5] *(fig 8)* showed several imperfections and complications: sliding down of the nail, malunions in varus, and frequently severe, external rotation with shortening, as well as proximal cephalic perforations within the articular space. It was improved by I. Kempf and S. Bitar [8] by manufacturing a distal 1.5-cm slot allowing controlled sliding of the nails *(fig 9)*.

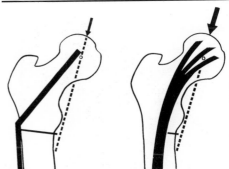

8 *Principle of Ender Nailing. In comparison with blade plate: shortening of the lever arm.*

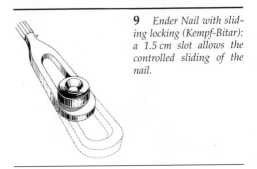

9 *Ender Nail with sliding locking (Kempf-Bitar): a 1.5 cm slot allows the controlled sliding of the nail.*

Nevertheless, the method is increasingly abandoned in developed countries because of prolonged knee pain, restriction of motion and no possibility of immediate, full weight-bearing in very unstable fractures.

However, due to its low cost, this method could be of interest in developing countries.

■ *Gamma Nailing*

Gamma Nailing *(fig 10A, B)*, developed in Strasbourg by Kempf, Grosse and Tagland [11], represents the latest development and advance in the treatment of trochanteric fractures; it is based on the principle of a closed procedure and interlocking nailing with sliding possibilities [9-11]. The Gamma Nail consists of an intramedullary nail, wider at the proximal end and narrower at the distal end, and a cervical lag screw, which is easily introduced by a targeting device and is also used for the distal interlocking. It is inspired by the Küntscher Y-nail *(fig 10B)*, which we modified by inverting the mechanical construction of the nail so that the lag screw passes through the intramedullary nail.

Implants *(fig 10A, B)*

● *Nails*

The standard nail. The standard nail is manufactured in Orthinox. It has a slight valgus and antecurvature with a proximal diameter of 17 mm, a distal diameter of 11, 12 or 14 mm and a length of 20 cm. The cervico-diaphyseal angulations are 125°, 130°, 135° and 140°. The distal part presents two holes for 6.28-mm self-tapping screws. The most frequently used diameter is 11 mm. For this reason, this standard nail is increasingly replaced by the "Trochanteric Nail", which is 11 mm in diameter, 18 cm

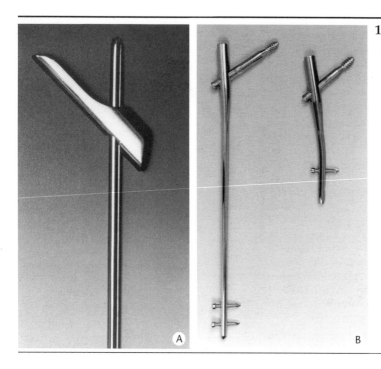

10 *A. Küntscher Y-Nail.*
B. Long Gamma Nail.
Trochanteric Gamma
Nail.

long and has one single distal interlocking hole. The proximal hollow part of the nail is threaded for introduction of a set-screw, which blocks the rotation and controls the sliding of the lag screw.

The long Gamma Nail. The proximal part has the same characteristics as the standard nail, with the same diameter and the same angulations. The distal part is an unslotted, rigid nail of 11 mm diameter, 32–44 cm in length, and has two distal holes for 6.28-mm self-tapping, interlocking screws.

- *Lag screw*

The lag screw exists in lengths from 80 to 130 mm. The proximal part presents four grooves for penetration of the tip of the set-screw.

- *Instrumentation*

The overall design of the instrumentation is similar to the ancillaries used in the conventional locking nailing technique: nail impactor, sighting devices, lag screw guide

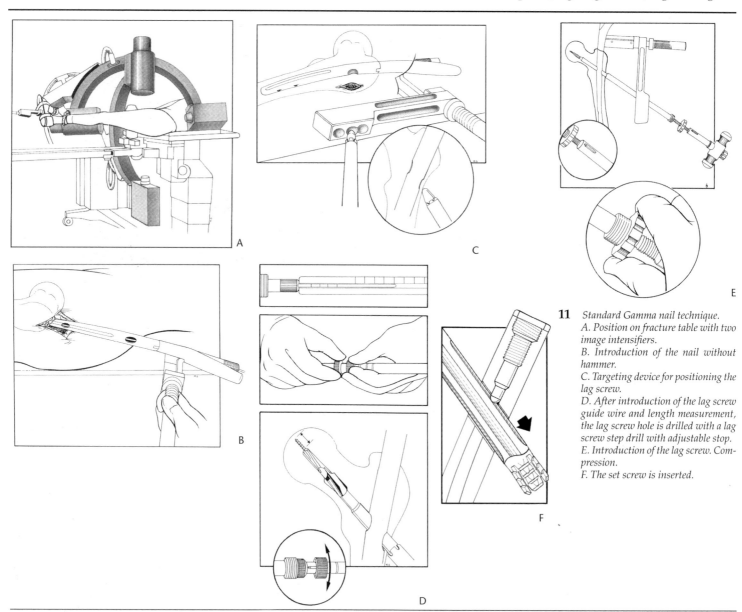

11 *Standard Gamma nail technique.*
A. Position on fracture table with two image intensifiers.
B. Introduction of the nail without hammer.
C. Targeting device for positioning the lag screw.
D. After introduction of the lag screw guide wire and length measurement, the lag screw hole is drilled with a lag screw step drill with adjustable stop.
E. Introduction of the lag screw. Compression.
F. The set screw is inserted.

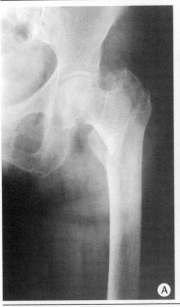 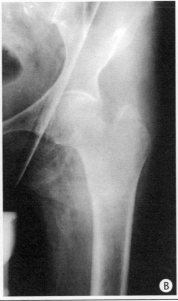 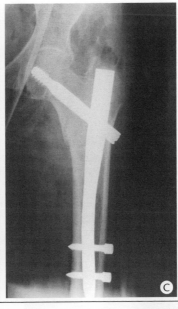

12 *A. Pertrochanteric fracture, Ender 4, A1.2.*
B. Perfect reduction.
C. Osteosynthesis with standard Gamma Nail.

wire with a 10-mm threaded tip, step drill for lag screw, lag screw driver, set-screw driver, etc.

Surgical techniques *(fig 11)*

● *Standard Gamma Nail*

— Preoperative planning on a true AP control X-ray of the fracture after reduction. Check the femoral neck angle and select the appropriate nail with the aid of the template.

— Place the patient in a supine position on a fracture table *(fig 11A)*. To allow good access to the trochanter major, bend the trunk on the side opposite the fracture and fix it with a thoracic support.

— One, or preferably two, if possible, image intensifiers can be used to check the frontal and lateral view.

— A 6- to 8-mm incision is made over the trochanteric region *(fig 11B)*. The fascia lata is divided. The entry point at the tip of the greater trochanter is enlarged with a pointed awl. The guide wire is inserted. Ream until 17 mm of the trochanteric region. The proximal part of the medullary canal of the femur is prepared using a reamer with a diameter 2 mm greater than the selected nail diameter.

— The selected nail is introduced by hand (without a hammer), avoiding any additional diaphyseal fracture, a frequent complication in the beginning *(fig 11B)*.

— The targeting device with the chosen angulation is fixed *(fig 11C)*. Through a small incision and with the help of guide sleeves and a pointed awl, the lag screw guide wire with a 10-mm threaded tip is screwed into the bone, whilst checking for an adequate position near the inner cortex of the neck in the frontal view, and strictly in the centre of neck and head in the lateral view. After transfer of the estimated length of the lag screw, the cannulated lag-screw step drill with an adjustable stop is inserted over the guide-wire with the lag screw on it, and driven into the bone *(fig 11D)*.

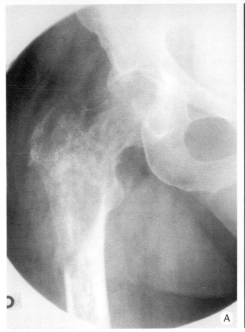 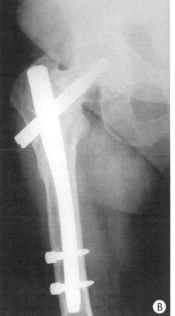

13 *A. Metastasis of mamma carcinoma.*
B. Result after 6 months after stabilisation with standard Gamma Nail.

— The lag screw, attached to a special screwdriver, is introduced over the guide wire. Once the introduction is complete, the screwdriver handle must be parallel with the targeting device to allow the set-screw tip to enter one of the four lag-screw grooves.

— If necessary, compression can be applied using the thumb-wheel on the screwdriver *(fig 11E)*.

— The set-screw is inserted and first tightened onto the lag screw, then finally backed off a quarter-turn to allow free sliding of the lag screw *(fig 11F)*.

— If distal locking is indicated, the same proximal target device is used. The bone is drilled through a double sleeve and without using the pointed awl: two 6.28-mm self-tapping screws for the standard nail, one screw for the trochanteric nail.

The indications for the standard Gamma Nail are all types of trochanteric fractures *(fig 12A, B, C)*, especially Ender type 6, 7 (Evans 2a, 2b) and short oblique type 8 (trochantero-diaphyseal); pathologic fractures *(fig 13A, B)*; or fracture in hips with coxa vara deformities and pseudarthrosis.

Postoperative care. From a strictly functional point of view, immediate weight-bearing is desirable in all types of fractures including the very unstable ones; however, this depends on the general condition of the patient.

Critics have pointed out the imperfection of the reduction in closed procedures, which theoretically could be better realised by open reduction. However, apart from the rare cases of irreducible Ender type 7

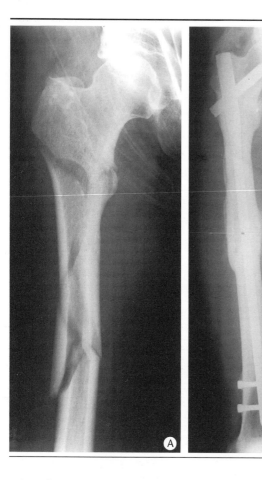

14 A. Trochanteric-diaphyseal fracture Ender 8, A1.3.
B. Long Gamma nail. Final result.

41 minutes (10–140 min). Spinal anaesthesia was performed in 90 cases and general anaesthesia in 31 cases. Repositioning was anatomic in 88 cases (71%), correct in 25 cases (20%), and poor in eight cases (7%). The mean irradiation time was 88 seconds. The most used implants had the following characteristics: angulation 130°; 100-mm long screw; a diameter of 12 mm, and more recently, 11 mm. The position of the lag screw was good in 86 cases (66%), acceptable in 33 cases (27%) and poor in eight cases (6.6%). Early weight-bearing (1 week) was achieved in 83.4% of the cases.

Peroperative complications included nine additional fractures, but this major complication totally disappeared after introducing the nail by hand without the use of a hammer. Six difficulties in performing distal locking were apparent; this disappeared with the use of a double guide sleeve.

Postoperative complications included six haematomas, three superficial infections, one deep infection and three phlebites.

The final results showed 15 exitus at three months (12.6%), zero nonunions, three malunions in rotation > 10° and 7 in varus > 10%.

In conclusion, the main advantages of the Gamma Nail are that, although it is a routine but demanding technique, it is applicable in all types of fractures without any additional fixation, it is a closed procedure, and it results in immediate full weight-bearing in all types of fractures.

subtrochanteric fractures with fixed flexion displacement of the proximal fragment, which need the help of a lever introduced through the wound to obtain the reduction, this criticism is untrue. In fact, the quality of closed reduction is as good as that of open reduction in the vast majority of cases. What is important is that the Gamma Nail, as for the DHS, the DHS-like devices and the Ender Nail, has a sliding capacity to guide the secondary collapse of unstable fractures. In most cases, it ends in a moderate malunion, for example, in slight varus and shortening, that very seldom requires a corrective osteotomy.

• *Long Gamma Nail*

The installation is the same as for the standard nail, but with transcondylar traction by Steinman pin placed as distally as possible under television control. Due to the rigidity of the unslotted 11-mm nail, it is necessary to ream until 13 mm. The nail is introduced without the use of a hammer. The longest nail is selected to perform the distal double-locking in good conditions without passing through large muscle masses.

This nail is indicated for all trochanteric and subtrochanteric fractures *(fig 14A, B)* with extension to the diaphyseal area, high diaphyseal femoral fractures, and associated fractures: trochanteric–mediodiaphyseal, distal metaphyseo–diaphyseal, pathological fractures and pseudarthrosis.

For the association cervical neck-diaphysis, we always prefer the combined Grosse-Kempf Nail with two or three additional cervical screws.

Postoperative care is the same as above and immediate weight-bearing in all types of fractures depends on the patient's general condition.

RESULTS

■ *DHS* [13]

In a series of 307 fractures of the trochanteric massif, Langlais et al [13] reported that 70% were unstable, repositioning was good in 90% of the cases, the screw was positioned in the centre of femoral head in 77% of the cases, and early weight-bearing was achieved in 65% of the patients.

Postoperative complications were superficial infection in three patients (1%), cut-out of the screw in three patients (1%) and loosening of the plate in three patients (1%).

The final results showed nonunion in three patients (1%) and mortality at three months (9%).

■ *Standard Gamma Nail* [10, 11]

A retrospective study of 121 cases out of 238 treated in the Traumatology Center of Strasbourg between May 1988 and November 1990 showed a predominance of unstable fractures (69%). The operation was always performed in the first 28 hours and the average duration of operation was

■ *Long Gamma Nail* [10]

For this new procedure, our own experience (138 cases of severe associated high energy fractures of the femur treated between 1990 and 1995) shows that the patients are much younger (mean age 46.6 years) and the operation is much longer and more aggressive than that for the standard Gamma Nail (65 minutes and blood transfusion in 106 patients).

The only complication was one additional fracture. Weight-bearing on the third day was possible in 78% of the cases. We noted several secondary and late complications: four deep sepsis, three of them cured by appropriate methods, four nonunions healed by renailing; three malunions in rotation; three in varus not reoperated for the moment; and seven exitus before the fifth month.

In summary, this operation is much longer, much more aggressive and has more serious complications.

PROSTHETIC REPLACEMENT

As in the treatment of femoral neck fractures, several authors (Vidal in France [18], Broos in Belgium [31]) have proposed prosthetic replacement in the treatment of trochanteric fractures, mainly with the same argument of the possibility of immediate, full weight-bearing.

Different types of prosthesis can be used. This is a much more aggressive procedure in elderly people than a conventional total hip replacement or an osteosynthesis. Thus, it appears unbiological and shocking to treat a fracture with such a mutilating procedure that almost always consolidates without problems if a technically correct and stable osteosynthesis is performed.

Surgeons in favour of this method obtain as good results as with more conservative methods. Broos [3] reported the following: average operating time for Bipolar prosthesis 42 minutes, long stem prosthesis 64 minutes; blood loss Bipolar prosthesis 276 mL, long stem prosthesis 726 mL. Results: 1 luxation in 102 endoprostheses compared with 13 mechanical failures in 14 Ender Nail and in 41 angled plates.

Nevertheless, we think that there are very restricted indications for prosthetic replacement, for example trochanteric fractures on severe painful coxarthrosis.

COMMENTS

Nonunions are very rare and can be treated either by re-osteosynthesis or valgisation-osteotomy.

Head necrosis is exceptional; total hip replacement is the solution.

Only severe malunions in young people require corrective osteotomies (valgisation, derotation, etc.)

Infection in the fracture site is one of the more catastrophic events and can lead to large resections and severe disability.

In pathological fractures, we prefer closed procedures, such as Gamma Nails and interlocking nails, which are less aggressive than open procedures with plates and cement (*fig 15*) and allow immediate and full weight-bearing.

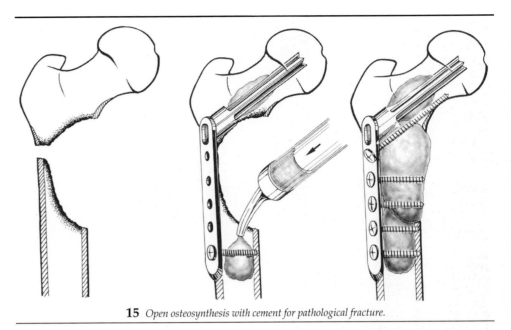

15 *Open osteosynthesis with cement for pathological fracture.*

Conclusions

Trochanteric fractures represent a major health problem in developed countries, where prevention is a major goal. For modern treatment, we see two "stars":
– in open procedures, all kinds of Hip Compression Screw;
– in closed procedures, the Gamma Nail.

References

[1] Babst R, Renner N, Biedermann M, Rosso R, Heberer M, Harder F et al. Clinical results using the Trochanter Stabilisation Plate (TSP): the modular extension for internal fixation of selected unstable intertrochanteric fractures. *J Orthop Trauma* 1998 ; 12 : 392-399

[2] Boyd HB, Griffin LL. Classification and treatment of trochanteric fractures. *Arch Surg* 1989 ; 58 : 853-856

[3] Broos PL, Willemsen PJ, Rommens PM, Stapparts KH, Gruwez JA. Pertrochanteric fractures in elderly patients. Treatment with a long-neck endoprosthesis. *Unfall chirurg* 1989 ; 92 : 234-239

[4] Decoulx P, Lavarde G. Les fractures de la région trochantérienne. In : 71ᵉ congrès français de chirurgie, Paris 1969. Paris : Masson, 1976 : 383-496

[5] Ender J. Per und Subtrochantäre Oberschenkelbrüche. *Hefte Unfallheilk* 1979 ; 106 : 2

[6] Evans EH. Treatment of trochanteric fractures of the femur. *J Bone Surg* 1949 ; 318 : 190-203

[7] Jensen JS. Classification of trochanteric fractures. *Acta Orth Scan* 1980 ; 51 : 803-810

[8] Kempf I, Bitar S. L'enclouage d'Ender, bilan et améliorations techniques. Le verrouillage coulissant. *Rev Chir Orthop* 1982 ; 68 : 199-205

[9] Kempf I, Dagrenat D, Karger C. Fractures de l'extrémité supérieure du fémur. *Encycl Méd Chir* (Éditions Scientifiques et Médicales Elsevier SAS, Paris), Appareil locomoteur, 14-076-A-10, 1993 : 1-28

[10] Kempf I, Taglang G, Favreul E. Le clou gamma. In : Cahiers d'enseignement de la SOFCOT. Paris : Expansion scientifique française, 1999 : n° 69

[11] Kempf I, Grosse A, Taglang G, Favreul E. Le clou Gamma dans le traitement à foyer fermé des fractures trochantériennes. Résultats et indications à propos d'une série de 121 cas. *Rev Chir Orthop* 1993 ; 79 : 29-40

[12] Küntscher G. Praxis der Marknagelung. Stuttgart : Friedrich K Schattauer, 1962

[13] Langlais F, Burdin TH, Jobard D, Lambotte JC, Simon P, Babin S. Ostéosynthèse par vis-plaque des fractures du massif trochantérien. In : Cahiers d'enseignement de la SOFCOT, Paris : Expansion scientifique française, 1999 : n° 69

[14] Müller ME, Allgöwer M, Willenegger H. Manual of internal fixation. Berlin : Springer-Verlag, 1991

[15] Müller ME, Nazarian S, Koch P. Classification AO des fractures du fémur. Paris : Springer-Verlag, 1987

[16] Ramadier JO, Teinturier J. Les fractures trochantériennes et juxtatrochantériennes. *Rev Chir Orthop* 1956 ; 42 : 795-782

[17] Reggazoni P, Ruedi T, Winquist R, Allgöwer M. The dynamic hip-screw. Berlin : Springer-Verlag, 1986

[18] Vidal J, Buscayret C, Goalard C. Prothèse massive de Vidal-Goalard. In : Cahiers d'enseignement de la SOFCOT. Paris : Expansion scientifique française, 1989 ; n° 12 : 104-111

Acetabular fractures

G Zinghi
A Moroni

Abstract. – *Acetabular fractures are difficult to diagnose and to treat. According to the spatial distribution of the skeletal injury, acetabular fractures can be classified as occurring on the vertical plane, on the horizontal plane and on multiple planes. Judet and Letournel radiographic views are indispensable for correct radiographic diagnosis. Two-dimensional and three-dimensional CTs are useful for planning the reduction manoeuvres and surgical approaches. Nonoperative methods for complex acetabular fractures are unreliable in restoring the articular surface. Surgical treatment is indicated in the majority of the cases. The goal is to anatomically reduce the fracture and to achieve a stable fixation. This allows early functional recovery. The main surgical approaches include the Kocher-Langenbeck, the ilioinguinal and the extended iliofemoral Letournel. Femoral head necrosis, infections and sciatic nerve palsy are the major complications. If the acetabulum is anatomically reconstructed, there is a high rate of excellent and good long term results.*

Keywords: hip, pelvic ring, acetabulum, fractures, classifications, surgical approaches.

Introduction

Acetabular fractures are difficult to diagnose and to treat. In this chapter, emphasis will be given to those fractures which require surgical treatment. These fractures are classified and treated according to a specific diagnostic and treatment protocol. The cases which require conservative treatment are outlined but will not be discussed. They include non-displaced fractures, fractures of the anterior column with minor displacement, posterior dislocation of the femoral head with detachment of a minor bone fragment, and infratectal transverse fractures.

Radiographic diagnosis

Radiographic diagnosis of acetabular fractures can be made on the three radiographic views originally described by Judet and Letournel [6-8, 10, 11]. Anteroposterior, iliac oblique, and obturator oblique radiographic views are necessary for the choice of treatment and the surgical approach. A thorough knowledge of pelvic anatomy is also necessary for the

Gianfranco Zinghi, M.D.
Antonio Moroni, M.D.
Third Department of Orthopaedic Surgery, Rizzoli Orthopaedic Institute, via G.C. Pupilli 1, 40136 Bologna, Italy.

radiographic diagnosis and surgical treatment of these fractures.

In the anteroposterior view, six major radiological landmarks of the acetabulum can be identified: the border of the anteroposterior wall of the acetabulum; the roof; the tear drop; the ilioischiatic line; the pelvic inlet (brim of the true pelvis); and the innominate line.

The obturator oblique view is used to study the anterior column. The following features can be identified: the pelvic brim (the fundamental line of the anterior column); elements of the articular surface, especially the posterior border; the obturator foramen; and the iliac wing.

The iliac oblique view is used to study the posterior column. The following features can be identified: the posterior border of the iliac bone, the anterior border of the acetabulum, and the iliac wing.

The three radiographic views described by Judet and Letournel are still the best way to diagnose an acetabular fracture. However, there are particular features that can only be studied by computed tomography (CT). These features include lesions of the sacroiliac joint, retained intra-articular bone fragments in the hip joint, and impacted cancellous bone fragments in the acetabular wall. Conventional CT is a useful tool for postoperative evaluation of the fractures.

Two-dimensional CT is indicated in both-column, high anterior column and high posterior wall fractures to evaluate the congruency between the femoral head and the roof.

Three-dimensional CT is especially recommended to select the surgical approach and the reduction manoeuvres when treating transverse, anterior wall, high anterior column and both-column fractures.

Surgical approach and reduction technique

Early in 1974, Judet and Letournel claimed that the basic treatment principles for displaced articular fractures also apply to displaced acetabular fractures [7]. The goal of treating displaced acetabular fractures should be the anatomical reduction of the articular surfaces, rigid internal fixation of the fracture fragments and early motion [1, 5, 9, 12-16, 19-21]. These goals can be achieved by adequate exposure of the acetabulum and firm internal fixation.

Given that the quality of the exposure and accuracy of the reduction are closely related, the choice of the surgical approach is important. Approaches that have been advocated are ilioinguinal, iliofemoral, extended iliofemoral, Kocher-Langenbeck, transtrochanteric, triradiate and modified extended iliofemoral.

Exposure of the entire acetabulum cannot be achieved through a single approach. The

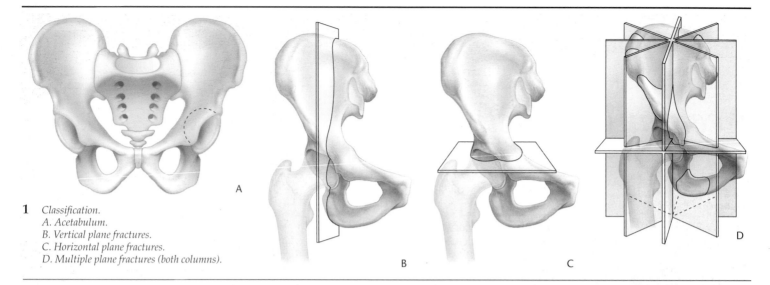

1 *Classification.*
A. Acetabulum.
B. Vertical plane fractures.
C. Horizontal plane fractures.
D. Multiple plane fractures (both columns).

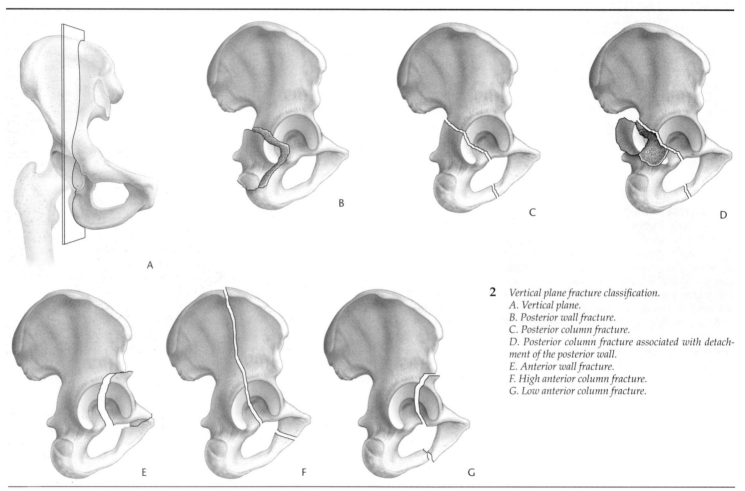

2 *Vertical plane fracture classification.*
A. Vertical plane.
B. Posterior wall fracture.
C. Posterior column fracture.
D. Posterior column fracture associated with detachment of the posterior wall.
E. Anterior wall fracture.
F. High anterior column fracture.
G. Low anterior column fracture.

three surgical approaches commonly used include Kocher-Langenbeck, ilioinguinal, and extended iliofemoral exposures.

KOCHER-LANGENBECK APPROACH

The Kocher-Langenbeck approach is indicated for the posterior column, posterior wall, some transverse, and the both-column fractures. Through this approach, the surgeon has access to the posterior column, the greater and lesser sciatic notch, all of the retro-acetabular surface, the subcotyloid groove, and the posterior part of the ischiopubic ramus.

The patient is anaesthetised and then transferred to the operating table. A urinary catheter is inserted with an aseptic technique prior to surgery. The patient is then placed in the prone decubitus position. Betadine solution is used for ten minutes to clean the affected site. The entire lower extremity, with the gluteal areas, is isolated with sterile drapes. The lower extremity is wrapped with a sterile bandage. An assistant keeps the hip extended and the knee flexed at 90 degrees to relax the sciatic nerve.

ILIOINGUINAL APPROACH

The ilioinguinal approach is indicated in

fracture types which are anterior to the tear drop, and in some transverse and both-column fractures. Through this approach, the surgeon has access to the whole medial aspect of the iliac wing, to the whole anterior column and to the pubic symphysis.

EXTENDED LETOURNEL ILIOFEMORAL APPROACH

The extended iliofemoral approach is indicated in the both-column, transverse, and late presented T-shaped fractures. Through this approach, the surgeon has access to the whole external surface of the

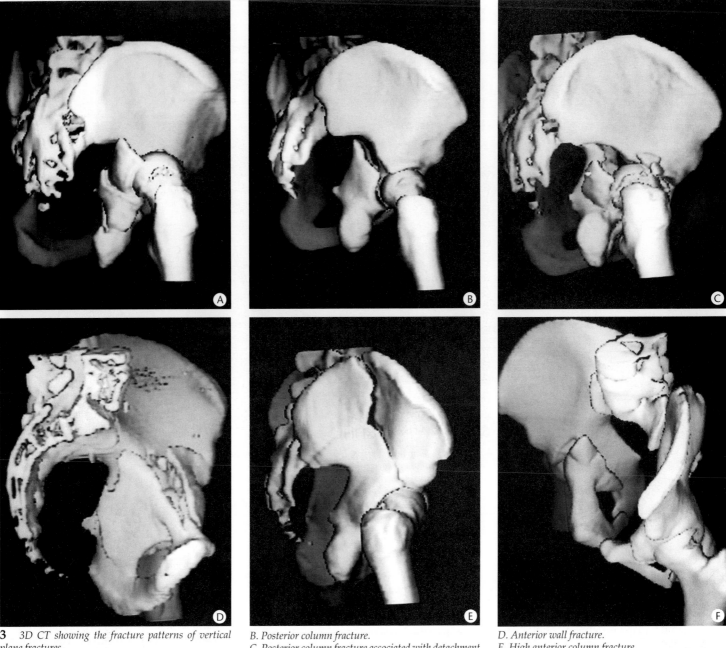

3 *3D CT showing the fracture patterns of vertical plane fractures.*
  A. Posterior wall fracture.

B. Posterior column fracture.
C. Posterior column fracture associated with detachment of the posterior wall.

D. Anterior wall fracture.
E. High anterior column fracture.
F. Low anterior column fracture.

innominate bone, the external aspect of the ilium, the posterior column until the sciatic tuberosity, the anterior column medially to the iliopectineal eminence, and the pelvic brim.

Classification

In 1964, Robert Judet et al [6] stated that classification of acetabular fractures must be simple and based on the elementary lesions of the acetabulum. According to this classification, acetabular fractures are classified as either elementary or associated. He listed four types of elementary fractures: fracture of the posterior lip, fracture of the ilioischial column, transverse fracture and fracture of the iliopublic column.

In 1974, Judet and Letournel [7] reclassified both elementary and associated acetabular fractures. Elementary fractures were subdivided into posterior wall fracture, pure posterior column fracture, anterior wall fracture, anterior column fracture, and transverse fracture. Associated fractures were subdivided into "T" fracture, posterior column fracture associated with posterior wall fracture, transverse fracture associated with posterior wall fracture, anterior column fracture associated with posterior hemitransverse fracture, and both-column fracture. This classification was slightly modified in 1981 by Letournel [11].

In 1990, Müller [17] published his AO Classification in which acetabular fractures are divided into types A, B and C in order to portray the increased severity of the fracture using an alphanumerical system. This classification was further elaborated by Tile in 1995 [21]. Tile classified acetabular fractures into Type A: partial articular fractures, one column involved; type B: partial articular fracture, transverse or T type fracture, both-columns involved; and type C: complete articular fracture, both-column fracture, floating acetabulum.

In 1996, the Orthopaedic Trauma Association (OTA) [18] presented a detailed classification based on Müller's AO-classification. The OTA classification groups acetabular fractures into type A: partial articular, involving only one column or wall; type B: partial articular and transverse; type C: complete articular involving both-columns. These fracture types are further subdivided numerically.

Based upon the projection of the fracture lines on different spatial planes, the authors slightly modified the Letournel classification. According to this classification, the acetabular fractures are subdivided into

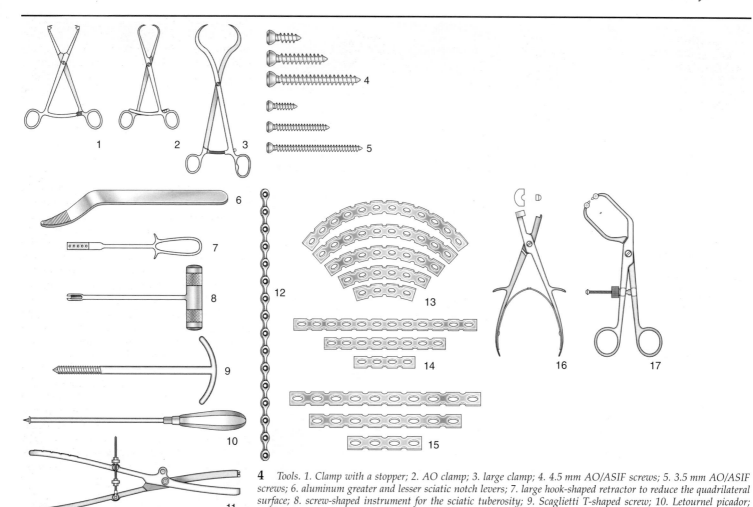

4 *Tools. 1. Clamp with a stopper; 2. AO clamp; 3. large clamp; 4. 4.5 mm AO/ASIF screws; 5. 3.5 mm AO/ASIF screws; 6. aluminum greater and lesser sciatic notch levers; 7. large hook-shaped retractor to reduce the quadrilateral surface; 8. screw-shaped instrument for the sciatic tuberosity; 9. Scaglietti T-shaped screw; 10. Letournel picador; 11. Farabeuf large clamp; 12. mouldable Citieffe plate; 13. narrow curved PCD plate; 14. straight, narrow PCD plate; 15. wide PCD plate; 16. Citieffe plate moulder; 17. Matta curved clamp.*

fractures on the vertical plane, horizontal plane and on multiple planes (*fig 1, 2, 3*).

This classification has the advantage of grouping together fractures which are treated with similar surgical approaches and fixation techniques. Each group has a specific diagnostic and treatment protocol. The horizontal plane is defined as any plane crossing the pelvis at right angles to the vertical axis of the body. The vertical plane is defined as any plane crossing the pelvis at right angles to the horizontal plane. A multiple plane fracture occurs when the fracture lines are projected onto more than one plane.

Preoperative planning

Emergency surgical treatment is indicated for irreducible dislocations [11]. In most cases, however, surgical treatment can be delayed until the patient's condition has stabilised and the necessary radiographic examinations are available. In cases of multiple trauma, preoperative tests are advisable to avoid general complications.

Surgical tools (fig 4)

The instruments employed in surgery include a set of reduction clamps and 3.5 and 4.5 mm AO/ASIF screws. Posterior column fractures can be reduced by traction on a hook-shaped retractor introduced in the greater sciatic notch and/or with large AO acetabular clamps. Anterior column fractures can be reduced with large acetabular clamps or Matta's curved clamps. In transverse fractures, the Farabeuf clamps anchored to 4.5 mm screws allow both reduction of the rotational displacements and compression of the fracture lines. Scaglietti's T-shaped screw inserted parallel to the longitudinal axis of the femoral neck is used to apply lateral traction on the quadrilateral surface. Letournel's picador is useful to reduce fragments of the anterior or posterior wall.

The bendable plates must correspond to the bone surface precisely. Narrow, curved or straight 3.5 mm screw dynamic compression plates (DCP) and wide 4.5 mm screw DCP plates are recommended. In addition, we frequently use Citieffe malleable plates with 3.5 screws. These plates can be moulded on the horizontal plane with a special clamp. During screw insertion it is not necessary to tap the drill holes. The screws can be inserted with a power drill and the last turns tightened manually.

Tools commonly used in acetabular fracture surgery are presented in fig. 4.

Fractures on the vertical plane

In this fracture group, the tear drop is a useful landmark for selecting the surgical approach and technique. Fractures on the vertical plane are classified as anterior or posterior to the tear drop. The fractures posterior to the tear drop include the posterior wall, posterior column, and posterior column associated with detachment of the posterior wall. The fractures anterior to the tear drop include the anterior wall, high anterior column, and low anterior column.

Posterior wall fractures

The posterior wall fractures are subdivided into simple and comminuted. In the simple fractures, the fracture line outlines a fragment involving the posterior wall at both the joint level and the quadrilateral surface. This fragment can be different in size. In comminuted fractures, there are multiple fragments and the femoral head has a tendency to dislocate posteriorly.

Judet and Letournel classified these fractures into two types: Type I and Type II fractures [7].

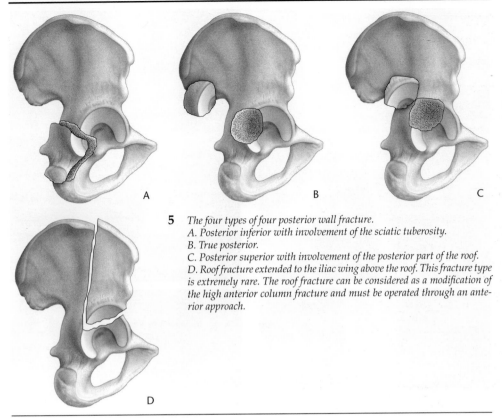

5   *The four types of four posterior wall fracture.*
A. Posterior inferior with involvement of the sciatic tuberosity.
B. True posterior.
C. Posterior superior with involvement of the posterior part of the roof.
D. Roof fracture extended to the iliac wing above the roof. This fracture type is extremely rare. The roof fracture can be considered as a modification of the high anterior column fracture and must be operated through an anterior approach.

the fracture. The fracture line affects the border of the posterior wall. In the obturator oblique view, the fragment is clearly visible with its typical claw shape. The iliac oblique view is not useful in this type of fracture. Conventional CT and 2-D CT may reveal loose or impacted bone fragments.

SURGICAL TREATMENT

Surgery is performed through the Kocher-Langenbeck approach. In type II fractures, care has to be given to identify and remove any loose fragments in the hip joint or fragments impacted in the adjacent cancellous bone. Impacted fragments must be reduced and any bone loss filled with autologous bone harvested from the trochanteric area. During this manoeuvre, preserve any soft tissue attachment to the basic fragments. After temporarily fixing the fragment with one or two Kirschner wires, interfragmentary fixation is performed with one or two 3.5 mm screws. In order to avoid screw penetration into the hip joint, the drill point must be directed tangentially to the joint. When the main fragment is split in two or more secondary fragments, the fixation is accomplished with a neutralisation 3.5 mm screw plate contouring the acetabulum from the sciatic tuberosity to the iliac bone above the acetabulum. Both 3.5 mm screw DCP plates or 3.5 mm screw Citieffe plates can be used (fig 6, 7).

Classification of posterior column fractures

The posterior part of the pelvis from the greater sciatic notch to the descending pubic ramus is involved in the posterior column fractures. We describe posterior column fractures, posterior column fractures anterior to the tear drop, and the slipped epiphysis of the posterior ramus of Y-shaped cartilage in childhood and adolescence on the basis of Judet and Letournel's classification [11] (fig 8, 9, 10).

TYPE I FRACTURES

Type I fractures are fractures with capsule laceration and separation of a part of the adjacent roof. The detached fragment is avascular and buried in the soft tissues. A common complication is necrosis of the detached fragment.

TYPE II FRACTURES

Type II fractures are fractures without capsule laceration. The fragment remains attached to the capsule and, hence, holds part of its blood supply.

In Type II fractures, the dislocating femoral head hits the acetabular margin and impacts minute fragments into the cancellous bone. The acetabulum may lose its rounded shape

due to subsequent partial or total resorption of the impacted cancellous bone fragments.

Other types of posterior wall fractures (fig 5) include posterosuperior fractures involving the posterior part of the roof; posteroinferior fractures partially involving the sciatic tuberosity; and roof fractures involving the iliac bone above the roof.

Posteroinferior fractures must be distinguished from the posterior column fractures. Note also that the roof fractures can be confused with the high anterior column fractures, due to their similar radiographic patterns. The roof fractures are preferably operated through an anterior approach.

In the anteroposterior view, only one of the six radiographic landmarks are involved by

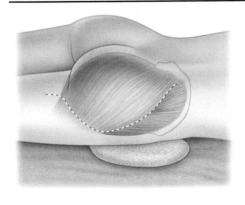

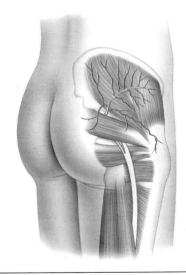

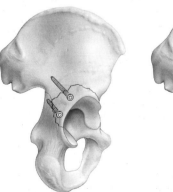

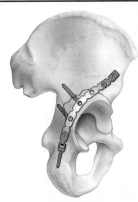

6   *Posterior wall fracture. The fragment was fixed with two interfragmentary screws. Then, a neutralisation plate contouring the posterior column from the sciatic tuberosity to the supra-acetabular surface was implanted.*

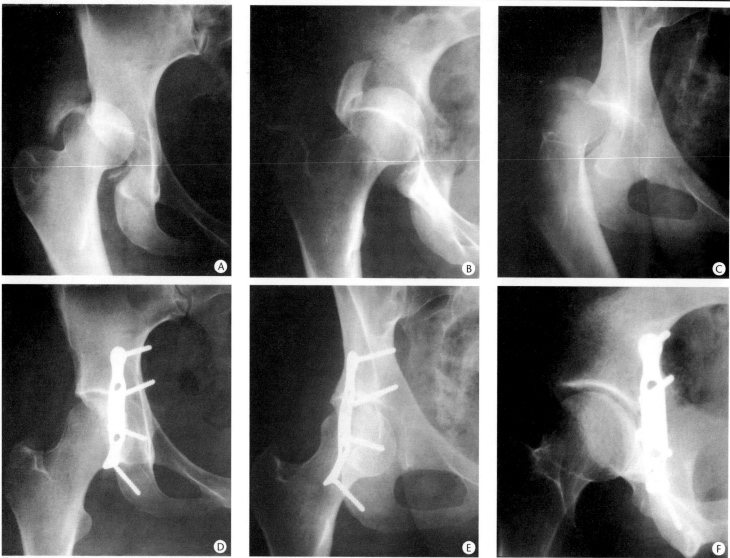

7 *Posterior wall fracture with Type I dislocation. Appearance before (A, B, C) and after fixation (D, E, F) which was performed with a four hole plate implanted through the Kocher-Langenbeck approach. The clinical and radiographic results were excellent.*

POSTERIOR COLUMN FRACTURES

The whole posterior column is detached in one fragment. The fracture line begins at the most proximal part of the angle of the greater sciatic notch, then crosses the posterior part of the acetabular surface, ending at the descending pubic ramus. Medially, the anterior two-thirds of the quadrilateral surface is involved between the greater sciatic notch and the obturator canal. Here the fracture line runs parallel to the innominate line; the tear drop is intact and maintains a regular contact with the innominate line.

POSTERIOR COLUMN FRACTURES ANTERIOR TO THE TEAR DROP

In its endopelvic part, the fracture line almost overlaps the innominate line and the initial part of the obturator canal, then it deviates distally, involving the tear drop area. In its outer pelvic part, the fracture line crosses the acetabulum at the level of the anterior half of the posterior part of the acetabular surface, involving the roof. Compared to the previous group, these fractures are more difficult to reduce.

SLIPPED EPIPHYSIS OF THE POSTERIOR BRANCH OF THE Y CARTILAGE *(fig 10)*

Rarely found in early adolescence, the slipped epiphysis line runs along the posterosuperior branch of the Y cartilage line that corresponds to the intermediate part of the greater sciatic notch. More distally, the fracture extends from the greater sciatic notch to the descending pubic ramus. The fragment, with the femoral head, is posteromedially displaced and rotated around a vertical axis.

RADIOGRAPHIC DIAGNOSIS

In posterior column fractures, radiographic diagnosis can be made with conventional X-rays. The anterior posterior radiographic view shows that the femoral head is driven medially with the fracture fragment. The obturator oblique view reveals integrity of the innominate line, discontinuity of the descending pubic ramus or of the sciatic tuberosity, and discontinuity of the posterior border of the acetabulum. In the iliac oblique view, the posterior column is displaced and driven medially to the tear drop.

In fractures anterior to the obturator canal, the tear drop either disappears or is displaced medially along with the posterior column. In slipped epiphysis in children and adolescents, the anteroposterior view shows a widening of the posterior side of the horizontal tract of the Y cartilage. 3D CT can be useful to evaluate the size and position of the detached fragment.

SURGICAL TREATMENT

Using the Kocher-Langenbeck approach, the landmarks useful for fracture reduction are the greater sciatic notch and the quadrilateral surface, both of which can be palpated with a finger inserted inside the pelvis. After cleaning the fracture ends of small fragments which may impede reduction, the reduction can be achieved without great difficulty.

The reduction is performed by traction on the fragment with a hook-shaped retractor, and by rotating it with Scaglietti's T-shaped screw inserted into the sciatic tuberosity. An AO acetabular clamp keeps the fragment reduced at the level of the greater sciatic

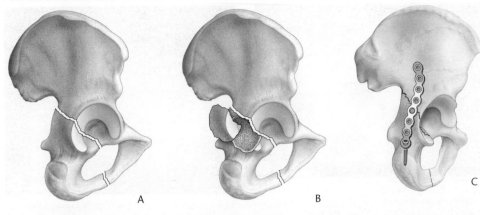

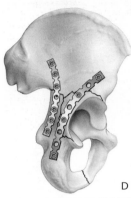

8 *Example of fixation in a posterior column fracture (A, C). DCP plate implanted across the fracture line from the sciatic tuberosity to the retro- and supra-acetabular surfaces. Example of fixation in a posterior column fracture with detachment of posterior wall (B, D). After reducing the fracture of the column, a long curved DCP plate crossing the fracture line is implanted close to the grater sciatic notch. Then the wall is fixed with inter-fragmentary screws and a long neutralisation plate.*

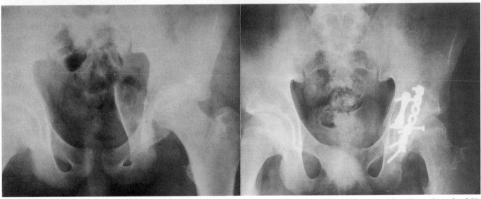

9 *Posterior column fracture associated with detachment of the posterior wall in a 18 year-old patient. Standard X-rays and 3D CT are shown. Note the dislocation of the femoral head. X-rays taken four years after surgery show a 3.5 mm screw fixing a small wall fragment, a long DCP plate extending from the sciatic tuberosity to the supra-acetabular surface, and a plate crossing the fracture line close to the greater sciatic notch.*

to the tear drop where significant rotational and traction forces must be applied.

The reduction of a slipped epiphysis is easier. In these cases, the main problem can be a difficulty in reducing the fragment. A thin chisel is used as a lever along with a holder to anatomically reduce the detached fragment. Fixation is achieved with a DCP plate with 3.5 mm screws inserted into the sciatic tuberosity and in the retro-acetabular part of the ilium.

Posterior column fractures associated with detachment of the posterior wall

In posterior column fractures associated with detachment of the posterior wall, the fracture patterns are similar to those seen in posterior column fractures. Fracture patterns associated with a posterior dislocation of the femoral head make the prognosis uncertain due to a high risk of subsequent necrosis of the femoral head.

RADIOGRAPHIC DIAGNOSIS

Conventional radiography shows the same radiographic patterns as in posterior column fractures without detachment of the posterior wall. CT scan may reveal intra-articular fragments in Judet's type II fractures. In case of doubt, 3D CT is necessary.

SURGICAL TREATMENT

The first phase of reduction for the posterior column is performed through the Kocher-Langenbeck approach. Reduction is checked by inserting a finger inside the pelvis. After the reduction of the posterior column is accomplished, the second phase starts with reduction of the posterior wall. Fixation is initiated by implanting interfragmentary screws. Then two narrow DCP plates are shaped to contour both the wall and the column from the supracetabular surface to the sciatic tuberosity (*fig 8, 9*).

Fractures anterior to the tear drop

One must distinguish between the anterior wall fractures, the high anterior column and low anterior column fractures which are frequently associated with a dislocation or displacement of the femoral head (*fig 11*).

Anterior wall fractures

Anterior wall fractures are similar to the posterior wall fractures. The detached fragments include the anterior horn of the

notch. If a step is palpated at the level of the quadrilateral surface, it is a sign of rotation of the fragment along its longitudinal axis. In this case, the reduction manoeuvre has to be repeated. Fixation is performed with two 3.5 mm AO interfragmentary screws

implanted tangentially to the quadrilateral surface. Fixation is then completed with a DCP plate with two screws implanted into the iliac bone above the acetabulum and two screws into the sciatic tuberosity. Reduction is far more difficult in the fractures anterior

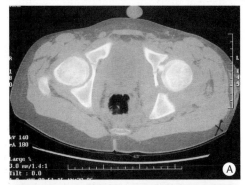

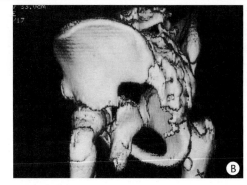

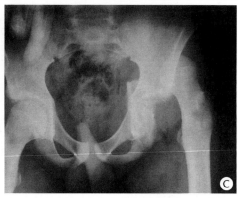

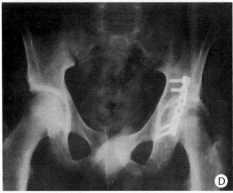

10 *Slipped epiphysis of the posterior branch of the Y cartilage in a 13 year-old patient. Standard X-rays show dislocation of the femoral head on admission. CT shows a retained fragment loose in the joint. X-rays taken one year after reduction and fixation show some ectopic bone formation. The patient is asymptomatic.*

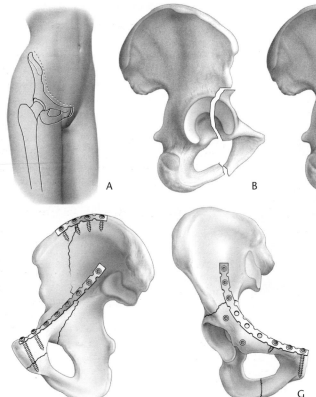

11 *Ilioinguinal approach. This approach is indicated for the treatment of anterior column fractures.*
A. Approach.
B. Anterior wall fractures. The detached fragments include the roof, the anterior horn of the articular surface, the anterior half of the quadrilateral surface, and the innominate line from the anterior inferior iliac spine to the ascending pubic ramus.
C. High anterior column fracture. The fracture line begins in the iliac crest and a large fragment including the anterior third of the iliac wing, the roof, the cotyloid fossa, and part of the descending pubic ramus is detached. The high anterior column fracture can be confused with a both-column fracture.
D. Low-anterior column fracture. The detached fragment extends from the interspinous notch to the descending pubic ramus and includes the roof, a large part of the articular surface and of the cotyloid fossa.
E, F, G. Examples of fixation performed on the three anterior column fracture types. Avoid screw penetration into the joint by using a wide surgical approach using long plates and contouring the plates carefully to the border of the anterior column.

articular surface, the anterior half of the quadrilateral surface, and the innominate line from the anterior inferior iliac spine to the ascending pubic ramus. The femoral head is completely or partially dislocated anteriorly following the displacement of the fragment.

The pelvic bone between the anterior inferior iliac spine and the ascending pubic ramus and the whole anterior wall are detached and split into one or more fragments. In most cases, the fragment is split along the innominate line and thus, the innominate line is discontinued at two points.

RADIOGRAPHIC DIAGNOSIS
Radiographic views disclose involvement of the anterior part of the acetabulum. The involvement of the iliac wing, the pubic angle and the descending pubic ramus is not visible. The anteroposterior view shows the involvement of the anterior border of the acetabulum and the innominate line. In many cases, the tear drop is no longer visible. The most useful radiographic view is the obturator oblique, which shows a large butterfly-shaped fragment with pointed edges along the innominate line. Conventional and 2D CT views show involvement of the anterior part of the roof. Three-dimensional CT reveals the anatomical patterns of the fragment. In the

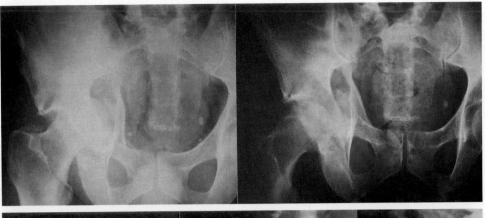

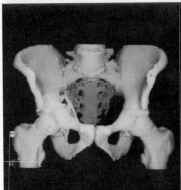 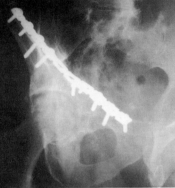 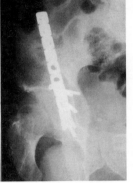

12 *Standard X-rays showing an anterior wall fracture in a 36 year-old patient before and after reduction of an anterior dislocation of the femoral head. Along the anterior column border, the typical butterfly image can be seen. 3D CT shows two fragments along the innominate line. The obturator oblique radiographic view shows a fixation screw tangent to the quadrilateral surface Five years after surgery there is an excellent joint line in both the obturator oblique and iliac oblique radiographic views.*

innominate line and the ascending pubic ramus can be exposed. These are the landmarks for the reduction. The fracture is reduced by operating mainly on the external window. The loose fragment, including the anterior part of the iliac wing and the roof, is almost always rotated externally. In order to disengage the fracture line that joins the iliac crest to the pelvic brim, we recommend either the use of the Cobb's periosteum stripper as a lever, or exertion of pressure from the inside towards the outside with Letournel's picador while two assistants exert a combined longitudinal and transversal traction on the lower limb. Exposure of the ascending pubic ramus is necessary not only in order to implant a long plate, but also to detect possible secondary fracture lines. The main plate (3.5 or 4.5 mm screw DCP plate) needs to be sufficiently long and has to closely follow the anterior column profile from the internal iliac fossa to the pubic spine. When necessary, additional plates can be implanted in the internal iliac fossa. The quality of reduction is checked on the iliac crest and along the innominate line; possible endopelvic fracture gaps can be checked and palpated with a finger.

differential diagnosis, note the resemblance of a transverse fracture associated with detachment of the anterior wall.

SURGICAL TREATMENT

Reduction manoeuvres performed through the ilioinguinal approach require the use of three windows: the internal iliac fossa, the innominate line and the ascending pubic ramus. Any dislocation of the femoral head should be reduced by applying traction onto a screw inserted into the femoral neck. Then the fragments should be reduced. The quality of the reduction is checked along the innominate line. Reduction manoeuvres can be difficult, and internal and external reduction forces exerted with Letournel's picador can be necessary. In order to maintain reduction, one can use acetabular clamps, Matta's curved clamps and one or two 2 mm AO wires. Long 3.5 mm interfragmentary screws are inserted perpendicularly to the quadrilateral surface close to the pelvic brim. It is also necessary to contour the whole anterior column with a moulded DCP plate. 3.5 or 4.5 mm screws are implanted proximally into the iliac fossa and distally into the ascending pubic ramus. Care should be taken not to implant screws in the area between the inferior anterior iliac spine and the iliopectineal eminence which corresponds to the acetabular roof. If a screw has to be inserted proximally to the iliopectineal eminence, the drill should be

pointed towards the tear drop to avoid penetrating the joint (fig 11, 12).

High anterior column fractures

In these fractures, the whole anterior part of the pelvic brim is involved. These fractures are difficult to treat. The fracture line begins at the iliac wing, descends longitudinally crossing the acetabulum and ends at the descending pubic ramus. The differential diagnosis should consider both-column fractures (type II) and also transverse fractures associated with high detachment of the anterior column.

RADIOGRAPHIC DIAGNOSIS

The most useful radiographic view is the obturator oblique showing the involvement of the iliac wing and the discontinuity of the innominate line at the ascending pubic ramus level. The femoral head is partially dislocated anteriorly. The iliac oblique view shows the involvement of the iliac wing. 2D CT is useful to study the roof on various sections from the ischiadic tuberosity to the tear drop. 3D CT helps the surgeon to ascertain the diagnosis.

SURGICAL TREATMENT

With the anterior ilioinguinal surgical approach, a wide area of the pelvic girdle, including the internal iliac fossa, the

Low anterior column fractures

In low anterior column fractures, the fracture line begins at the interspinous notch, and involves the quadrilateral surface and the anterior horn of the articular surface ending in the descending ramus of the pubis. These fractures are easy to reduce because the fracture line runs transversally and the bone spikes in the fracture ends can help identify the reduction points.

RADIOGRAPHIC DIAGNOSIS

An anterior posterior radiographic view shows discontinuity of the iliopubic line and of the anterior border of the acetabulum. The tear drop has disappeared. The most useful radiographic view for this type of fracture is the obturator oblique which discloses the fracture line along the innominate line. This view also shows the partial or total anterior dislocation of the femoral head. 3D CT provides a perfect view of the endopelvic pattern of the fracture line.

SURGICAL TREATMENT

Reduction can be performed through the external window of the ilioinguinal approach, by flexing the hip and inserting a lever in the obturator canal. In order to disengage the fracture line, one can use a thin chisel inserted between the displaced fracture fragments. The reduction is frequently stable and can be maintained with a curved DCP plate contouring the pelvic brim. The plate must be fixed with 3.5 screws. Again, penetrating the joint with the screws must be avoided.

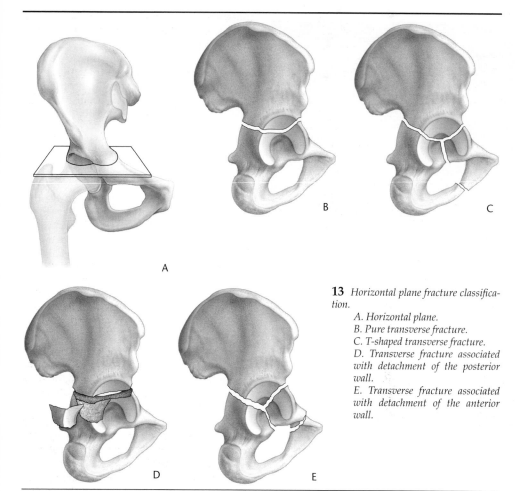

A

13 *Horizontal plane fracture classification.*

A. Horizontal plane.
B. Pure transverse fracture.
C. T-shaped transverse fracture.
D. Transverse fracture associated with detachment of the posterior wall.
E. Transverse fracture associated with detachment of the anterior wall.

need to be operated on. Through a posterior surgical approach, fractures with slight dislocation are easily reduced with either an acetabular clamp anchored with two 4.5 mm screws inserted proximally and distally to the fracture line or with a Farabeuf clamp anchored with two 4.5 mm screws.

In our series, the Kocher-Langenbeck approach has resulted in a high percentage of poor reductions in fractures with dislocation. In fact, through the posterior approach, although the Farabeuf clamp permits a good exertion of reduction strength, it is not easy to control the rotation and the sagittal displacement of the inferior fragment.

The 3D CT anterior endopelvic view reveals that the distal fracture fragment usually is displaced posteriorly and medially. A very similar displacement occurs in Chiari's osteotomy.

SURGICAL TREATMENT

Recently, we have operated many transverse fractures through an ilioinguinal approach, guided by 3D CT images; the results obtained have been excellent. Reduction manoeuvres were performed through the external window, flexing the hip at 90°, by retracting the iliopsoas muscle and inserting a lever medially to the pelvic brim. To reduce the fracture, longitudinal traction is applied to the limb by a screw temporarily inserted into the femoral head. Furthermore, an acetabular clamp should be used to grasp the loose sciatic fragment and the iliac fragment (the latter still attached to the pelvis) across the two sides of the innominate line.

In posterior fixation, a 3.5 mm screw DCP plate is sufficient to stabilise the fracture. Screws should be implanted across the tuberosity of the ischium, where they have excellent hold, and the retro-acetabular surface. In the case of anterior fixation, the plate must contour the border of the anterior column (*fig 15, 16*).

T-shaped fractures

In T-shaped fractures, a vertical fracture line which splits the distal fragment in two parts, anterior and posterior, is added to the horizontal fracture line. As in transverse fractures, the horizontal fracture line begins at the anterior inferior iliac spine, the interspinous notch or the greater sciatic notch, and ends in the anterior border of the pelvis between the anterior superior iliac spine and the anterior inferior iliac spine at different heights (*fig 17*). The horizontal component of the fracture splits the acetabulum into a proximal half that includes the roof and a distal half which includes the two fragments of the ischiopubic component. This can resemble the patterns of a transtectal, juxtatectal or infratectal fracture.

Horizontal plane fractures (fig 13)

These fractures are classified as: pure transverse, T-shaped, transverse with detachment of the posterior wall, and transverse with detachment of the anterior wall.

Pure transverse fractures

The fracture line begins at the greater sciatic notch, crosses the pelvic brim horizontally and continues to the anterior border of the acetabulum, between the anterior superior iliac spine and the anterior inferior iliac spine. The proximal fracture fragment including the roof remains in contact with the sacrum while the distal fracture fragment is displaced by the trauma. Fracture line obliquity can vary.

The acetabulum can be involved by the fracture at different levels. According to Judet and Letournel's classification, three types of fractures can be distinguished. In the transtectal fracture, the weight-bearing part of the roof is involved by the fracture. In the juxtatectal fracture, the junction of the acetabular fossa and the articular surface is involved by the fracture. In the infratectal fracture, the two horns of the articular surface are involved by the fracture. Transtectal fractures involve the greater

sciatic notch. Infratectal fractures involve the lesser sciatic notch. Juxtatectal fractures involve the anterior inferior iliac spine, which is frequently split into two parts by the fracture. Given the relationship between the acetabulum and the femoral head, pure transverse fractures can be subdivided into either fractures without dislocation, when the femoral head is still in contact with the roof, or fractures with dislocation, when the femoral head is medially displaced. In fractures with slight dislocation, the acetabulum tends to become ovoid in shape and incongruent. This can lead to secondary osteoarthritic changes. In fractures with gross dislocation, the distal fragment, anteriorly and medially displaced, is followed by the femoral head (*fig 14*).

RADIOGRAPHIC DIAGNOSIS

Only the expert orthopaedic surgeon can correctly diagnose these fractures with conventional Letournel radiographic views. From high quality radiographs, it is necessary to identify the fragment position and to plan the reduction manoeuvre and choice of surgical approach accordingly. 2D CT scans allow the study of the relationship between the femoral head and the roof, and the extent of ovoid-shaped deformity of the acetabulum.

Aside from infratectal fractures which do not involve the weight-bearing part of the roof, all transverse fractures with displacement

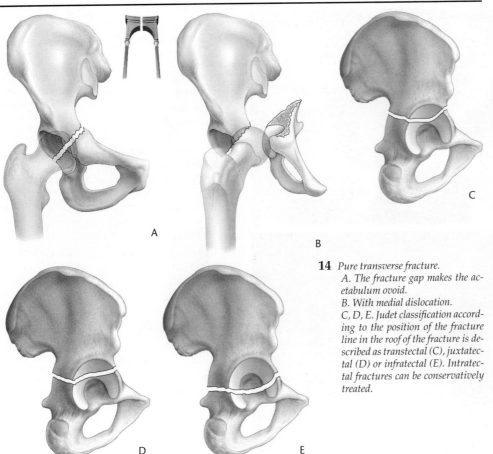

14 *Pure transverse fracture.*
A. The fracture gap makes the acetabulum ovoid.
B. With medial dislocation.
C, D, E. Judet classification according to the position of the fracture line in the roof of the fracture is described as transtectal (C), juxtatectal (D) or infratectal (E). Intratectal fractures can be conservatively treated.

cases, the displacement of the femoral head can cause a partial dislocation or a posterior dislocation.

RADIOGRAPHIC DIAGNOSIS

The diagnosis of these fractures must be accurate in order to choose the appropriate surgical approach. The correct diagnosis can be difficult if only conventional radiographs are available. The CT, 2D CT and 3D CT are useful to precisely diagnose the type of fracture.

SURGICAL TREATMENT

In T-shaped fractures, the reduction and fixation of the posterior fragment is not difficult. One can easily reduce and fix this fragment through the Kocher-Langenbeck approach. Fixation of the posterior fragment must be performed with short screws (maximum 2 or 2.5 cm long screws) in order to avoid compromising the anterior fixation, when necessary.

A secondary operation through an ilioinguinal approach is necessary if a residual displacement of the anterior fragment is palpated beyond the greater sciatic notch or is seen on intraoperative radiographs.

As in the posterior column fractures, the reduction is performed along the greater sciatic notch, applying traction and rotation with a hook-shaped retractor. To maintain the reduction, an AO acetabular clamp can be used. To evaluate the quality of the reduction, it is necessary to palpate with a finger the posterior part of the quadrilateral surface. For the fixation, one can use 3.5 mm cortical interfragmentary screws and a standard narrow AO DCP plate crossing the retro-acetabular surface from the sciatic tuberosity to the supra-acetabular surface.

The anterior reduction is performed through an ilioinguinal approach. Reduction of the anterior column is accomplished combining flexion, longitudinal and lateral traction manoeuvres with a Scaglietti screw inserted into the femoral neck. Fixation requires the use of long plates. Screws must not be implanted into the roof from the anterior-inferior iliac spine to the iliopectineal eminence (*fig 18, 19*).

According to the pattern of the vertical shaft (the stem of the T), three fracture types can be distinguished. Type I occurs when the stem of the T crosses the cotyloid fossa and the obturator canal, splitting the descending pubic ramus in half. Type II occurs when the stem of the T runs obliquely and posteriorly, crossing the posterior part of the obturator canal, the ischium or the ischium's posterior aspect. The most frequent type of this fracture group involves the posterior horn of the articular surface and the posterior half of the ischium, leaving intact the obturator canal. Type III occurs when the stem of the T runs anteriorly, crossing the anterior part of the obturator canal until the pubic spine.

The femoral head dislocates medially, posteriorly or anteriorly according to the obliquity of the stem of the T. These dislocation patterns are important radiographically and prognostically. If the horizontal fracture line is transtectal (high transverse), the acetabulum becomes ovoid and its congruency with the femoral head is lost. If the fracture line is juxtatectal, the two distal fragments are medially displaced along with the femoral head; this maintains the congruency of the joint (medial dislocation). In type II T-shaped fractures, the femoral head follows the posterior displacement of the sciatic fragment. This can also occur in type III T-shaped fractures (anterior dislocation or anterior partial dislocation).

The T-shaped fracture can be associated with a detachment of the posterior wall; in such

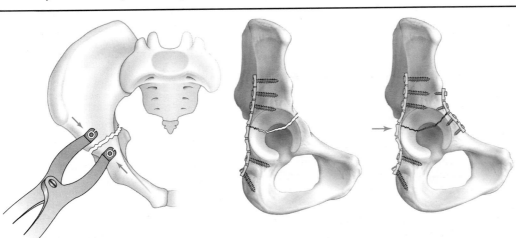

15 *In transverse fractures, fixation is performed through a posterior approach. An additional anterior approach may be necessary to secure the rounded shape of the acetabulum.*

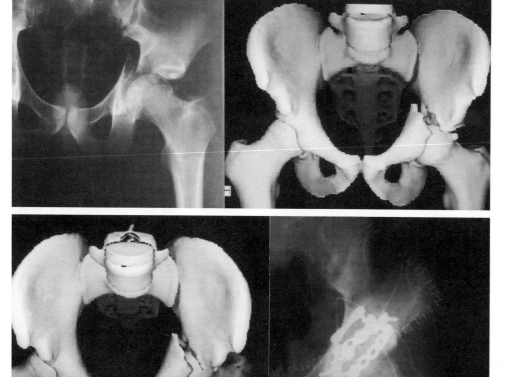

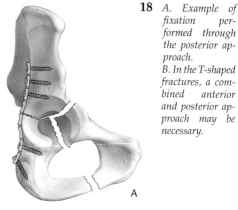

18 *A. Example of fixation performed through the posterior approach.*
B. In the T-shaped fractures, a combined anterior and posterior approach may be necessary.

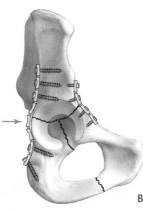

16 *Juxtatectal fractures with medial dislocation in a 26 year-old patient. The comminuted jagged fracture line helps the reduction. These fractures are better reduced through an anterior approach. In this patient, reduction and fixation were performed through the ilioinguinal approach followed by the posterior approach.*

dislocation is posterior, there is little displacement of the distal fragment. If the dislocation is medial, there is severe displacement and the roof is no longer in contact with the femoral head.

Transverse fractures with detachment of the posterior wall

The main fracture line is a transverse fracture. The associated posterior wall fracture can be either Type I or Type II [7]. At the time of trauma, the dislocation of the femoral head is always posterior. The medial dislocation that is sometimes associated with this fracture is the result of a previously reduced posterior dislocation. In this fracture type, it is important to detect a previous posterior dislocation by X-rays taken

immediately after the trauma. After a posterior dislocation, necrosis of the femoral head is very frequent. According to Judet and Letournel [7], the main pattern of this fracture type is the dislocation of the femoral head which follows the displacement of the posterior wall.

RADIOGRAPHIC DIAGNOSIS

The main fracture line alters the vertical and oblique landmarks in all the radiographic views, while the obturator canal remains intact, as in most tranverse fractures. If the

SURGICAL TREATMENT

The Kocher-Langenbeck posterior approach permits complete exposure of both the transverse fracture line and the wall fragments. In fractures with little displacement, anatomical reduction is followed by fixation with a narrow DCP plate positioned 0.5 cm from the posterior pelvic brim. In fractures with severe displacement and medial dislocation of the femoral head, a combined anterior (ilioinguinal) and posterior (Kocher-Langenbeck) approach may be necessary; analysis of the 3D CT images will guide in selecting the approach. Reduction

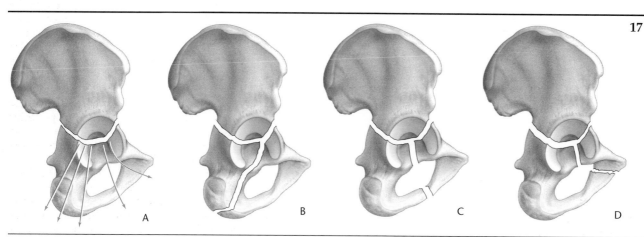

17 *A. The T-shaped fracture is very similar to the transverse fracture. The only difference is that the distal fragment is split in two from the vertical fracture line.*
B. Posterior T-shaped fracture.
C. Medial T-shaped fracture.
D. Anterior T-shaped fracture.

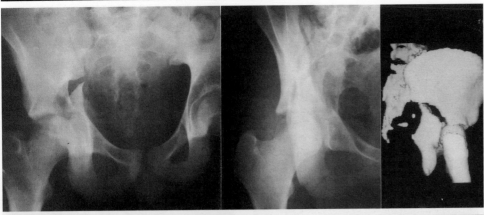

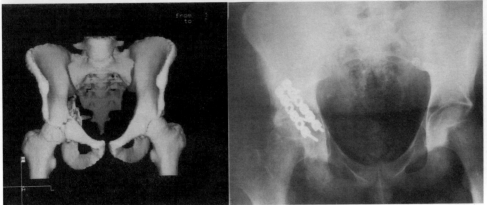

19 *T-shaped transverse fracture in a 36 year-old patient. The 3D CT does not show the fracture line at the ischium level. In this case, a perfect reduction was obtained through the Kocher-Langenbeck approach. Fixation was accomplished with two DCP plates.*

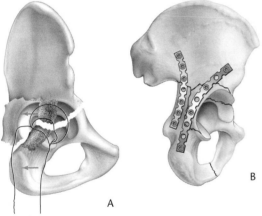

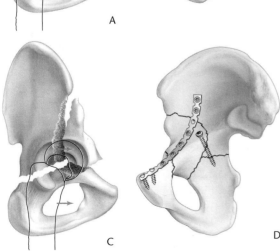

20 *A, B. Transverse fracture associated with posterior wall detachment. A posterior approach is advocated. In some cases, an associated fixation by an anterior approach may be necessary.*
C, D. Transverse fracture associated with a detachment. An ilioinguinal approach is advocated. To prevent the acetabulum from becoming ovoid, an additional fixation by a posterior approach may be necessary.

manoeuvres, fixation, and plate positioning are the same as in the pure transverse fractures with medial dislocation *(fig 20, 21).*

Transverse fractures with detachment of the anterior wall (or anterior column)

When an incomplete transverse fracture is associated with detachment of a large fragment of the anterior wall or anterior column the femoral head is partially or totally dislocated anteriorly.

RADIOGRAPHIC DIAGNOSIS

These fractures are rare. Conventional CT and 3D CT are useful to identify the anterior fragment and the magnitude of anterior dislocation of the femoral head. 2D CT is important to study the roof when a detachment of the high anterior column is associated with the transverse fracture.

SURGICAL TREATMENT

The reduction of the anterior wall and/or of the anterior column should be performed through an ilioinguinal approach, using the medial and the intermediate window. Given that the radiographic patterns of these fractures are the same as in the corresponding elementary fractures, the surgical manoeuvres are also the same. If the posterior part of the fracture line is undisplaced, surgery is performed through an anterior approach. Conversely, if it is displaced, a secondary posterior approach may be needed *(fig 22).*

Both-column fractures

Apart from the transitional forms of difficult classification, both-column fractures have been classified in two types [7]. In the first type, the iliac wing fracture line extends from the greater sciatic notch to the interspinous notch, isolating the joint. In the second type, the iliac wing fracture line runs longitudinally from proximal to distal, dividing the acetabulum into two parts from the greater sciatic notch to the iliac crest.

The hemipelvis is divided into three parts: a stable iliac fragment still in contact with the sacrum, and two unstable fragments that correspond to the anterior and posterior columns [7]. The anterior column includes most of the joint (roof, anterior half of the posterior acetabular surface and anterior horn of the articular surface). The posterior column includes the posterior half of the retro-acetabular surface and the posterior horn. Beyond the obturator canal, the fracture can separate both columns at the descending pubic ramus, the ascending pubic ramus, or at the level of the quadrilateral surface. The reduction of these fractures is difficult, even for experienced surgeons, because the acetabular roof cannot be used as a landmark, as the fragments

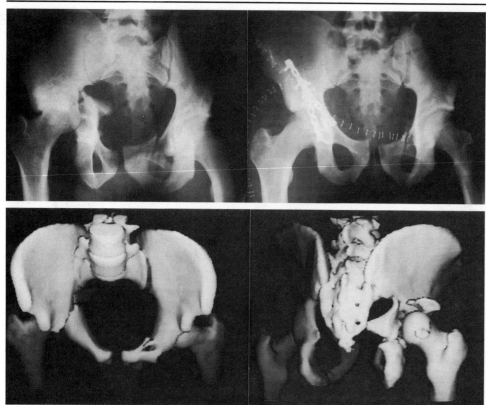

21 *Transverse fracture associated with a detachment of the posterior wall, treated by combined anterior and posterior approaches.*

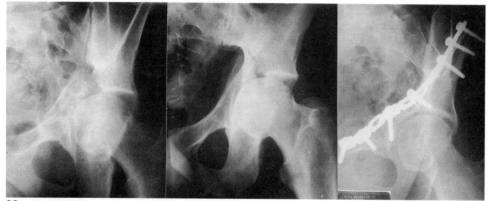

22 *Transverse fracture associated with a detachment of the anterior wall. In the obturator oblique view, the typical butterfly image of the anterior wall fractures is visible. X-rays taken four years before surgery show a 4.5 mm DCP plate contouring the anterior column from the internal iliac fossa to the pubic quadrilateral surface.*

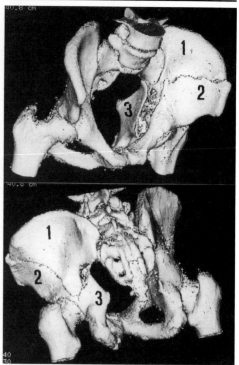

23 *Inlet and outlet 3D CT views in a both-column fracture. The posterior iliac fragment (1) is the stable fragment of the fracture still connected to the sacrum. The anterior iliac fragment (2) is loose and variable in size. It includes the anterior third of the iliac crest, the anterior border of the pelvis and the anterior part of the roof. The distal fragment (third fragment) belongs to the posterior column. The lower part of the greater sciatic spine, the lesser sciatic notch and the sciatic tuberosity are visible.*

have to be reduced and fixated to the part of the iliac bone which remains attached to the sacrum.

RADIOGRAPHIC DIAGNOSIS

In conventional radiographic views, the greater sciatic notch appears interrupted (the arch sign or Judet's curved line) and a large ilioischiadic fragment, with an irregular and/or double-edged fracture line comprising the posterior column, is driven medially inside the pelvis. The obturator oblique view shows the spur sign caused by an overlap between the iliac wing fragment and the anterior column which is externally rotated and medially displaced. The iliac oblique view shows the pattern of the iliac wing fracture line and often a medial, rotational displacement of the roof. The

radiographic signs for the diagnosis of both-column fractures are listed in order of importance as follows: Judet curved line sign, spur sign, iliac wing fracture, total or partial roof involvement. The false congruency sign described by Judet and Letournel on standard radiographic views is due to the rotation of the main fracture fragments along the femoral head which is medially and partially dislocated [7]. False congruency signs can be shown on both the horizontal and vertical plane by conventional CT and 2D CT, respectively. Two-dimensional CT shows the extent of the roof comminution on sections taken from the sciatic tuberosity to the tear drop. This is very important for the prognosis of the fracture (acetabular necrosis, osteoarthritic changes). Three-dimensional CT outlet and inlet views show fine details of all the

anatomo-radiographic patterns of the fractures previously listed and their positions. Outlet iliac views show that the fracture generally consists of three major fragments: the posterior iliac fragment (first fragment), the anterior iliac fragment (second fragment), and the distal fragment (third fragment). This distinction is very important for the surgical reduction manoeuvres (*fig 23*).

The posterior iliac fragment corresponds to the stable component of the iliac fragment which remains in contact with the sacrum.

The anterior iliac fragment (second fragment) is loose and varies in size. It includes the anterior third of the iliac crest, the anterior border of the pelvis (from the superior anterior iliac spine to the superior inferior iliac spine), and the anterior part of the roof.

The distal fragment (third fragment) is also loose and belongs to the posterior column. It includes the lower part with the greater sciatic notch, the sciatic spine and the lesser sciatic tuberosity.

In the endopelvic 3D CT view, the stable part (first fragment) is connected to the sacrum and can be studied until the innominate line; the part of the fragment which includes the posterior part of the quadrilateral surface is not visible.

The second fragment, which corresponds to the roof, is laterally rotated along the sagittal axis and is adjacent to the first segment. This

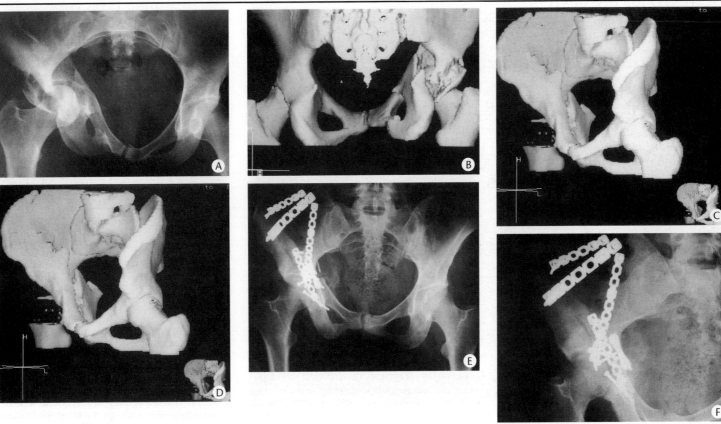

24 *Both-column fracture in a 45 year-old patient. A, B. Note the curved line sign that Judet interpreted as an interruption of the innominate line. C, D. On the contrary, 3D CT posterior view shows that the curved line is caused by an interruption of the greater* *sciatic notch. E, F. Post-operative X-rays taken after fixation performed through the combined anterior and posterior approach.*

explains the feature of the spur sign in conventional radiographic views. The second fragment may include another fragment, the fourth type fragment, which corresponds to the anterior part of the roof and/or of the anterior wall. This fragment remains in contact with the femoral head when it is dislocated. This view also shows that the femoral head is uncovered and is driven proximally. This feature is present even if conventional radiography indicates "apparent good congruency".

SURGICAL TREATMENT

Through the Kocher-Langenbeck approach, it is possible to reduce the posterior column fracture along the greater sciatic notch. This leads to the disappearance of Judet's curved line. The posterior approach can be proximally extended to expose both the retro- and supra-acetabular surfaces. The posterior column must be reduced and attached to the stable iliac fragment.

The extended Letournel iliofemoral approach gives control of any both-column fracture type. In our series [22], however, we found a very high incidence of complications (infection, acetabular necrosis and femoral head necrosis). Therefore, this approach is no longer used at our centre.

Through the ilioinguinal approach, one can widely expose the anterior column, working in the external window.

The key to reduction of the anterior column fracture (first type fracture) is based on two surgical manoeuvres which must be performed in the external window. The second fragment must be released from the stable part by applying longitudinal traction and inserting a thin lever between the fracture ends. If the manoeuvre is successful, the spur sign disappears. This is repeated until a stable anatomical reduction is achieved. In doing so, the Letournel picador is very useful to apply compression on the second fragment. The reduction of the second fragment (and occasionally the fourth fragment) is important to restore the dome shape of the acetabulum.

The most difficult task is to reconstruct the concave aspect of the internal iliac fossa. The second fragment must be reduced to the first fragment at the level of the iliac crest. A useful landmark is the superior anterior iliac spine. The presence of a fourth fragment can complicate reduction. In such a case, one should work alternatively in the intermediate and lateral windows.

For fixation, two curved DCP plates can be used. One must be inserted into the internal iliac fossa between the sacroiliac joint and the second fragment. The other plate is placed between the sacroiliac joint and the ileopectineal eminence along the innominate line or until the pubic spine, depending on the fracture type, working alternatively through the three windows. At this stage, traction is applied to a T-shaped Sciaglietti screw inserted into the femoral neck. The posterior column is reduced with one or two curved Matta clamps. Fixation should be performed with two long 4.5 mm cortical screws. One screw is inserted perpendicularly to the quadrilateral surface, or to the posterior edge of the pelvic brim. The second screw is inserted in the lateral window pointing towards the first screw, aiming at the lower part of the second fragment and the posterior part of the quadrilateral surface.

If intraoperative Judet and Letournel radiographic views show complete reduction of all fractures, surgery can be completed by closing the wound. If the posterior column has not been reduced at the level of the greater sciatic notch, as revealed by a persistent Judet curve line sign, it is necessary to remove the two cortical screws, repeat the reduction and, if necessary, resort to an additional posterior approach.

Exposure at the level of the intermediate and medial windows allows to reduce the secondary fracture line along the ascending pubic ramus, to check the quadrilateral surface by a finger inserted endopevically, and to apply a long, curved plate from the internal iliac fossa to the pubic spine (*fig 23, 24*).

Dislocations of the femoral head

Some fracture types can be associated with an anterior, medial or posterior dislocation of the femoral head.

POSTERIOR DISLOCATION

The posterior dislocation incidence is high (32% in our series). Medial dislocation represents 5% of the cases, whereas anterior dislocation is very rare (about 1%). Posterior dislocation can be present in posterior wall fractures, posterior column fractures, posterior column fractures associated with detachment of the posterior wall, transverse fractures associated with detachment of the posterior wall, and in T-shaped fractures with posterior oblique fracture line or associated with detachment of the posterior wall. When a posterior dislocation occurs, it is likely that the femoral head will undergo a partial or total, early or late necrosis. The femoral head necrosis rate and its seriousness are inversely proportional to a timely reduction. Rates from 2% to 40% are reported [1, 7, 8, 10]. Surgical treatment must be prompt due to the high rate of femoral head necrosis. In our series, the highest incidence of femoral head necrosis (12%) was observed in the posterior column fractures, isolated or associated with a detachment of the posterior wall.

MEDIAL DISLOCATION

If imaging techniques (conventional Judet and Letournel radiographic views and 3D CT) show a posterior wall fracture associated with the transverse fracture line, the medial dislocation should be considered a sign of a previous posterior dislocation that was reduced. Thus, the patient should be informed of the possible risk of femoral head necrosis, regardless of the adequacy of the treatment. The same risks apply to T-shaped fractures with a longitudinal stem.

ANTERIOR DISLOCATION

Anterior dislocation or partial anterior dislocation can be associated with fractures of the anterior wall, the high anterior column, the low anterior column, and transverse fractures associated with the detachment of the anterior wall or of the anterior column. According to the literature, the incidence of femoral head necrosis after an anterior dislocation of the femoral head is unknown [11]. In our series, there was no necrosis in recent fractures and only one case in an old malunited fracture of the anterior wall.

Drains

Correct placement of drains is necessary to allow drainage and to prevent infection. In the Kocher-Langenbeck approach, we generally use two drains, one medial to the greater sciatic notch, the other in the soft tissues between the superficial and deep muscular layers. In the ilioinguinal approach, a drain is placed inside the pelvic brim, another two in the Retzius space and in the inguinal canal.

Antibiotic and anti-thromboembolic prophylaxis

We recommend antibiotic prophylaxis beginning the day before surgery and continuing for five days postoperatively. We recommend antithromboembolic prophylaxis ending at weight-bearing.

Postoperative treatment

Active and passive range of motion of the limb begin at three or four days after surgery. Weight-bearing with the use of crutches begins two weeks after surgery and full weight-bearing at three months after surgery.

Inveterate fractures

Fractures surgically treated beyond three weeks after trauma are considered as inveterate fractures. Beyond this limit, an acetabular fracture is difficult to treat because callous formation makes the reduction manoeuvres difficult. Rigid time limits are difficult to establish. Patients suffering from head trauma may present with abundant callus formation very early, even from the first week. On the other hand, elementary fractures affecting the posterior column can be reduced without major difficulty even at four weeks.

If a displaced acetabular fracture is not reduced, this can result in severe functional impairment. Malunion with articular incongruency frequently results in post-traumatic osteoarthritis. This is common in both-column fractures and in horizontal plane fractures, in general. In many untreated fractures, the acetabulum becomes ovoid. This causes a slow occurrence of osteoarthritic changes, particularly in the transverse fractures without dislocation and in posterior column fractures.

Nonunion is very rare (we have seen only five cases in our series) and is usually the consequence of an untreated transverse fracture with medial dislocation. According to Letournel and Judet [11], the time limit for the treatment of an inveterate fracture ranges between three weeks and three months. Beyond this limit, one should define it as a deformity.

Complications

MORTALITY

517 patients, all operated by the same surgeon (G.Z.), were studied to evaluate the postoperative complications. Deaths due to pulmonary embolism were 2.8% of our series, 12.8% due to venous embolism in the lower limb and 9% due to pulmonary infarction.

WOUND INFECTION

With the Kocher-Langenbeck approach, the infection rate was 3.8%; it rose to 16% in cases operated with Letournel's extended iliofemoral approach, the use of which we discontinued 10 years ago. There were no major problems with the ilioinguinal approach. In all infections, careful and extensive debridement of the infected tissues was performed; both the necrotic bone and the hardware were removed and cleansed with betadine for 8 to 10 days. Bacteriology showed *Staphylococcus aureus* in 60% of the cases, *Pseudomonas* in 38% and *Enterococcus* in 2%.

MALPOSITION OF SCREWS

A screw penetrating the joint may compromise the clinical result and must be removed as soon as possible. While in some cases there is no pain, in other cases there is flexion contacture of the hip and reduction of the abduction and rotation range of motion. Letournel and Judet reported that this complication is rare if the fixation technique is accurate and performed by experienced surgeons [11]. In our series, however, postoperative CT showed screws penetrating the joint in 5.6% of the cases, mostly after the anterior approach. The removal of the screws resulted in a clinical improvement in 50% of the cases.

INJURY TO THE SCIATIC NERVE

Little has been mentioned in the literature about post-traumatic palsy of the sciatic nerve, its cause and clinical sequelae. Though various authors, including Decoulx [3], studied sciatic nerve palsy in high energy trauma of the pelvis, its pathogenesis and frequency still remain unclear. Palsy is encountered in 10 to 20% of the patients. In 1916, Putti identified the area posterior to the acetabulum as a critical point for the sciatic nerve [22]. The peroneal nerve is more susceptible to injury when the femoral head dislocates. However, there are cases in which there is no palsy and the sciatic nerve appears damaged, and cases in which there is palsy and the sciatic nerve appears intact. In our series, only 11.1% of the surgically examined palsies showed nerve damage. Decoulx stated that the nerve can be traumatised both at the greater sciatic notch level and on the level of the lumbosacral trunk [3]. This may explain the variety of clinical symptoms. The peroneal nerve and roots usually suffer more damage than the tibial nerve roots; only the latter will recover.

Postoperative palsies have a completely different pathogenesis and clinical symptoms. In our series, its incidence was 3.8% although we paid attention to keeping the knee flexed during surgery performed through the Kocher-Langenbeck approach. In all the cases of our series, only the peroneal nerve was involved. There was a spontaneous and complete recovery within 6 to 14 months. We think that intraoperative palsies are caused by a compression damage of the nerve during surgery.

ECTOPIC OSSIFICATION

Ectopic bone formation only occurred with the Kocher-Langenbeck approach. Brooker's grade I to III ectopic bone formation occurred in 7.3% of our series and were mostly found after a serious contusion of the soft tissues or cranial trauma [2].

SUDECK'S ATROPHY

Sudeck's atrophy appears in 15% of the operations performed through the combined ilioinguinal and Kocher-Langenbeck approach. In all cases, it disappeared with the prescription of progressive weight-bearing and anabolic treatment.

FEMORAL HEAD NECROSIS

Femoral head necrosis occurred in 12% of all posterior dislocations. Combined necrosis of the femoral head and acetabulum occurred in 8% of our series and was observed in comminuted fractures of the posterior wall, in transverse fractures associated with the detachment of the posterior wall, or in both-column fractures. Femoral head necrosis can be partial or total. Partial femoral head necrosis involves the external anterior superior part of the head and results in an asymptomatic deformity. Total femoral head necrosis results in severe pain, limping and functional impairment. Acetabular necrosis, either associated or isolated, adds to the severity of symptoms.

Results

In 1974, Judet and Letournel stated that 85% of anatomical reductions remain asymptomatic even at long-term follow-up periods [7]. In the remaining 15%, progressive osteoarthritic changes were due to cartilage necrosis or postoperative complications even when reduction was anatomical. These changes are caused by a lack of blood supply to one or both articular surfaces. If reduction of the fracture is not anatomic, the incidence of osteoarthritic changes is high and the percentage of positive results is very low. Thus, an anatomical reduction must be the goal of surgical treatment. The reduction must be evaluated during surgery and confirmed with postoperative radiographs. A reduction may appear perfect during surgery, but when postoperative X-rays are scrutinised, some details of the fracture complex do not appear to have been restored. It is important to develop an adequate diagnostic protocol, comprising fracture type, the selection of the appropriate surgical approach to facilitate reduction, radiographic exposure and cost of treatment.

We evaluated 371 surgically-treated fractures operated with a minimum follow-up of 2 years and maximum follow-up of 15 years. In 81% of the patients, surgery was performed within 3 weeks after trauma; in 19% of the cases, surgery was performed beyond the three week period. In our series, the quality of the surgical reduction and long-term radiographic results were evaluated according to Matta's score [12-14]. Ectopic bone formation was evaluated according to Brooker [2]. Harris' Hip Score was used to evaluate the functional results [4]. Reduction was evaluated as anatomic in all the fracture lines in 81% of fresh fractures and in 27% of the late-presented fractures. We observed that the quality of reduction was strictly dependent on the complexity of the fracture. The highest rates of anatomic reductions were obtained in the posterior wall fractures and posterior column fractures. The lowest rates of anatomic reductions were obtained in transverse fractures and both-column fractures. In 87% of the cases, there were excellent and good clinical and radiographic results. Reduction was not anatomical in 29% of the cases. The non-anatomical reductions were classified according to Matta's four groups: Group I - femoral head in contact with the roof; Group II - incongruency between the femoral head and the roof; Group III - medial dislocation of the femoral head; and Group IV - false congruency [12-14]. Matta I, II and III groups occurred in horizontal plane fractures, Group IV in both-column fractures. In the non-anatomical reductions, the percentage of excellent and good results was 24%, mainly in cases where the femoral head remained in contact with the roof. In the other cases, the results were poor; we never observed an acceptable clinical result in cases associated with a false congruency.

References

[1] Baumgaertner MR. Fractures of the posterior wall of the acetabulum. *J Am Acad Orthop Surg* 1999 ; 7 : 54-65

[2] Brooker AF, Bowerman JW, Robinson RA, Riley LH Jr. Ectopic ossification following total hip replacement, *J Bone Joint Surg Am* 1973 ; 55 : 1629

[3] Delcoulx P, Delcoulx J, Duquennoy A, Spy E, Lob G. L'origine radiculaire des paralysies sciatiques par luxation-fracture de la hanche. *Rev Chir Orthop* 1971 ; 57 : 355-373

[4] Harris WH. Traumatic arthritis of the hip after dislocation and acetabular fractures: treatment by mold arthroplasty. An end-result study using a new method of result evaluation. *J Bone Joint Surg Am* 1969 ; 51 : 737

[5] Helfet DL, Borrelli J, Dipasquale T, Sanders R. Stabilization of acetabular fractures in elderly patients. *J Bone Joint Surg Am* 1992 ; 74 : 753-760

[6] Judet R, Judet J, Letournel E. Fractures of the acetabulum: classification and surgical approaches for open reduction. *J Bone Joint Surg Am* 1964 ; 46 : 1615

[7] Judet R, Letournel E. Les fractures du cotyle. Paris : Masson, 1974

[8] Letournel E. Acetabulum fractures: classification and management. *Clin Orthop* 1980 ; 151 : 81

[9] Letournel E. Voie latérale dans le traitement des fractures du cotyle. *Acta Orthop Belg* 1984 ; 50 : 381-390

[10] Letournel E. Traitement chirurgical des fractures du cotyle. *Encycl Méd Chir* (Éditions Scientifiques et Médicales Elsevier SAS, Paris), Techniques chirurgicales - Orthopédie-traumatologie, 44-520, 1991 : 1-30

[11] Letournel E, Judet R. Fractures of the acetabulum. Berlin : Springer-Verlag, 1981

[12] Matta JM, Anderson LM, Epstein HC, Hendricks P. Fractures of the acetabulum. A retrospective analysis. *Clin Orthop* 1986 ; 205 : 230-240

[13] Matta JM, Mehne DK, Roffi R. Fractures of the acetabulum. Early results of a prospective study. *Clin Orthop* 1986 ; 205 : 241-250

[14] Matta JM, Merritt PO. Displaced acetabular fractures. *Clin Orthop* 1988 ; 230 : 83-90

[15] Mears DC, Rubash HE. Extensile exposure of the pelvis. *Contemp Orthop* 1983 ; 6 : 21

[16] Moroni A, Caja VL, Sabato C, Zinghi, G. Surgical treatment of both-column fractures by staged combined ilioinguinal and Kocher-Langenbeck approaches. *Injury* 1995 ; 26 : 219-224

[17] Müller ME, Allgower M, Schneider R, Willeneger H. AO manual on internal fixation. Heidelberg : Springer-Verlag, 1990

[18] Orthopaedic Trauma Association. *J Orthop Trauma* 1996 ; 10 (suppl 1) : 71-75

[19] Routt ML Jr, Swiontkowski MF. Operative treatment of complex acetabular fractures. *J Bone Joint Surg Am* 1990 ; 72 : 897-904

[20] Senegas J, Liorzou G, Yates M. Complex acetabular fractures: a transtrochanteric lateral surgical approach. *Clin Orthop* 1980 ; 151 : 107-112

[21] Tile M. Fractures of the pelvis and acetabulum. Baltimore : Williams and Wilkins, 1995

[22] Zinghi GF, Bungaro P, Specchia L, Rollo G, Sabetta E. Fratture e complicanze. Padova : Piccin, 1998

Fractures and dislocations of the pelvic ring

T Pohlemann
A Gänsslen
H Tscherne

Abstract. – Because pelvic fractures are rare injuries, the understanding of the bony and peripelvic anatomy, as well as special definitions of the injury mechanism, the diagnostics and the classification of the injury, are all of major importance. These provide the basis for a general treatment algorithm. In cases of a combination of haemodynamic instability with pelvic instability, an emergency protocol based on pelvic stabilisation (C-clamp) together with surgical haemostasis by pelvic tamponade is described. In the other situations, the indication for surgical stabilisation is based on the amount of residual stability (classification). In stable pelvic ring injuries, usually no fixation is required. With residual posterior stability (B-type injury), an anterior stabilisation alone is sufficient, whereas in combined disruptions (translational or C-type injuries), a combined anterior and posterior pelvic ring stabilisation is necessary to allow maximal safety for anatomical healing. For each fracture pattern, specific methods of stabilisation are recommended for reliable results.

Keywords: pelvis, pelvic ring trauma, fractures, dislocation, injury classification, stabilisation techniques, emergency treatment.

Introduction

Pelvic injuries are rare injuries when compared to fractures in other body regions. Their overall incidence is estimated at about 3% of all fractures, or 19 - 37 injuries/100,000 persons/year [2, 11, 17, 18, 26]. In multiply-injured patients, the incidence rises to about 25%, and in the subgroup of traffic-related fatalities, a pelvic fracture was detected in 42% of the cases [21, 34]. A pelvic injury must therefore be looked upon as an indicator of major trauma until associated injuries can definitely be excluded. The close correlation of the pelvic girdle to the intrapelvic neurovascular, hollow-visceral and urogenital structures may lead to a wide range of severe complications and late sequelae if not diagnosed and treated early. Evaluation, emergency treatment, definitive diagnosis, decision making and therapy are therefore a continuous process in which the principle goals must be not only to ensure the survival of the patient, but also to achieve the optimal anatomical and functional restoration. The use of an elaborated standard protocol for the evaluation and treatment of these frequently disabling injuries is highly recommended.

Anatomy

OSTEOLIGAMENTOUS STRUCTURES

The pelvic ring is a stiff osteoligamentous ring structure, and the pelvic joints (sacroiliac joints and pubic symphysis) allow only very limited movement under load. Most of the load transfer is transmitted through the posterior ring structures, giving them the key role in providing pelvic stability. The pelvic bones have no intrinsic stability and therefore the integrity of the ligamentous structures is essential for the preservation of structural firmness (fig 1).

SOFT TISSUES

Besides the osteoligamentous integrity, the large number of pelvic organs and soft tissues play an important role, affecting both the acute (e.g. haemorrhage) and the late (e.g. neurological, urological injuries) prognosis. A clear understanding of the structures at potential risk is necessary for the treatment of pelvic fractures.

The most frequent vascular injuries occur to the dense paravesical and presacral venous plexus within the small pelvis. Whereas a spontaneous haemostasis may be expected in all stable fracture types, gross instability of the pelvic girdle can lead to life-threatening blood loss caused by disruption of all compartment borders. The growing haematoma can rapidly occupy the complete retroperitoneal space up to the diaphragm [32]. Significant arterial bleeding is encountered in only 10-15% of the cases as a major source of haemorrhage, mainly due to rupture of branches of the internal iliac arteries [1, 10].

Injuries to the urogenital system occur in about 6% of all cases, predominantly as extraperitoneal bladder injuries or ruptures of the male urethra after internal rotation type injuries [22].

Injuries to the rectum are rare (2% of all cases), but are associated with a high mortality, especially when they are diagnosed late and intrapelvic and ischiorectal abscesses and sepsis occur [22].

A shearing force, frequently seen after crush injuries or over-roll accidents, can lead to extensive degloving injuries of the peripelvic subcutaneous tissues. If not treated immediately by incision and evacuation, those so-called Morel-Lavallé lesions can result in extended skin and soft tissue necrosis with the later need for major plastic reconstruction [7].

Tim Pohlemann, Prof. Dr. med, Direktor.
Axel Gänsslen, M.D.
Abteilung für Unfall-, Hand- und Wiederherstellungschirurgie, Chirurgische Universitätsklinik, 66421 Homburg/Saar, Germany
Harald Tscherne, Prof. Dr. med. emeritus.
Medizinische Hochschule Hannover, Unfallchirurgische Klinik, Carl Neuberg Str. 1, 30625 Hannover, Germany.

All references to this article must include: Pohlemann T, Gänsslen A and Tscherne H. Fractures and dislocations of the pelvic ring. Editions Scientifiques et Médicales Elsevier SAS (Paris). All rights reserved. Surgical Techniques in Orthopaedics and Traumatology, 55-410-A-10, 2000, 11 p.

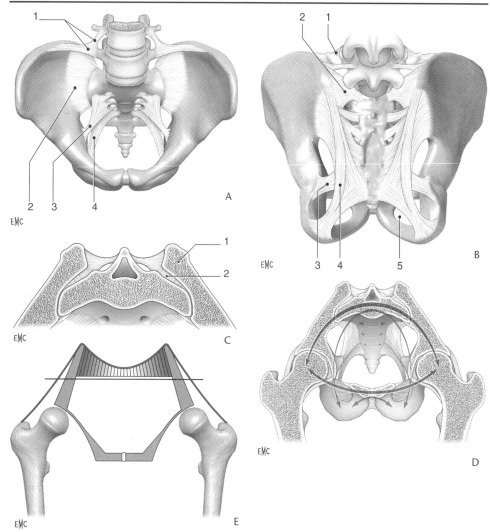

1 *Pelvic ring structure with ligaments, demonstrating the principle of ligamentous attachments. The stabilising structures are located mainly in the posterior pelvic ring. It constitutes a keystone for load transmission from the lumbar spine to the hip joints. The sacrum is suspended by ligaments between the posterior iliac bones.*

A. Anterior view 1. Lig. iliolumbale; 2. Ligg. sacroiliaca ventralia; 3. Lig. sacrospinale; 4. Lig. sacrotuberale.

B. Posterior view. 1. Lig. iliolumbale; 2. Ligg sacroiliaca dorsalia; 3. Lig. sacrospinale; 4. Lig. sacrotuberale; 5. foramen obturatum (membrana obturatoira).

C. Sacrum is suspended by ligaments between the posterior iliac bones. 1. Spina iliaca posterior; 2. lig. sacroiliaca interossea.

D, E. Load transmission from the lumbar spine to the hip joints.

Table I. – Incidence and mortality after different types of pelvic injuries. (*Data from the German Multicenter Study Group I (n = 1722) [22]).

	Type A*	Type B*	Type C*	Complex*	Complex (HB<8g/dL)	Hemi-pelvectomy
n =	728	305	143	160	29	12
Mortality	3.7 %	13.2 %	18.9 %	21.3 %	55.2 %	58.3 %

TERMINOLOGY AND DEFINITIONS

The combination of an osteoligamentous injury with concomitant visceral, urogenital and neurovascular soft tissue injury has a significantly increased mortality and is therefore defined as a complex pelvic injury *(table I)* [1]. In cases where a life-threatening haemorrhage results in unstable haemodynamics, the lethality is further increased. Patients with an estimated blood loss of more than 2000 mL therefore require specific immediate attention. Complete disruption of the major neurovascular structures at the level of the pelvis may be defined as a traumatic hemipelvectomy [23]. Although limb salvage can be achieved, restoration of the lower extremity function cannot be expected due to the neurological injury.

Mechanism of injury

A large number of injury mechanisms can lead to a pelvic fracture. In the last century, Malgaine already identified the significance of combined anterior and posterior pelvic ring disruptions. However, a clear understanding of the specific mechanisms required to create specific pelvic fractures was a long time in coming. Pennal and Sutherland, after intensive studies, focused on three main force vectors which consistently lead to a specific fracture pattern [20]. The first two primary force vectors are compression forces in the AP and lateral directions. The AP compression force leads to an external rotation of one or both hemipelves, whereas a lateral compression leads to an internal rotation with impaction, usually preserving intact pelvic floor ligaments. They also defined a vertical shear injury which leads to complete disruption of all stabilising structures of the anterior and posterior ring. As the orientation of the pelvic ring cannot be well defined, this type of injury should be called a "translational injury" to include shear injuries in all directions. With several modifications and refinements, these three mechanisms are still the basis for the presently used evaluation and classification of pelvic ring injuries. Further developments added the amount of residual stability to the classification [19] and, at present, efforts are being made to include prognostic factors (secondary displacement) for a better differentiation in transient types.

Classification

More than 40 classification systems or major modifications have been published over the last 30 years. Pelvic injury can comprise multiple lesions of the anterior and/or posterior ring, and of the right and/or left side; many anatomical regions may be involved and a great variety of fractures may ensue. Information as a basis for decision making can be extracted from the injury mechanism, as stated by Pennal, Buchholz, Burgess and others [3, 4, 20, 28] or, even more important, from the residual stability left after the injury [30]. In addition, an anatomical representation of the fracture pattern is required for selection of implants and procedures [12].

The basis for the present AO classification of pelvic injuries is a combination of the evaluation of the injury mechanism and the resulting stability/instability of the pelvic ring [20, 31]. There is a continuous transition from stability to instability. For practical reasons and as a basis for indications, three different grades of stability/instability are differentiated *(fig 2)* [28]:

– **Stable**: The mechanical ring structure of the pelvic ring remains intact (A-type injury, incidence: 50-70% of patients).

– **Partially unstable**: Partial posterior, rotational instability after anteroposterior or lateral compression injuries (B-type injuries, incidence: 20-30% of patients).

– **Unstable**: Combined anterior and posterior, vertical instability (C-type, incidence 10-20% of patients).

In addition to these three basic types (A, B, C), subgroups and specific modifiers can be

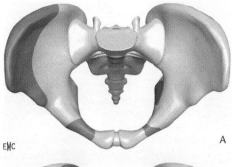

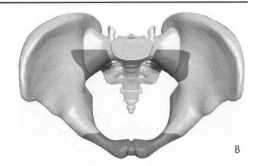

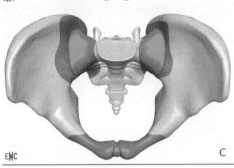

2 *AO classification of pelvic ring injuries. Three different grades of stability/instability are differentiated.*
A. Type A: rotationally and vertically stable lesions.
B. Type B: rotationally unstable and vertically stable lesions.
C. Type C: rotationally and vertically unstable lesions.

added to describe virtually every injury or injury combination. This detailed alphanumeric notation is especially recommended for scientific purposes [25].

Differentiation between a partial or complete posterior instability (B- or C-type) can be difficult. The primary evaluation must be reverified and followed by a revision of the classification and the therapeutic decisions, if necessary.

For daily use, a comprehensive combination of the stability-instability status of the pelvis (A, B, C) together with an anatomical description of the fracture pattern allows reliable decision making.

Diagnosis

The aim of the diagnostic work-up is the immediate detection of life-threatening injuries to serve as the basis for surgical decision-making about further therapy. In particular, because unstable pelvic ring injuries are frequently associated with multiple injuries, specific primary treatment algorithms should be used.

CLINICAL EXAMINATION

Clinical evaluation of the patient should include information about the accident mechanism, to estimate the direction and the magnitude of the force transmitted. A close inspection should concentrate on obvious signs of injury such as haematomas, open wounds, progressive swelling (vascular injury?) and blood loss from the urethra, the rectum or the vagina. A neurological examination should be completed as soon as possible, as these patients frequently require intubation and respirator ventilation, which prevents further neurological evaluation. The pulses of the legs must be verified. The physical examination of the pelvis includes a manual anteroposterior and lateral compression of the pelvic ring. Any pathological movement indicates pelvic instability. If the pelvis is unstable, a repetition of the manual examination should be avoided to prevent further induction of blood loss.

RADIOLOGICAL EXAMINATION

It is not possible to assess the pelvic ring by physical examination alone. The diagnosis is based mainly on a radiological examination *(fig 3)*. The first film is the standard AP projection of the pelvis. It is mandatory in all cases of suspected pelvic injury and in all multiply-injured patients. This is technically simple and allows decision-making about emergency procedures in almost 90% of the cases. Two special projections must be added to supply the necessary three dimensional information. With a caudad ("inlet") and cephalad ("outlet") projection, an anteroposterior and cranial-caudal displacement of the hemipelvis can be detected. A CT examination is added in all cases where a posterior lesion, a sacral

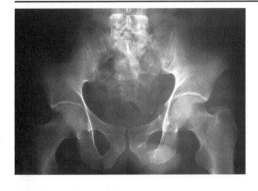

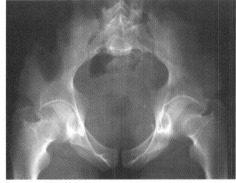

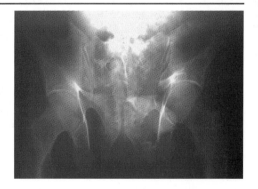

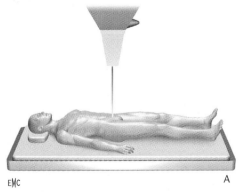

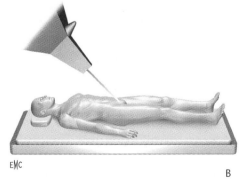

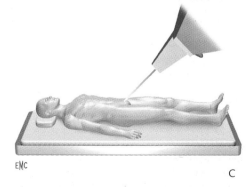

3 *Radiographic projections for evaluation of pelvic ring injuries:*
A. Pelvis AP projection and resulting radiograph.

B. Caudad projection (inlet view) and resulting radiograph.

C. Cephalad projection (outlet view) and resulting radiograph.

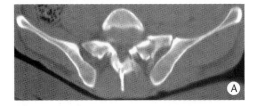
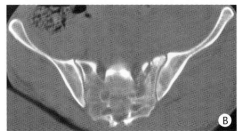
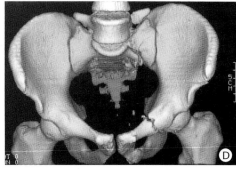

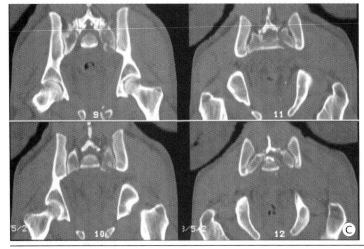

4   *CT examination of the injury shown in figure 3.*
A. Axial CT at the cranial level of the sacroiliac joint.
B. Axial CT at the caudal level of the sacroiliac joint.
C. Multiplanar reformation: frontal cut.
D. 3-D reconstruction.

fracture or an acetabular fracture cannot be excluded (*fig 4*). By means of modern CT imaging techniques, nearly every possible spatial plane can now be reconstructed for detailed examination of the fracture pattern. CT is not indicated in emergency situations, and in most cases it can be delayed until the general condition of the patient is stabilised.

ADDITIONAL DIAGNOSTIC MEASURES

In cases of a complex pelvic trauma, additional examinations must be added to exclude or closely define urological injuries (cystogram, intravenous pyelogram, contrast CT, sonography), intra-abdominal injuries (sonography, CT), genital or holovisceral injuries. In rare cases of arterial injury, angiography might be required.

Principles of treatment

The primary goal in the assessment of pelvic fractures is the detection or exclusion of injury-induced haemodynamic instability, the clinical and radiological assessment of the grade of mechanical stability of the pelvic ring, and the diagnosis of soft tissue and organ injuries. Diagnosis of an unstable pelvic injury with profuse bleeding must lead to immediate surgical resuscitation procedures, preferably according to the algorithm described later.

In the vast majority of cases, however, circulation is only minimally influenced by the pelvic injury.

INSTABILITY OF THE PELVIC RING COMBINED WITH HAEMODYNAMIC INSTABILITY

Several treatment protocols for haemorrhage control have been published, advocating a wide variety of methods. No single method can provide complete control of the situation. Therefore, only a combination of interventions (early pelvic stabilisation followed by surgery, if necessary) arranged in a priority-orientated algorithm can provide a beneficial impact on patient survival. Due to constant improvement of this protocol, a decrease in mortality after complex pelvic fractures has been observed at our institution over the last 20 years.

■ *Treatment protocol*

A standardised protocol for primary clinical treatment is used for all multiply-injured patients. It is based on three simple decisions to be made within 30 minutes after admission (*fig 5*). Whereas the rare case of profuse pelvic bleeding requires immediate surgical intervention, there will be time for the majority of patients to undergo a primary diagnostic evaluation (clinical examination, pelvis AP-radiograph and ultrasound examination of the abdomen). If the haemorrhage is due to pelvic instability, an emergency stabilisation of the pelvic girdle is performed immediately. The use of the pelvic C-clamp allows effective stabilisation as early as 10-15 minutes after admission in the emergency room (*fig 6*). If this device is not available, immediate application of simple external fixators or even traction may be used. Frequently, the mechanical stabilisation will reduce the amount of pelvic blood loss, but it will not provide complete haemostasis. If 10 to 15 minutes after application the patient's haemodynamics are still unstable, a surgical intervention with exploration of the pelvic retroperitoneum must be performed.

■ *Technique of pelvic packing*

The patient is positioned supine and the entire abdomen and pelvis are draped. If no or only minimal intraperitoneal free fluid has been detected on primary and control ultrasound examinations, a midline incision of the lower abdomen is used, leaving the peritoneum intact. If the intraperitoneal haemorrhage is considerable, as is frequently seen in internal rotation impacts, the incision is extended and a laparotomy is performed.

In the majority of cases, the pelvic fasciae are already disrupted by the injury and direct access through the right or left paravesical space to the presacral region is possible without further dissection. Primary orientation includes the control of arterial bleeding, either by clamping, ligature or vascular repair. In mass bleeding, a transient clamping of the infrarenal part of the aorta can be helpful (laparotomy required). In the majority of cases, however, a specific source of bleeding cannot be identified, as haemorrhages arise from the venous plexus and the posterior fracture site. In B-type injuries (open-book injuries), the sources of bleeding are generally located close to the anterior pelvic ring; in C-type injuries, the origin of bleeding is most frequently located in the presacral region. Haemorrhage is controlled by application of tight presacral and paravesical packing (*fig 7*). Tamponades can only be effective if sufficient stability of the posterior pelvic ring is present (C-clamp). If a major displacement of the posterior lesion is still present (check by palpation), the reduction is optimised by clamp loosening and manual reduction before the tamponades are reapplied.

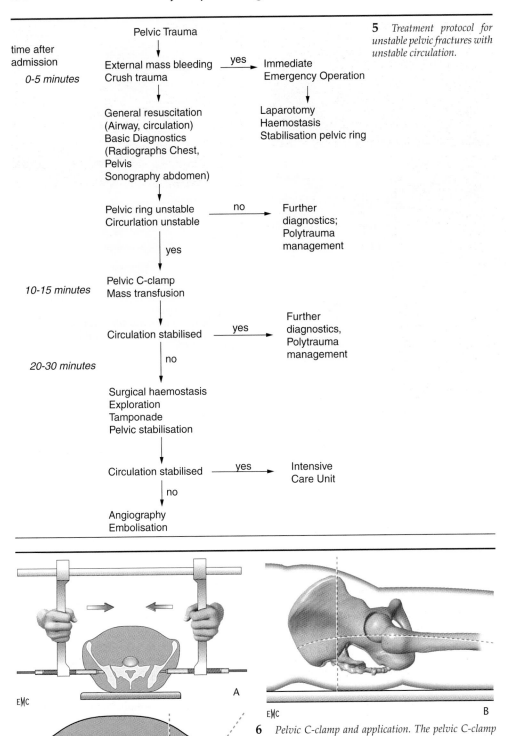

time after admission
0-5 minutes

Pelvic Trauma

External mass bleeding
Crush trauma → yes → Immediate Emergency Operation

General resuscitation (Airway, circulation)
Basic Diagnostics (Radiographs Chest, Pelvis Sonography abdomen)

Laparotomy
Haemostasis
Stabilisation pelvic ring

Pelvic ring unstable
Circurlation unstable → no → Further diagnostics; Polytrauma management

yes

10-15 minutes
Pelvic C-clamp
Mass transfusion

Circulation stabilised → yes → Further diagnostics, Polytrauma management

no

20-30 minutes
Surgical haemostasis
Exploration
Tamponade
Pelvic stabilisation

Circulation stabilised → yes → Intensive Care Unit

no

Angiography
Embolisation

5 *Treatment protocol for unstable pelvic fractures with unstable circulation.*

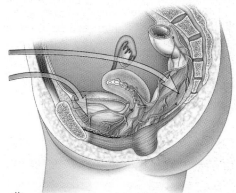

7 *The technique of pelvic packing. The predominant bleeding sites (paravesical and presacral venous plexus) are packed with a variable number of cloth pads.*

the early stage (e.g. suprapubic urine drainage, insertion of a transurethral catheter and suture of the bladder after urological injuries, or diverting colostomy with wash-out and drainage in rectal injuries).

The cloth pads used for the pelvic tamponades are left for 24-48 hours and are removed or replaced in planned second look revisions.

Angiography and embolisation are recommended if a significant pelvic blood loss persists, even after tamponade.

UNSTABLE PELVIC RING WITH STABLE HAEMODYNAMICS

A detailed evaluation of the nature of the pelvic ring injury is a prerequisite for correct decision making about surgical stabilisation techniques. A complete diagnostic work-up must be completed before definitive treatment decisions can be made.

■ *Indications for surgical intervention*

– A-type: Surgical stabilisation is not required. Functional treatment will not lead to further displacement. The treatment consists of short bed-rest and early ambulation. The indication for open reduction and internal stabilisation is exceptional (e.g. open or displaced iliac crest fractures, displaced pubic rami fractures and avulsion fractures in young professional athletes).

– B-type: Stabilisation of the anterior pelvic ring provides sufficient stabilisation for early ambulation with partial weight-bearing. As early differentiation between the B-type injury and the C-type injury can be misleading, especially in minimally displaced lateral compression type fractures with a transforaminal sacral fracture line, radiological controls have to be made 8 and 14 days after injury or after ambulation to ensure that no secondary posterior displacement of the hemipelvis has occurred.

– C-type: A combined posterior and anterior stabilisation is required for anatomical reduction and healing.

6 *Pelvic C-clamp and application. The pelvic C-clamp consists of two sidearms that move along a crossbar. The free end of each sidearm has an opening which accepts a threaded bolt with an inner bore that allows a Steinmann pin with a minimum length of 250 mm to pass through it. The Steinmann pin allows the device to be anchored to the obliquely oriented surface of the posterior ilium (A). The skin must be incised at the intersection between the femur axis and a perpendicular line from the anterior superior iliac spine (B). The optimal insertion point is demonstrated in a frontal cut through the pelvis (C).*

The anterior pelvic ring is stabilised at the end of the procedure, either by internal fixation with a symphysis plate or by using a simple external fixator (transpubic instabilities).

Additional organ injuries are repaired according to general surgical rules. Care has to be taken to adjust further surgery to the patient's general condition. In a few cases, only emergency procedures are advisable in

Each region of the pelvic ring in which an instability (not only a fracture line!) can be diagnosed should be addressed by surgical stabilisation. Whether the completed stabilisation is suitable for early ambulation must be decided individually. In a unilateral injury, mobilisation with partial weight-bearing of the injured side is usually possible after use of the recommended techniques.

■ *Instruments, implants and timing*

Pelvic surgery includes complicated procedures in an anatomical region with a high risk potential (vascular injuries, neurological injuries, organs, soft tissues, etc.). Detailed surgical planning is therefore strongly recommended. Pelvic surgery is specialist surgery and a transfer of the patient has to be considered if only limited personal experience is available.

The following hospital resources are mandatory:

– availability of therapy in a postoperative intensive care unit;

– availability of sufficient blood replacement;

– strategies of haemorrhage minimisation (operative technique, cell saver);

– experienced operation team with adequate assistance;

– standard orthopaedic and special pelvic instruments.

The timing for surgery depends on the patient's general condition. As a high percentage of these patients suffer from multiple injuries, early stable fixation will not only facilitate nursing care, but will also have a favourable effect on the clinical outcome. In patients with stable haemodynamics, definitive surgery should be completed within 14 days (preferably within 3 days) after injury. After 14 days, the difficulty of anatomical reduction is significantly increased, leading to a high rate of malreductions. To prevent disabling malunions and nonunions, which represent complex problems for late surgical correction, early decisions for anatomical reduction and stabilisation should be made.

■ *External versus internal fixation*

The discussion about indications for external or internal stabilisation in the different types of pelvic injuries is not yet completely finished. Multiple studies have shown the limited value of external fixators alone for the definitive treatment of C-type injuries [29]. On the other hand, the external fixator has a place in the emergency treatment of pelvic instabilities and can be used as an additional fixation device in certain fracture patterns. Therefore, the methods of external and internal fixation complement each other.

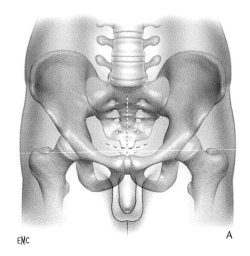

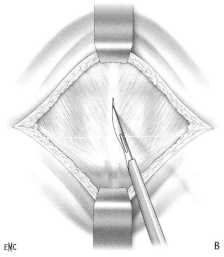

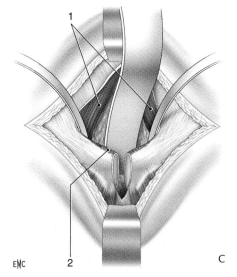

8 *Pfannenstiel approach to the pubic symphysis.*
A. Orientation and skin incision.
B. Dissection of the rectus attachments.
C. Complete exposure. 1. m. rectus abdominis; 2. traumatic avulsion.

Internal fixation

There exists a large variety of techniques for internal stabilisation of pelvic fractures. The methods described have resulted in reliable results in all cases where the indication and technique were correct. The approaches described allow open reduction and internal fixation of the anterior and, partially, of the posterior pelvic ring. All fixations with the exception of the sacrum can be addressed with the patient supine, allowing in many cases the simultaneous exposure of the anterior and posterior rings to facilitate anatomical reduction.

SURGICAL APPROACHES

Various exposures are described for internal stabilisation of the pelvic ring. In our hands, three exposures are sufficient for a complete stabilisation of all fractures involving the pelvic ring (except acetabular fractures). These are the Pfannenstiel incision for exposure of the pubic symphysis, the anterolateral approach to the iliac fossa, and a dorsal approach to the sacrum in the prone position.

■ *Exposure of the pubic symphysis*

A Pfannenstiel incision is used to expose the pubic symphysis (*fig 8*). The patient is in the supine position. Draping includes the posterior iliac crest, when a combined posterior (sacroiliac joint) and anterior stabilisation is required. The leg of the predominantly injured side is draped free to allow for easier reduction. Landmarks are the pubic tubercles and the midline. A transverse incision about 1 cm cranial of the pubic symphysis is made. The dissection is made through a longitudinal split of the rectus muscles in the linea alba. The rectus attachments are saved in as far as possible. Usually one side is disrupted by the injury anyhow. On the other side, less than two-thirds to one-half detachment is strongly recommended to prevent the later occurrence of hernia. Further dissection is made bluntly by pushing the bladder posteriorly through the space of Retzii. The exact orientation of the dorsal surface of the symphysis can be ensured by palpation. The insertion of blunt pelvic Hohmann retractors prevents bladder injuries.

When closing the wound, a tight fixation of the detached or ruptured rectus insertions to the bone (with transosseus sutures when required) and to the opposite rectus muscle is necessary to minimise the danger of abdominal wall hernias.

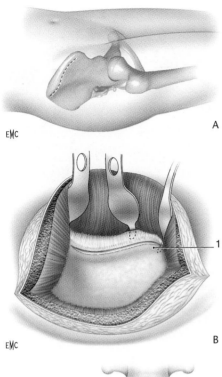

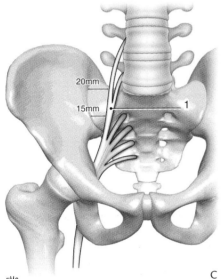

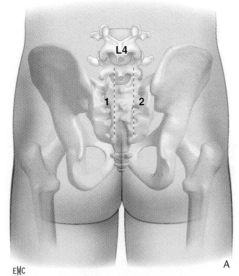

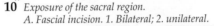

10 *Exposure of the sacral region.*
A. Fascial incision. 1. Bilateral; 2. unilateral.

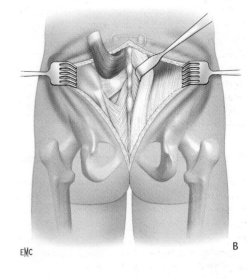

B. Complete exposure.

9 *Anterolateral approach to the iliac fossa.*
A. Orientation and skin incision.
B. Exposure of the sacroiliac joint. 1. Linea termina-lis.
C. Overview of structures at risk (note the close relation of the lumbosacral trunk to the sacroiliac joint). 1. Truncus lumbosacralis.

■ Exposure of the iliac wing and the sacroiliac joint

The exposure used for internal stabilisation of sacroiliac joint dislocations and fracture-dislocations, as well as fractures of the iliac wing, is referred to as the anterior-lateral approach to the fossa iliaca [27] or the first window of the ilioinguinal approach [12] (fig 9). The patient is positioned supine. The following landmarks must be identified: the anterior superior iliac spine and the iliac crest extending to the posterior superior spine. The incision should start 1-2 cm posterior to the anterior superior iliac spine to prevent injury to the lateral cutaneous femoral nerve. It follows the iliac crest

posteriorly about 1 cm distal to it. The incision should extend as far posterior as possible to allow optimal overview. The insertion of the abdominal wall muscles is dissected in the tendinous section close to the crest. The origin of the iliacus muscle is stripped subperiostally in continuity, allowing a complete exposure of the inside of the iliac wing. In the case of a sacroiliac joint dislocation, the disrupted joint can easily be exposed. For anterior plating, additional dissection must be performed to reach the lateral part of the sacrum. Care has to be taken to avoid an iatrogenic injury to the lumbosacral trunk (L5 nerve root) which extends anteriorly as close as 1 cm to the joint line. A careful complete elevation of the sacral fibres of the anterior sacroiliac ligaments and the periosteum is required. The insertion of Hohmann retractors into the lateral part of the sacrum allows sufficient exposure for inspection of the sacroiliac joint, reduction and insertion of the implants.

In cases of an associated symphysis disruption, this area is simultaneously exposed through a Pfannenstiel incision to facilitate anatomical reduction.

Closure of the wound is easy, as all structures fall back when the retractors are removed. A tight suture of the attachments of the abdominal wall muscles, preferably to the tendinous portion of the abductor muscle origin, is performed.

■ Exposure of the sacrum

The patient is positioned prone on a regular radiolucent operating table. Intraoperative fluoroscopic control with inlet and outlet views is desirable, but not mandatory for the procedure. Draping is performed with access to the following landmarks: both posterior iliac crests, the spinal process of L4 and the upper end of the rima ani. The exact position of the skin incision is varied according to the fracture pattern (fig 10).

For transforaminal and transalar sacrum fractures, a longitudinal incision is made between the posterior iliac crest and the medial sacral crest. The lumbosacral fascia is incised close to its origin at the spinal process L4 and L5 and the medial sacral crest. With a sharp dissector or a cautery knife, the muscle is elevated from the sacrum. If a more extensive exposure of the lateral sacral region is necessary, the complete muscle mass can be elevated by dissecting its lateral attachment to the posterior iliac crest. Care has to be taken to keep the soft tissues moist during the entire procedure.

For central and bilateral sacrum fractures, a longitudinal incision close to the central sacral crest is used. The above-described deep preparation can be extended to both sides of the sacrum. This allows the complete posterior aspect of the sacrum to be exposed using a single incision.

FIXATION TECHNIQUES

■ Disruption of the pubic symphysis

The standard method of stabilisation of symphysis disruption is open reduction and internal fixation (ORIF) with a 4-hole dynamic compression plate (4.5 mm DCP) (fig 11). For small individuals, a 3.5 mm DCP or AO reconstruction plates may be used as well. To achieve optimal stability, care must be taken to position the plate screws in a cranio-caudal direction, allowing the longest possible bone-screw contact for optimal holding power.

■ Fractures of the pubic rami

Pubic rami fractures usually heal well due to an extensive muscle envelope, which provides sufficient stability of the fracture as early as approximately three weeks after injury. The strong periosteum, ligaments and muscle coverage provide additional stability

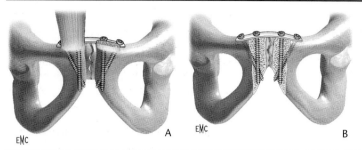

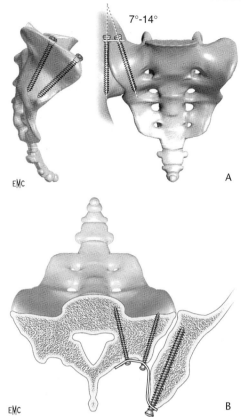

11 *Position of symphysis plate.*
A. The symphysis plate is placed behind the rectus attachments.
B. The lateral screws are positioned oblique to and the medial screws parallel to the pubic symphysis for optimal screw length (50-70 mm).

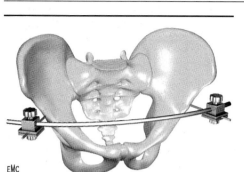

12 *Stabilisation of transpubic instabilities by external fixation. For anterior stabilisation of a B-type injury with transpubic instability, or in addition to posterior internal fixation of a C-type lesion, a simple two pin supra-acetabular external fixator is sufficient.*

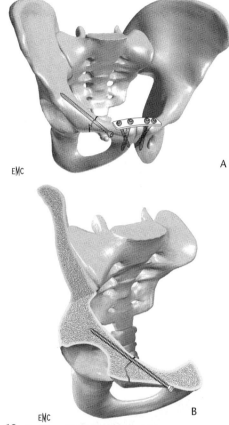

13 *Position of the intraosseous pubic screw.*
A. This type of fixation is only used when an additional pubic symphysis disruption is present and therefore an open reduction has to be performed. The intraosseous pubic screw can be inserted without extension of the Pfannenstiel approach.
B. Note the close relationship to the hip joint. The use of intraoperative flouroscopy is mandatory. If technical difficulties arise, the method of fixation should be changed to external fixation.

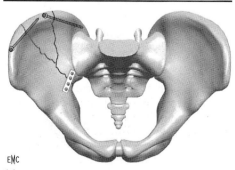

14 *Stabilisation of the iliac wing. Modified by the individual fracture pattern plates (3.5 reconstruction plates or DC plates) are used in the region of the iliac wing, whereas 3.5 mm lag-screws can be used in the region of the iliac crest.*

15 *Anterior plating of the disrupted sacroiliac joint. Anterior plates are used for stabilisation of sacroiliac dislocations or fracture-dislocations with minor fragments. Care must be taken to avoid injury to the lumbosacral trunk (L5-nerve root).*
A. Direction of screw insertion.
B. Implants in place.

in most cases. Surgical stabilisation is therefore only necessary if wide diastasis of the fracture or severe displacement of the pubic rami is present, or if after stabilisation of posterior lesions (C-type injuries) the anterior ring has to be stabilised. The standard device is a simple two pin external fixator (fig 12).

In combination with plate fixation of a symphysis disruption, a fracture of the pubic bone can be stabilised by the use of an intrapubic screw (fig 13). Care has to be taken to avoid penetration of the screws into the hip joint. The intraoperative use of an image intensifier is therefore recommended. In case of technical problems, especially in emergency situations, the use of the external fixator is preferred.

■ *Fractures of the iliac wing*

Transiliacal fractures have a wide variety of fracture patterns, and individualised planning of the internal fixation is therefore required. In the region of the iliac crest, lag screws (3.5 mm) are sufficient in most cases. At the region of the pelvic brim, 3.5 mm DC or reconstruction plates are used (fig 14).

■ *Instability of the sacroiliac region*

Sacroiliac instability can occur with either a disruption of the sacroiliac joint (sacroiliac dislocation) or as fracture-dislocations involving either the ilium (transiliacal) or the sacrum (transsacral).

The authors' preferred method is an anterior plate fixation (fig 15). In the majority of cases, the reduction is made easier, as the anterior lesion (e.g. symphysis disruption) can be exposed simultaneously. The supine position has additional advantages in

polytrauma situations where patient monitoring and other simultaneous operations are facilitated.

An excellent orientation is provided by inspection of the sacroiliac joint, and the screw holes can be drilled into the sacrum under direct vision. Two standard narrow 4.5 DC plates are preferred as implants. An angle of 60-90° between the plates enables iliac fixation in the dense bone at the pelvic brim and the dorsal iliac crest. Injury to the lumbosacral trunk (L5) must be avoided by careful dissection, as this structure is as close as 1.5 cm in the region of the ventral sacroiliac joint.

If a sacroiliac fracture-dislocation exists, internal stabilisation depends upon the fracture configuration. Combinations of screw and plate fixation using the anterolateral approach are preferred.

An alternative technique is transiliosacral lag screw fixation with the patent in a supine or prone position. The use of an image intensifier proposed by Matta and Saucedo [15] is recommended to minimise the risk of iatrogenic injuries to the sacral plexus (fig 16).

■ *Fractures of the sacrum*

The surgical treatment of sacral injuries is still under discussion. A specific problem is

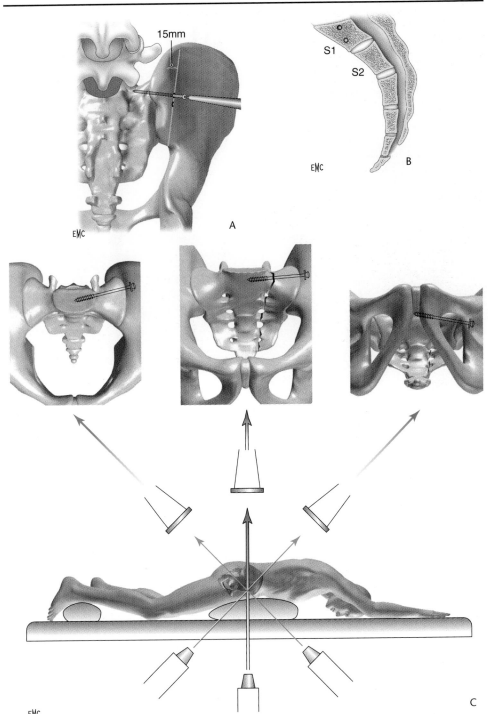

16 *Transiliosacral lag screw stabilisation. This technique can be used for pure sacroiliac dislocations and for sacrum fractures. A closed technique is recommended only when an absolutely anatomical reduction can be achieved before screw insertion.*
  A. Orientation and starting points for transiliosacral lag screw fixation.
  B. Position of the screw at the level S1.
  C. For insertion, permanent fluoroscopy control in AP, inlet and outlet projections is required.

External fixation

External fixation of the pelvic ring as the definitive and sole treatment is sufficient only in B-type injuries or as a supplement to posterior internal fixation in C-type injuries. However, external fixations play an important role in emergency stabilisation of the pelvic ring. In our own setting, emergency external fixation is used when a C-clamp stabilisation is either contraindicated or unavailable. The preferred insertion site for the external fixator pins is the supra-acetabular region. As these pins provide excellent holding power, one pin at each site is usually considered to be sufficient, especially when only supplementary stabilisation after a posterior ORIF is required. When choosing the iliac crest as the insertion site, a minimum of 2-3 pins on each side is recommended to compensate for possible misplacements and the reduced holding power in the thin bone of the iliac wing.

Postoperative treatment

The goal of pelvic stabilisation is the early mobilisation of the patient. The methods of fixation described (presuming the operative technique was correct) will provide sufficient stability for mobilisation under partial weight-bearing.

Radiographic controls should be made after mobilisation to check for late displacement due to errors in classification (B or C-type injury?) or technical mistakes. The length of partial weight-bearing is limited to 6 weeks in B-type injuries and 8-10 weeks after C-type injuries.

Implant removal is recommended 6-12 months after surgery when the pelvic joints (pubic symphysis and sacroiliac joint) have been transfixed.

Complications

Complications after pelvic injuries can include the whole variety of surgical complications (table II). Preventive measures are as follows:

– As pelvic injuries are accompanied by a high rate of thromboembolic complications [5, 16, 18, 25], prophylaxis has to be administered continuously, supplemented with the necessary preoperative screening procedures (colour-coded Doppler ultrasound, magnetic resonance venography and conventional venography to detect occult venous thrombus formation).

– To minimise the risk of infections, in addition to precise surgical technique, the administration of perioperative antibiotics is recommended [14, 22, 29]. Postoperative haematomas should be revised immediately after detection.

the combination of pelvic instability with a fracture pattern directly involving the cauda equina. A high rate of neurological complications therefore must be expected.

Treatment should be based on the early detection of risk factors for potential damage of the neural elements (displaced fractures, neurological deficits on clinical examination, fragment interference with nerve roots in CT-scans) and proceed to adequate stabilisation of the injury.

In our own protocol, unstable sacrum fractures are exposed by a posterior approach allowing direct visualisation of the fracture line and decompression of the sacral plexus [24]. For direct plate fixation, safe zones of the sacrum are used (fig 17). Alternative techniques for stabilisation are the use of transiliosacral lag screws (fig 16), ilioiliacal plate fixations (fig 18), internal fixators and the application of ilioiliacal sacral bars. Regardless of the chosen method of fixation, a complete decompression and the absolute anatomical reduction of the sacrum with stable fixation must be ensured.

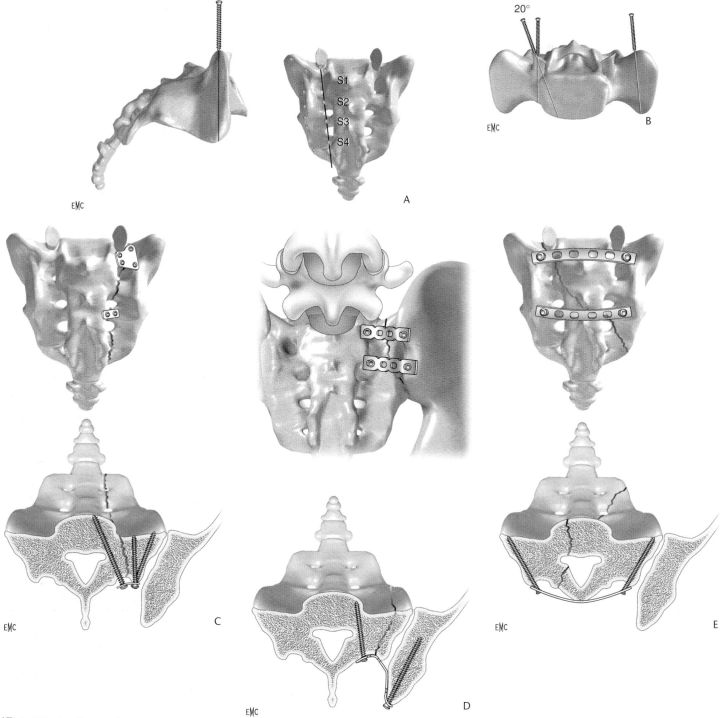

17 *Stabilisation of sacrum fractures with plates. In cases of neurological deficit, decompression of the nerve roots through the opened fracture line with removal of bone fragments is necessary.*

A. Entry points for screw insertion in the sacrum. Lateral to the foramen, screws can be inserted in every region. In the line of the foramen, screws can only be placed in the middle distance between two foramens perpendicular to the posterior lamina.

B. The orientation of the drill has to be adjusted to the specific sacral geometry.
C. Plate fixation of a transforaminal fracture.
D. Plate fixation of a transalar fracture with small lateral fragment.
E. Fixation of a central fracture.

– Iatrogenic neurological [6, 33] and vascular injuries have to be prevented by exact planning and knowledge of anatomy and approaches.

– In the majority of cases, complications result from inadequate primary diagnosis and misjudgement of the injury classification, leading to inadequate indications and choice of stabilisation methods. An exact preoperative analysis and a complete understanding of the nature of the injury are the key for successful surgical treatment with anatomical healing [9, 21].

Results

Pelvic fractures, especially the unstable types, lead to a high rate of late sequelae. Recent studies, including a multicenter study, have shown that with the use of standard indications and the described techniques, a rate of over 80% of anatomical reconstructions could be achieved, even after C-types injuries [22]. In contrast, the rate of clinically good and excellent results is still less than 60% in these cases. Several studies have shown a correlation between the long-term outcome and the quality of reduction (*table III*). Henderson [8] stated that all patients having a posterior residual displacement over 1 cm after nonoperative treatment of a C-type injury reported daily sensations of pain, compared to 56% when

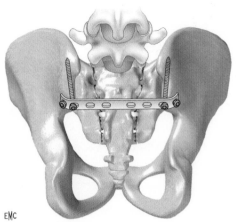

EMC

18 *Posterior stabilisation by an ilio-iliacal plate. In cases of severe comminution, bilateral fractures, or in cases where screw and plate fixation does not provide sufficient stability, an ilio-iliacal plate fixation can be used as a salvage procedure. The disadvantage is that extensive dissection is required for application of the plate.*

Table II. – Incidence of complications after pelvic ring injuries.

Complications	Author	Incidence
deep vein thrombosis	Montgomery, 1995 [16] Geerts, 1994 [5]	35-60%
pulmonary embolism	O'Malley, 1990 [18] Poole, 1992 [25]	2-10%
infection (ORIF)	German Multicenter Study Group, 1997 [22] Tile, 1995 [29]	2-14%
infection (external fixation)	German Multicenter Study Group, 1997 [22] Leung, 1992 [14]	0-33%
iatrogenic nerve injury	Vecsei, 1984 [33] Gorczyka, 1996 [6]	1-15%
secondary displacement (anterior fixation of type C injuries)	Hofmann, 1986 [9] Pohlemann, 1994 [21]	52-65%

Table III. – Results and outcome after pelvic injuries. (Data from the German Multicenter Study I, *Pelvic Outcome Store* [22]).

	Type A	Type B	Type C	Complex
pain (none or slight)	87%	79%	70%	36%
nerve deficit	4%	14%	34%	31%
urological disturbances	14%	9%	8%	28%
clinical score* (excellent & good)	81%	84%	79%	46%
radiological score* (good)	100%	91%	71%	66%
pelvic outcome* (excellent)	46%	35%	21%	11%

The Pelvic Outcome Score consists of two basic features: the clinical result (analysis of pain, neurological and/or urological deficit, functional limitations, maximum 4 points) and the radiological result (analysis of permanent anterior/posterior displacement, maximum 3 points).

the remaining displacement was less than 1 cm, and 18% after anatomical healing [8]. The results of the German Multicenter Study Group I [22] showed that in the group of good and excellent results, a residual displacement of over 5 mm was present only in 3.5% of the cases, whereas in the group of moderate and poor results, a displacement of 5 mm or more was present in 28%, leading to the presumption that a residual posterior displacement of 5 mm is a critical value.

The cause of pelvic disability can be a long-term nerurological or/and urological deficit. In addition, unspecified pain in the posterior pelvic ring or low back pain is frequently encountered. Further studies must be conducted to clarify the origins of these com complaints. Whether they can be addressed by surgical means cannot be stated at the moment.

References

[1] Bosch U, Pohlemann T, Haas N, Tscherne H. Klassifikation und Management des komplexen Beckentraumas. *Unfallchirurg* 1992 ; 95 : 189-196

[2] Brooker A, Edwards C. External Fixation: The current state of the art. Baltimore : Williams and Wilkins, 1979

[3] Bucholz R. The pathological anatomy of Malgaigne fracture-dislocations of the pelvis. *J Bone Joint Surg Am* 1981 ; 63 : 400-404

[4] Burgess AR, Eastridge B, Young JW, Ellison T, Ellison P, Poka A et al. Pelvic ring disruption: effective classification systems and treatment protocols. *J Trauma* 1990 ; 30 : 848-856

[5] Geerts W, Coren K, Jay R, Chen E, Szalai J. A prospective study of venous thromboembolism after major trauma. *N Engl J Med* 1994 ; 331 : 1601-1606

[6] Gorczyca J, Conner J. A beginner's experience with percutaneous iliosacral screws. In: Abstractband, Fractures of the pelvis and acetabulum. 3rd International Consensus, Pittsburgh, 1996 : 1-96

[7] Hak D, Olsen S, Matta J. Management of the Morel-Levallé lesion. In: Abstractband, Orthopaedic trauma association. 12th Annual Meeting, 1996

[8] Henderson R. The long-term result of nonoperatively treated major pelvic disruption. *J Orthop Trauma* 1989 ; 3 : 41-47,

[9] Hofmann G, Bredow J. Spätergebnisse der Beckenringverletzungen-Behandlung mit dem Fixateur externe. *Hefte Unfallheilkunde* 1986 ; 181 : 612-618

[10] Huittinen V, Slätis P. Postmortem angiography and dissection of the hypogastric artery in pelvic fractures. *Surgery* 1973 ; 73 : 454-462

[11] Kjaer I, Jansen J, Rotwit L, Hansen B, Hansen L, Frend K. Epidemiology of pelvic fractures in a Danish country. In: Abstractband, Fractures of the pelvis and acetabulum. 3rd International Consensus, Pittsburgh, 1996

[12] Letournel E. Annotation to pelvic fractures. *Injury* 1978 ; 10 : 145-148

[13] Letournel E. The treatment of acetabular fractures through the ilioinguinal approach. *Clin Orthop* 1994 ; 292 : 62-76

[14] Leung K, Chien P, Shen W, So W. Operative treatment of unstable pelvic fractures. *Injury* 1992 ; 23 : 31-37

[15] Matta J, Saucedo T. Internal fixation of pelvic ring fractures. *Clin Orthop* 1989 ; 242 : 83-97

[16] Montgomery KD, Geerts WH, Potter HG, Helfet DL. Thromboembolic complications in patients with pelvic trauma. *Clin Orthop* 1996 ; 329 : 68-87

[17] Mucha P, Farnell M. Analysis of pelvic fracture management. *J Trauma* 1984 ; 24 : 379-386

[18] O'Malley KF, Ross SE. Pulmonary embolism in major trauma patients. *J Trauma* 1990 ; 30 : 748-50

[19] Orthopaedic Trauma Association, Fracture and dislocation compendium. *J Orthop Trauma* 1996 ; 10 : 71-75

[20] Pennal G, Tile M, Waddell J, Garside H. Pelvic disruption: assessment and classification. *Clin Orthop* 1980 ; 151 : 12-21

[21] Pohlemann T, Bosch U, Gänsslen A, Tscherne H. The Hannover experience in management of pelvic fractures. *Clin Orthop* 1994 ; 305 : 69-80

[22] Pohlemann T, Gänsslen A, Hartung S. Beckenverletzungen/Pelvic Injuries. Hefte zu "Der Unfallchirurg", Heft 266, 1997

[23] Pohlemann T, Paul C, Gänsslen A, Regel G, Tscherne H. Die traumatische Hemipelvektomie. Erfahrungen aus 11 Fällen. *Unfallchirurg* 1996 ; 99 : 304-312

[24] Pohlemann T, Tscherne H. Fixation of sacral fractures. *Tech Orthop* 1995 ; 9 : 315-326

[25] Poole G, Ward E, Griswold J, Muakkassa F, Hsu H. Complications of pelvic fractures from blunt trauma. *Am Surg* 1992 ; 58 : 225-231

[26] Ragnarsson B, Jacobsson B. Epidemiology of pelvic fractures in a Swedish county. *Acta Orthop Scand* 1992 ; 63 : 297-300

[27] Ragnarsson B, Olerud C, Olerud S. Anterior square-plate fixation of sacroiliac disruption. *Acta Orthop Scand* 1993 ; 64 : 138-142

[28] Tile M. Pelvic ring fractures: should they be fixed? *J Bone Joint Surg Br* 1988 ; 70 : 1-12

[29] Tile M. Fractures of the pelvis and acetabulum. Baltimore : Williams and Wilkins, 1995

[30] Tile M, Burry C, Poigenfürst J. Pelvis. In : Müller ME, Allgöwer M, Schneider R, Willenegger H eds. Manual of Internal Fixation. Berlin : Springer-Verlag, 1991 : 485-500

[31] Tile M, Pennal G. Pelvic disruptions: principles of management. *Clin Orthop* 1980 ; 151 : 56-64

[32] Trentz O, Bühren V, Friedl H. Beckenverletzungen. *Chirurg* 1989 ; 60 : 639-648

[33] Véscei V, Kuderna H, Grosse A, Hofmann G. Indikationen und Ergebnisse bei der Anwendung des Fixateur externe zur Versorgung von Beckenbrüchen und -verrenkungen. *Hefte Unfallheilkd* 1984 ; 164 : 228-233

[34] Voigt G. Untersuchungen zur Mechanik der Beckenfrakturen und Luxationen. *Hefte Unfallheilkd* 1965 ; 85 : 1-92

[35] Young JW, Burgess AR, Brumback RJ, Poka A. Pelvic fractures: value of plain radiography in early assessment and management. *Radiology* 1986 ; 160 : 445-451

Proximal femoral and pelvic fracture in children

AJ Kaelin
D Ceroni

Abstract. – Most children's fractures heal quickly without complication, but there is a high incidence of complications in pelvic and hip fractures in the growing child. These lesions occur after high energy trauma and are associated with head, abdomen, urinary, nerve and thoracic injuries which can be life-threatening. Pelvic fractures, once the accurate diagnosis has been made, have a favourable outcome with simple treatment. Hip fractures need extensive treatment, often open reduction and internal fixation, and are followed by frequent complications.

This chapter presents the epidemiology, diagnosis, classification, treatment and complications of pelvic and hip fracture in children.

Keywords: pelvis, fracture in children, hip, proximal femoral fracture in children.

Proximal femoral fractures in children

Upper femoral fractures in children are very rare in comparison to adults. They represent less than 1% of all fractures in the growing period. This type of fracture can occur at any age, but the highest incidence is between 11 and 12 years. The sex ratio is 3 to 1 in favour of boys. The treatment differs from that in adults, because children tolerate immobilisation better, thus traction or a spica cast can be used, depending on the fracture type and the age of the patient.

FEMORAL NECK PARTICULARITIES IN CHILDREN

At birth, a single large block of cartilage constitutes the femoral neck, the femoral head and the greater and lesser trochanter. Progressively, the ossification nuclei appear (femoral head at 4 months, greater trochanter at 3 years, lesser trochanter at 8 years). The cervical and trochanteric epiphyseal lines become discoid and ultimately give 30% of femoral growth. A great deal of remodelling takes place in the femoral neck during growth. The cancellous bone in the femoral neck in children is harder and denser than in the adult. As a result, the fracture lines are smoother and no impaction occurs [3, 4, 11, 19].

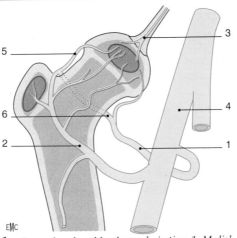

1 *Femoral neck and head vascularisation. 1. Medial circumflex artery; 2. lateral circumflex artery; 3. ligamentum teres artery; 4. arteria femoralis profunda; 5. posterosuperior retinacular system; 6. posteroinferior retinacular system.*

The vascularity of the femoral neck and head is particularly at risk from both fracture and operation, due to the intra-articular situation of the epiphysis and the pattern of the terminal arterial branches which run on the surface of the bone and are easily damaged *(fig 1)*. Ratliff [17] describes 3 types of necrosis, depending on the location of the vascular lesion:

– Type A: diffuse necrosis of the entire epiphysis and proximal femoral neck due to interruption of the blood supply from the lateral epiphyseal, metaphyseal and nutrient vessels.

– Type B: metaphyseal necrosis due to interruption of the blood supply from the superior metaphyseal vessels with preservation of the lateral epiphyseal vessels.

– Type C: femoral epiphyseal necrosis (superior half) produced by a lesion of the lateral epiphyseal vessels *(fig 2)*.

MECHANISM OF INJURY

Most femoral neck fractures occur as the result of high energy trauma (80%), such as falls from a great height or road traffic accidents. They are often (35%) accompanied

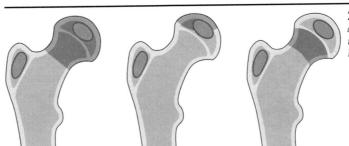

2 *Ratliff classification for head and neck necrosis after fracture in children. From left to right A, B, C.*

André J Kaelin, M.D.
Dimitri Ceroni, M.D.
Unité d'Orthopédie Pédiatrique, Hôpital des Enfants, 1211 Geneva 14, Switzerland.

All references to this article must include: Kaelin AJ and Ceroni D. Proximal femoral and pelvic fracture in children. Editions Scientifiques et Médicales Elsevier SAS (Paris). All rights reserved. Surgical Techniques in Orthopaedics and Traumatology, 55-410-B-10, 2001, 6 p.

by head, thoracic or abdominal injuries, as well as pelvic or other long bone fractures. High energy axial falls produce varus forces that cause cervicotrochanteric or transtrochanteric fracture. Road traffic accidents involve children mainly as pedestrians. They are commonly hit by the automobile bumper at the level of the trochanter, and the horizontal forces produce a valgus deformity. Since the femoral head is locked in the acetabulum, the fracture is usually located at the epiphyseal line or at the transcervical level. Acetabular and pelvic fractures are often associated with transverse forces [3, 4, 11, 19]. When a hip fracture occurs after a history of trivial trauma, the possibility of a pathological fracture (unicameral bone cyst, aneurysmal bone cyst, fibrous dysplasia, osteogenesis imperfecta, neuromuscular diseases) or a child abuse situation should be considered. Stress fractures can occur following overuse in sport, exercise without proper training or pathological fragility of the bone, as in juvenile osteoporosis and in mild forms of osteogenesis imperfecta. During traumatic delivery, epiphyseal subcapital fracture can occur, mimicking a congenital hip dislocation. Fracture avulsion of the greater or lesser trochanter can occur after a violent and sudden isometric muscle contraction.

CLINICAL SYMPTOMS AND DIAGNOSIS

Usually the diagnosis is not difficult. A severe injury is followed by hip pain. The patient is unable to walk or to bear weight. The affected limb is held in flexion and slight adduction. In a displaced fracture, the shortening is 1 to 2 cm and active mobilisation is not possible. Palpation is often painful posterior to the greater trochanter and swelling may be noted in the inguinal area.

The diagnosis is established by anteroposterior pelvic and lateral hip X-rays. The femoral head remains in the acetabulum and the proximal femur is displaced proximally, anteriorly and in external rotation.

CLASSIFICATIONS

Femoral neck fractures are classified according to their anatomical location. Delbet cited by Colonna [6] developed a system of four types (*fig 3*).

Type 1: Acute traumatic transepiphyseal fracture, anatomically like a Salter-Harris type 1. It should not be confused with a acute slipped epiphysis. This is the rarest lesion and occurs in 8% of true femoral neck fractures. It is often associated with a hip dislocation, which dramatically increases the risk of femoral head necrosis. Obstetrical femoral neck fractures are mostly of Type 1 and they could be mistaken for congenital dislocation due to the lack of head ossification. Ultrasonic examination provides

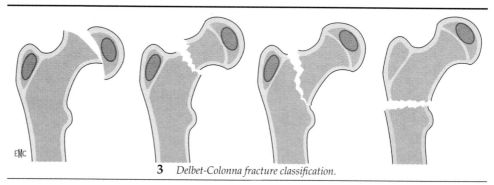

3 *Delbet-Colonna fracture classification.*

accurate imaging showing the femoral head in the acetabulum and the dislocated metaphysis.

Type 2: Transcervical fractures are the most frequent (49%). The lateral fragment can be of variable size. There is no posterior comminution as in adult fractures. Those with a more horizontal fracture line have a better prognosis than those with a vertical fracture line, according to Pauwels' principles. The risk of head necrosis is high.

Type 3: Cervicotrochanteric or basicervical fractures are observed in 43% of the cases. The greater trochanter usually remains with the distal fragment. Femoral neck necrosis is frequent, but the vascularity of the head is preserved.

Type 4: Intertrochanteric fractures are rare in children. They are not true femoral neck lesions. The risk of necrosis is low.

Avulsion fractures of the greater or the lesser trochanter occur after sudden muscular contraction in children around puberty [21].

TREATMENT

The treatment of femoral neck fracture in children is not a true emergency. Reduction and stabilisation either by conservative or surgical techniques must be performed in optimum conditions by a trained medical team [3, 4, 11, 19].

■ *General principles*

Orthopaedic (closed) reduction is performed on a orthopaedic table in the prone position under general anaesthesia and muscular relaxation. Gentle axial traction is followed by abduction and internal flexion. Perfect reduction is checked by an X-ray. These conditions are mandatory before proceeding to cast immobilisation or percutaneous pinning.

Percutaneous osteosynthesis is the preferred fixation. Kirschner wires are used when the epiphyseal line must be crossed and cannulated screws for metaphyseal fixation. Angulated plates, nails and compression screws must be avoided because of their size and the high density of metaphyseal bone in children.

One or two Kirschner pins or screws provide sufficient stability.

Open reduction is reserved for failure of closed reduction and for fractures associated with hip dislocation.

The surgical approach must preserve the vascularity supply to the neck and head and the integrity of the greater trochanter epiphyseal line.

INDICATIONS AND TREATMENT BY FRACTURE TYPE (*fig 4*)

■ *Delbet-Colonna Type 1*

Obstetrical fractures are immobilised in overhead traction for ten days, then kept in abduction for 2 to 3 weeks (double draping, Pavlik harness) [10].

Minimally displaced (less than 25%) fractures in non-walking children are treated by a spica cast for 4 to 6 weeks. Position: flexion 50°, abduction 20°-30°, neutral rotation.

Patients older than 1 year need closed reduction under anaesthesia followed by percutaneous transepiphyseal pinning (Kirschner wires are left protruding in the subcutaneous layer) and a spica cast for eight weeks. Accurate X-ray evaluation is mandatory before mobilisation, due to the high rate of necrosis and delayed union.

In pre-adolescent and adolescent patients, cannulated screws are used, followed by a long period of non-weight-bearing.

When closed reduction is impossible or in the case of fracture with hip dislocation, an open reduction must be carried out. The surgical approach is determined by the direction of the dislocation. The location of the dislocated head must be determined by X-ray or CT-scan. An anterior approach (Smith-Peterson or Watson-Jones) is used for anterior dislocation, a posterior approach (Moore or modified Gibson) for posterior dislocation. The head is reduced first by gentle manipulation, then the fracture fixation can be performed under direct vision [3, 4, 11, 19].

■ *Delbet-Colonna Type 2*

Transcervical fractures are the most frequent. Nondisplaced fractures can be treated conservatively by spica cast in small children and by traction in patients older than 7 years. For fractures in adolescents, percutaneous fixation by two cannulated cancellous screws is used. For every patient, ultrasound imaging is used to detect the pressure of a haemarthrosis which should be evacuated by needle aspiration in order to decrease the risk of head necrosis.

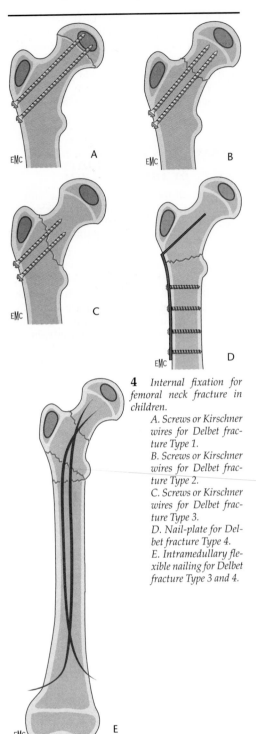

4 *Internal fixation for femoral neck fracture in children.*

A. Screws or Kirschner wires for Delbet fracture Type 1.

B. Screws or Kirschner wires for Delbet fracture Type 2.

C. Screws or Kirschner wires for Delbet fracture Type 3.

D. Nail-plate for Delbet fracture Type 4.

E. Intramedullary flexible nailing for Delbet fracture Type 3 and 4.

Dislocated fractures are first reduced on a traction table in abduction and internal rotation; internal fixation is mandatory due to the risk of secondary displacement. The osteosynthesis is performed by percutaneous fixation using 2 cannulated cancellous screws, which should not cross the epiphyseal plate. Spica cast or traction are applied for a period of 6 to 8 weeks. Delbet-Colonna Type 2 fractures have a high risk of neck necrosis (11% to 50%), thus weight-bearing is only allowed when full bony consolidation is seen on the X-ray.

Screws are not removed before a year after primary surgery, unless secondary treatment is necessary for femoral neck necrosis.

Delbet-Colonna Type 3

For nondisplaced and displaced cervicotrochanteric fractures, internal fixation is recommended because of the very high risk of secondary displacement. For displaced fractures, reduction is obtained using a traction table. In small children, percutaneous internal fixation is obtain by two cannulated screws. A spica cast is applied for 6 weeks. In preadolescent patients when the greater trochanteric epiphyseal plate is closed, a nail plate can be used as in adults, without postoperative immobilisation. Femoral neck necrosis for Delbet-Colonna Type 3 fractures is more frequent in the growing child than in cervicotrochanteric fractures in the adult.

Delbet-Colonna Type 4

Intertrochanteric and subtrochanteric fractures are not true femoral neck fractures and are followed by fewer complications. In nondisplaced fractures in children younger than 5, rapid bone healing is obtained in 3 to 4 weeks in a spica cast. Older children are immobilised for 6 to 8 weeks [13]. In preadolescence, internal fixation is done by flexible intramedullary nailing [16]; if the epiphyseal plates are closed, the same fixation is used as in adults.

In a displaced fracture, after reduction on a fracture table, internal fixation is performed by percutaneous screws, intramedullary nails or blade plates as in adults, depending on the age and the fracture pattern. In younger children and if there is a lack of compliance, a spica cast is used for 6 weeks.

Lesser and greater trochanter fractures [21]

Lesser trochanter avulsion, displaced or nondisplaced, is treated by bed rest for 6 to 8 days in order to control the pain, then by progressive mobilisation, stretching and strengthening exercises.

Nondisplaced greater trochanter fractures are treated non-operatively (as for lesser trochanter fractures). Displaced fractures should be fixed surgically using a tension band technique. Dissection in the posterior area of the greater trochanter must be carried out with great care to avoid damage to the posterior circumflex artery which provides the blood supply to the femoral head.

Stress fracture

Stress fractures in preadolescents are very rare. They occur only in over-trained athletes or in children with pathological bone fragility. Fractures in compression are treated conservatively; transverse fractures must be stabilised by internal fixation [20].

COMPLICATIONS

Avascular necrosis of the neck or of the femoral head is the most common complication of femoral neck fractures in children [3, 4, 7, 9, 19]. Delbet-Colonna Types 1 to 3 have a rate of avascular necrosis from 11% to 87%. The risk of necrosis increases with the displacement of the fracture and in association with hip dislocation. The use of an inappropriate surgical approach, or too-large or too-numerous implants, are also a factor risk. Decreased uptake shown on bone pin-hole radioisotopic scanning is the earliest sign of necrosis. In children, X-ray signs are evident by 2 months after trauma. Long-term prognosis depends on the Ratliff classification: Type 1 has a worse prognosis than types 2 and 3. The prognosis is better in young children with a small area of necrosis. Conservative treatment is always the first choice: physical therapy, bed rest, traction and non-weight-bearing. In children younger than 10 years, metal removal and an abduction orthosis must be considered. Once the full extent of the area of necrosis is established, treatments range from osteotomy to arthoplasty and hip arthrodesis. Chondrolysis has been reported in conjunction with femoral head necrosis [9].

Coxa vara and nonunion (6% to 10%) are mostly seen after conservative treatment. Coxa vara has the potential for spontaneous correction if there is sufficient growth remaining. In coxa vara with an angle of less than 100°, valgus osteotomy is indicated. For nonunion, the treatment must be performed as soon as it is recognised, by a subtrochanteric valgus osteotomy bringing the fracture line horizontal. Stable internal fixation is always used; bone grafts can speed up the healing process [3, 4, 7, 9, 19].

Premature epiphyseal closure occurs due to physeal damage following the trauma, necrosis or surgical treatment, and causes leg length discrepancies in younger children. It can be managed by contralateral distal femoral epiphysiodesis. Greater trochanter overgrowth is treated by growth arrest at this site [3, 4, 7, 9, 19].

Fractures of the pelvis in children

GENERAL CONSIDERATIONS

Pelvic fractures are uncommon in children, but they can have a high incidence of complications. Because of the greater plasticity of the bone and the increased flexibility of the sacroiliac joint and symphysis pubis in the child, greater force is required to fracture a child's pelvis than an adult's. Pelvic fractures generally result from high energy trauma [2], which is why they are associated with other injuries to neurovascular structures, abdominal viscera and the genitourinary system. When a fracture of a child's pelvis is seen radiographically, it is important to remember that soft tissue injuries may be present and that the treatment of these injuries should take priority over management of the fracture. Even if most pelvic fractures in

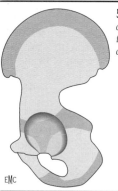

5 *Schematic lateral view of a child's pelvis, showing the triradiate cartilage and other growth cartilage.*

children require minimal treatment of the fracture itself, aggressive treatment, usually operative, can be necessary to control massive blood loss and to avoid late functional complications that could be debilitating throughout life. Complications in pelvic fractures are essentially associated with concomitant injuries that occur immediately and lead to a high mortality rate [1]. However, fractures through the triradiate cartilage can cause growth arrest and a progressive abnormal development of the acetabulum; failure to reduce acetabular fractures can cause early degenerative change.

ACETABULUM DEVELOPMENT

Between the pelvic ossification centres, a residual area of hyaline cartilage (triradiate cartilage) remains where the three anlages are juxtaposed *(fig 5)*. This triradiate cartilage divides the acetabulum into three sectors, so that the ilium contributes superiorly, the pubis anteroinferiorly and the ischium posteroinferiorly. During growth, the three juxtaposed ossification centres act as the metaphysis of tubular bones and permit acetabular development. Thus, fractures through the triradiate cartilage can have exactly the same complications with regard to growth as transphyseal fractures of tubular bones.

CLASSIFICATION OF CHILDREN'S FRACTURES

Several classifications of pelvic fractures in children have been described and many are based on the following questions. Does the fracture break the pelvic ring and if so, is instability present? Does the fracture concern the acetabulum, and if so, is the fracture associated with hip dislocation, with joint instability or with a lesion of the triradiate cartilage? Key and Conwell's classification [15] takes these criteria into account and is helpful concerning the choice of treatment.

■ *Classification of Key and Conwell*

I. Fractures without a break in the continuity of the pelvic ring.
   A. Avulsion fractures.
      1. Anterior superior iliac spine.
      2. Anterior inferior iliac spine.

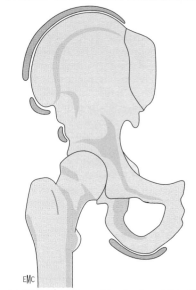

6 *Location of pelvic avulsion fracture; 70 to 75% of such fractures involve the anterior superior iliac spine and the ischial tuberosity.*

      3. Ischial tuberosity.
   B. Fractures of the pubis or ischium.
   C. Fractures of the wing of the ilium.
   D. Fractures of the sacrum or coccyx.
II. Single break in the pelvic ring.
   A. Fracture of two ipsilateral rami.
   B. Fractures near or subluxation of the symphysis pubis.
   C. Fractures near or subluxation of the sacroiliac joint.
III. Double break in the pelvic ring.
   A. Double vertical fractures or dislocation of the pubis (straddle fractures).
   B. Double vertical fractures or dislocation (Malgaigne).
IV. Fractures of the acetabulum.
   A. Small fragment associated with dislocation of the hip.
   B. Linear fracture associated with undisplaced pelvic fracture.
   C. Linear fracture associated with hip joint instability.
   D. Fracture secondary to central dislocation of the acetabulum.

AVULSION FRACTURES OF THE PELVIS *(fig 6)*

These injuries usually occur in sportive adolescents and are caused by powerful muscular contraction on a developing apophysis. Most avulsion fractures involve the anterior superior iliac spine and the ischial tuberosity; however, avulsions of the anterior inferior iliac spine and of the iliac crest have been described. Usually, the treatment consists of a short period of rest during the period of acute pain, followed by partial weight-bearing for some weeks. Excessive callus formation can arise after healing, especially of ischial avulsions, but it rarely needs to be excised. In cases with

significant displacement, it has been reported that open reduction with internal fixation of the avulsed apophysis does not improve the results. The treatment of such injuries should be conservative and the patient advised not to return to athletic activities too early, in order to avoid new injury.

FRACTURES WITHOUT A BREAK IN THE CONTINUITY OF THE PELVIC RIM

These are all the fractures that cause only a partial, not continuous, break in the pelvis ring, which remains totally stable. Among such injuries, fractures of the pubic or ischial rami are the most common, together with fractures of the sacrum and coccyx. Fracture of the wing of the ilium may be caused by direct trauma to the ilium, which generally occurs in pedestrian motor-vehicle accidents. Even if such fractures commonly show only minor displacement, it is important to remember that they indicate high energy trauma. Treatment of a child with such a lesion is always dictated by the associated injuries. Bed rest in the most comfortable position until symptoms subside is all that is necessary for the treatment of the fracture. This is followed by progressive weight-bearing until pain is completely resolved. Attempts at reduction should be avoided, even in sacral or coccygeal fractures, because they rarely achieve a stable reduction and complications such as a tear in the rectum can occur [4].

SINGLE BREAK IN THE PELVIC RING

Fractures of two ipsilateral rami, fractures near or subluxation of the symphysis pubis, or fractures near or subluxation of the sacroiliac joint, constitute single breaks in the pelvic ring which may occur in children because of the mobility of the sacroiliac joint and the symphysis pubis. However, if significant displacement is present, then a second injury in the pelvic ring should be sought [4]. Considerable force is necessary to cause such injuries and other associated fractures or soft tissue damage should be expected. Short-term bed rest followed by progressive weight-bearing on crutches is often all that is necessary. Unilateral traction rarely improves alignment of the fracture or subluxation of the symphysis pubis, but a pelvic sling can be indicated for any such cases. Finally, the fractures almost always unite with adequate remodelling even of the most displaced fractures [4].

DOUBLE BREAKS IN THE PELVIC RING *(fig 7)*

Double breaks of the pelvic ring always follow high-velocity trauma, and associated injuries are common. By definition, the pelvis or a part of the pelvic ring is unstable, leading to a floating fragment (bilateral fractures of both the inferior and superior

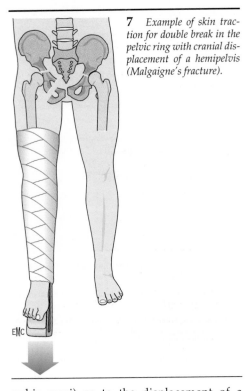

7 *Example of skin traction for double break in the pelvic ring with cranial displacement of a hemipelvis (Malgaigne's fracture).*

pubic rami) or to the displacement of a hemipelvis (Malgaigne's fracture). Unstable fractures of the pelvic ring in children are usually treated conservatively [18]. The treatment guidelines for such fractures are based on the extent and the direction of the displacement. If there is only cranial displacement, skeletal traction or even skin traction in a small child can be used [4]. If lateral displacement is severe, closed manipulation in the lateral decubitus position and spica casting or pelvic sling can be used. External or internal fixation should be used only when conservative methods fail. The use of the external fixator has been recommended in unstable pelvic fractures to control massive blood loss and to permit early mobilisation in polytraumatised children [8]. In older adolescents, treatment can follow the guidelines for the treatment of adult fractures, including internal or external fixation for fracture stabilisation and early mobilisation [4]. The long-term results of unstable pelvic fractures depend on the presence or absence of low back pain, which is strongly correlated with pelvic asymmetry [18]. Pelvic asymmetry is caused by the healing of unstable fractures in malposition and is responsible for symptomatic scoliotic deformations of the lumbar spine.

ACETABULAR FRACTURES

Fractures of the acetabulum are rare in children and occur only in particular situations. Small fragment fractures, generally involving the posterior rim of the acetabulum, can occur with dislocations of the hip. Linear fractures of the acetabulum involving the triradiate cartilage are possible in pelvic fractures with a break in the pelvic ring. Large fractures of the superior dome of the acetabulum are generally caused by forces transmitted along the femur and result in instability of the hip joint and in a lesion of the triradiate cartilage. Finally, central fracture dislocation of the hip can occur in children, often with gross disruption of the triradiate cartilage [4]. The aim of treatment for acetabular fractures in children is the same as for all articular fractures: to restore joint congruity, to maintain articular stability and to realign the triradiate cartilage. In fractures associated with traumatic hip dislocation, closed reduction of the dislocation is usually sufficient. If reduction appears incongruous, entrapment of osseous or cartilaginous fragments or even an inverted labrum must be suspected, and open reduction of the hip is recommended to remove the interposed structures from the articulation [4]. Logically, the surgical approach should depend on the direction of the traumatic dislocation. When fractures of the acetabulum are not displaced and associated with pelvic fractures, treatment of these lesions have priority. If the pelvic fractures are stable, bed rest and extended non-weight-bearing are generally the recommended treatment in order to prevent displacement of the acetabular fragments. If the pelvic fractures appear unstable or if the child is unreliable, skeletal or skin traction may be necessary. The goal of the treatment of displaced acetabular fractures in children is to obtain anatomical congruity of the weight-bearing acetabular fragments. This can be obtained by skeletal traction on the ipsilateral extremity, but open reduction is usually required, especially when residual displacement is greater than to 2 mm [14]. Central fracture-dislocation in children is associated with poor results, regardless of the type of treatment. Surgical treatment does not improve the results.

Open reduction and internal fixation seem to promote massive heterotopic bone formation. Distal and lateral skeletal traction can reduce the forces transmitted by the femoral head to the acetabulum, and such treatment appears to be the most convenient for most central fracture-dislocations in children. However, open reduction and internal fixation should be considered, especially for older adolescents, if reduction with skeletal traction is not acceptable [4].

ASSOCIATED INJURIES

As most pelvic fractures in children are caused by pedestrian motor-vehicle accidents, various associated lesions can occur, many of which are not related to the pelvic fracture itself. These include craniocerebral lesions, major thoracic injuries, such as pneumothorax, haematopneumothorax or ruptured diaphragm, and lesions in the abdomen (splenic, liver and kidney lacerations). Vertebral fractures or long bone fractures can also occur during the accident. Other associated injuries are closely related to the pelvic fracture fragments, which can cause tearing, stretching or crushing of soft tissue contents within the pelvis. Vascular injuries due to pelvic trauma are unusual in children [5]. Massive blood loss in the child occurs more commonly from solid visceral injury than from pelvic vascular disruption [12]. Generally, haemorrhage due to injury of large vessels within the abdominal cavity can be controlled surgically. Retroperitoneal bleeding with hypotension is difficult to control surgically, and usually requires angiography with a selective embolisation. Indications for angiography are 4 or more units of blood transfusion within 24 hours, or a half blood mass less in one hour [12]. Finally, external fixation can be useful to reduce and stabilise the pelvis in order to control massive blood loss [8]. Ruptured urethra and bladder are less commonly associated with pelvic fractures in children. If any signs of urinary tract disruption are present, a cystourethrogram should be performed, followed if necessary by an intravenous pyelogram. Neurologic involvement due to local direct injury to nerves is uncommon after pelvic fractures in children. The neurologic injuries are generally not permanent, but can cause very disabling causalgia.

References ➤

References

[1] Allouis M, Bracq H, Catier P, Babut JM. Serious pelvic traumatisms in children. *Chir Pediatr* 1981 ; 22 : 43-50

[2] Bryan WJ, Tullos HS. Pediatric pelvic fractures: review of 52 patients. *J Trauma* 1979 ; 19 : 799-805

[3] Canale ST, Beaty JH. Hip fractures and dislocation. In : Canale ST ed. Operative pediatric orthopedics. St Louis : CV Mosby, 1995 : 965-981

[4] Canale ST, Beaty JH. Pelvic and hip Fractures. In : Rockwood CA, Wilkins KE, Beaty JH eds. Fractures in children. Philadelphia : Lippincott-Raven, 1996 : 1109-1193

[5] Canarelli JP, Collet LM, Ricard J, Boboyono JM. Vascular complications in pelvic injuries in children. *Chir Pediatr* 1988 ; 29 : 233-241

[6] Colonna PC. Fractures of the neck of the femur in children. *Am J Surg* 1929 ; 6 : 793-797

[7] Davison BL, Weinstein SL. Hip fractures in children: a long-term follow-up study. *J Pediatr Orthop* 1992 ; 12 : 355-358

[8] Engelhardt P. Malgaigne pelvic ring injury in chilhood. *Orthopade* 1992 ; 21 : 422-426

[9] Forlin E, Guille JT, Kumar SJ, Rhee KJ. Complications associated with fracture of the neck of the femur in children. *J Pediatr Orthop* 1992 ; 12 : 503-509

[10] Forlin E, Guille JT, Kumar SJ, Rhee KJ. Transepiphyseal fractures of the neck of the femur in very young children. *J Pediatr Orthop* 1992 ; 12 : 164-168

[11] Hughes OH, Beaty JH. Fractures of the head and neck of the femur in children. *J Bone Joint Surg* 1994 ; 76 : 283-292

[12] Ismail N, Bellemare JF, Mollitt DL, Di Scala C, Koeppel B, Teppas JJ 3rd. Death from pelvic fracture: children are different. *J Pediatr Surg* 1996 ; 31 : 82-85

[13] Jeng C, Sponseller PD, Yates A, Paletta G. Subtrochanteric femoral fractures in children. Alignment after 90°-90° traction and cast application. *Clin Orthop* 1997 ; 441 : 170-174

[14] Judet R, Judet J, Letournel E. Fractures of the acetabulum: classification and surgical approaches for open reduction. *J Bone Joint Surg Am* 1964 ; 46 : 1615-1646

[15] Key JA, Conwell HE. Management of fractures, dislocations and sprains. St Louis : CV Mosby, 1951

[16] Métaizeau JP. Ostéosynthèse chez l'enfant. Montpellier : Sauramps Médical, 1988 : 77-84

[17] Ratliff AH. Fractures of the neck of the femur in children. *J Bone Joint Surg* 1962 ; 44 : 528-542

[18] Schwarz N, Posch E, Mayr J, Fischmeister FM, Schwarz AF, Ohner T. Long-term results of unstable pelvic ring fractures in children. *Injury* 1998 ; 29 : 431-433

[19] Sinet A, Damsin JP, Carlioz H. Fractures de l'extrémité supérieure du fémur chez l'enfant. *Encycl Méd Chir* (Éditions Scientifiques et Médicales Elsevier SAS Paris), Techniques chirurgicales - Orthopédie-traumatologie, 44-625, 1984

[20] St Pierre P, Staheli LT, Smith JB, Green NE. Femoral neck stress fractures in children and adolescents. *J Pediatr Orthop* 1995 ; 15 : 470-473

[21] Theologis TN, Epps H, Latz K, Cole WG. Isolated fractures of the lesser and greater trochanter. *Injury* 1997 ; 28 : 363-364

Dysplasia dislocation of the hip: conservative treatment and open reduction

A Dimeglio
D Moukoko

Abstract. – The pathology of developmental dislocation of the hip covers diverse entities from benign dysplasia to severe irreducible dislocated hips. Treatment is a question of nuance and skill. Each hip represents a specific case and not all will require treatment – certain benign forms recover spontaneously, whereas certain severe forms do better left untreated: two dislocated hips are better than two stiff ones. The most severe complication is avascular necrosis, of which the devastating effects must be kept in the clinician's mind during each step of treatment. Very early diagnosis and treatment will provide the best results and lower the risk of complications.

The first steps of treatment begin with identification of the intra- and extra-articular obstacles. Treatment must be initiated as soon as the diagnosis of dysplasia dislocation of the hip (DDH) has been made. Younger infants can be treated easily with the Pavlik harness, using ultrasonography as a guide. However, this is a highly demanding technique. Failure of the harness must be promptly identified, after which traction, adduction tenotomy and a hip spica cast may be considered. A hip arthrogram is the most valuable tool in assessing concentric reduction of the hip. If non-operative treatment is unsatisfactory, open reduction is required. In very young patients, the medial approach has its place. The anterolateral approach is widely used, especially after the failure of a previous medial exposure and for older infants where several reconstructive steps can be implemented in one stage.

Keywords: hip, dysplasia dislocation of the hip, open reduction, closed reduction, Pavlik harness, hip spica cast, hip arthrogram, avascular necrosis.

General principles

THERAPEUTIC PRINCIPLES

The incidence of significant dysplasia dislocation of the hip (DDH) is approximately 2 per 1,000 live births. The incidence of unstable hips is about 8 per 1,000, but 50% of these settle and stabilise in the first few weeks of life, and would do so even without treatment. In reality, DDH comprises a large spectrum of diverse afflictions with a gradient of increasing severity:

– dysplastic unstable hip;

– subluxable hip;

– dislocatable hip;

– dislocated reducible hip;

– dislocated irreducible hip.

Alain Dimeglio, M.D.
Didier Moukoko, M.D.
Paediatric Orthopaedic Department, CHU Lapeyronie, 371, avenue du Doyen Gaston Giraud, 34295 Montpellier cedex 5, France.

The first objective in the management of DDH is to achieve concentric reduction at the earliest age possible. The earlier treatment is initiated, the easier it is to restore the anatomy completely [4]. The first few weeks are the golden period. Femoro-acetabular concentricity achieved very early guarantees harmonious growth leading to anatomical normality.

The second objective is to avoid aseptic necrosis and physeal injury which may lead to deformity in the upper femur, acetabular dysplasia, and premature degenerative arthritis. Avascular necrosis (AVN) is a severe complication, its devastating effects becoming apparent only years later [1, 7, 21]. The exact time of the vascular trauma is often unknown, but as a rule it is of iatrogenic origin. Avascular necreosis a more serious complication than loss of reduction, as the latter is reversible.

The third objective is to facilitate the resolution of dysplasia, which leads to degenerative joint disease. The later treatment is initiated, the less potential there is for acetabular and femoral head remodelling. Surgery becomes necessary, either to achieve concentric reduction or to correct the axis and coverage. The risk of complications is greater.

UNDERSTANDING THE OBSTACLES

Treatment of a dislocated hip cannot be undertaken without understanding the different obstacles that prevent reduction. In the reducible dislocated hip, the displacement of the femoral head leads to both local and regional anatomical modifications – capsular, muscular and osteo-articular. Initially functional, they rapidly become structural. Time is against the surgeon. As the dislocation is perpetuated, the obstacles become fixed. These obstacles are identified as being either extra-articular or intra-articular [16, 22, 27].

■ *Extra-articular obstacles*

The adductor longus: its retraction is reliably identified by the gradual loss in the hip of passive abduction as the dislocation ages. It is all the more severe as the child becomes older and as the head is increasingly displaced proximally. Its

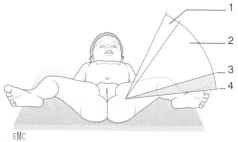

1 *Ideal hip abduction should be located between 2 extreme points to avoid insufficient abduction which could lead to redislocation or excessive abduction compromising the vascularity of the femoral head. 1. Zone of redislocation (adduction); 2. safe zone (Ramsey); 3. comfortable abduction limit; 4. maximal abduction.*

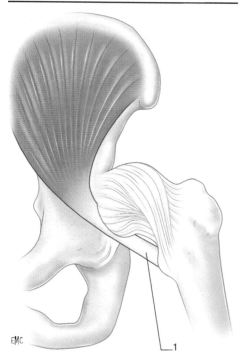

2 *The tight iliopsoas tendon (1) is an obstacle to concentric reduction. It can be overcome by hip flexion or iliopsoas tenotomy.*

retraction limits the descent of the head under the limbus when the lower limb is in a straight position. Furthermore, spontaneous hip abduction is limited, and the safe zone becomes too narrow to maintain reduction. Ramsey defines the safe zone as the zone of hip abduction in which the femoral head remains reduced within the acetabulum, incurring minimal risk of avascular necrosis due to an unduly forced position [19] *(fig 1)*.

The iliopsoas: its retraction is simultaneously a cause and a consequence of the ascent of the femoral head to a high proximal position. It prevents the "descent" of the head under the limbus. Furthermore, as the muscular-tendinous junction crosses the anterior face of the hip joint, its retraction exerts a posteriorly oriented pressure on the anterior capsule, "dislocating" the head. This leaves a mark on the anterior capsule which with time becomes structural and produces the isthmic contracture of the capsule *(fig 2)* [5]. Its

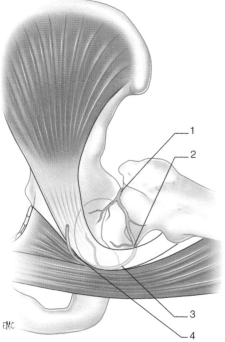

3 *The medial circumflex femoral artery risks compression with excessive abduction. Four sites are vulnerable. From distal to proximal, it can be compressed between the greater trochanter and the acetabular labrum (1); the iliopsoas tendon and the femoral neck (2); the iliopsoas tendon and the acetabular labrum; (3) the iliopsoas tendon and the pectineus muscle (4).*

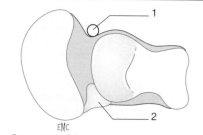

4 *Contracture of the medial capsule anteriorly, due to pressure by the iliopsoas tendon, mirrors the inverted labrum posteriorly. 1. Iliopsoas tendon; 2. labrum.*

anatomical intimacy with the anterior and posterior circumflex arteries creates a risk for the proximal femoral vascularisation of the dislocated hip, as well as of the reduced hip with a tight retracted iliopsoas *(fig 3)*.

■ *Intra-articular obstacles*

An antero-medial constricted capsule is demonstrated on the hip arthrogram by an hourglass-shaped appearance. Due to long-standing pressure of a tightly retracted iliopsoas muscle as it crosses the anterior aspect of the hip, this can lead to a fibrous adhesion of the inner anterior capsule to the acetabulum ridge itself *(fig 4)*.

The transverse acetabular ligament prevents concentric reduction by forcing the head upwards and considerably reduces the diameter of the acetabular cavity.

The ligamentum teres is elongated and enlarged, representing a voluminous tissue mass interspersed between the femoral head and the depth of the acetabular cavity *(fig 5)*.

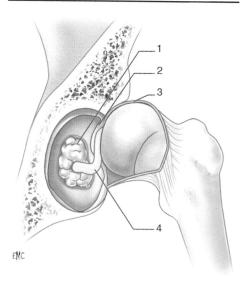

5 *Intra-articular obstacles include the ligamentum teres femoris and the fibro-fatty tissue. 1. Fibro-fatty tissue; 2. inverted limbus (acetabular labrum); 3. joint capsule; 4. ligamentum teres femoris.*

An inverted labrum is described as an intra-articular obstacle which may be suspected when there is a supra-lateral shadow on the AP arthrogram. However, in non-teratological congenital dislocation of the hip (CDH), Ponseti demonstrated that the limbus was atrophic, everted and adherent to the inner capsule [16]. The defect observed on the arthrogram would correspond to a thickening of the acetabular hyaline cartilage responsible for the Ortolani reductional "click".

The inversion of the limbus, however, is iatrogenic. Attempts at lowering a superiorly migrated femoral head can produce a compression on the superolateral surface of the limbus, leading to its inversion [3]. This phenomenon is aggravated by abducting the hip during traction before the femoral head reaches a position underneath the limbus [14].

The diameter of the acetabulum is limited sagittally by the neolimbus posteriorly and by capsular constriction anteriorly; it is limited axially by the neolimbus superiorly and the transverse acetabular ligament inferiorly.

The proximal femur becomes deformed, with head flattening and coxa valga which prevent concentricity.

Hip reduction can overcome these obstacles with time. If the femoral head presents well under the limbus and faces the acetabulum, and reducing soft tissue forces are balanced around the reduction axis, the head will penetrate the deepest parts of the acetabulum. This is the rationale for closed reduction advocated by the French school, even in late-diagnosed dislocations [3]. A more drastic position is adopted by the Anglo-Saxon school, which recommends surgically moving aside of any obstacles which might prevent a perfect concentric reduction [26].

Indications for treatment

Management of the dislocated hip requires a thoughtful and analytical approach. In each age range, certain generalisations are helpful.

AT BIRTH (NEONATE)

There is widespread agreement that the best time to diagnose and treat instability is the neonatal period; although some cases of hip instability will resolve spontaneously, those which persist untreated will be more difficult to manage at a later age.

The rationale for treatment at this age is that the hip is not in a proximally high position. If the hip is positioned in flexion and some degree of abduction, the dislocation reduces and the instability will disappear promptly in most cases. Immobilisation is not the goal of the treatment and is difficult to achieve, as babies move a great deal, even in a cast. Consequently, rigid braces and forced abduction must be avoided.

Triple diapers and abduction diapers have no place in the treatment of DDH in the newborn. They do not produce flexion, and the amount of abduction is completely unpredictable. They give the family a false sense of security and are generally ineffective.

The Pavlik harness is indicated when the hip is dislocatable or dislocated [15]; the gradual reduction is monitored by ultrasonography. This is the most commonly-used device.

FROM 1 TO 4 MONTHS

Before the age of four months, hip instability regresses with the Pavlik harness in 90% of the cases. The decision to stop full-time wear is made when the hips have been stable on clinical examination for 4 to 8 weeks and ultrasonography is normal. An abduction orthosis is then indicated to allow the dysplasia to resolve. The older the child when treatment is begun, the longer the harness must be worn.

Ultrasonography is a complementary tool to the harness. It is an excellent way to document progress towards completion of a successful reduction; it allows monitoring of the acetabular development during treatment and the gradual dynamic stabilisation of the hip joint.

In difficult irreducible hips, if the hip does not reduce after one week, with evident obstacles to the reduction or persistent instability, the harness should be discontinued and other forms of treatment considered: progressive traction, closed reduction, arthrography, adductor tenotomy, and hip spica casting.

Failure of the Pavlik harness should be recognised early and trigger an imaging study. Ultrasonography or MRI are helpful in identifying obstacles [24].

FROM 4 TO 24 MONTHS

After the fourth month, the Pavlik harness loses some of its effectiveness, and closed reduction becomes the treatment of choice, usually preceded by skin traction [17]. The goal of traction is the gradual stretching of the retracted soft tissue structures, which facilitates reduction and decreases hyper-pressure on the reduced femoral head, potentially a source of avascular necrosis. It avoids the stretching and extrinsic compression of the circumflex arteries produced by a sudden reduction and forced stabilising positions. It decreases the need for open reduction [30]. The direction of traction varies widely – overhead, longitudinal, with or without abduction – as does its duration. Usually three weeks are necessary, followed by a gentle closed reduction performed under general anaesthetic. At that time, the stability of the hip is assessed and a hip arthrogram is carried out. If the range of unforced abduction (safe zone) is insufficient, a tenotomy of the adductor muscles is performed to facilitate the stabilisation.

Concentric hips are immobilised in a spica cast, whereas failure to obtain concentric and stable reduction indicates an open reduction. The position of stability should be greater than 90 degrees of hip flexion, 30-40 degrees of abduction, and neutral to slightly internal rotation. Applying the plaster cast is a therapeutic act in itself and should not be left to the inexperienced surgeon without supervision. Cast application obeys strict rules, and should be undertaken with meticulous precision to avoid losing the reduction obtained. Cast changes should be performed under general anaesthetic. After 6 weeks, when full abduction is present with no clinical instability and perfect reduction is demonstrated on X-rays, the new cast can be applied for six more weeks.

If there is a doubt about stability, the arthrogram should be repeated. The hip must not be forced into a non-physiological position to maintain reduction, as this would significantly increase the risks of proximal growth disturbances. Closed reduction must be discontinued if gross instability persists or if a concentric reduction cannot be obtained.

Open reduction must then be considered, taking all obstacles into account:

– adductor tightness (long adductor tenotomy);

– iliopsoas contracture (musculo-tendinous junction lengthening);

– capsular laxity (plication);

– ligamentum teres hypertrophy (excision);

– hypertrophy of the fibro-fatty tissue (removal);

– an inverted limbus in non-teratologic DDH is seldom a problem, and we strongly advise against its removal.

Reduction can be accompanied by complementary osteotomies to address adjacent morphological problems:

– acetabular insufficiency: after the age of 2, a pelvic osteotomy can improve the coverage of the femoral head [20];

– high proximally displaced hip: a femoral shortening osteotomy for decompression can be considered at any age;

– excessive femoral anteversion: a derotation femoral osteotomy can be performed.

The medial approach exposes the hip joint directly over the site of the obstacles to reduction, and dissection and blood loss are minimal, reducing the risk of postoperative stiffness. However, access is deep and difficult; capsule laxity cannot be addressed and therefore the risk of re-dislocation is high; and the circumflex medial artery runs the risk of trauma, leading to secondary avascular necrosis [23].

Thus the medial approach is best reserved for younger infants, when capsulorrhaphy is not anticipated. In a successfully maintained reduction, the capsule spontaneously tightens. When the medial approach fails, a second chance exists to reduce the hip by the anterolateral exposure.

This approach is most widely used to reduce the hip joint, especially in older infants. It allows greater visibility of the entire hip during surgery, and the possibility of performing a capsulorrhaphy and pelvic osteotomy if necessary. However, dissection is more extensive and there is more risk of postoperative stiffness. A posterior approach has been described, but is seldom used [29].

AFTER 24 MONTHS

After 24 months, the anatomical lesions are more severe, reducing the success of closed management. Non-operative treatment associating pre-reduction traction and a hip spica cast has been reported with a good success rate, but in 75% of the cases secondary surgery was required to correct osseous dysplasia of the proximal femur and/or of the acetabulum.

One-stage surgical correction associates open reduction, a femoral shortening osteotomy and a pelvic osteotomy (Salter or Pemberton).

Long-term results depend on the deformities of the femoral head and acetabulum: it is difficult to recover several months of abnormal growth.

In late discovered forms (after the age of 8), especially with bilateral involvement, the hips have to be "abandoned". It is better to have two dislocated hips than two stiff ones.

TERATOLOGICAL HIPS

These occur at the earliest stages of pregnancy. They may be isolated or associated with multiple malformations

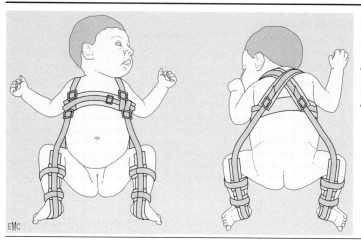

6 *The Pavlik harness maintains a non-forced position with 90° flexion and spontaneous gravity abduction. It is a powerful tool, but is potentially dangerous as is can lead to AVN in the case of forced abduction.*

(Larsen's syndrome). Anatomical lesions are very severe, the hip is irreducible, and closed reduction is destined to failure. Surgical treatment is controversial: bilateral forms can be left untreated, favouring mobility. Surgery is difficult and leads to poor results in 50% of cases, with 20% redislocation and 50% AVN.

Specific techniques

PAVLIK HARNESS

Treatment by the Pavlik harness is complex. It must be considered as a gradual orthopaedic reduction, to be monitored meticulously and managed by the paediatric orthopaedic surgeon. It is not the vocation of the paediatrician to prescribe it. This technique, described in 1957 [15], is based on a philosophy of:

– preserving beneficial hip motion;

– maintaining the centring position of the femoral head. The relaxation of the iliopsoas muscle is produced by hip flexion;

– gradual abduction is obtained by the weight of the thighs, avoiding an unduly forced position, thus decreasing the risks of vascular compromise and its resulting avascular necrosis.

It is a dynamic flexion abduction orthosis. Its goal is to maintain the abduction stability in the safe zone. If spontaneous abduction is too limited, an adductor tenotomy can be associated with the treatment.

The indications are unstable, dislocatable, dislocated reducible hips before the age of 4 months. As the child ages and soft tissue contractures develop along with secondary changes in the acetabulum, the success rate of the Pavlik harness decreases.

■ *Technique* (fig 6)

The thoracic belt should be placed at nipple level. The shoulder straps should cross in the centre of the back so that they do not slide off the shoulders. The anterior strap buckles should be located at the child's anterior axillary line to produce pure hip

flexion. Placement of the straps too far medially produces hip flexion, abduction and lateral rotation. The proximal leg straps should be placed just distal to the knee to prevent bowstringing which would result in internal rotation and adduction of the hip. The posterior straps should not pull the hip into forced abduction, but should simply prevent adduction. Excessive abduction increases the risk of AVN. Even a slight abduction forced against the retracted adductor or iliopsoas muscles will exert compressive forces between the head and acetabulum, impairing micro-vascularisation.

The hips are generally positioned between 80-110 degrees of flexion and 45-60 degrees of abduction. The femoral head must be directed toward the triradiate cartilage; its position should be confirmed by ultrasonography. The surgeon should be present during the scan and feel the tactile sensation of reduction.

■ *Management*

The harness should be worn full-time until stability is obtained, as determined by negative Barlow and Ortolani tests and a dynamic ultrasound study. In the meantime, the patient is examined twice a week and the straps are adjusted to accommodate growth. The family is instructed in the care of the child including bathing, diapering and dressing.

Ultrasonography is performed at the initial step of treatment, monitors the progression of reduction and is repeated after each major adjustment in the harness until stabilisation is confirmed.

■ *Persistent dislocation*

– If the dislocation is superior, additional flexion is indicated.

– If the dislocation is inferior, a decrease in flexion is necessary.

– If the dislocation is lateral, the situation is observed initially. As long as the femoral head is directed towards the triradiate cartilage, as confirmed by ultrasonography, the head may gradually penetrate the acetabulum.

■ *Harness failure*

This should be recognised early. Obstacles must be identified and seen at ultrasonography. An arthrogram can also be useful and, in complex cases, the acetabulum can be studied by MRI [24]. In Type III, the labrum is inverted and closes the isthmus. Reduction is impossible and pursuing Pavlik treatment is useless and dangerous. If the hip is not reduced within eight days, there is no need to continue treatment, and closed reduction should be considered.

The Pavlik harness is a powerful and reliable tool, leading to 90% reduction and stabilisation of DDH [9]. However, this apparatus is difficult to handle. Several problems have been identified with its use, of which the most common are:

– failure to obtain reduction, related to improper use by the physician;

– failure to recognise the lack of reduction for many weeks;

– poor harness design which allows the hips to adduct and externally rotate with hip flexion.

■ *Complications*

Avascular necrosis – the most disastrous – can be secondary to forced abduction or persistent use of the harness despite failure of reduction. Inferior dislocation of the hip and transient femoral nerve palsy are both due to excessive flexion.

■ *Contraindications*

Contraindications are high proximal displacement of the femoral head, irreducible hips and teratologic hips. These situations should lead to an alternative treatment, closed or open reduction.

TRACTION: A SUBJECT OF CONTROVERSY

Traction treatment is used for children with dislocations diagnosed between four months and two years, and also for whom initial harness and splint management has failed. Children in this age group have a dislocated hip on examination that is not reducible.

Traction aims to achieve three goals:

– to facilitate or obtain the reduction;

– to decrease the need for open reduction;

– to decrease the risk of avascular necrosis.

There are three different philosophies concerning the use of traction:

For the **conservatives** (fig 7), traction plays a major role in the process of closed reduction. It follows strict rules, based on a 3-stage procedure: 1) lowering the femoral head below the limbus by progressively increasing weight longitudinally; followed by 2) gradual abduction, placing the femoral neck horizontally; and 3) compensation of femoral anteversion by an equal amount of

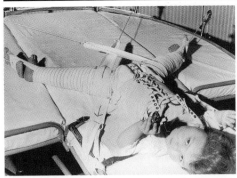

7   *Conservative traction treatment can be extremely complex with 3-dimensional control of limb placement. This method shows a high success rate and minimal AVN risk. However, it is a long and demanding process.*

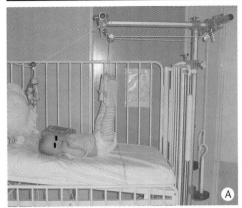

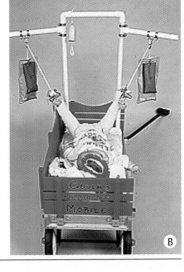

8   *A. Hip flexion produces relaxation of the iliopsoas tendon, thus reducing the anterior capsular obstacle.*
B. Home traction, popular in the USA, decreases the cost of hospitalisation.

internal rotation in order to place the femoral head in the axis of reduction.

The hip spica cast will be applied in this exact position.

This technique has proved very efficient, even in late treated hips, with a minimal risk of AVN [3, 14]. However, the traction must be methodical, rigorous and adjusted. Those who have modified the rules by decreasing the treatment have progressively removed its meaning.

According to the **nihilists,** such as Weinstein, there is no objective evidence in the medical literature that traction affects any of the intra- or extra-articular obstacles to reduction [10, 27]. The need for open reduction depends more on what is considered to be a satisfactory reduction than on whether or not pre-reduction traction is used.

As for the incidence of avascular necrosis, the literature, at best, can be summarised as inconclusive. The supposed gradual stretching effect of traction can be reproduced acutely by femoral shortening during an open reduction [8]. The most consistent feature producing avascular necrosis is excessive pressure on the femoral head – for this reason, this group is unwilling to use the femoral head to "force" the obstacles to concentric reduction. If gentle closed reduction does not result in concentric reduction, obstacles must be surgically removed.

The **liberal approach** is our choice. The traction modalities are numerous. As concerns the direction of traction, overhead traction *(fig 8A)* has the disadvantage of not stretching the iliopsoas muscle; however, it releases the pressure of its tendon over the anteromedial capsule, which could prevent reduction. Semi-flexed hips (45 degrees), associated with a slight flexion of the knees, release the tension on the hamstring muscles, allowing descent of the femoral head. Longitudinal traction gradually stretches the tight iliopsoas, and to a lesser degree the adductors. Traction in abduction (particularly in extreme abduction) carries the risk of avascular necrosis. Weight is gradually increased based on skin tolerance, which must be checked daily.

The duration of traction will be long if the aim is to gradually reduce the hip, and short if the aim is to prepare the hip for closed reduction under anaesthetic or for open reduction.

Skin traction is preferred to skeletal traction which has become unpopular due to numerous complications associated with the distal femoral pin: site infection, growth plate injury and fractures.

Hospital skin traction has its disadvantages: hospital-acquired afflictions, family and psychological disruptions and high cost. It is, however, our preferred treatment because it can be constantly adjusted and dosed under medical control.

Home traction is popular in the USA *(fig 8B)*. It can be carried out overhead or with 45 degrees of hip flexion [2]. A special vehicle is made and delivered to families. Traction is maintained for 20 hours out of 24, with a weight of 1 kg at first, increased gradually to 2.5 kg.

With an adequate period of traction (from three to six weeks), most hips presenting in this age group may then undergo closed reduction by a gentle Ortolani manoeuvre in the operating room. Traction stretches the soft tissues and places the dislocated hip in a more manageable position. It may aid in loosening soft tissue contractures, facilitating later closed reduction. It is important to avoid an iatrogenic forced position which may lead to AVN.

HIP ARTHROGRAMS

The arthrogram has been widely used in the management of DDH, as the contours of nonossified structures in the joint can be made opaque. However, due to its invasive character, and the development of new high-performance imaging techniques such as ultrasonography, MRI and dynamic MRI [24], the trend is for its gradual replacement. Nevertheless, it is still a very valuable tool for the surgeon, since it allows dynamic analysis of the joint. In our opinion, it is an integral part of closed reduction.

■ *Indication*

Hip arthrograms are helpful in determining some of the anatomical intra- and extra-articular obstacles to reduction. They also help to determine if a congruous reduction has been obtained.

■ *Techniques*

The approach can be antero-medial, antero-lateral, or infero-medial.

We use the infero-medial approach. The examination is carried out under general anaesthetic. The entire hip and lower extremity are draped in a sterile fashion to allow manipulation and posturing of the hip under image intensifiers.

A needle is introduced into the genito-crural crease, posterior to the adductor longus tendon. It is directed toward the inferior hip capsule in the horizontal plane (aiming at the ipsilateral axilla) under image intensifier control. After the needle contacts the bone at the junction between the neck and the head, the needle is drawn back by 2 mm and 2 cc of saline solution are injected. Drawing the needle back out completely confirms the intra-articular position of the needle point. Then 1 to 2 cc of opaque dye are injected and the diffusion of the contrast medium is facilitated by moving the hip.

Dynamic studies are then performed under image intensifier in neutral, abduction and a combination of abduction and internal rotation.

■ *Results*

Arthrograms offer valuable information about the pathological conditions that prevent concentric or stable reduction of the hip.

An enlarged ligamentum teres can be identified, but more often it appears with the enlarged fibro-fatty tissue to fill the depth of the acetabular cavity. The transverse acetabular ligament is observed to be prominent and increased in thickness. The hourglass constriction of the capsule,

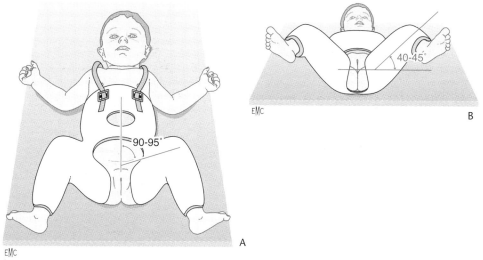

9 *The child is placed on a spica frame, resting on the sacrum with the posterior chest wall at the shoulder level. Hip position: abduction 45°, flexion 90°. A small towel is placed in front of the abdomen, to be removed after spica application. A 5 cm stockinet is rolled from the nipple line to the ankle. Felt pads are applied over the proximal and distal ends of the spica and over bony points and knees; a last piece joins both groins via the gluteal folds, over the iliac crest in front of the abdomen.*
A single layer of 10 cm plaster roll is applied from the nipple line to the ankles, reinforced by splints from nipple line to sacrum (preventing posterior sliding of the femoral head); from the inguinal area, around the gluteal region, iliac crest, abdomen and symmetrically on the opposite side; from nipple line to the knee, holding hip flexion and abduction; over the knee to maintain flexion. A second layer of 10 cm plaster roll is applied to cover this structure.
   A. Hip flexion is 90° to 95°. It appears to be more because of the shape of the soft tissues of the thigh.
   B. The abdomen is maintained at 45°. Excessive abduction compromises the femoral head vascularity and therefore must be avoided.

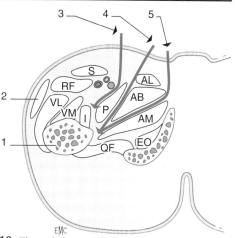

10 *The medial approach allows direct access to the hip joint and its obstacles; however the visual field remains limited. 1. Femur; 2. ligamentum teres femoris; 3. Weinstein approach; 4. Ludloff approach; 5. Ferguson approach.*

creating an isthmus, can be an indirect sign of a tight iliopsoas tendon compressing the anteromedial capsule. The incongruity between the femoral head and acetabulum is often misleading. The cavity of the acetabulum appears small due to all of the above-mentioned obstacles.

The shape of the femoral head is difficult to assess since the ligamentum teres interferes, giving a false impression of deformation or a false impression of sphericity.

An inverted acetabular labrum is infrequent. It is often a misinterpretation of a shadow at the supero-lateral ridge of the acetabulum which originates in the hyaline cartilage [16] and which, as a rule, is not an obstacle to reduction.

Studying the adequacy of the reduction provides prognostic criteria. Interposition of soft tissues does not allow concentric reduction and increases the need for secondary bone procedures. According to Tanaka, if the acetabular floor shows more than 3.5 mm of thickness, this indicates soft-tissue interposition [25]. If this does not disappear within 6 weeks, a secondary procedure is required. Race and Herring studied the medial dye pool and found that more than 7 mm on the initial post-reductional arthrogram indicated the need for open reduction [18]. The arthrogram must normalise within 6 weeks to confirm that concentricity has been achieved.

CLOSED REDUCTION

This consists of three weeks of hospital skin traction to bring down the femoral head. Skin tapes should be applied above the knee to the thigh level to distribute the traction forces over a large skin area.

Overhead traction should be used until nine months of age. In older infants, hip flexion should be used at 45 degrees, with the knee slightly flexed at 25 degrees.

Under general anaesthetic, closed reduction and arthrography are performed in the operating room. An adductor tenotomy can be associated in the case of adductor contracture; it can be performed percutaneously. The goal is to obtain symmetrical abduction in both hips. Then the cast is applied. This is a crucial step. The cast must hold the hips in the required abduction to maintain stability and concentricity of the hips. It must offer support under the greater trochanteric area to avoid posterior slippage of the femoral head [11] (fig 9).

In children with hip dislocation up to the age of two, closed reduction after preliminary traction must be attempted. Some authors recommend this approach up to three years of age [5]. After 18 months, the immobilisation required to obtain a stable hip is long (6 months), and after closed reduction the risk of acetabular dysplasia at this age is high, necessitating secondary surgery.

Zionts has reported a series of closed reductions [30]: 75% of the children treated between one and three years of age were treated effectively and with success by preliminary traction and reduction under general anaesthetic, associated in some cases with adductor tenotomy. Of the hips treated by closed reduction, 66% (two-thirds) required complementary surgery to treat residual dysplasia; after 18 months of age, the percentage was 74%.

OPEN REDUCTION

Open reduction must be considered in cases of failure of closed reduction with persistent instability or persistent lateralisation of the femoral head.

It can be performed by the medial approach or by the anterolateral approach. In many centres in the USA, open reduction is performed as soon as the failure of closed reduction is observed. In France and the U.K., the vast majority of paediatric surgeons prefer to differ the procedure until after the age of one, when the bony nucleus centre begins to appear. This strategy is based on the reduced vulnerability of the ossified head to AVN [21]. However, this wasted time will have induced growth deformities – aspherical head, insufficient cotyle, and more organic retractions.

■ *Medial open reduction*

This is not a new idea. Ludloff described this approach as early as 1908 [12]. Since this description, some modifications have been suggested by different authors (fig 10). Ludloff approached the hip in a plane between the abductor brevis and the pectineus. Ferguson approached the hip in a plane between the adductor brevis and the adductor magnus [6]. Weinstein and Ponseti modified Ludloff's approach and entered the hip capsule via a plane between the femoral bundle and the pectineus muscle [28]. This anteromedial approach provides better exposure, but great care must be taken not to damage the medial femoral circumflex artery which lies in the operative field. Medial open reduction is used extensively up to the age of one year. Between the ages of 1 and 2 years, its use is more controversial because capsulorrhaphy of the lateral part of the capsule cannot be carried out through this approach, and subluxation and redislocation are therefore more likely. Few centres use medial open reduction after the age of two years.

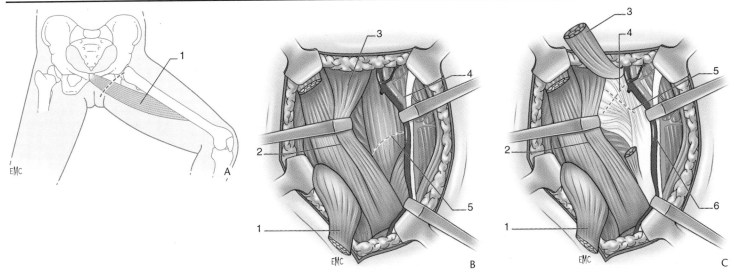

11 A. Medial approach - transversal skin incision 2 cm distal to the groin crease.
1. Adductor longus m.
B. Careful retraction of the vascular bundle. Beware the risk of AVN of the femoral head due to lesions of the medial femoral circumflex artery. 1. Adductor longus m. detached and retracted; 2. adductor brevis m.; 3. pectineus m. retracted medially;

4. femoral vessels and nerve retracted laterally; 5. section of iliopsoas tendon.
C. T-shaped incision of the capsule allows exposure of all intra-articular obstacles.
1. Adductor longus m.; 2. adductor magnus m.; 3. pectineus m. retracted medially; 4. transverse cut; 5. capsule incised along axis of femoral neck; 6. femoral vessels and nerve retracted laterally.

Advantages: This provides a direct approach over the area where the intra- and extra-articular obstacles to reduction are located, minimal dissection, and minimal postoperative stiffness. Blood loss is minimal (usually less than 20 ml) and both hips can be operated on safely – if necessary, in the same procedure. There is no injury to the hip abductors and to the growth plate of the iliac crest, both of which can be injured during a standard anterior approach to the hip. The scar is cosmetically acceptable and well hidden. In case of failure, an anterolateral approach constitutes a second chance.

Disadvantages: Capsulorrhaphy is impossible. The visual field is limited and there is a risk of lesions to the circumflex artery.

Contraindications: Teratologic hip and redislocation of previously operated hips.

Technique (fig 11)

The patient is installed in the supine position; the entire lower extremity and hemi-pelvis are draped free to allow mobility of the hip and knee during surgery. The perineal area must be draped out of the field.

With the hip flexed (70°), abducted and laterally rotated, make a transverse incision of about 6-8 cm parallel to the groin crease, 2 cm distally, centred over the anterior margin of the adductor longus tendon (fig 11A). Skin and subcutaneous tissues are incised down to the deep fascia, taking care not to injure the saphenous vein.

The fascia in incised longitudinally, over the adductor longus muscle. The adductor longus is isolated, sectioned at its insertion on the pelvis, and allowed to retract distally. The anterior branches of the obturator nerve on the surface of the adductor brevis muscle

can be observed. The neurovascular bundle is gently retracted superiorly. The anterior branch of the obturator nerve is kept in sight. The sheath overlying the pectineus muscle will be opened sharply, and its superior and inferior borders identified (fig 11B).

The interval between the pectineus muscle and the femoral neurovascular bundle is identified and bluntly dissected. The medial femoral circumflex vascular bundle can be seen in the field and must be carefully preserved.

The lesser trochanter and iliopsoas tendon are easily palpated in the inferior aspect of the wound. The iliopsoas tendon is isolated, sectioned sharply, and allowed to retract (fig 11B).

In order to expose the capsule, the femoral bundle must be gently retracted superiorly, and the pectineus muscle inferiorly. Elevate the fatty tissue and bursa over the tendon, and continue to dissect proximally to expose the inferomedial aspect of the femoral head (fig 11C).

Use a T-incision on the capsule, with the long limb along the femoral neck, to expose the transverse acetabular ligament, the fibro-fatty tissue and the ligamentum teres.

The ligamentum teres is grasped and delivered into the wound. The leg is rotated to bring this attachment into view. It must then be excised to facilitate the reduction. The ligamentum teres is sectioned at its base along with the transverse acetabular ligament, thus opening up the "horseshoe" of the acetabulum and increasing its diameter. The fibro-fatty tissue is removed completely. The neolimbus is never an obstacle to reduction and should never be excised.

With this approach, reduction of the hip is now possible, and care can be taken to

assess the best position of the hip for postoperative immobilisation. A capsulorrhaphy cannot be performed later.

The hip joint capsule is left open. The deep fascia and skin are closed. There is no need for a drain.

Immobilise with hip flexion around 90 degrees, and abduction at 45 degrees in the position of best congruency.

A "micro-medial" approach has been described. It consists in fact of a tenotomy of the adductor longus and of the iliopsoas through a medial exposure. Reduction can be attempted without capsulotomy. If concentricity is restored (carefully assessed by an arthrogram), the hip spica cast can be applied after skin closure.

The capsule has the ability to retract spontaneously, rendering capsulorrhaphy useless in younger patients (before age 1), provided the reduction is maintained. The acetabulum has the potential to develop many years after open or closed reduction. The younger the patient, the more rapid the acetabular development.

■ *Anterolateral open reduction*

Anterolateral reduction is the standard method of open reduction for older children with DDH (after 12-15 months). As it is a more extensive procedure, it has not been popular for younger children (under six months) in the past. Reduction was often delayed until the child was older and bigger. Many centres use this as the only method of open reduction. It still relies on an adequate concentric reduction of the hip to stimulate acetabular development, but it is not a guarantee against AVN [13].

Advantages: This approach provides excellent visual control of all pathological features of the dislocated hip, the possibility of removing capsular adhesions on the iliac

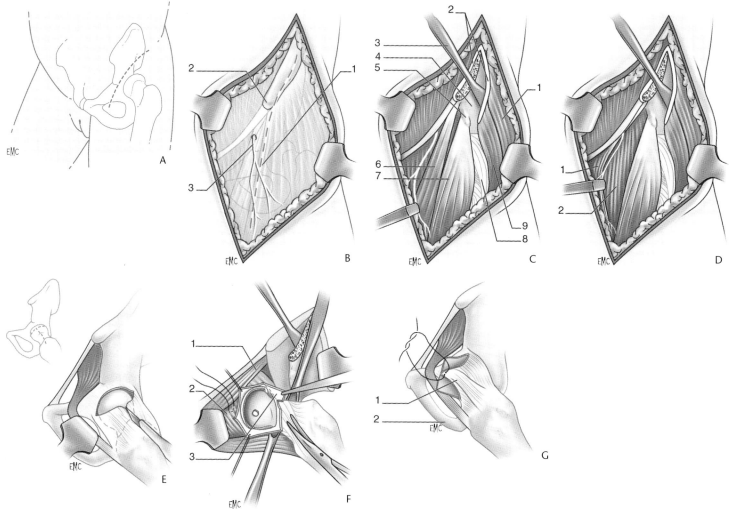

12 *A. The bikini incision is situated in the hip flexion crease for cosmetic reasons.*
B. Iliac crest exposure. Note the position of the femoral cutaneous nerve to avoid injury. 1. Incision of fascia lata; 2. anterosuperior iliac spine; 3. injury to the lateral femoral cutaneous nerve must be avoided.
C. Gentle subperiosteal exposure of the iliac crest with meticulous haemostasis will avoid heavy blood loss. 1. Gluteus medius and minimus elevated subperiostally from the ilium to the level of the sciatic notch; 2. iliac apophysis split; 3. periosteal elevator; 4. ilium; 5. anteroinferior iliac spine; 6. sartorius m.; 7. rectus femoris m.; 8. capsule of hip; 8. tensor fasciae latae m.

D. Hip flexion and abduction allow identification and division of iliopsoas. 1. Sartious m. retracted; 2. iliopsaos.
E. T-shaped incision of the capsule must allow exposure of the transverse acetabular ligament.
F. Excision of redundant capsule. 1. Iliopsaos m.; 2. superior ramus of pubis; 3. redundant triangular portior of capsule excised.
G. Capsule closure must be adjusted to provide primary stability without restraining hip motion. 1. Superolateral part of capsule sutured tautly to superior ramus of pubis; 2. position of hip: abduction, flexion and medial rotation.

wing over the acetabular ridge, and performing capsulorrhaphy. Additional procedures such as pelvic osteotomy can be performed during the same surgery.

Disadvantages: In case of failure or relapse, no favourable alternative is available. This is a "single chance" procedure. There is a greater risk of postoperative stiffness. A bilateral hip procedure is not advisable.

Technique *(fig 12)*

The anterior approach is based on the anterolateral approach described by Smith Peterson. Salter described a modification of the skin incision to make it more cosmetically acceptable. The "bikini incision" is situated in the hip flexion crease.

With the patient in the full lateral position so that the affected hip is up, the entire lower extremity and hemi-pelvis are draped free to allow mobility of the hip and knee during surgery. The perineal area must be draped out of the field. The patient is then turned to lie in a supine position.

Make a transverse skin incision of about 7 to 10 cm, centred 2 to 2.5 cm below the anterosuperior iliac spine in the hip flexion crease, prolonged for a few cm in the groove between the tensor fasciae latae laterally and the sartorius medially *(fig 12A)*.

Incise the deep fascia and gradually pull the skin up over the iliac crest, which becomes exposed *(fig 12B)*.

Develop the interval between the sartorius and the tensor fasciae latae, which will reveal the lateral femoral cutaneous nerve proximally. It emerges 2 cm distal to the anterosuperior iliac spine. Take care to keep it medial with silicone tubing.

The sartorius-tensor interval should be separated by blunt dissection. Open a groove laterally between the tensor fasciae latae muscle and the sartorius and rectus femoris muscles medially. This will expose the fatty tissue covering the front of the hip capsule. Incise sharply the cartilaginous iliac apophysis to split it longitudinally as far as the bone. Strip the periosteum off the outer

table, pulling the tensor and abductors laterally, and off the inner table, retracting the iliac muscle *(fig 12C)*.

Divide the sartorius from its insertion on the anterosuperior iliac spine. Both the straight and reflected heads of the rectus femoris are divided and reflected distally by a combination of sharp and blunt dissection. To expose the capsule, divide and clean the pericapsular fat and fibrous tissue. The capsule should be peeled gradually from the fibro-fatty attachments, from the iliac muscle fibres medially, and from the gluteus medius and minimus laterally.

It is important to inspect the iliac wing over the acetabulum for adherence of the capsule, which results in a false acetabulum. Strip the capsule of the ilium down to the true acetabulum. Do not remove the articular cartilage.

The hip can then be flexed, abducted and rotated laterally to expose the iliopsoas tendon *(fig 12D)*. This should be divided to allow the hip to be reduced without tension that could result in avascular necrosis or redislocation. Care should be taken to identify and protect the femoral nerve which is situated near the tendon.

The capsule is incised using a T-shaped incision, the long limb along the femoral neck, the short limb parallel to the acetabular rim, from back to front carried out towards the transverse acetabular ligament, which must be sectioned *(fig 12E)*. The acetabulum is often difficult to identify; it appears to be shrunk to the size of a thimble.

The ligamentum teres preventing anatomic concentric reduction of the hip should be excised, as well as the fibro-fatty tissue.

The femoral head should be reduced into the acetabulum. This should be easily done with the hip flexed at 30-40 degrees and rotated internally slightly. All the obstacles must be removed to identify the real acetabulum and to study the congruency between femoral head and acetabular cavity. Femoral anteversion is difficult to assess.

This is followed by a capsulorrhaphy. This is a crucial step – if too tight, it will result in stiffness; if too loose, it will fail in stabilising the femoral head in the depth of the acetabulum. We excise the segment of redundant capsule in an "orange segment" shape *(fig 12F)*. The divided edges are sutured firmly from side to side, taking care to stretch distally the external side, then eliminate the dislocation pouch *(fig 12G)*.

The two halves of the iliac apophysis are sutured back together over the iliac crest. Failure to reinsert perfectly the gluteus medius will lead to post-operative limping. The sartorius is reinserted back to the anterior superior iliac spine. The rectus femoris is not reinserted to its origin, to avoid hip flexion contracture. The wound is closed in a routine manner over suction drainage.

An anteroposterior radiograph is taken to check the concentricity of reduction.

The spica cast is applied with flexion between 60-70 degrees, abduction between 40-45 degrees, and internal rotation between 0-25 degrees. Knee flexion is at 45 degrees to relax the hamstrings.

Postoperative care: Drainage is removed at 48 hours. A one-cut CT scan is performed through the acetabulum to check for concentricity in the early postoperative period. Cast removal is between 4 and 6 weeks, followed by a hip abduction splint full-time during 6 to 12 weeks, and then only at night.

ASSOCIATED OSTEOTOMIES

Complementary bony procedures can be performed, such as a pelvic osteotomy (Salter), femoral shortening, or femoral derotation.

Anterolateral reduction with a Salter pelvic osteotomy is used extensively in some centres for children over 18 months. It is a method of addressing the acetabular dysplasia and the reduction of the dislocated hip at the same time. The advantage is that there are very few secondary operations required for acetabular dysplasia. The disadvantage is that it requires a more involved and theoretically more difficult operation, and Salter osteotomy may be unnecessary in about 40% of the cases.

■ *Open reduction and femoral osteotomy*

If a significant internal rotation is necessary to stabilise the femoral head into the acetabulum due to excessive femoral anteversion, a femoral derotation osteotomy can be performed at the same time. The osteotomy site in the subtrochanteric area aims to compensate for the internal rotation. The goal is to place the knee and foot in the normal walking axis.

If reduction is difficult because the femoral head is too high, a femoral shortening can be associated. The older the patient, the higher the disruption – and the greater the indication for femoral shortening to reduce the trans-articular tension that could result in avascular necrosis.

References

[1] Bucholz RW, Ogden JA. Patterns of ischemic necrosis of the proximal femur in nonoperatively treated congenital hip disease. In : The hip. Proceedings of the sixth open scientific meeting of the Hip Society. St Louis : CV Mosby, 1978 : 43-63

[2] Camp J, Herring JA, Dworezynski C. Comparison of inpatient and outpatient traction in developmental dislocation of the hip. *J Pediatr Orthop* 1994 ; 14 : 9-12

[3] Carlioz H, Filipe G. The natural history of the limbus in congenital dislocation of the hip: An arthrographic study. In : Tachdjian MO ed. Congenital dislocation of the hip. New York : Churchill Livingstone, 1982 : 247-262

[4] Catterall A. The early diagnosis of congenital hip dislocation of the hip. *J Bone Joint Surg Br* 1994 ; 76 : 515-516

[5] Daoud A, Saighi-Bououina A. Congenital dislocation of the hip in the older child. *J Bone Joint Surg Am* 1996 ; 78 : 30-40

[6] Ferguson AB Jr. Primary open reduction of congenital dislocation of the hip using a median adductor approach. *J Bone Joint Surg Am* 1973 ; 55 : 671-689

[7] Gage JR, Winter RB. Avascular necrosis of the capital femoral epiphysis as a complication of closed reduction of congenital dislocation of the hip. *J Bone Joint Surg Am* 1972 ; 54 : 373-388

[8] Galpin RD, Roach JW, Wenger DR, Herring JA, Birch JG. One-stage treatment of congenital dislocation of the hip in older children, including femoral shortening. *J Bone Joint Surg Am* 1989 ; 71 : 734-741

[9] Grill H, Bensahel H, Canadell J, Dungl P, Matasovic T, Vizkelety T. The Pavlik harness in the treatment of CDH: report on a multicenter study of the European Paediatric Orthopaedic Society. *J Pediatr Orthop* 1988 ; 8 : 1-8

[10] Kahle WK, Anderson MB, Alpert J, Stevens PM, Coleman SS. The value of preliminary traction in the treatment of congenital dislocation of the hip. *J Bone Joint Surg Am* 1990 ; 72 : 1043-1047

[11] Kumar SJ. Hip spica cast application for the treatment of congenital dislocation of the hip. *J Pediatr Orthop* 1981 ; 1 : 97-99

[12] Ludloff K. The open reduction of the congenital hip dislocation by an anterior incision. *Am J Orthop Surg* 1913 ; 10 : 438

[13] Morcuende JA, Meyer MD, Dolan LA, Weinstein SL. Long-term outcome after open reduction through an anteromedial approach for congenital dislocation of the hip. *J Bone Joint Surg Am* 1997 ; 79 : 810-817

[14] Morel G, Briard JL. Progressive gradual reduction of the dislocated hip in the child after walking age. In : Tachdjian MO ed. Congenital dislocation of the hip. New York : Churchill Livingstone, 1982 : 373-383

[15] Pavlik A. Stirrups as an aid in the treatment of congenital dysplasias of the hip in children. By Arnold Pavlik, 1950. *J Pediatr Orthop* 1989 ; 9 : 157-159

[16] Ponseti IV. Morphology of the acetabulum in congenital dislocation of the hip. *J Bone Joint Surg Am* 1978 ; 60 : 586-599

[17] Pous JP, Dimeglio A, Daoud A. Que reste-t-il de l'extension continue dans le traitement de la luxation congénitale de hanche ? *Rev Chir Orthop* 1979 ; 65 : 327-332

[18] Race C, Herring JA. Congenital dislocation of the hip: An evaluation of closed reduction. *J Pediatr Orthop* 1983 ; 3 : 166-172

[19] Ramsey PL, Lasser S, MacEwen GD. Congenital dislocation of the hip. Use of the Pavlik harness in the child during the first six months of life. *J Bone Joint Surg Am* 1976 ; 58 : 1000-1004

[20] Salter RB, Dubos JP. The first fifteen year's personal experience with innominate osteotomy in the treatment of congenital dislocation and subluxation of the hip. *Clin Orthop* 1974 ; 98 : 72-103

[21] Salter RB, Kostuik J, Dallas S. Avascular necrosis of the femoral head as a complication of treatment for congenital dislocation of the hip in young children: a clinical and experimental investigation. *Can J Surg* 1969 ; 12 : 44-61

[22] Seringe R. Dysplasies et luxations congénitales de hanche. *Encycl Méd Chir* (Éditions Scientifiques et Médicales Elsevier SAS, Paris), Appareil locomoteur, 15-226-A-10, Pédiatrie, 4-007-E-10, 1998 : 1-29

[23] Staheli LT. Medial approach open reduction for congenitally dislocated hips: A critical analysis of forty cases. In : Tachdjian MO ed. Congenital dislocation of the hip. New York : Churchill Livingstone, 1982 : 295-303

[24] Suzuki S, Kashiwagi N, Seto Y, Mukai S. Location of the femoral head in developmental dysplasia of the hip: three dimensional evaluation by means of magnetic resonance imaging. *J Pediatr Orthop* 1999 ; 19 : 88-91

[25] Tanaka T, Yoshiashi Y, Miura T. Changes in soft tissue interposition after reduction of developmental dislocation of the hip. *J Pediatr Orthop* 1994 ; 14 : 16-23

[26] Weinstein SL. Closed versus open reduction of congenital hip dislocation in patients under 2 years of age. *Orthopaedics* 1990 ; 13 : 221-227

[27] Weinstein SL. Traction in developmental dislocation of the hip: Is its use justified? *Clin Orthop* 1997 ; 338 : 79-85

[28] Weinstein SL, Ponseti IV. Congenital dislocation of the hip: open reduction through a medial approach. *J Bone Joint Surg Am* 1979 ; 61 : 119-124

[29] Wilkinson JA. Congenital displacement of the hip joint. New York : Springer-Verlag, 1985

[30] Zionts LE, MacEwen GD. Treatment of congenital dislocation of the hip in children between the ages of one and three years. *J Bone Joint Surg Am* 1986 ; 68 : 829-846

Pelvic osteotomies in the treatment of congenital dislocation and subluxation of the hip (developmental dysplasia of the hip: DDH)

T Vízkelety
G Szőke
JA Fixsen

Abstract. – *Malrotation of the acetabulum is common in developmental dysplasia of the hip (DDH). Pelvic osteotomy can be used to correct this malrotation. The type of pelvic osteotomy which is appropriate depends on the age of the patient and the nature of the deformity or malposition of the acetabulum. The indications, surgical technique, post-operative management and complications of innominate (Salter) osteotomy and pericapsular (Pemberton) pelvic osteotomy are described. The role of double and triple pelvic osteotomies is discussed. The surgical technique, post-operative management and complications of triple (Tönnis) pelvic osteotomy are described in detail.*

Keywords: hip, developmental dysplasia of the hip (DDH), pelvic osteotomies, innominate osteotomy (Salter), pericapsular osteotomy (Pemberton), triple osteotomy (Tönnis).

Innominate osteotomy

INTRODUCTION

Osteotomy of the innominate or hip bone, which comprises the ilium, ischium, pubis and acetabulum by a horizontal osteotomy above the level of the acetabulum was popularised by Salter in 1961 [16]. The principal of innominate osteotomy is simply to redirect the acetabulum to provide improved anterior and lateral cover of the femoral head (*fig 1, 2*).

INDICATIONS FOR INNOMINATE OSTEOTOMY

Salter in his original paper suggested the following indications [16]:

– For congenital dislocation, he considered it should be the primary operation combined with closed or open reduction of the hip from the age of 18 months to 6 years.

– For congenital subluxation, he considered it should be the primary operation from 18 months up to early adult life.

– He also suggested it was indicated as a secondary treatment for residual or recurrent

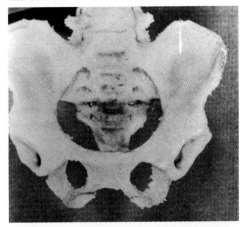
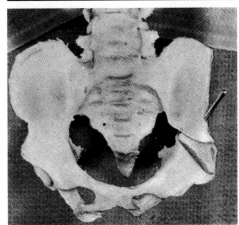
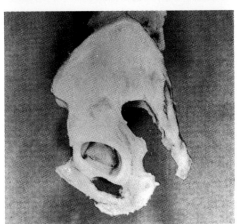
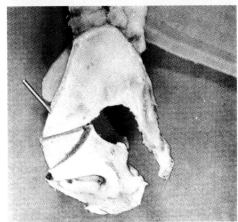

1 *Dissected pelvis of a two and a half-year old girl: AP and lateral views. (Reproduced with permission from Salter RB. Innominate osteotomy in the treatment of congenital dislocation and subluxation of the hip. J Bone Joint Surg Br 1961; 43: 518-539.)*

2 *An osteotomy through the left innominate bone has been performed to demonstrate the redirection of the entire acetabulum. (Reproduced with permission from Salter RB. Innominate osteotomy in the treatment of congenital dislocation and subluxation of the hip. J Bone Joint Surg Br 1961; 43: 518-539.)*

Tibor Vízkelety, Dr.Sc., Professor.
George Szőke, M.Sc.(Oxon), Ph.D., Lecturer, Orthopaedic Department of Semmelweis Medical University, Budapest, Hungary.
John A Fixsen, M.A. M Chir. FRCS, Department of Orthopaedic Surgery, Great Ormond Street Hospital for Children NHS Trust, Great Ormond Street, London WC1N 3JH, United Kingdom.

dislocation or subluxation after other methods of treatment had failed. Nowadays many surgeons would consider the procedure from the age of one year, provided the pelvis was of reasonable size, and would use double or triple osteotomy over the age of 8-10 years.

The essential prerequisites for successful innominate osteotomy are:

– Complete reduction of the femoral head into the acetabulum.

– Congruity between the joint surfaces.

– Good range of hip motion.

The technique of innominate osteotomy is basically the same for both hip dislocation and subluxation. In the presence of hip dislocation, if closed reduction is unsuccessful, open reduction has to be performed together with release of the iliopsoas tendon prior to the innominate osteotomy. This will make the operation time considerably longer. In children over the age of six, innominate osteotomy may have to be combined with femoral osteotomy and shortening [3]. In adolescence and early adult life, double or triple pelvic osteotomies are required, as it becomes increasingly difficult to satisfactorily reposition the acetabulum without dividing the bones below as well as above the level of the acetabulum.

In Salter's original description, continuous skin or skeletal traction was used for dislocation of the hip. The length of time on traction depends on the age of the child and on the height of the dislocation [16]. There has been considerable discussion in recent years about the value of such traction. Many surgeons now prefer not to use traction in younger children and prefer femoral osteotomy with shortening, combined with open reduction and innominate or other pelvic osteotomy in older children above the age of 3-4 years. Following a period of traction, Salter described releasing any residual adduction contracture by subcutaneous adductor tenotomy under general anaesthesia and attempting gentle closed reduction. He advised arthrography at this stage to assess the completeness of reduction. If the reduction was not satisfactory, then arthrotomy was necessary, combined with innominate osteotomy in patients over the age of 18 months. The original technique was described by Salter for combined open reduction and innominate osteotomy [16]. With experience, this combined operation should not take longer than 1-1.5 hours. Blood transfusion is not usually necessary but an intravenous infusion is indicated.

Innominate osteotomy on both sides of the same pelvis should not be performed at the same time, as this would in effect disconnect the distal part of the pelvis on both sides from the proximal portion, leading to an unstable situation and inability to control the rotation of the distal pelvic fragments on the two sides.

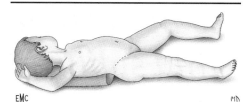

3   *Supine position and skin incision. (Redrawn with permission from Salter RB. Innominate osteotomy in the treatment of congenital dislocation and subluxation of the hip. J Bone Joint Surg Br 1961; 43: 518-539.)*

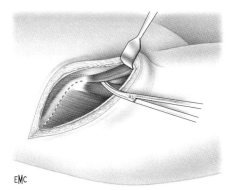

4   *Incision in the iliac apophysis and gap between tensor fasciae lata laterally and the sartorius and rectus femoris medially. (Redrawn with permission from Salter RB. Innominate osteotomy in the treatment of congenital dislocation and subluxation of the hip. J Bone Joint Surg Br 1961; 43: 518-539.)*

SURGICAL TECHNIQUE

The patient lies in the supine position with a sandbag under the trunk on the side of the operation, to tilt the trunk and pelvis up on the operated side. The limb is draped so that it can be moved freely during the operation and the operative site is covered with Opsite® or an equivalent adhesive surgical drape. If the adductor muscles are tight and have not been released previously, a subcutaneous adductor tenotomy of the adductor longus is performed.

■ *Exposure*

The skin incision starts below the middle of the iliac crest and runs forward beneath the anterior superior iliac spine to the mid-point of the inguinal ligament *(fig 3)*. This incision heals well as it is in Langers' lines and also in a hidden area (the so-called bikini incision). The interval between the tensor fasciae lata laterally and the sartorius muscle and rectus femoris muscle medially is developed *(fig 4)*. It is important to identify and avoid damage to the lateral femoral cutaneous nerve during the proximal part of this dissection. The iliac apophysis is split vertically from the mid-point of the iliac crest, to the anterior superior iliac spine and then down to the anterior inferior iliac spine. The lateral part of the apophysis with the periosteum and the attached muscles is then stripped down to the sciatic notch posteriorly and to the superior rim of the acetabulum. This space is packed with a gauze swab. If, in the case of a dislocation, the capsule of the hip has become adherent

to the lateral aspect of the ilium above the acetabulum, then it should be freed by a periosteal elevator. Blunt dissection between the capsule and the abductor muscles will provide satisfactory exposure of the anterior and lateral portion of the hip capsule. The reflected head of the rectus femoris muscle is a useful guide to the lateral rim of the acetabulum

■ *Open reduction*

In the presence of dislocation, an open reduction is necessary. The capsule should be opened by a T-shaped incision which provides wide exposure of the acetabulum. The detachment or tenotomy of the iliopsoas muscle gives a good view into the inferior part of the acetabulum. Any excessive fibro-fatty tissue is removed. The capsule must be opened down to and including the transverse ligament to allow the femoral head to be replaced satisfactorily in the acetabulum. The state of the ligamentum teres is variable, but if it is hypertrophied it may need to be removed. Similarly the state of the limbus may be very variable from absent to grossly hypertrophic. If possible, the limbus should not be removed but should be everted over the femoral head. It may be necessary to resect a small part of the rim of the limbus or to make radial cuts in it to allow the femoral head to be satisfactorily reduced. The iliopsoas muscle is always invariably tight when the head has been reduced, and it should be lengthened by dividing the tendon at or below the pelvic rim.

■ *Position of stability*

The position of maximum stability of the femoral head in the acetabulum is now assessed. The simplest way of doing this is to consider flexion, abduction and internal rotation. Zadeh et al [31] have made an important contribution to the concept of a "Test of Stability". They suggest that innominate osteotomy is indicated if flexion or flexion with abduction is required to achieve stability [31]. However, if significant flexion is not required, but greater than 30° of abduction and/or internal rotation are necessary, then a femoral osteotomy is preferable. Finally, in the situation where more than 30° of flexion, abduction and internal rotation are necessary, this is the indication for a femoral and an innominate osteotomy to be combined. Sometimes it is necessary to shorten the femur for stability.

■ *Osteotomy*

Once satisfactory reduction of the hip has been achieved, the inner wall of the ilium is exposed subperiostally. Bone wax may be necessary if there is significant bleeding from the bone at this stage. The sciatic notch is exposed and the periosteum gently lifted from it, due to the proximity of the sciatic nerve and superior gluteal artery. Bone levers are placed subperiostally in the sciatic

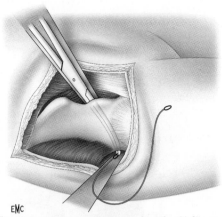

5 *The cartilage apophysis is split. The Gigli saw is passed subperiosteally around the sciatic notch with curved forceps. (Redrawn with permission from Salter RB. Innominate osteotomy in the treatment of congenital dislocation and subluxation of the hip. J Bone Joint Surg Br 1961; 43: 518-539.)*

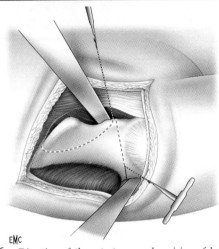

6 *Direction of the osteotomy and excision of bone wedge. (Redrawn with permission from Salter RB. Innominate osteotomy in the treatment of congenital dislocation and subluxation of the hip. J Bone Joint Surg Br 1961; 43: 518-539.)*

notch and a Gigli saw passed subperiosteally through the sciatic notch using curved forceps *(fig 5)*. A horizontal osteotomy of the ilium is then performed above the acetabulum, exiting at the anterior inferior iliac spine *(fig 6)*. A wedge-shaped piece of bone is then cut from the anterior portion of the iliac bone in the region of the anterior superior iliac spine. The distal fragment of the osteotomy is then displaced forwards and laterally making sure that good bone contact persists posteriorly between the two fragments and the triangular wedge of bone positioned to hold the distal fragment in the new position. Towel forceps can be helpful in obtaining displacement of the distal fragment. Salter originally used one K-wire to hold the position *(fig 7)* but most surgeons now prefer two K-wires inserted from the iliac crest across the wedge of bone into the distal fragment above the acetabulum. In the case of a hip dislocation, the hip is now reduced and a careful capsulorrhaphy performed excising excess capsule, so that the hip is firmly held in the

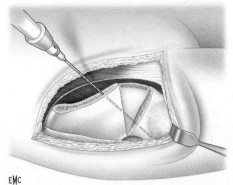

7 *Insertion of the wedge-shaped bone graft and fixation by a single K-wire. (Redrawn with permission from Salter RB. Innominate osteotomy in the treatment of congenital dislocation and subluxation of the hip. J Bone Joint Surg Br 1961; 43: 518-539.)*

acetabulum. The apophysis is sutured with strong sutures. The K-wires are bent over and divided below the skin. Suction drainage can be used if the surgeon prefers this and the skin is closed with a subcutaneous suture. Salter originally described stainless steel wire but the authors prefer an absorbable subcutaneous suture such as Dexon® reinforced with Steristrips®.

POST-OPERATIVE MANAGEMENT

The hip is immobilised in a hip spica in approximately 30° of flexion, abduction and slight internal rotation. The knee is flexed to diminish any tension on the hamstrings. In small children, it may be wise to extend the spica to above the knee on the opposite side to control the pelvis adequately. The hip spica is normally maintained for at least six weeks, when radiographs are taken to check that the osteotomy has healed and the reduction has been maintained. The K-wires may then be removed under general anaesthesia and gentle active movements encouraged. Partial weight-bearing with crutches is indicated until a good range of movement has been obtained. Long term follow-up at least until skeletal maturity is necessary.

RESULTS

Salter presented his early results 1-3 years after operation. He found 24 excellent hips out of 25, but admitted that such early results can be misleading in DDH [16].

Salter and Dubos published their personal experience in 1974 with an average follow-up of five and half years [18]. In the younger age group, from one and a half to four years of age, the operation gave excellent and good radiographic results in 93.6 % according to the Severin classification. However, in the age group from 4-10 years, the good and excellent results fell to 56.7 %.

In 1988, Waters et al [29] reported the results in 29 hips, with an average follow-up of 9 years and 3 months but a range from 3 years to 14 years, in which all the patients

had either good or excellent radiographic results. Similarly, in 1998 Mellerovicz et al [10] also had satisfactory results after an average follow-up of 9.5 years.

In 1985, Heine and Felske-Adler, however, reported unsatisfactory results. This appeared to be related to previous conservative or surgical treatment, or was associated with avascular necrosis [3]. Moulin and Morscher in 1988 reported a follow-up of 24 years and showed that around the age of 11 years, the shape of the acetabulum appears to stabilise [12]. They suggested that the ideal age to perform an innominate osteotomy was between the ages of 2 and 4 years. Exceptionally, the operation could be performed later if the acetabular angle was not greater than 40°.

Windhager et al (1990) suggested that the results depended on the age and pre-operative status of the patients [30]. However, by contrast Saleh et al (1995), in an interesting prospective study comparing the pelvic remodelling after Salter osteotomy in immature and mature patients, showed that in immature patients remodelling of the pelvic deformity occurs very quickly, but that despite such remodelling the redirection of the acetabulum is maintained with no deterioration in the change of the CE (centre edge) angle. When the procedure is carried out in the mature pelvis, no such remodelling occurs in the short term, but it is still possible to achieve a gratifying improvement in the CE angle. The shift of the spinous process of the ischium towards the mid-line significantly interferes with the width of the birth canal, as seen on the AP radiograph. Their study was not continued for long enough to determine whether long term remodelling occurs in the mature pelvis [15].

McCarthy et al (1996) reported good results from innominate osteotomy performed for acetabular dysplasia in 31 hips, in adolescents and adults. The average age at operation was 22 years and the average follow-up 5 years, with a range from 2 to 14 years [8]. Huang and Wang (1997) reported a comparative study of non-operative treatment compared with operative treatment by open reduction and innominate osteotomy in two groups of children aged between 13 and 17 months. They concluded that treatment time was significantly shortened and there were fewer complications and redislocations in the operated group. However, the follow-up time in both groups was short [5]. In 1994, Pope et al described the use of both innominate and Chiari type pelvic osteotomies to correct acetabular abnormalities in cerebral palsy. The age of the patients ranged from just under 3 years to 15.5 years and a significant improvement in the centre edge angle and the acetabular index was shown [14]. However, nowadays most surgeons dealing with quadriplegic (total body involvement) cerebral palsy would reconstruct the hip using a combination of femoral osteotomy and the Dega type acetabuloplasty.

COMPLICATIONS

Salter [16] in his original article described a superficial wound infection and avascular necrosis of the femoral head in one of the 25 patients treated. He pointed out that it was essential to obtain a concentric reduction of the hip in the acetabulum at the time of operation. During operation, care should be taken to avoid damage to the sciatic nerve or the superior gluteal artery. Injury to the lateral cutaneous nerve of the thigh can cause troublesome numbness on the lateral side of the thigh, particularly in older patients. It is essential when displacing the distal fragment anteriorly and laterally that the posterior corner of the distal fragment remain in contact with the proximal fragment and the bone wedge does not displace. For this reason, many surgeons prefer two K-wires rather than the original single K-wire described by Salter.

Tönnis (1990) found that the occurrence of avascular necrosis (osteochondritis, AVN) after open reduction was 8.4 % in his data collected from the German literature [27]. This increased to 10.3 % after innominate osteotomy or other forms of acetabuloplasty. The incidence following intertrochanteric femoral osteotomy in this series was 22.2 %, but decreased to 5.5 % if the femoral osteotomy was combined with shortening.

Fixsen in 1987 [2] reported 10 cases of anterior and posterior redisplacement of the hip after innominate osteotomy. Posterior displacement was much more difficult to deal with successfully. The exact cause of the redisplacement was difficult to determine, but he agreed with Tachdjian [23] that it was likely to be a poorly executed osteotomy, a lax capsulorrhaphy or excessive anteversion. The advent of improved methods of assessing the acetabulum three-dimensionally has shown that it is possible to retrovert the acetabulum after innominate and other pelvic osteotomies, thereby uncovering the femoral head posteriorly and predisposing it to posterior displacement.

Pericapsular (Pemberton) pelvic osteotomy

INTRODUCTION AND INDICATIONS

Pericapsular osteotomy of the ilium for treatment of congenital subluxation and dislocation of the hip was described by Pemberton in 1965 [13]. Pemberton considered that in both the dislocating and the subluxing hip the acetabulum was relatively large in relation to the size of the femoral head. This meant that in order to adequately stabilise the hip, the acetabulum should be literally wrapped around the femoral head to prevent it from moving in relation to it. It

was particularly important to prevent displacement of the femoral head forward and laterally beneath the anterior inferior iliac spine. The open triradiate cartilage is the only flexible structure around which the size and shape of the acetabulum could be changed and Pemberton used this as a hinge for his osteotomy. Initially Pemberton suggested that his operation could be used from the age of 1 to 18 months up to closure of the triradiate cartilage at 12-14 years. However, subsequently, Coleman in an important review of pericapsular (Pemberton) and innominate (Salter) osteotomies [1] suggested that pericapsular (Pemberton) osteotomy should be used under the age of 6, as the smaller and less flexible triradiate cartilage in the older child led to less satisfactory results.

TECHNIQUE

Pemberton originally described a standard Smith-Peterson approach but the "bikini" type incision described by Salter allows much better healing of the scar. As in innominate osteotomy, the iliac apophysis is exposed and split, taking care not to damage the lateral cutaneous nerve of the thigh and the gap between the sartorius and the tensor fascia lata clearly displayed. The muscles are raised from both the inner and outer cortex of the ilium down to the sciatic notch and two curved retractors are inserted subperiostially taking great care not to damage the sciatic nerve or the superior gluteal vessels. In Pemberton's original series, the capsule was not opened unless there was difficulty in obtaining a closed reduction. Subsequently he recommended opening the capsule to inspect the femoral head and to remove any interposed soft tissues. A curved osteotomy is performed with a narrow curved osteotome through the outer cortex of the ilium, starting just above the anterior inferior iliac spine *(fig 8)*. The osteotomy is performed about 5 mm above the insertion of the capsule and runs backwards parallel to it. The osteotome is driven backwards under direct vision until it can be seen to be well in front of the retractor in the sciatic notch. At this point the blade of the osteotome will not be visible when it is inserted further and it is important that the tip of the instrument be directed in such a manner that it cannot enter the sciatic notch but will reach the ilio-ischial limb of the triradiate cartilage at its mid portion, about half way between the anterior margin of the sciatic notch and the posterior margin of the acetabulum. The inner cortex is cut with the same narrow curved osteotome, starting again from the anterior inferior iliac spine. If the surgeon wishes the femoral head coverage to be more anterior, then the level of the cut is at the same level as the cut in the outer cortex. If the surgeon wishes to direct the acetabulum more laterally, the cut should be inferior on the inner cortex of the ileum to that on the outer cortex. Again, the cut on

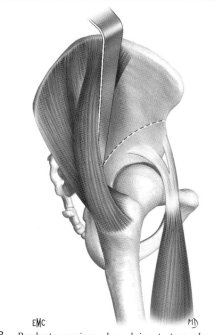

8 *Pemberton pericapsular pelvic osteotomy showing the line of the osteotomy cut in the outer cortex of the ilium.*

the inner table is made with a narrow curved osteotome and the cutting edge of the osteotome will disappear from view in front of the sciatic notch as it is driven the last 5-10 mm so as to reach the triradiate cartilage on the inside of the pelvis. It is important not to cut into the sciatic notch and break the pelvic ring so that the osteotomy remains stable and can be hinged on the triradiate cartilage. After both cortices have been cut, a broad osteotome is used to divide the cancellous bone, and the iliac portion of the acetabular roof can then be turned down over the reduced femoral head, opening a gap of about 20 mm in the average small child. A wedge-shaped block of bone from the anterior superior iliac spine is cut and fitted into the gap to hold the acetabular roof in its new position *(fig 9)*. Pemberton suggested cutting a groove in each side of the osteotomy to hold the bone graft, which is usually secure without any form of internal fixation such as a Kirschner wire. If the capsule has been opened it is then closed and a careful capsulorrhaphy performed, particularly if there is excess capsule. The iliac apophysis is then sutured and suction drainage commonly employed. The wound is closed in layers and a control X-ray taken.

POST-OPERATIVE MANAGEMENT

A 1 ½ hip spica is applied with the leg in slight abduction, flexion and internal rotation. Pemberton recommended two months in the hip spica following which, if a control X-ray was satisfactory, the spica could be removed and mobilisation with partial weight-bearing using crutches encouraged.

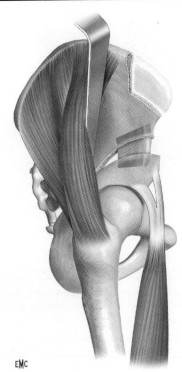

9 *Pemberton pericapsular osteotomy showing insertion of the wedge-shaped bone graft.*

COMPLICATIONS

Tachdjian, in his book on congenital dislocation of the hip published in 1982 [22], states that Pemberton's osteotomy is an excellent procedure for treating a deficient acetabulum in that it allows as much correction as needed to adequately cover the femoral head. However, it can cause stiffness of the hip following surgery. It also temporarily causes a deformity in the acetabular subchondral bone in about 60% of cases. A serious complication is acetabular growth disturbance or arrest, particularly if the bone cut extends into the triradiate cartilage. As in all surgery around the infant hip, avascular necrosis can occur. Tachdjian considered that Pemberton's osteotomy was much more difficult to perform than the Salter type innominate osteotomy, but allowed for a greater degree of correction of the acetabulum, particularly anteriorly.

Triple pelvic osteotomy

INTRODUCTION AND INDICATION

The Salter innominate osteotomy and Pemberton pericapsular osteotomy are insufficient to correct a seriously dysplastic or malpositioned acetabulum over the age of 8-10 years. Double pelvic osteotomy [4, 21] and triple pelvic osteotomy [4, 7, 20] have been described to correct the position of the acetabulum and cover the femoral head satisfactorily over the age of 8-10 years. Triple osteotomy is much more commonly used and will therefore be described.

The principle of triple osteotomy is to divide the acetabulum both through the ilium and

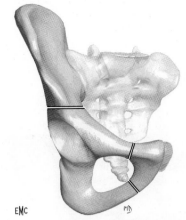

10 *Drawing of Le Cœur type triple osteotomy.*

through the ischium and the pubis so that in older patients satisfactory reorientation of the acetabulum can be achieved. Several methods and approaches have been described. Le Cœur in 1964 [7] was probably the first to describe a triple pelvic osteotomy. He divided the superior and inferior pubic ramus near the symphysis and the ileum above the acetabulum *(fig 10)*.

Hopf (1966) suggested both double and triple osteotomies [4]. The latter differed from that described by Le Cœur only in that the divisions of the pubis and the ischium were made nearer to the acetabulum. Sutherland and Greenfield published their experience of double osteotomy in 1977 [21].

Steel published his technique of triple osteotomy in 1973, which again was very similar to the method of Hopf but suggested an easier approach to the ischium [19, 20]. Tönnis described his form of triple osteotomy in 1981 [28]. The aim of his modification was to divide the bones as close as possible to the acetabulum and thus achieve an easier and more satisfactory correction of the acetabular malposition. The operation is performed through two or three separate skin incisions, as this makes the procedure both safer and easier to perform.

SURGICAL TECHNIQUE (TÖNNIS METHOD)

The operation is performed under image intensifier with a translucent operating table. The procedure is carried out in two parts. For the first part, to divide the ischium, the patient is in the prone position. For the second part, to divide the pubis and ilium, the patient is in the supine position. The skin preparation and draping of the patient is best carried out with the patient lying on his side with the operative side uppermost. The skin is prepared from the umbilical level to the knee on the operative side and then draped to the mid-line of the body anteriorly and posteriorly. An adhesive translucent skin drape, such as Opsite®, is then used to cover the operative site and the thigh down to the knee before the patient is turned into the prone position. An oblique incision in the direction of the fibres of the gluteus

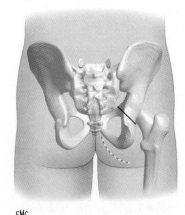

11 *Triple pelvic osteotomy (Tönnis). Diagram showing the pelvis; the dotted line indicates the site of the posterior oblique incision for the exposure of the ischial ramus.*

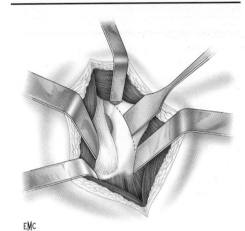

12 *Triple pelvic osteotomy (Tönnis). Exposure and division of the ischium with an osteotome.*

maximus muscle is made above the ischial tuberosity *(fig 11)*. The muscle fibres are separated by blunt dissection and the ischial tuberosity and sacrotuberous ligament exposed. Care should be taken not to extend the dissection too far proximally to avoid damage to the inferior gluteal artery and nerve. The underlying fascia is exposed. The obturator internus muscle and the gemelli are exposed proximal to the ischial tuberosity and divided in order to expose the ischial ramus. The ramus is then exposed subperiosteally from the ischial tuberosity to the sciatic notch. A blunt retractor is then placed in the sciatic notch to retract the gluteal vessels and nerves proximally and the sciatic nerve upwards and laterally. Retractors are then placed medially and laterally around the ischial ramus, taking care to preserve the sacrotuberous ligament and the sacrospinous ligament, as these are important in stability of the spine. The ischium is then divided with an osteotome directed from lateral to medial and slightly inclined towards the centre of the body *(fig 12)*. It is useful to have practised this manœuvre on the bony skeleton prior to performing this part of the operation. It is essential that the osteotomy be complete, particularly on the inner side of the ischial ramus.

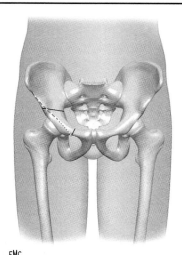

13 *Triple pelvic osteotomy (Tönnis). Drawing to show the skin incision and the site on the innominate bone of the iliac and pubic osteotomies.*

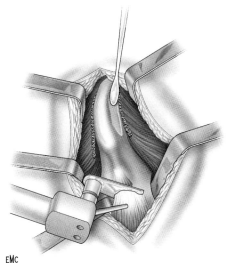

15 *Triple pelvic osteotomy (Tönnis). Initial cut in the ilium using an oscillating saw.*

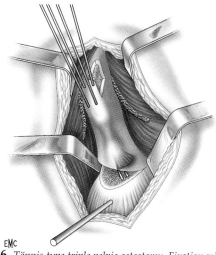

16 *Tönnis type triple pelvic osteotomy. Fixation with Kirschner wires (2.5 mm) in a fan-like manner.*

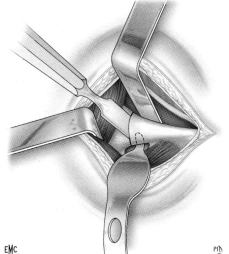

14 *Triple pelvic osteotomy (Tönnis). Exposure and osteotomy of the pubic ramus.*

The wound is then closed and the patient turned into the supine position. Initially both the iliac and the pubic osteotomies were done through a single incision (fig 13), but Tönnis then found it easier to use two incisions, a small medial incision to divide the pubis and an anterolateral incision for the ilium. A small skin incision is made parallel to the inguinal ligament where the pubic bone is easily palpable, just medial to the psoas tendon. The psoas muscle, femoral vessels and nerves are retracted laterally and the pubis exposed subperiostially. It is osteotomised parallel to and as close as possible to the hip joint (fig 14).

Osteotomy of the ilium is carried out through an anterolateral "bikini" type incision popularised by Salter. The muscles are detached from the iliac crest and the iliac wing down to the sciatic notch which is exposed subperiostially and retracted with blunt retractors of the Hohmann type. In Steel's osteotomy, the ilium is divided transversely with a Gigli saw, but to aid rotation it is easier if the osteotomy is made obliquely from cranial laterally to caudal medially. The site of the osteotomy can be identified by image intensification. Prior to performing the osteotomy, a Steinmann pin (4 mm in diameter) is drilled into the ilium in the oblique plane of the osteotomy 1 cm above the acetabular roof and 1.5 cm distal to the planned osteotomy, which is carried out 2.5 cm above the acetabulum. The osteotomy line is then marked with an osteotome and the osteotomy performed at a safe distance from the capsule and acetabulum to avoid damage to blood vessels. The first part of the osteotomy can be made with an oscillating saw but an osteotome should be used in the sciatic notch (fig 15).

The three osteotomies have now been completed and the acetabulum should be easy to rotate using the Steinmann pin as a handle to pull the acetabular fragment downwards and rotate it laterally. If the acetabular fragment is pulled too far forward it will limit flexion, and if the hip shows decreased medial rotation, then the acetabulum should be rotated inwards. Once the acetabulum has been satisfactorily positioned, there will be a gap in the anterior portion of the iliac osteotomy which is filled with bone graft taken from the iliac crest in the region of the anterior superior iliac spine.

The position of the acetabulum is checked again with the image intensifier and stabilised with usually four Kirschner wires (1.8 mm to 2 mm in diameter) inserted from the iliac crest. These wires should diverge in a fan-like manner into the medial and lateral frontal and posterior parts of the acetabulum (fig 16). The ends of the pins are bent over and cut to length. They are retained for 3-4 months.

POST-OPERATIVE MANAGEMENT

Post-operatively a hip spica is applied for six weeks. The hip should not be immobilised in external rotation. To avoid stiffness even in adults the spica should be removed at 6 weeks and gentle non-weight-bearing exercises encouraged until bony union has been obtained.

COMPLICATIONS

Tönnis reported one transient peroneal nerve palsy, probably due to pressure from the hip spica and one slight weakness of the quadriceps muscle. Transient weakness of the gluteus maximus muscle was seen on several occasions. Other authors have reported post-operative myositis ossificans and paresis [19, 20, 24, 26]. This is major surgery on the pelvis and can be associated with significant blood loss, even in expert hands. There is a considerable risk of damage to major nerves and blood vessels around the hip and in the pelvis. It is advisable that such surgery be undertaken by a surgeon having wide experience of surgery of the pelvis in the child, adolescent and adult.

References

[1] Coleman SF. The incomplete pericapsular (Pemberton) and innominate (Salter) osteotomies: a complete analysis. *Clin Orthop* 1974 ; 98 : 116-123

[2] Fixsen JA. Anterior and posterior displacement of the hip after innominate osteotomy. *J Bone Joint Surg Br* 1987 ; 69 : 361-364

[3] Heine J, Felske-Adler C. Ergebnisse der Behandlung der kongenitalen Hüftluxation durch offene Reposition und Beckenosteotomie nach Salter. *Z Orthop* 1985 ; 123 : 273-277

[4] Hopf A. Hüftpfannenverlagerung durch doppelte Beckenosteotomie zur Behandlung der Hüftgelenkdysplasie und subluxation bei Jugendlichen und Erwachsenen. *Z Orthop* 1966 ; 101 : 559-586

[5] Huang SC, Wang JH. A comparative study of nonoperative versus operative treatment of developmental dysplasia of the hip in patients of walking age. *J Pediatr Orthop* 1997 ; 17 : 181-188

[6] Kamegaya M, Shinohara Y, Shinada Y, Moriya H, Koizumi W, Tsuchiya K. The use of a hydroxyapatite block for innominate osteotomy. *J Bone Joint Surg Br* 1994 ; 76 123-126

[7] Le Cœur P. Correction des défants d'orientation de l'articulation coxofémorale par ostéotomie de l'isthme iliaque. *Rev Chir Orthop* 1964 ; 51 : 211

[8] McCarthy JJ, Fox JS, Gurd AE. Innominate osteotomy in adolescents and adults who have acetabular dysplasia. *J Bone Joint Surg Am* 1996 ; 78 : 1455-1461

[9] McKay DW. Congenital dislocation of the hip. In : Tachdjian MO ed. Edinburgh : Churchill Livingstone, 1982

[10] Mellerovicz HH, Matussek J, Baum C. Long-term results of Salter and Chiari hip osteotomies in developmental hip dysplasia. *Arch Orthop Trauma Surg* 1998 ; 117 : 222-227

[11] Monod A, Filipe G. Les ostéotomies triples du bassin chez l'enfant. *Rev Chir Orthop* 1989 ; 75 : 524-531

[12] Moulin P, Morscher E. Langzeitresultate der Beckenosteotomie nach Salter. *Orthopäde* 1988 ; 17 : 479-484

[13] Pemberton PA. Pericapsular osteotomy of the ilium for treatment of congenital subluxation and dislocation of the hip. *J Bone Joint Surg Am* 1965 ; 47 : 65-68

[14] Pope DF, Bueff UH, Deluca PA. Pelvic osteotomies for subluxation of the hip in cerebral palsy. *J Pediatr Orthop* 1994 ; 14 : 724-730

[15] Saleh JM, O'Sullivan ME, O'Brien TM. Pelvic remodelling after Salter osteotomy. *J Pediatr Orthop* 1995 ; 15 : 342-345

[16] Salter RB. Innominate osteotomy in the treatment of congenital dislocation and subluxation of the hip. *J Bone Joint Surg Br* 1961 ; 43 : 518-539

[17] Salter RB. Role of innominate osteotomy in the treatment of congenital dislocation and subluxation of the hip in the older child. *J Bone Joint Surg Am* 1966 ; 48 : 1413-1439

[18] Salter RB, Dubos JP. The first fifteen years' personal experience with innominate osteotomy in the treatment of congenital dislocation and subluxation of the hip. *Clin Orthop* 1974 ; 98 : 72-103

[19] Steel HH. Congenital dislocation of the hip. In : Tachdjian MO ed. Edinburgh : Churchill Livingstone, 1982

[20] Steel HH. Triple osteotomy of the innominate bone. *J Bone Joint Surg Am* 1973 ; 55 : 343-350

[21] Sutherland DH, Greenfield R. Double innnominate osteotomy. *J Bone Joint Surg Am* 1977 ; 59 : 1082-1091

[22] Tachdjian MO. Pemberton's innominate osteotomy, indications, technique, results, pitfalls and complications. In : Tachdjian MO ed. Congenital dislocation of the hip. Edinburgh : Churchill Livingstone, 1982 : 542-554

[23] Tachdjian MO. Salter innominate osteotomy to derotate the maldirected acetabulum. In : Tachdjian MO ed. Congenital dislocation of the hip. Edinburgh : Churchill Livingstone, 1982 : 567-594

[24] Tönnis D. Die angeborene Hüftdysplasie und Hüftluxation im Kindes und Erwachsenenalter. Berlin : Springer-Verlag, 1984

[25] Tönnis D. Die angeborene Hüftdysplasie und Hüftluxation. Berlin : Springer-Verlag, 1984 : 309-321

[26] Tönnis D. Congenital dislocation of the hip. In : Tachdjian MO ed. Edinburgh : Churchill Livingstone, 1982

[27] Tönnis D. Surgical treatment of congenital dislocation of the hip. *Clin Orthop* 1990 ; 258 : 33-40

[28] Tönnis D, Behrens K, Tscharani F. Eine neue Technik der Dreifachosteotomie zur Schwenkung dysplastischer Hüftpfannen bei Jugendlichen und Erwachsenen. *Z Orthop* 1981 ; 119 : 253-263

[29] Waters P, Kurica K, Hall J, Micheli LJ. Salter innominate osteotomies in congenital dislocation of the hip. *J Pediatr Orthop* 1988 ; 8 : 650-655

[30] Windhager R, Lack W, Schiller CH, Kotz R. Die Beckenosteotomie nach Salter in der Behandlung der kongenitalen Hüftluxation und Hüftdysplasie unter besonder Berücksichtigung der Beckenkippung. *Z Orthop* 1990 ; 128 : 575-583

[31] Zadeh HG, Catterall A, Hashemi-Nejad A, Perry RE. Test of stability as an aid to decide the need for osteotomy in association with open reduction in developmental dysplasia of the hip. *J Bone Joint Surg Br* 2000 ; 82 : 17-27

Acetabuloplasties and shelf operations

G Bollini
M Jacquemier
JL Jouve

Abstract. — *There are two major techniques to improve cover of the femoral head. Shelf operations involve extending the acetabular roof without altering its slope while acetabuloplasties can improve the orientation of the acetabular roof by performing a supra-acetabular osteotomy. After describing the surgical approach to this region, the individual techniques for both shelf operations and acetabuloplasties are detailed.*

© 2001, Editions Scientifiques et Médicales Elsevier SAS. All rights reserved.

Keywords: hip, congenital dysplasia, shelf operation, acetabuloplasty.

Introduction

Many operations have been developed to improve acetabular cover, and Salter's classification is used when discussing these techniques [11].

A shelf operation uses a bone graft to extend the roof of the acetabulum. It is extra-articular and does not alter the inclination of the acetabulum. The shelf can be constructed either by using a free bone graft, or by translation of the local bone structure as in a Chiari osteotomy.

An acetabuloplasty alters the slope of the roof of the acetabulum by an incomplete osteotomy which retains a hinge to allow the necessary displacement to be made. Various techniques are available and the optimal position is then maintained by inserting a bone graft.

Colonna's capsular arthroplasty [4] involves deepening the acetabular cavity, and nowadays is really only used as a salvage procedure.

Only acetabuloplasties and shelf procedures which use a bone graft are described. Shelf operations are really only used in older children whose acetabulae have little re-modelling potential, or when it seems unlikely that there will be adequate spontaneous development of the roof. Acetabuloplasties are more useful when acetabular roof growth has not been achieved and there is still a likelihood of

Gérard Bollini, M.D.
Michel Jacquemier, M.D.
Jean-Luc Jouve, M.D.
Orthopaedic Department, CHU Timone Enfants, 264, rue Saint-Pierre, 13385 Marseille, France.

useful further development. The object is to obtain both an immediate plastic improvement followed by secondary re-modelling which will improve acetabular orientation owing to the reorientation of the acetabular ephiphysis. Correction of malposition can be made in one, two or three directions according to the technique used. All these procedures differ from pelvic osteotomies which change the orientation of the entire acetabulum to improve cover of a previously well-reduced femoral head. The choice of technique depends on careful determination of the exact orientation of the acetabulum and of any associated lack of cover of the femoral head by bone scan or by MRI. This will then allow the best procedure to be chosen to correct the lack of femoral head cover.

The supra-acetabular region

PATIENT POSITION

With the patient supine and a pillow under the buttock to present the iliac crest, a support is placed against the opposite greater trochanter. It is important to be able to use an image-intensifier or portable X-ray machine during the operation. It is also important to leave the iliac crest exposed, with the field extending two fingers' breadth distal to the anterosuperior iliac spine: two fingers above the crest of the ilium and two fingers posterior to the summit of the crest. The lower limb should be prepared so that it can be manipulated during the operation.

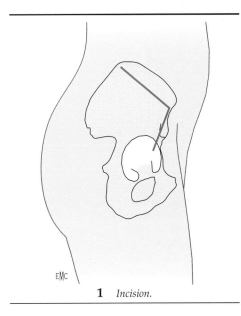

1 *Incision.*

SURGICAL APPROACH

The skin incision is parallel to and runs one or two centimetres below the iliac crest. It should be made in an anterior direction and start below the summit of the crest *(fig 1)*. At the anterosuperior iliac spine it turns down towards the middle of the femoral head. Proximally, the abdominal muscles are retracted inwards and diathermy is used to mobilise their attachment from the outer part of the exposed iliac crest *(fig 2)*. The cartilage of the crest is incised vertically, and divided in two so that both sides of the ilium can be exposed sub-periosteally *(fig 3)*. Anteriorly, it is important to identify the cutaneous femoral nerve which may be found in various positions; it can usually be identified two or three centimetres distal to the anterosuperior iliac spine between the

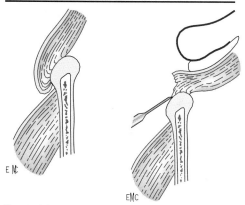

2   *Mobilisation of the abdominal muscles and the iliac crest.*

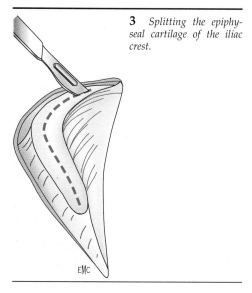

3   *Splitting the epiphyseal cartilage of the iliac crest.*

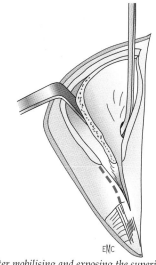

4   *After mobilising and exposing the superior portion of the two iliac fossae, the gluteus minimus fascia is incised.*

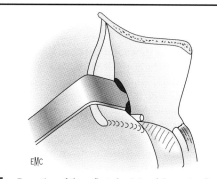

5   *Resection of the reflected origin of the rectus femoris.*

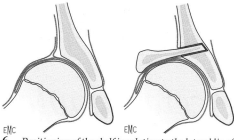

6   *Positioning of the shelf in relation to the lateral lip of the acetabular roof. It is important to avoid any step between the shelf and the lateral lip.*

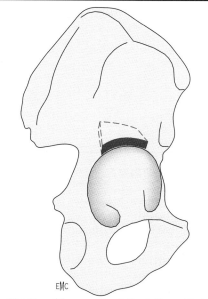

7   *Situation of the groove in relation to the acetabulum.*

sartorius and the tensor fascia lata. With the nerve retracted medially, the space between the fascia lata and the sartorius is opened to expose the tendon of the rectus femoris. A branch of the anterior supra-acetabular artery often has to be dealt with at this stage. The tendon of the rectus femoris is exposed proximally to delineate its two components: the straight head and the reflected head. The antero-inferior iliac spine is also identified. The periosteum between the two anterior iliac spines is then incised to allow further stripping of both sides of the ilium. Usually, it is unnecessary to detach the origin of the tensor fascia lata muscle. The fascia covering the gluteus medius is incised vertically and the muscle retracted posteriorly (*fig 4*). The periosteum covering the external surface of the iliac wing proximal to the reflected head of rectus femoris is also divided. A flap consisting of the gluteus minimus can then be retracted posteriorly and this will allow exposure of the reflected head of the rectus femoris (*fig 5*). This tendon is usually extracapsular but it can be covered by a fold of the joint capsule. This tendon is resected (*fig 5*) as it is of little, if any, use when fixing a graft or shelf in position and its loss does not appear to cause any significant disability. The edge of the acetabulum can then be palpated deep to the bed of this tendon, and

the capsule is dissected superiorly and anteriorly, taking care not to disturb its posterior part.

CLOSURE

The periosteal flap and gluteus minimus are replaced, and the two halves of the iliac crest are sutured together. The tendon of the tensor fascia lata is also repaired. Drainage is not usually indicated, and closure is completed by suture in two layers.

Shelf operations

The technique described was published in 1954 by Salmon [10].

PREPARATION OF THE GROOVE TO RECEIVE THE BONE GRAFT

It is essential that the inferior surface of the graft extend into the lateral margin of the acetabulum without creating a step (*fig 6*). Therefore, it is wise to use an image intensifier to identify the correct site, and then to mark this with a pin or a needle. The inferior margin of the groove should follow anteriorly and posteriorly the curve of the perimeter of the acetabulum for about one third of its length, and it should be

about 6-7 mm in depth (*fig 7*). The direction in the frontal plane should be slightly oblique (from lateral to medial, and from inferior to superior). In the horizontal plane, it should be slightly oblique from lateral to medial as well as from inferior to superior in order to ensure firm fixation of the graft. The groove should extend to the medial cortex of the ilium. Diathermy can be used to mark the borders of the groove which is then created with a hammer and chisel, taking great care to ensure correct orientation of the chisel. A curette is then used to clear the groove, to ensure that the graft can be easily but firmly inserted.

PREPARATION OF THE GRAFT

A free graft consisting of both cortices is taken from the iliac crest. A graft with only one cortex can be used if the crest is very thick. Its shape is fashioned according to the curvature of the lateral cortex, and will depend on the size of the femoral head that is to be covered; this can be determined using an image intensifier. Usually the graft is trapezoidal with a large base formed by the crest of the ilium. Its apex, which will be inserted into the groove, is the inferior and thinnest part of the graft. Its length should be equal to the length of the intra-osseus part of the shelf plus the necessary length to cover the femoral head adequately without

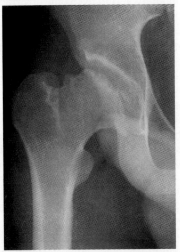

8 *Polyepiphyseal dysplasia: preoperative view at 16 years old.*

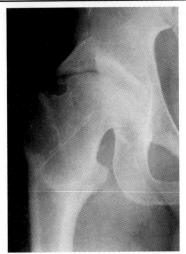

9 *View at 20 years old - four years postoperatively. (Shelf operation and femoral valgus osteotomy.)*

interfering with abduction. The thickness of the graft should correspond to the size of the groove; it is sometimes fashioned using a bone nibbler. It is also helpful to shape it to match the groove by performing purely cortical osteotomies on its inferior surface and then bending it appropriately. This must be done very carefully to avoid a complete fracture. It is always useful to harvest a graft in such a manner that a further graft can be raised if there is any problem with the original.

The graft is introduced firmly but carefully, avoiding any compression of its lateral border. Good fixation can usually be produced and there are no indications to add further bone grafts or any metallic support "above" the graft. Closure starts with replacement of the periosteal flap and the gluteus minimus. The two edges of the iliac crest are sutured as is the tensor fascia lata.

No drainage is necessary unless there has been extensive bleeding from the groove. Final closure is performed in two layers (*fig 8, 9*).

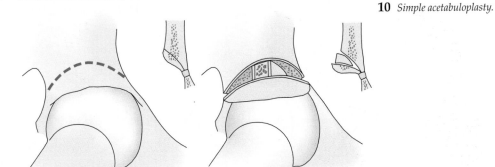

10 *Simple acetabuloplasty.*

OTHER METHODS OF FIXING THE SHELF

The technique described above produces a stable shelf and no plaster immobilisation is required, but other shelf procedures require reinforcement. In fact, these additional measures can be used with Salmon's technique if the surgeon deems them necessary. Castaing [2] described the use of a reinforcing buttress, a second shelf which necessitates a small groove in the lateral cortex. Tightening the screw gives greater or lesser support to the buttress. Roy Camille [9] advises a "Y" plate inserted upside down, with two limbs adapted to fit and to support the shelf and, in particular, to prevent any superior migration.

POST-OPERATIVE MANAGEMENT

After dressing the wound, both legs are put in skin traction for three weeks and no 90° hip flexion (or sitting) is allowed. Physiotherapy is prescribed for the muscles of the lower limbs, and non-weight-bearing walking starts after one month. Normal walking starts two months after the operation.

COMPLICATIONS AND PROBLEMS

– Too high a position of the groove and hence of the shelf. It is most important to avoid this situation, but if it does occur the operation must be repeated with correct siting of the shelf. The thickness of the graft may be insufficient, and this will entail the use of a supplementary graft placed above the shelf. Inadequate fixation of the shelf will also necessitate one or other of the procedures already described.

– Fracture of the graft from over-bending. If there is good fixation then nothing need be done. If not, a bone graft will be necessary.

– Instability of the shelf: this requires supplementary fixation and stabilisation.

– Secondary migration of the shelf. If this is due to poor impaction of the graft, then further stabilisation as already described will be necessary.

Acetabuloplasty

We describe:

– A simple acetabuloplasty, unicortical, and involving simple bending from medial to lateral of the acetabular roof, hinged on the horizontal branch of the "Y" cartilage.

– A simple acetabuloplasty, unicortical, involving simple bending from medial to lateral of the acetabular roof, hinged on the internal cortex of the ilium: Dega's osteotomy [5, 6].

– A complex acetabuloplasty, bicortical, with displacement in three planes of the acetabular socket using an incomplete iliac osteotomy (Pemberton [8]).

SIMPLE ACETABULOPLASTY

The description is based on the techniques of Zanoli [12] and Bertrand [1], as modified by Mubarak [7]. The site of the osteotomy is marked on the lateral cortex (*fig 10*) and is two centimetres above the lip of the acetabulum, curved anteroposteriorly and extending anteriorly to just above the antero-inferior iliac spine. It runs posteriorly for a similar distance. A hammer and chisel (straight and curved) are used at the upper pole of the osteotomy and an image intensifier is required to identify the middle of the horizontal limb of the "Y" cartilage. The point of entry and the direction and progress of the chisel are followed by fluoroscopy, and when the horizontal limb is reached, the first chisel (or osteotome) is left in place, and a second instrument is used to make the same cut both anteriorly and posteriorly. The anterior and posterior margins of the cortex of the ilium are simply incised. A larger osteotome is then used to displace inferiorly and laterally the inferior part of the osteotomy using the horizontal limb of the "Y" cartilage as a hinge. The resulting gap is held open with a laminar spreader while two or three bicortical comma-shaped iliac bone grafts of appropriate size are taken from the iliac crest and inserted into the opened osteotomy.

11 *Dega's acetabuloplasty.*

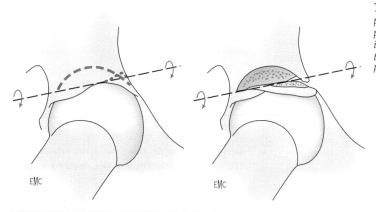

12 *Pemberton's acetabulo-plasty. The two cuts are practically at the same level in order to produce good anterior cover of the femoral head.*

DEGA'S ACETABULOPLASTY [6]

After exposing the two sides of the ilium, the osteotomy is situated 5 mm above the lip of the acetabulum *(fig 11)* so as to produce a thin inferior fragment. On the outer surface of the ilium, the osteotomy starts just above the antero-inferior iliac spine and passes posteriorly, parallel to the superior margin of the acetabulum as far as the sciatic notch. A straight and narrow osteotome introduced at the superior aspect of the acetabulum is directed to a point about 5 mm above the horizontal limb of the triangular cartilage. The osteotomy is completed anteriorly and posteriorly in the same direction. A larger osteotome is then used to displace the distal part of the osteotomy inferiorly so as to both lower the roof and modify its slope. A bicortical iliac graft is then placed in the opened osteotomy.

PEMBERTON'S ACETABULOPLASTY [8]

A blunt Hohmann retractor is placed in the sciatic notch and another on either side of the ilium. This exposes the anterior two thirds of the wing of the ilium. The osteotomy is then performed separately in each iliac cortex. In the lateral cortex it starts just above the antero-inferior iliac spine *(fig 12)* and passes backwards, parallel to the superior lip of the acetabulum until it reaches to within 1 to 1.5 cm anterior to the sciatic notch which it is important not to divide. The posterior border of the osteotomy should be at the level of the lateral retractor separation of the muscles of

the external iliac fossa, and half-way between the sciatic notch and the posterior lip of the acetabulum. When the course of the osteotomy has been marked, it is carried out using a curved osteotome. On the medial iliac cortex, it starts at the same point as on the lateral cortex, and follows the same direction. Posteriorly, it should stop short of the sciatic notch, and its exact direction will depend on the size of the femoral head to be covered. If the uncovered area is anterior, the roof of the acetabulum should be displaced inferiorly, and the extent of the medial posterior end of the osteotomy should be the same as that made posteriorly and laterally. If the uncovered area is more lateral, the medial posterior osteotomy end should be more anterior in relation to the iliopubic part of the "Y" cartilage. After dividing the lateral and medial cortices, a larger and curved osteotome is used to divide the intramedullary bone. This instrument is then used to move and bend the inferior fragment of the osteotomy in the required direction. A bicortical iliac comma-shaped graft is then placed in the opened osteotomy.

POSTOPERATIVE MANAGEMENT OF ACETABULOPLASTIES

Although these osteotomies are inherently stable, it is wise to immobilise children in order to prevent too early weight-bearing. This is best effected with a hip spica cast for four to six weeks. Weight-bearing can then commence. Physiotherapy is used to restore

joint mobility and to overcome any transient lack of buttock muscle activity.

COMPLICATIONS AND PROBLEMS OF ACETABULOPLASTIES

Problems can arise from incorrect direction of the osteotomy.

In simple acetabuloplasties performed with image intensification, complications are rare. Penetration of a limb of the "Y" cartilage by a chisel or osteotomy can be responsible for producing epiphysiodesis of this structure with resulting progressive extrusion of the femoral head.

With Dega's operation it is difficult to correct any malorientation of the osteotomy once this has been made and therefore it is essential to use image intensification during this part of the procedure.

In Pemberton's osteotomy, it is difficult to decide before operation how deep to make the medial osteotomy, and this must depend on the local morphology.

Displacement of the distal fragment is often aided by the use of a self-retaining retractor, but care must be taken not to damage the cortex to which this is applied.

Indications

It is impossible to prepare a simple table of the indications for this type of surgery, but it is important to carefully consider the condition of the specific hip joint.

THE STATE OF THE ACETABULUM

In the frontal plane the magnitude of any bone dysplasia should be assessed from an anteroposterior radiograph of the pelvis, and any cartilage dysplasia by MRI.

In the horizontal plane there are two important features to note: the orientation of the acetabulum by measuring its anteversion and the site of any uncovering of the head.

The degree of congruence or incongruity of the hip joint must be assessed.

AGE

The age of the child is important as this relates to the potential for remodelling of the acetabulum. Coleman [3] has shown the efficacy of acetabuloplasty performed under the age of six years.

AETIOLOGY

– In acetabular dysplasia with congenital dislocation, the fault is more anterior and lateral.

– With dysplasia associated with spasticity, the acetabular deficiency is more general, and particularly posterior.

– In spina bifida the deficiency is general.

– In Legg-Calvé-Perthes disease, it is the excessive width of the femoral head and its deformation which are responsible for lack of cover.

GENERAL EFFECTS OF OSTEOTOMIES AND ACETABULOPLASTIES

Acetabuloplasties tend to decrease the volume of the acetabulum.

Shelf operations tend to increase the volume of the acetabulum.

These factors must be taken into account when choosing which type of operation should be performed.

AGE FOR SPECIFIC PROCEDURES

– Shelf operations are performed between ten years and adulthood.

– Acetabuloplasty

– simple: from two to six or seven years;

– Pemberton: from two to eight or ten years;

– Dega: from two to six or seven years.

REQUIREMENTS

Acetabuloplasty with an open "Y" cartilage will diminish the volume of the acetabulum but the joint must be congruent.

Shelf operation with a closed "Y" cartilage will increase the volume of the acetabulum with an incongruous hip joint.

COVER PRODUCED ACCORDING TO PROCEDURE

– Simple acetabuloplasty: predominately lateral and anterior cover.

– Dega acetabuloplasty: predominately anterior and lateral cover.

– Pemberton acetabuloplasty: lateral and anterior cover.

– Shelf operation: antero-lateral cover.

CONTRAINDICATIONS

Acetabuloplasties when the hip is neither centred nor "centrable" (notably Legg-Calvé-Perthes disease).

References

[1] Bertrand P, Guias H, Benard HM. Réflexions sur les butées dans les subluxations de la hanche. *Rev Chir Orthop* 1964 ; 50 : 123-131

[2] Castaing J, Lama E. Technique du greffon appuyé dans la butée ostéoplastique de la hanche. *Ann Chir* 1962 ; 16 : 1765-1767

[3] Coleman S. The incomplete pericapsular (Pemberton) and innominate (Salter) osteotomies. A complete analysis. *Clin Orthop* 1974 ; 98 : 116-123

[4] Colonna PC. Capsular arthroplasty for congenital dislocation of the hip, a two stage procedure. *Surg Gynecol Obstet* 1936 ; 63 : 677-682

[5] Dega W. Contributo allo studio clinico della riconstruzione del tetto cotiloideo. Atti del XXIII. Congresso della Soc. Italiana di Ortopedia. Bologna 15-17, X, 1932

[6] Dega W. Development and clinical importance of the dysplastic acetabulum. In : Progress in orthopaedic surgery 2. Acetabular dysplasia. Berlin : Springer-Verlag, 1978 : 47-72

[7] Mubarak SJ, Valencia FG, Wenger DR. One-stage correction of the spastic dislocated hip: use of pericapsular acetabuloplasty to improve coverage. *J Bone Joint Surg Am* 1992 ; 74 : 1347-1357

[8] Pemberton PA. Pericapsular osteotomy of the ilium for treatment of congenital subluxation and dislocation of the hip. *J Bone Joint Surg Am* 1965 ; 47 : 65-86

[9] Roy-Camille R. Butée ostéoplastique armée de hanche. Technique permettant la marche au 21ème jour. *Presse Méd* 1968 ; 76 : 273-275

[10] Salmon M, Acquaviva J, Corti P. Arthroplastie extracapsulaire de la hanche. Quelques résultats radiologiques. *Rev Chir Orthop* 1954 ; 40 : 120-121

[11] Salter RB. Innominate osteotomy in the treatment of congenital dislocation and subluxation of the hip. *J Bone Joint Surg Br* 1961 ; 43 : 518-539

[12] Zanoli R. L'osteotomia del tetto del cotile nelle sua reconstruzione osteoplastica. *Atti Mem Soc Lom Chir* 1937 ; 5 : 211-214

Chiari osteotomy of the hip

W Schwägerl
P Zenz

Abstract. – The Chiari osteotomy of the hip is a supra-acetabular rotatory displacement osteotomy. The femoral head and the joint capsule are medialised and covered by the undersurface of the osteotomised os ilium. Better coverage of the femoral head and a reduction of the resultant exertion of force on the joint lead to better hip function and decrease of pain.

The indications are acetabular dysplasia of the young and adult patient, coxa magna and all forms of adult osteoarthritis of dysplastic hips.

Exact planning and performance of the osteotomy are the keys to the success of this method. The site, direction and shape of the osteotomy are described in detail, as well as modifications of the technique, additional procedures and the management of complications.

Since its introduction in 1953, this operation has proven to be a secure, reproducible and lasting solution in treating congenital dysplasia of the hip.

© 2000, Editions Scientifiques et Médicales Elsevier SAS. All rights reserved.

Keywords: hip, congenital dislocation of the hip, Chiari osteotomy, osteotomy, pelvic osteotomy, Perthes' disease.

Introduction

The Chiari osteotomy is a supra-acetabular rotatory displacement osteotomy. Chiari developed this surgical technique 45 years ago, pursuing the goal of covering the femoral head by enlarging the capacity of an insufficient acetabular roof [3]. This became necessary in cases of primary hip dysplasia, when there was a discrepancy between acetabular capacity and size of the femoral head. The same phenomena may appear following Perthes' disease.

Rationale of the procedure

The distal fragment of the osteotomy is displaced medially. This movement ameliorates and changes the situation of the hip in different ways:

– Creation of a new roof with an enlarged capacity of the acetabulum and a better distribution of pressure throughout the joint.

W Schwägerl, M.D.
Peter Zenz, M.D.
Otto Wagner Spital, Orthopädisches Zentrum, Sanatoriumstr. 2, A-1145 Wien, Austria.

– According to Pauwels' law [13], the load of the hip joint is decreased due to shortening of the lever arm of the body weight (*fig 1*).

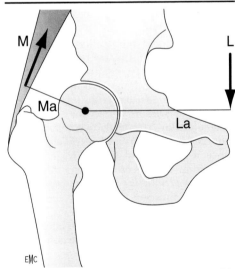

1 *According to Pauwels' Law of weight-bearing of the hip joint, in the one-legged stance, the equilibrium of the pelvis can be maintained only if the muscle force (M) is great enough to counteract the body weight (L). Since M x Ma = L x La (law of balance), a short femoral neck (Ma) increases the load of the hip joint and may lead to an insufficiency of the force of the abductor muscles (M), leading to a Trendelenburg limp. Under normal conditions, the lever arm of the body weight (La) is three times greater than the lever arm of the muscle force (Ma).*

– Due to the interposition of the capsule between the iliac bone and the femoral head, fibrocartilaginous tissue develops out of the interposed capsule.

– The greater trochanter comes closer to the iliac bone; this weakens the gluteus muscles. The reversal of lost muscular balance is achieved through postoperative rehabilitation.

In summary, the most important result is the enlarged capacity of the acetabulum, along with better distribution of pressure throughout the joint. A fibrocartilaginous tissue layer develops out of the interposed joint capsule between the femoral head and the newly formed acetabular roof.

Clinical interest of the operation

The biomechanical improvements result in a decrease of pain and a better walking and moving ability for the patient, at the cost of lower gluteus muscle power. Therefore, the importance of postoperative rehabilitation is crucial [16].

Preoperative requirements

INSTRUMENTS

The operation is performed on an extension table. The uninvolved coxal bone is fixed at the middle peg of the extension table, while the involved hip should be allowed good mobility. An image intensifier is brought over the opposite side and focused above the hip to be operated. The involved leg is set up in slight outward rotation and in 10-15° abduction. The instruments required are: narrow straight and narrow curved raspatories; two radiolucent retractors, an obliquely-cut chisel, K-wires and a drill.

PREOPERATIVE RADIOGRAPHS

Preoperative planning includes an AP overview of the pelvic region, a false profile, as well as two functional radiographs, one in maximum abduction and one in maximum adduction.

These views should answer the following questions:

– Is the femoral head well-seated within the dysplastic hip. Is it lateralised, or lateralised and ascended?

This will influence the starting point and direction of the osteotomy. Usually, the osteotomy will ascend in a 7° angle. The higher the femoral head has slipped, the less the angle should be, to avoid injuring the sacroiliac joint. Sketching the entire operation plan on the radiograph, including the intended line of the osteotomy on the AP view, provides a better idea of the ideal localisation and direction of the osteotomy.

The adducted functional radiograph indicates whether an additional valgus rotation osteotomy is necessary to reduce possible pressure points between a badly-shaped femoral head and the newly-created acetabular roof.

– Is the pelvic osteotomy the indication of choice or would a simple varus derotation osteotomy of the femoral shaft have sufficient effect?

This would be the case if, in addition to good congruence between femoral head and acetabulum, a sufficient roof can be found in the abducted functional radiograph, as well as a sufficient frontal roof in the false profile radiograph.

PREOPERATIVE PLANNING

Evaluation of the preoperative X-rays allows sketching the exact localisation of the osteotomy, contouring the acetabular rim on the AP view. As a rule, an ascension of 7° is the ideal direction. Sufficient medialiation should be pursued. Stabilisation of the osteotomy must be ensured. Care must be taken to avoid muscle injury, since additional trauma would be hard on the gluteal muscles, already affected by their postoperative relaxation.

Surgical technique

INCISION

The skin incision parallels the iliac crest 2 cm below its course. The incision starts 4 cm posterior from the anteroposterior iliac spine and extends distally in a curved manner, heading in a lateral dorsal direction at the end. It should have a length of 12-13 cm. This incision avoids injuring the lateral femoral cutaneous nerve.

FURTHER DISSECTION

A longitudinal transection of the fascia is performed distally from the superior iliac spine. The layer between the tensor fasciae latae and the sartorius muscle is dissected free, using the curved preparation scissors. After ligature of the crossing vessels, the anterior part of the hip joint is exposed. The periost is incised at the iliac crest. It is reflected along with the head of the sartorius from the lateral wall of the ilium to medial, using a straight raspatory. Under control of the image converter, the dissection with a curved raspatory continues subperiostally until the greater sciatic notch is reached. A radiolucent retractor is inserted into the now exposed inner pelvic brim down to the greater sciatic notch. A curved raspatory then aims for the greater sciatic notch, but this time from the outer pelvic brim and after being inserted between the small gluteus muscle and the joint. The raspatory is replaced by another radiolucent spatula. Both spatulas should now be in contact while holding the pelvic brim both from inside and outside. The image intensifier should be consulted for confirmation.

Using the curved preparation scissors, the indirect head of the rectus femoris is reflected ventrally, cranially and 3 cm dorsally, and then transected up to its head as dorsally as possible with a single cut of the straight scissors across the line of the acetabular rim. This leads to a relaxation of the rectus tendon and exposes a gap between capsule and tendon large enough to perform the osteotomy from this point. This approach allows maximum sparing of the gluteus muscles. If necessary, the ventral portion of the gluteus muscles can be elevated subperiostally from the lateral wall of the ilium; 3 to 4 cm should be sufficient.

OSTEOTOMY *(fig 2)*

For the first osteotomy cut, a chisel is applied along the cranial pole of the femur head between the capsule and the relaxed head of the rectus femoris until it reaches the bony parts of the acetabular rim. The image converter should confirm the optimal entry point for the osteotomy 3-5 mm above the joint capsule. If the position differs, the chisel has to be repositioned. If the entry point is altered by an osteophyte, this could cause the chisel to deviate either cranially or

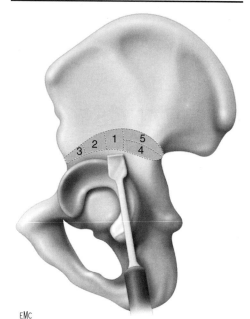

EMC

2 *Site of the osteotomy in 5 planes, according to the orientation of the chisel.*

caudally. Cranial deviation forms a step, an inconvenience which can be tolerated, but which should be avoided if possible. A caudal deviation, on the other hand, must be avoided by all means. Otherwise, the osteotomy would enter the joint and immediately deteriorate the result of the operation. In difficult cases with osteophytes, opening the capsule and finding the entry point under clear visualisation may be helpful. It is recommended to fragmentise the osteophyte beforehand, using a small chisel, and then to introduce a K-wire into the intended entry point. Drilling should be angled 7° upwards.

The osteotomy is then performed with an obliquely-cut chisel underneath the K-wire. The asymmetric cut of the chisel pushes it steadily against the K-wire, allowing a straight osteotomy in spite of an osteophyte. For reference, the opposite anterosuperior iliac spine may be aimed at to determine the correct direction of the osteotomy. This also corresponds to the required 7°, provided there is a regular femoral head position. For the first osteotomy cut, it is suggested to make use of the K-wire support, even in cases without osteophytes.

The second osteotomy cut is performed still under the rectus tendon, but further ventrally. In reference to the first cut, the chisel is tilted 20° ventrally and moved ahead one length of its width. Simultaneously, the chisel handle is lowered by 30°.

Still remaining under the rectus tendon, the third osteotomy cut is performed after another tilt of 20° ventrally and another lowering of the handle by 20°. This completes the transection of the frontal acetabular roof to the anteroinferior iliac spine. The lowering of the handle is of great importance, since the chisel edge otherwise penetrates the anteroinferior iliac spine. The osteotomy, which is now accomplished cranially and to the front, must still be completed dorsally.

The fourth osteotomy cut extends from the cleft of the first cut dorsally along the lateral iliac wall, aiming exactly at the spatula sitting in the sciatic notch. By keeping towards this aiming point, penetration of the sacroiliac joint can be prevented, due to a flattening of the cutting direction angle when approaching the retractor.

The fifth cut is performed in the same manner, parallel to the fourth cut, again extending from the cleft of the first cut, but this time osteotomising the medial iliac wall. The protection intended by the introduction of the spatula is controlled by the assistant surgeon who holds the spatula and therefore feels contact with the progressing chisel edge.

The osteotomy is now completed. The image converter should now indicate a spontaneously created medialisation step of about 10 mm. If this is not the case, the osteotomy must be checked by reintroducing the chisel carefully and sliding it from front to back in search of remaining bony bridges. After transection of these remains, it should be possible to lift off the osteotomy easily and widely with the chisel placed in the cleft of the first cut. A look into the image converter allows confirmation.

MEDIALISATION *(fig 3A)*

The leg, with the knee joint bent 45°, is abducted by the assistant, while the surgeon places it in extension. This creates the necessary medialisation pressure on the acetabulum. It is displaced medially along the osteotomy. The results of this movement can easily be noted when introducing a finger into the lower pelvis. It is advisable to have another assistant stabilising the opposite pelvic bone manually during the manoeuvre. Using chisels with straight blades creates a polygonal cutting plane which prevents the osteotomy edges from drifting off dorsally in the course of the medialisation manoeuvre. If this happens anyway, an assistant has to reposition the dislocated osteotomy from underneath the covering sheet by applying pressure on the ischial tuberosity, while the surgeon stabilises the iliac crest. If the angle of the osteotomy is too flat, medialisation can be accomplished by insertion of a chisel into the osteotomy in order to lever it down medially. The handle has to be lowered distally and the medialiation manoeuvre is repeated as described above. As soon as a sufficient covering effect (Chiari effect) is achieved, i.e. the femoral head is well covered in the neutral position, the osteotomy is transfixed with 3 K-wires.

TRANSFIXATION *(fig 3B)*

Transfixation is performed across the medium gluteus muscle. The first K-wire is drilled starting from a point situated two

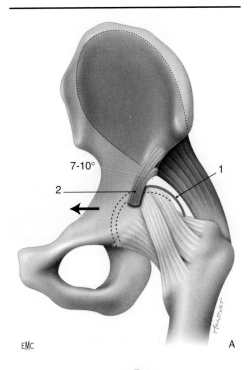

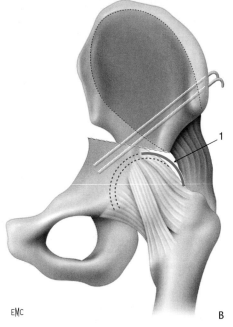

3 *Direction, completion and transfixation of the osteotomy. The weakening of the abductor muscles is due to the medialisation and cranialisation of the femoral head. The interposed capsule lies under the newly formed acetabulum. 1. Capsule; 2. m. rectus femoris.*

fingers behind the anterosuperior iliac spine and from there vertically two fingers in a dorsal direction, through the gluteus muscle and into the posterior bony pillar. The second K-wire is drilled in parallel to the first K-wire and 2.5 cm in the dorsocranial direction. If the medialisation is considerable, the K-wires may cross the gap outside the bone, which is not regarded as an inconvenience. An optional third K-wire can be drilled into the frontal bony pillar. Under image converter control, the femoral head is abducted, adducted and rotated. If the position of the osteotomy persists throughout this manoeuvre, the transfixation

can be qualified as stable. The K-wires are bent off and cut at the level of the muscle stratum, facilitating their recovery in the subcutaneous tissues for removal.

CLOSING THE WOUND

A no. 12 Redon drain is introduced into the lower pelvis, the reflected sartorius muscle is sutured over the iliac crest to the head of the tensor fasciae latae, and the wound is then closed layer after layer. The postoperative situation is documented by radiography.

During this operative technique, which has changed only slightly since Chiari, the gluteal muscles are left completely intact. Chiari used to immobilise the osteotomy for 3 weeks after surgery by means of a pelvic cast. Thanks to the transfixation technique, rehabilitation can start as of the first postoperative day.

Postoperative treatment

Active and passive physical therapy begins from the first day on, including intensive gluteal training. Walking activity should start on the third to fifth day postoperatively, with partial loading (25-30 kg) only 5 weeks after surgery. Then follows a radiographic control and change to full weight-bearing. Intense gluteal training has to be kept up for at least 8 months. The K-wires can be removed 3 months postoperatively.

Intraoperative complications

Stronger haemorrhages cease when the osteotomy is sufficiently medialised. This applies particularly in the case of haemorrhage from the gluteocranial artery. So far, other major vessels have not been reported as sources of haemorrhage.

Excessive displacement with central dislocation is extremely unusual. Restoration begins by screwing a femoral head extractor, such as that used for total hip arthroplasty, into the greater trochanter. It is then pulled laterally under adduction and forced extension of the leg. After successful repositioning, the osteotomy is transfixed as described above.

Postoperative complications

PSEUDOARTHROSIS

The incidence of pseudoarthrosis is extremely low. Chiari did not mention it at all. Amongst the patients of the Vienna orthopaedic clinic [4, 5, 6, 9, 17], there has only been one case. In the case of pseudoarthrosis, the same approach is chosen: the affected tissue is removed and the denuded bone is refilled with graft from the iliac crest. This is followed by K-wire transfixation (two K-wires in the frontal pillar, one in the posterior pillar). Alternatively, the use of two or three compression screws may be advantageous.

ECTOPIC OSSIFICATION

Ectopic ossifications can develop in the area of the head of the rectus muscle on the inferior spine. They can reach a degree where flexion becomes painful, handicapping the patient. In this case, they should be removed. The exostosis is dissected free and chiselled off using the same approach. Effective prophylaxis can be provided by Indomethacin [14].

LESIONS OF THE SCIATIC OR PERONEAL NERVE

Lesions of the sciatic or peroneal nerve (due to compression or haematoma) are extremely rare and usually recover within 6-8 weeks after conservative treatment.

LESIONS OF THE LATERAL FEMORAL CUTANEOUS NERVE

These can be avoided by the proper skin incision.

Alternative techniques

Schwägerl and Zenz [15] have developed the transtrochanteric approach. This approach aims for better visibility over the osteotomy site by temporary osteotomy of the greater trochanter and its cranial reflection. In this manner, the outside pelvic rim is dissected free without transection of muscles. Additionally, the curved line of the osteotomy can be much better visualised during the entire course of the operation, thus allowing more control over the procedure. The possibility of subsequent lateral and distal shifting of the trochanter enables strengthening of the gluteus muscles and therefore prevents possible permanent disability. Fixation of the shifted trochanter is achieved by two lag screws, which are removed one year after the operation. This approach is particularly indicated in the presence of an initial high trochanter position, muscle insufficiency or when the osteotomy has to be oriented at a steeper angle. However, even without these indications, the advantages prevail over the possible disadvantages, which are the necessity of screw removal and a possibility of pseudoarthrosis. As regards the operation technique, it should be pointed out that the medial osteotomy spatula must be inserted above the rectus muscle between the anterosuperior and the anteroinferior iliac spines.
Duquennoy and his colleagues [7] have significantly modified the original technique.

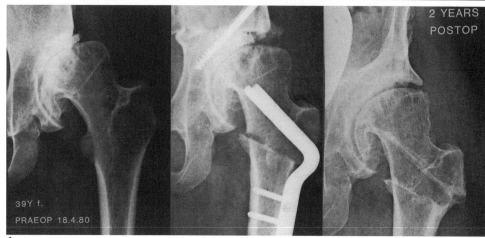

4 *Preoperative, postoperative and two-year result after a Chiari osteotomy of the left hip. The operation was combined with a valgus intertrochanteric osteotomy in the presence of a large inferior osteophyte. Osteosynthesis by one lag screw.*

Two-thirds of the medium gluteus muscle are reflected and the osteotomy is performed from ventral to dorsal. This method uses four introduced K-wires and is performed in the dorsal segment with a round chisel. A compression screw is used for transfixation. Morscher and Hefti [11] modified the approach by chiselling off the iliac spine and reflection of the abdominal muscles. The bony head of the tensor fasciae latae is reflected, as well as the indirect head of the rectus muscle, and an L-shaped capsulotomy is carried out. A 15° ascending osteotomy of the bony pelvic brim is performed using a straight chisel.

Additional operations

VALGUS ROTATION OSTEOTOMY

This additional procedure is required when a flattened femoral head is likely to cause an overloaded pressure point under the new acetabulum. If a functional radiograph in the maximal adducted position indicates a flattened femoral head, one can expect a congruent relationship between the femoral head and the new acetabulum after a combination of pelvic and valgus rotation osteotomy. Better strengthening of the gluteus muscles is an additional advantage of the valgus effect (*fig 4*).

VARUS DEROTATION OSTEOTOMY

This additional operation is seldom necessary. It is indicated when the preoperative functional radiograph in the abducted position shows a femoral head deformity with better congruence to the acetabular roof than in the normal position. Less gluteus muscle power as well as a leg shortening effect have to be taken into account at the same time.

Indications

Lateral and frontal acetabular dysplasia of the young patient:

– with a concentrically seated femoral head;

– with a lateral position;

– with a lateral and ascended position (-2 cm).

Coxa magna following Perthes' disease [1, 5].

All forms of adult osteoarthritis of dysplastic hips [4, 7]:

– with insufficiency of the lateral frontal acetabular roof;

– with insufficiency only of the lateral acetabular roof, if the functional radiographs in the abducted position show no improvement of the head position. Sufficient frontal coverage paired with an improvement of the head position in abducted functional radiographs would be an alternative indication for femoral varus derotation osteotomy.

Neuromuscular disorders: cerebral palsy, meningocele, etc. with unstable hips.

Limitations

The following circumstances indicate the limits of the possibilities of pelvic osteotomy or may even present a contraindication:

– Advanced osteoarthritis of the dysplastic hip.

– Loss of joint mobility. A minimum of 90° of preoperative flexion is mandatory.

– Clinical signs of labral lesions (especially detachment) verified by contrast MRI.

– Necrotic zones inside the acetabulum detected radiographically and verified by MRI or scintigraphy.

– The patient's age usually does not limit the indication for the operation. It is only the quality of the cartilage and the clinical mobility status that count when looking for methodological limits. In addition to the indication, total hip arthoplasty should be taken into consideration, depending on individual factors (work, habits, weight, muscle quality). The best results are achieved through pelvic osteotomy in juvenile patients or young adults having various forms of acetabular dysplasia, who cannot expect significant improvement by undergoing femoral shaft osteotomy alone. Additionally, the pelvic osteotomy improves shape and containment conditions for a follow-up endoprosthetic acetabulum implant operation. Clinical results are more favourable in patients under 40 years of age [10].

– When presented with a lateral subluxated hip ascended more than 2 cm, it should be very critically determined whether the direction of the osteotomy will involve the sacroiliac joint. A horizontal osteotomy may be performed, but handicaps the prognosis of joint recovery, mainly due to insufficient relief of the intra-articular pressure. A

descending osteotomy direction is obviously not recommended. A preoperative sketch indicating the possible direction of the osteotomy can clearly answer these questions.

– When arthrotic changes appear after Perthes' disease, the indication also depends on the radiologically-proven quality of the remaining cartilage. If secondary arthrotic changes outweigh the joint incongruency, performance of a pelvic osteotomy is no longer indicated.

– Narrowing of the bony pelvic cavity and the pelvic outlet after Chiari's osteotomy can interfere with normal childbirth and Caesarean section could be necessary, especially after a bilateral procedure [8].

Conclusions

The long-term results described by various authors [2, 9, 17] and verified within our own material (over a period of 25 years) undoubtedly confirm the positive effects of the supra-acetabular displacement osteotomy developed by Chiari – provided that the access is muscle-sparing, the osteotomy technique is exactly performed, and that medialisation is sufficient. These results, together with the small number of possible complications, add to the great interest of this technique for patients and surgeons, especially given the the limited long-term experience with highly complex and risky triple osteotomies.

References

[1] Bennett JT, Mazurek RT, Cash JD. Chiari's osteotomy in the treatment of Perthes' disease. *J Bone Joint Surg Br* 1991 ; 73 : 225-228

[2] Böhler N, Eyb R, Moll-Schüller E. 35 Jahre Beckenosteoto-mie nach Chiari – Analyse der Miberfolge. *Mitteilungsblatt der DGOT* 1986 ; 3 : 73-74

[3] Chiari K. Beckenosteotomie als Pfannendachplastik. *Wiener Med Wschr* 1953 ; 103 : 707-770

[4] Chiari K. Die Beckenosteotomie in der Behandlung der Coxarthrose. *Beitr Orthop Traumatol* 1968 ; 15 : 163-168

[5] Chiari K. Medial displacement osteotomy of the pelvis. *Clin Orthop* 1974 ; 98 : 55-71

[6] Chiari K, Schwägerl W. Pelvic osteotomy: indications and results. *Rev Chir Orthop Reparatrice Appar Mot* 1976 ; 62 (5) : 560-568

[7] Duquennoy A, Migaud H, Gougeon F, Fontaine C, Guire C. Chiari's osteotomy in the adult. Apropos of 70 cases. *Rev Chir Orthop* 1987 ; 73 (5) : 365-376

[8] Kotz R, Slancar P. Beckenosteotomie unf Geburt. *Z Orthop* 1973 ; 111 : 797-800

[9] Lack W, Windhager R, Kutschera HP, Engel A. Chiari pelvic osteotomy for osteoarthritis secondary to hip dysplasia. Indications and long-term results. *J Bone Joint Surg Br* 1991 ; 73-B : 229-234

[10] Migaud H, Duquennoy A, Gougeon F, Fontaine C, Pasquier G. Outcome of Chiari pelvic osteotomy in adults. 90 hips with 2-15 years' follow-up. *Acta Orthop Scand* 1995 ; 66 (2) : 127-131

[11] Morscher E, Hefti F, Judet TH, Ficat P, Thomas BJ, Salvati EA, Pellicci PM, Wilson PD, Roy Camille R, Roy-Camille R, Laurin CA, Riley Jr. Traitement chirurgical des lésions non trauma-tiques de la hanche. Atlas de Chirurgie Orthopédique (Tome 3), membre inférieur. In : ed. Masson, Paris : 1992

[12] Nishina T, Saito S, Ohzono K, Shimizu N, Hosoya T, Ono K. Chiari pelvic osteotomy for osteoarthritis. The influence of the torn and detached acetabular labrum. *J Bone Joint Surg Br* 1990 ; 72 (5) : 765-769

[13] Pauwels F. Atlas zur Biomechanik der gesunden und kranken Hüfte Springer, Berlin : 1973

[14] Randelli G, Romano CL. Prophylaxis with indomethacin for heterotopic ossification after Chiari osteotomy of the pelvis. *J Bone Joint Surg Br* 1992 ; (9) : 1344-1346

[15] Schwägerl W, Zenz P. Der trastrochantäre Zugang zur Bec-kenosteotomie nach Chiari. [abstract. 383] *Z Orthop* 1998 ; 135 (5)

[16] Shiba N. Biomechanics of the Chiari pelvic osteotomy. *Nippon Seikeigeka Gakkai Zasshi* 1991 May; 65 (5) : 337-348

[17] Windhager R, Pongracz N, Schönecker R, Kotz R. The Chiari pelvic osteotomy for congenital dislocation and subluxa-tion of the hip in children and adults. A review of the results of twenty to thirty –four years. *J Bone Joint Surg Br* 1991 ; 73 : 890-895

The Bernese periacetabular osteotomy

M Weber
R Ganz

Abstract. – The aim of the Bernese periacetabular osteotomy is to improve the deficient coverage of the femoral head in residual hip dysplasia in the skeletally-mature patient. Through a series of osteotomies close to the joint, the acetabulum is completely freed to be reoriented and fixed in an optimal position. Prerequisites are the absence of major degenerative changes, and an improved coverage and good congruency on an AP view of the pelvis with the hip in 20-30° of abduction. Contraindications are dislocated hips, a femoral head seated in a secondary acetabulum, worsening of the congruency in the abduction view and advanced arthrosis. A modified Smith-Petersen approach is used. The osteotomy is performed in five steps. Soft tissue attachments are carefully preserved. Reorientation is assessed with intra-operative AP views of the entire pelvis. Fixation is achieved with three 3.5-mm screws. Immediate partial weight-bearing is allowed. No external fixation is used. Eight weeks postoperatively, satisfactory healing is checked radiographically. Then, abductor muscle strengthening is encouraged while patients rapidly progress to full weight-bearing.
The first group of 75 patients was followed for 10 to 14 years. Pain and limp were significantly improved. In 82% of the cases, the hip joint was preserved and it functioned well in 73% of the patients. Negative factors for a good long-term outcome were advanced age of the patients, pre-existing arthrosis and insufficient correction.

Keywords: hip, dysplasia, periacetabular osteotomy.

Introduction

Residual dysplasia of the hip after skeletal maturity can lead to pain and limp for various reasons. The unfavourable lever arm results in rapid fatigue of the abductor muscles. The anterolateral subluxation of the femoral head overloads and damages the labrum [15], and this can progress to early degeneration of the hip joint [1, 4, 9, 19, 20, 21, 30].

The deficient and mal-oriented coverage of the femoral head can be corrected by augmentation or reorientation of the acetabulum. The Chiari pelvic osteotomy [3] or the shelf procedures [18] enlarge the acetabular surface, but they do not supply hyaline cartilage to the weight-bearing zone and do not improve congruency. Salter's pelvic osteotomy [25] does not allow sufficient correction in the adult patient. The double osteotomy of Sutherland and Greenfield [31] and triple osteotomy of Steel [29] cannot be rotated freely, as their cuts are distant to the acetabulum. The size of the acetabular fragment and the connection to the

sacropelvic ligaments limit the amount of correction. The double osteotomy of Hopf [11] is intra-articular in the distal part of the joint. Triple osteotomies close to the joint have been described by Le Coeur [17], Tönnis [32, 33] and Carlioz [2]. They allow extensive reorientation, but they alter the shape of the true pelvis and require strong fixation because of the resulting pelvic discontinuity. The spherical osteotomies of Nishio [24], Wagner [35], Eppright [6] and Ninomiya and Tagawa [23] allow sufficient lateral and anterior correction, but the medialisation of the joint is difficult to obtain. Furthermore, it is difficult to adjust for anteversion/retroversion. Since the radiological tear drop remains unchanged, these osteotomies are intra-articular by definition. Finally, they jeopardise the vascularity of the acetabular fragment because of the close proximity of the osteotomy to the joint. The perfusion will then be limited to the arteria acetabularis and the scarce contributions of the capsular vessels.

These disadvantages have led to the following technique, which was developed in 1983 and described by Ganz et al in 1988 [8]. Since its introduction, only minor modifications have been added. To date, this

technique has been used in over 700 cases. Other centres of hip surgery have adopted this technique, mainly using the ilioinguinal approach (North America). Today, most surgeons use the modified Smith-Petersen approach again, since several cases of serious complications (thrombosis of the femoral artery) [13, 14] have occurred with the ilioinguinal approach.

Surgical procedure

The principle of the operation is to mobilise an acetabular fragment through a series of osteotomies close to the joint, then reorient and stabilise the fragment in an ideal position. The advantages of the following technique include the possibility of performing all five osteotomies through one single approach. It is possible to achieve extensive amounts of correction while respecting the vascularity of the fragment and the continuity of the posterior pelvic column. This allows minimal osteosynthesis and immediate partial weight-bearing without additional external fixation. The intact posterior column protects the sciatic nerve to a certain extent. Since the patient population consists mostly of young women,

Martin Weber, M.D.
Reinhold Ganz, M.D., Professor and Chairman.
Department of Orthopaedic Surgery, University of Bern, Switzerland.

it is important to know that the shape of the true pelvis is not altered; thus the osteotomy presents no obstacle to normal birth [7]. The disadvantages are the requirements for a high standard of three-dimensional anatomical knowledge, precision and carefulness. It is difficult to correct errors in the course of the procedure. This periacetabular osteotomy is not indicated for acetabular dysplasia with open physes and for patients with moderate to severe arthrosis. As a prerequisite, a radiological AP view of the hip in 20-30 degrees of abduction (without external rotation) should show improved acetabular coverage and congruency. In certain pathomorphologies, the need for a concomitant intertrochanteric osteotomy to optimise the positioning of the femoral head must be considered [10].

Contraindications are a dysplastic hip in a high dislocation, a femoral head seated in a secondary acetabulum, worsening of the congruency in the abduction view, moderate to severe arthrosis, and patient age over 50 years (relative contraindication).

SPECIAL INSTRUMENTS

Besides a standard set of retractors and osteotomes for pelvic osteotomies, the following special instruments are needed: blunt pelvic retractor with a double curve, angled pelvic osteotome with a 15 and 20 mm blade, adjustable leg positioning device.

Operative procedure

The operation is performed with the patient supine on a radiolucent operating table allowing an intraoperative AP view of the entire pelvis. General or spinal/epidural anaesthesia is suitable. The entire leg and hemipelvis are prepared. The leg needs to remain mobile. Free access to the entire pelvic crest and the proximal half of the thigh is necessary.

The approach is a modification of the iliofemoral approach developed by Smith-Petersen in 1917 and 1949 [27, 28], which is described in extenso in the literature [5, 12]. The skin incision starts at the iliac crest approximately in the middle between the anterior and the posterior superior iliac spine *(fig 1)*. It courses along the iliac crest to the anterior spine, onto the proximal thigh where it continues in a slight bow laterally. The interval between the musculus sartorius and musculus tensor fascia latae is entered inside the muscle sheet of the tensor muscle in order to protect the nervus cutaneus femoris lateralis. The superior anterior iliac spine is osteotomised and flipped medially *(fig 2)*. The musculus obliquus externus abdominis is released subperiostally and elevated off the inner surface of the iliac wing together with the musculus iliacus. The dissection continues along the crista interspinosa until the tendinous origins of

the rectus femoris are identified and released *(fig 3)*. They are retracted medially. The anterior joint capsule is freed of the musculus ilio-capsularis until the bursa ilio-pectinea is opened. The psoas tendon can then be elevated and a pointed Hohmann retractor can be inserted into the superior pubic ramus, 1.5 - 2 cm medially to the eminentia ilio-pectinea *(fig 4)*. This manoeuvre is aided by flexion/adduction of the leg, thus releasing tension of the soft

tissues. The anterior joint capsule is then further dissected in a distal direction by elevation of the musculus ilio-capsularis and psoas tendon until the end of the capsule posterior-inferiorly is reached. At the inferior end of this interval, the infracotyloid groove of the os ischium is palpated between the musculus obturator externus and the capsule using a blunt instrument *(fig 5)*. The 15-mm angled pelvic osteotome is inserted along the palpating instrument, onto the ischium

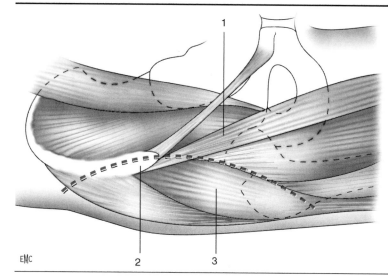

1 *Skin incision and superficial anatomy. 1. M. sartorius; 2. spina iliaca anterior superior; 3. m. tensor fasciae latae.*

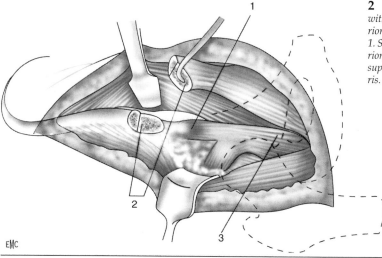

2 *Intermediate layers with osteotomy of the anterior superior iliac spine. 1. Spina iliaca anterior inferior; 2. spina iliaca anterior superior; 3. m. rectus femoris.*

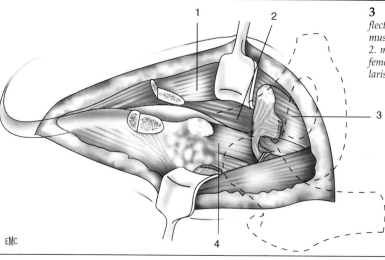

3 *Deep layers with reflected rectus femoris muscle. 1. M. sartorius; 2. m. iliacus; 3. m. rectus femoris; 4. m. ilio-capsularis.*

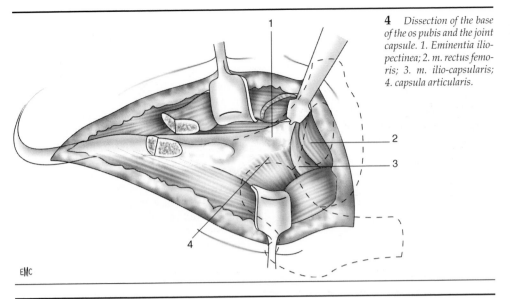

4   *Dissection of the base of the os pubis and the joint capsule. 1. Eminentia ilio-pectinea; 2. m. rectus femoris; 3. m. ilio-capsularis; 4. capsula articularis.*

EMC

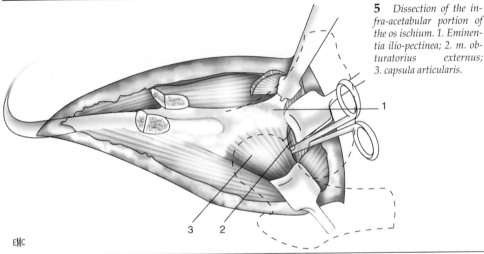

5   *Dissection of the in-fra-acetabular portion of the os ischium. 1. Eminen-tia ilio-pectinea; 2. m. ob-turatorius externus; 3. capsula articularis.*

EMC

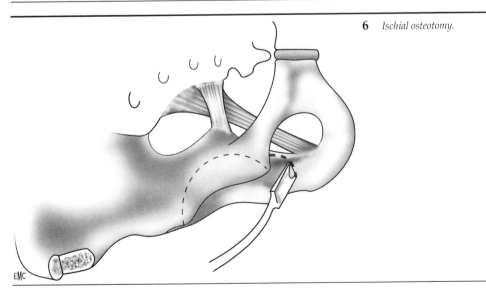

6   *Ischial osteotomy.*

EMC

limited exposure of the outer table of the pelvis is needed. At mid-distance between the superior and inferior anterior iliac spine, the musculus gluteus minimus is elevated off the bone, first sharply, then bluntly, until a blunt pelvic retractor can be inserted into the foramen ischiadicum majus. At the inside of the pelvis, the periosteum along the anterior surface of the anterior acetabular wall is incised and reflected medially. Once the entire quadrilateral surface is freed, a pelvic retractor is inserted onto the inner base of the spina ischiadica. This allows visualisation of the entire space down to the sacrospinal ligaments. The osteotomy is then outlined on the inner pelvic side using a 10-mm osteotome *(fig 8)*. The cut begins immediately below the osteotomised superior anterior iliac spine and runs in a dorsal direction; 1.5 cm before reaching the linea terminalis, it angles 110-120 degrees distally in the direction of the spina ischiadica. These latter figures can vary due to individual anatomy. It is important to preserve a posterior bridge of about 1 cm to the foramen ischiadicum maius and to leave enough supra-acetabular bone on the fragment to allow safe anchorage of a Schanz screw, which will be needed for manipulation of the fragment. The first step of the osteotomy is then cut with the oscillating saw. The second part is performed from the inside of the pelvis with angled and straight osteotomes *(fig 9)*. The first 15-20 mm of bone are osteomised, and the remaining distance is performed as a controlled fracture in the direction of the spina ischiadica. Since the subchondral bone and the rim of the foramen ischiadicum maius are very dense, the fracture will not enter the joint or the foramen. The fragment can be levered, using the osteotome in the second posterior part of the osteotomy until the fracture starts to propagate. A Schanz screw is inserted into the inferior anterior iliac spine and the supra-acetabular bone. With this screw and a laminar spreader inserted in the posterior osteotomy, the fragment can then be slightly elevated *(fig 10)*. The angled osteotome (20-mm blade) is inserted 4 cm below the linea terminalis at an angle of 50 degrees to the quadrilateral surface, in the direction of the end point of the first (ischial) osteotomy. It is advanced cautiously while the resistance of the acetabular fragment diminishes. Complete release is achieved internally, rotating the fragment by levering the Schanz screw in a medial direction while maximally opening the spreader.

The acetabular fragment is now freed completely and can be reoriented. Since dysplastic hip joints are frequently lateralised, it is important to rotate the acetabular fragment around the head and to medialise the joint as needed. If a supra-acetabular gap develops while rotating the fragment, then usually the soft tissue continuity inferiorly at the ischium needs to be further released. Sometimes the pubic

(fig 6). Its position can be verified fluoroscopically. It will then be advanced through two thirds of the ischium, taking care to cut the medial cortex without slipping off laterally, since the sciatic nerve can be damaged. It is therefore advisable to bring the leg into slight abduction. For the second osteotomy, the leg is adducted to relax the medial soft tissues. The base of the os pubis is dissected subperiostally. A blunt retractor on either side will protect the obturator vessels and nerve. The osteotomy is performed with a 15-mm osteotome, just medial to the eminentia ilio-pectinea, perpendicularly to the long axis of the os pubis and 45 degrees from lateral to medial *(fig 7)*.

The supra- and retroacetabular osteomy is roof-shaped and consists of two steps. Very

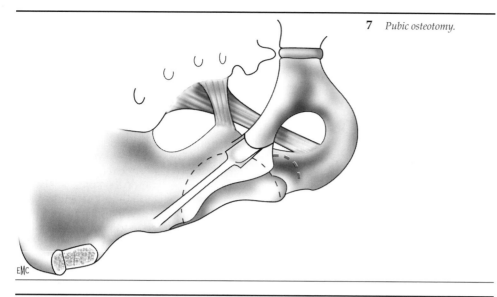

7 *Pubic osteotomy.*

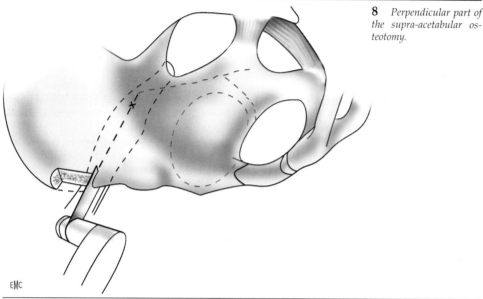

8 *Perpendicular part of the supra-acetabular osteotomy.*

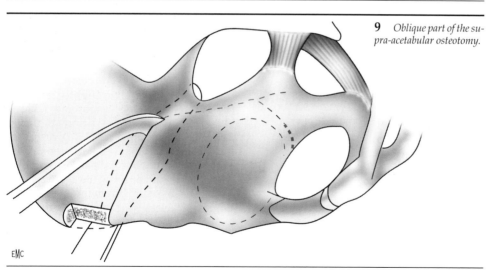

9 *Oblique part of the supra-acetabular osteotomy.*

possible. The edges of the anterior and posterior wall need to be balanced and should meet at the lateral edge. The centre of the femoral head must be at a correct distance from the linea ilio-ischiadica.

Only rarely is it necessary to add an intertrochanteric osteotomy (varus, extension). This is decided intraoperatively if the femoral head remains off centre and an abduction view shows reduction of the joint.

While waiting for the radiograph, an anterior T-shape capsulotomy is performed and the labrum is inspected [22]. Mobile tears are resected or repaired. A large os acetabuli will be fixed with a screw. The hip joint is then brought into flexion and internal rotation to verify a sufficient range of motion free of anterior impingement. If necessary, the anterolateral offset of the femoral head/neck junction is improved.

Definitive fixation of the acetabular fragment is accomplished using 3.5-mm cortical screws (*fig 11*). Two screws are inserted from the iliac crest; one anteroposterior screw is used from the anterior inferior spine in the direction of the sacroiliac joint. In osteoporotic bone, a short 3.5-mm reconstruction plate is used. Excess bone is removed from the acetabular fragment and inserted into the gaps.

The pars directa of the tendinous origin of the rectus femoris is reinserted to bone with non-resorbable sutures; the pars reflecta is repaired with the same suture material. The musculus ilio-capsularis is readapted to its bed with resorbable sutures. The fascial layers are closed with running sutures. The anterior superior iliac spine is reduced and fixed with a 2.7-mm screw. The abdominal wall muscles are reinserted onto the iliac crest.

Post-surgical care

The leg is placed in a foam splint. Prophylaxis against ectotopic ossification is not routinely used. The patient is mobilised on the second postoperative day. Weight-bearing of 5 kg is allowed. Straight leg raising is not permitted during six weeks because of the repaired muscle origins. At eight weeks post-operatively, the radiograph will show satisfactory bony healing. Progression to full weight-bearing and strengthening of the abductor muscles are then encouraged. At three months, patients can walk without crutches provided that the abductor muscles are sufficiently trained.

Special circumstances

The principal danger is an intra-articular osteotomy. In cases of an ovoid acetabulum with a high-riding femoral head, the first incomplete ischium osteotomy can accidentally enter the inferior border of the

osteotomy needs to be checked. The main correction is accomplished through anterior-distal rotation, which usually improves the lateral coverage as well. The corrected position is maintained by temporary fixation with 2.5 mm Kirschner wires having a threaded tip.

A radiographic AP view of the entire pelvis is then taken. It is important to verify the absence of rotation of the pelvis (the os coccyx must point strictly to the symphysis). The reduction of the acetabular fragment is then judged. The weight-bearing zone of the acetabulum must be as close to horizontal as

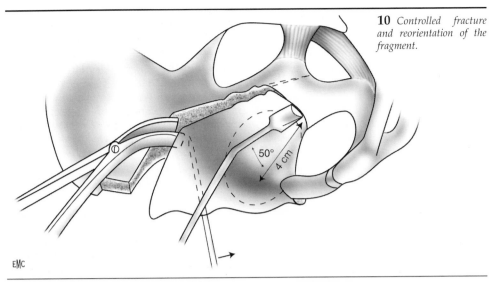

10 *Controlled fracture and reorientation of the fragment.*

osteotomy can also enter the joint if performed too far anteriorly. The latter osteotomy and the ischial osteotomy can damage the sciatic nerve.

Complications

Secondary loss of correction is the most important postoperative complication. If the acetabular fragment is not well balanced, the femoral head can re-sublux. Early full weight-bearing will tilt the fragment into overcorrection and possibly a protrusio of the femoral head can develop. In large corrections, a pseudarthrosis of the pubic osteotomy can develop; this is usually not symptomatic. Heterotopic ossifications occurred in the early periods of clinical application of this osteotomy. Since currently the abductors are not completely released but only tunnelled (over 3 cm along the iliac crest), no relevant heterotopic ossification has been observed, although no prophylaxis is administered. The 4.5-mm screws occasionally had to be removed because of the prominent screw heads. Since changing to 3.5-mm screws, this has no longer been observed.

Results

The results concerning the first group of patients with 75 periacetabular osteotomies were published in 1988 [8]. These patients were followed for 10-14 years. Pain and ambulatory capacity were improved significantly. In 58 cases (82%), the hip joint was preserved, and it functioned well in 73% of the cases. Negative factors for good long-term outcome were advanced age of the patients, moderate to severe pre-existing arthrosis and insufficient operative correction [26, 34]. Excluding these cases, the rate of very good results was 83%.

An in-depth analysis of the complications [14], based on 508 periacetabular osteotomies showed that 85% of the problems occurred during the first 50 osteotomies, indicating an significant learning curve. Eleven osteotomies entered the joint postero-inferiorly; two intra-articular osteotomies occurred posterosuperiorly. In 6 cases, the osteotomy fractured into the foramen ischidiadicum maius; one patient subsequently developed a migration of the acetabular fragment. Four of the fixations were unstable, one resulting in a loss of reduction, necessitating reoperation. Problems resulted from seven overcorrected and four undercorrected osteotomies. Undercorrection resulted in recurrence of the preoperative symptoms; overcorrection bears the danger of protrusio of the femoral head. Three cases of avascular necrosis of the acetabular fragment were observed. This complication is no longer seen, as the abductors are no longer taken down.

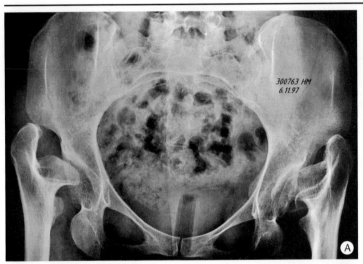

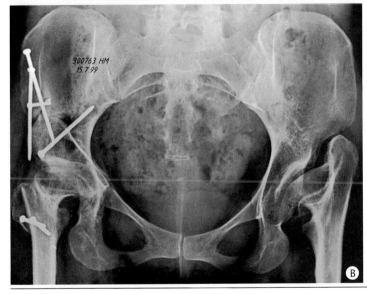

11 *34 year old female with severe bilateral acetabular dysplasia and Perthes-like deformity of both proximal femurs after conservative treatment of DDH in childhood.*
A. Preoperative hip morphology with more pain on the right side where the femoral head is subluxing.
B. Nearly two years after periacetabular osteotomy combined with trochanteric distal advancement and relative lengthening of the superior neck contour. On the right side, the patient has regained a stable and painfree hip. She is scheduled for the same procedure on the left side.

acetabulum. The pubic osteotomy should not be performed unless the pubic ramus has Berren completely protected with blunt retractors (obturator nerve and vessels). The osteotomy has to be medial to the eminentia ilio-pectinea. The periosteum needs to be incised, because otherwise the fragment cannot be sufficiently mobilised later. If the first cut of the supraacetabular osteotomy is too close to the joint, the vascularity of the fragment originating from the superior gluteal artery is endangered and the anchorage for the Schanz screw will be insufficient. The second part of the superior osteotomy can fracture into the foramen ischiadicum maius if it runs too close to the foramen; if it is too far distal, it can fracture into the joint. The third step of the superior

Problems specifically related to the approach are rare. They include 4 cases of relevant heterotopic ossification in the abductors. Dysaesthesias of the nervus cutaneous femoris lateralis occurred in about 30% of the patients, comparable to the rates that are described with the ilioinguinal approach [13, 14]. Over time, they usually improve and are well tolerated. The distal part of the incision crosses the Langer lines and frequently leads to large scar formation. Scar correction had to be performed only once.

Conclusion

The periacetabular osteotomy is a very technically-demanding operation with a high potential for correction. In-depth knowledge of the pelvic and hip anatomy is mandatory. Cadaver dissection and trial osteotomies are highly recommended. Large amounts of correction can be achieved. The fixation is minimal and immediate partial weight-bearing without external fixation is possible. The shape of the true pelvis is not altered. The potential for complications is high, although these have been rare in our experience after the first 50 osteotomies. Owing to this potential for complications, we feel that an orthopaedic surgeon wishing to perform this operation safely and to achieve adequate correction should do a minimum of 15-20 periacetabular osteotomies per year. Attempts at computer-assisted osteotomy and correction are promising [16]. Provided that patients are properly selected, this osteotomy can give long-lasting relief of the symptoms due to residual dysplasia of the hip, with minimal morbidity and simple rehabilitation.

References

[1] Aronson J. Osteoarthritis of the young adult hip: etiology and treatment. *Instr Course Lect* 1986 ; 35 : 119-128

[2] Carlioz H, Khouri N, Hulin P. Ostéotomie triple juxtacotyloïdienne. *Rev Chir Orthop* 1982 ; 68 : 497-501

[3] Chiari K. Ergebnisse mit der Beckenosteotomie als Pfannendachplastik. *Z Orthop Ihre Grenzgebiete* 1955 ; 87 : 14-26

[4] Cooperman DR, Wallenstein R, Stulberg SD. Acetabular dysplasia in the adult. *Clin Orthop* 1983 ; 175 : 79-85

[5] Crenshaw AH. Surgical techniques and approaches. In : Canale ST ed. Campbell's operative orthopaedics. St Louis : CV Mosby, 1998 : 82-84

[6] Eppright RH. Dial osteotomy of the acetabulum in the treatment of dysplasia of the hip. *J Bone Joint Surg Am* 1975 ; 57 : 1172-1172

[7] Flückiger G, Eggli S, Kosina J, Ganz R. Geburt nach periacetabulärer Osteotomie. *Orthopäde* 2000 (accepted for publication)

[8] Ganz R, Klaue K, Vinh TS, Mast JW. A new periacetabular osteotomy for the treatment of hip dysplasias. *Clin Orthop* 1988 ; 232 : 26-36

[9] Harris WH. Etiology of osteoarthritis of the hip. *Clin Orthop* 1986 ; 213 : 20-33

[10] Hersche O, Casillas M, Ganz R. Indications for intertrochanteric osteotomy after periacetabular osteotomy for adult hip dysplasia. *Clin Orthop* 1998 ; 347 : 19-26

[11] Hopf A. Hüftpfannenverlagerung durch doppelte Beckenosteotomie zur Behandlung der Hüftgelenkdysplasie und Subluxation bei Jugendlichen und Erwachsenen. *Z Orthop Ihre Grenzgebiete* 1966 ; 101 : 559-586

[12] Hoppenfeld S, DeBoer P. Surgical exposures in orthopaedics. In : The anatomic approach. Philadelphia : JB Lippincott, 1984 : 302-316

[13] Hussell JG, Mast JW, Murphy SB, Howie DW, Ganz R. A comparison of different surgical approaches for the periacetabular osteotomy. *Clin Orthop* 1999 ; 363 : 64-72

[14] Hussell JG, Rodriguez JA, Ganz R. Technical complications of the Bernese periacetabular osteotomy. *Clin Orthop* 1999 ; 363 : 81-92

[15] Klaue K, Durnin CW, Ganz R. The acetabular rim syndrome. *J Bone Joint Surg Br* 1991 ; 73 : 423-429

[16] Langlotz F, Bächler R, Berlemann U, Nolte LP, Ganz R. Computer assistance for pelvic osteotomies. *Clin Orthop* 1998 ; 354 : 92-102

[17] LeCœur P. Corrections des défauts d'orientation de l'articulation coxo-fémorale par ostéotomie de l'isthme iliaque. *Rev Chir Orthop* 1965 ; 51 : 211-212

[18] Love BR, Stevens PM, Williams PF. A long term review of shelf arthroplasty. *J Bone Joint Surg Br* 1980 ; 62 : 321-325

[19] Murphy SB, Ganz R, Müller ME. The prognosis of untreated dysplasia of the hip. *J Bone Joint Surg Am* 1995 ; 77 : 985-989

[20] Murphy SB, Kijewski PK, Millis MB, Harless A. Acetabular dysplasia in the adolescent and young adult. *Clin Orthop* 1990 ; 261 : 214-223

[21] Murphy SB, Millis MB, Hall JE. Surgical correction of acetabular dysplasia in the adult. *Clin Orthop* 1999 ; 363 : 38-44

[22] Myers SR, Eijer H, Ganz R. Anterior femoroacetabular impingement after periacetabular osteotomy. *Clin Orthop* 1999 ; 363 : 93-99

[23] Ninomiya S, Tagawa H. Rotational acetabular osteotomy for the dysplastic hip. *J Bone Joint Surg Am* 1984 ; 66 : 430-436

[24] Nishio A. Transposition osteotomy of the acetabulum in the treatment of congenital dislocation of the hip. *J Jpn Orthop Assoc* 1956 ; 30 : 482-484

[25] Salter RB. Innominate osteotomy in the treatment of congenital dislocation and subluxation of the hip. *J Bone Joint Surg Br* 1961 ; 43 : 518-539

[26] Siebenrock KA, Schöll E, Lottenbach M, Ganz R. Bernese periacetabular osteotomy. A minimal follow-up of 10 years. *Clin Orthop* 1999 ; 363 : 9-20

[27] Smith-Petersen MN. A new supra-articular subperiosteal approach to the hip joint. *Am J Orthop Surg* 1917 ; 15 : 592-595

[28] Smith-Petersen MN. Approach to and exposure of the hip joint for mold arthroplasty. *J Bone Joint Surg Am* 1949 ; 31 : 40-46

[29] Steel HH. Triple osteotomy of the innominate bone. *J Bone Joint Surg Am* 1973 ; 55 : 343-350

[30] Stulberg SD, Harris WH. Acetabular dysplasia and development of osteoarthritis of the hip. In : The hip. Proceedings of the Second Open Scientific Meeting of the Hip Society. St Louis : CV Mosby, 1975 ; 82

[31] Sutherland DH, Greenfield R. Double innominate osteotomy. *J Bone Joint Surg Am* 1977 ; 59 : 1082-1091

[32] Tönnis D. Eine neue Form der Hüftpfannenschwenkung durch Dreifachosteotomie zur Ermöglichung späterer Hüftprothesenversorgung. *Orthop Praxis* 1979 ; 15 : 1003-1005

[33] Tönnis D. Congenital dysplasia and dislocation of the hip in children and adults. 1987 Berlin : Springer-Verlag, 1987

[34] Trousdale RT, Ekkernkamp A, Ganz R, Wallrichs SL. Periacetabular and intertrochanteric osteotomy for the treatment of osteoarthrosis in dysplastic hips. *J Bone Joint Surg Am* 1995 ; 77 : 73-85

[35] Wagner H. Korrektur der Hüftgelenksdysplasie durch die sphärische Pfannendachplastik. In : Chapchal G ed. Beckenosteotomie-Pfannendachplastik. Stuttgart : Thieme, 1965 : 68-69

Legg-Calve-Perthes disease

A Catterall

Abstract. — The operative procedures related to the surgical management of children with Perthes' disease are identified and discussed. The indications for the various procedures are defined in terms of the pathology and clinical course of the disease, and the child requiring treatment is identified in terms of "at risk" signs. Various operative procedures can be considered, and the indications can be further defined by the use of the dynamic athrogram.

Keywords: paediatric hip, Perthes' disease, "head at risk" signs, femoral head, innominate osteotomy, lateral shelf acetabuloplasty.

Introduction

Despite the fact that Perthes' disease was recognised as a distinct entity over 90 years ago, its treatment still remains controversial [5, 18]. The pendulum of change in treatment has varied from all cases requiring treatment to a nihilistic view which suggests that, as it is a benign condition, no treatment is required. In recent years the concept of treatment for selected indications has becoming recognised [14]. Children over 8 years at presentation and those with "at risk" signs will require treatment in the early stages of the disease as will those with pain and hinge abduction in the late stages [17].

The pathology of femoral head deformity

Four processes may be recognised in the morphological changes in Perthes' disease [9]. There is a growth disturbance in cartilage which affects both the articular cartilage and the growth plate. There is evidence of an epiphyseal infarct, which involves a variable amount of the bony epiphysis. The infarct may have occurred on more than one occasion and is associated with fracture and crushing of the bony trabeculae in the

Anthony Catterall, M. Chir FRCS, Emeritus Consultant Orthopaedic Surgeon, Royal Medical Orthopaedic Hospital, London, United Kingdom.

weight-bearing area of the femoral head. Thirdly, there is a process of repair. The fourth is the presence of abnormal movement [8, 16].

The impact of the first three processes depends on the morphology of the femoral head at the time the insult occurs. In the younger child, there is a greater proportion of cartilage in the femoral head and the changes observed will be mainly an overgrowth of cartilage with some bony deformity. In the older child, where there is a greater proportion of epiphyseal bone within the femoral head, the effect of the crushing and fracture of the bony trabeculae will be more important, as an early change in head shape will occur.

During the course of the disease, following the infarction of the bony epiphysis, the articular cartilage thickens, particularly on the medial and lateral aspects of the femoral head. This results in a coxa magna. In the growth plate, there is inhibition of growth under the epiphyseal bone affected by the infarction. This growth disturbance tilts the femoral head on the long axis of the neck. In the epiphysis, there is evidence of recurrent bone infarction, which may or may not involve the whole epiphysis. In the weight-bearing part of the femoral head, fracture of the avascular trabeculae produces deformity and flattening of the femoral head which, particularly in the older child, may be associated with an anterolateral subluxation of the femoral head from the acetabulum. The process of repair re-establishes the normal growth processes within the femoral

head. It removes loose necrotic bone and allows union of the subchondral fracture. The subsequent re-ossification allows reconstitution of the subchondral bone plate and a resumption of the normal growth processes on the surface of the femoral head. Where the femoral head remains within the acetabulum, it usually stays round but if subluxation occurs, marked deformity may result.

On the clinical side, these three processes are usually associated with a fourth abnormality, an alteration of movement. There is a global and progressive loss of movement, particularly in the ranges of abduction and internal rotation. As a result of this, the femoral head begins to assume an adducted position with uncovering of the anterolateral segment. Where there is overgrowth of the anterolateral portion of the femoral head or a dysplastic anteverted acetabulum, this anterolateral segment comes to lie outside the confines of the bony acetabulum. Its lateral edge now begins to deform the femoral head, producing a dent in its soft load-bearing area. Attempted abduction in these circumstances changes from a movement of pure rotation of the femoral head within the acetabulum to one of hingeing of the flattened outer aspect of the femoral head on the lateral lip of the socket. This phenomenon is called "hinge abduction" [7, 12, 17]. The act of hingeing inhibits growth and ossification of the lateral aspect of the acetabular roof and induces a secondary acetabular dysplasia which further exacerbates the problem. The effect of this unstable movement is to induce a

Table I. – Signs of the "head at risk".

Clinical Signs
1. Progress of loss of movement.
2. The sign of "flexion with abduction".
3. Adduction contraction.
4. The heavy child.

Radiological Signs
1. Gage's sign.
2. Calcification lateral to the epiphysis.
3. Diffuse metaphyseal reaction.
4. Lateral subluxation.
5. Horizontal growth plate.

Table II. – Contraindications to treatment.

Early Stages
1. Group I cases.
2. Groups II, III not "at risk".

Late Stages
1. Cases where healing is established.
2. Cases where serious femoral head deformity is present without "hinge abduction".

Table III. – Indications for definitive treatment.

Early Stages
1. All "at risk" cases.
2. Groups II, III over 7 years.
3. Group IV cases where serious deformity has not occured.

Late Stages
1. Pain with hinge abduction.
2. Persisting fixed deformity.

Table IV. – Principles of treatment.

1. Restoration and maintenance of movement.
2. Reduction of forces through the hip joint.
3. Correction of subluxation.
4. Revascularisation of the necrotic bone with union of the subchondral fracture.

reactive synovitis in which spasm of the psoas and adductor muscles predominates, exacerbating the adducted position of the femoral head, which now becomes a fixed subluxation. Continuing overgrowth laterally, in the presence of this fixed subluxation, results in an irregular flattened femoral head. The irregularity is the result of pressure by the lateral edge of the acetabulum on the outer aspect of the femoral head.

Clinical recognition of femoral head deformity

In the early stages of femoral head deformity, there is a reduction in hip movement, particularly adduction and rotation. The adducted position of the leg results in an apparent shortening of the leg. As the hip starts to flex from this adducted position, it moves into the position of flexion and abduction because of the shape of the femoral head and the loss of rotation. This sign of "flexion with abduction" is present early during the process of femoral head deformity and is one of the "at risk signs" (table I) [4]. Treatment by restoring the normal axis of movement in the early stages will reverse the progression of the deformity, but persistence of the sign of flexion with abduction always implies progressive change. In the established condition, patients present with pain, limp and shortening.

Natural history

Many early reviewers justified treatment on the grounds that all cases did badly in the long-term. Some reports, however, suggested that good results could occur where the whole epiphysis was not involved in the process. A later report of untreated cases [4] highlighted the relatively benign nature of the condition. Fifty-eight percent achieved a good result without treatment. The prognosis was proportional to the degree of radiological involvement of the epiphysis, and radiological groups suggested assessing the degree of involvement. The concept of the "head at risk" was developed to identify cases which would do badly without treatment. These reflect both the clinical and radiological

features of progressive head involvement and are set out in table I. The prognosis was also proportional to the age of onset of the disease with poor results occurring in the older child. Approximately one-third of cases improved in the long-term by remodelling. The most important associated factors were the age of onset, the congruity of the joint at the time of healing and the range of abduction. The outlook for girls is less favourable than for boys. Stulberg et al [20] reported the long-term prognosis in relation to the shape of the femoral head at the time of healing. The highest incidence of osteoarthritis is seen in diseases starting over the age of 9 years, with a deformed femoral head occurring in a round acetabulum - "the square peg in a round hole".

Indications for and principles of treatment

Given the benign natural history of the condition, it is important to have indications for treatment so that unnecessary therapy can be avoided. In terms of the described pathology and the short- and long-term prognostic factors, the contraindications and indications for treatment are set out in tables II and III. Conservative treatment in which the child is free of any restrictive therapy is indicated where the growth disturbance is mild or where it has already occurred in cases presenting late in the disease. Definitive treatment will be required where the growth disturbance is likely to be severe (in all at risk cases and in the older child), or where deformity in the late stages is associated with pain and the phenomenon of hinge abduction. Treatment should not be delayed in the older child. The final indication is the child with a persistant fixed deformity, as such a hip will develop unstable movement in the long-term.

With an understanding of the pathology and the process of femoral head deformity, the principles of treatment may be defined

(table IV). These are the restoration and maintenance of movement, the reduction of forces through the hip joint, the correction of subluxation, and revascularisation of necrotic bone with union of the subchrondral fracture. Normal movement is required to prevent progressive deformity of the femoral head and to encourage remodelling. Abduction of the leg has two effects on the hip: first to reduce the forces through the joint [13] and second, to reposition the uncovered anterolateral aspect of the femoral head within the remodelling influence of the acetabulum. This reduction of forces through the joint should promote revascularisation of the infarcted bone and the re-establishment of normal growth. In addition, removing the abnormal forces from the lateral cartilaginous aspect of the acetabulum will allow it to resume a more normal appearance and growth. Where the volume of necrotic bone is large, as in the older child, a period of immobilisation may be required to allow revascularisation of this necrotic bone to prevent further trabecular fracture and collapse of the femoral head. When these principles are applied in the early and late stages of the disease, different methods of treatment will result. In the early stages, where the predominant pathology is cartilage overgrowth, restoration of movement, with the femoral head repositioned or contained within the acetabulum, is the method of choice. In the later stages, when serious deformity of the femoral head has occurred or healing is already established, restoration of movement with the joint congruous in the neutral position of weight-bearing allows the best long-term remodelling and prevents the long-term effects of hinge abduction. Containment is therefore a method of treatment, not a principle.

Assessment of growth disturbance and congruity of the joint (fig 1)

As there is no preventive treatment available, the child must be assessed on his/her first and subsequent visits and the decision made as to whether his progress is satisfactory: "doing well" or "doing badly" (table V) [2, 21]. Between these two situations, there are cases where there is clinical doubt ("don't knows"). These children require further investigation. Such an assessment must initially be clinical, supported by radiological examinations where appropriate. On each occasion, the stage of the disease must be recognised.

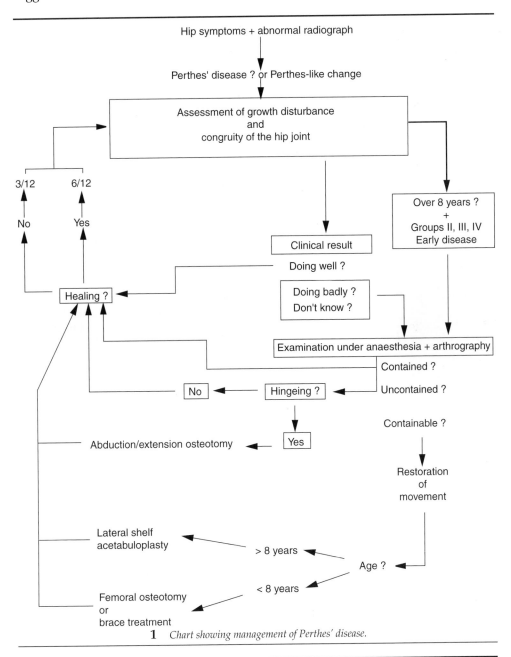

1 *Chart showing management of Perthes' disease.*

Perthes' disease. There is one essential investigation, the dynamic arthrogram, which defines the treatment required.

THE DYNAMIC ARTHROGRAM

■ *Indications*

A dynamic arthrogram is indicated in all cases where definite operative treatment is being planned as well as in unexplained pain in the hip.

■ *Procedure*

This is a dynamic assessment, performed under short general anaesthesia to look at the shape of the femoral head and the way the hip moves. It is of particular value in demonstrating the presence of unstable movement and the best position of congruity between the femoral head and the acetabulum. An image intensifier is essential for screening the hip in movement and for the assessment of head shape.

■ *Investigation*

This is undertaken in three stages.

Assessment of fixed deformity.

An examination under anaesthesia is performed to assess the extent of the fixed deformities present and the range of movement. This is compared to the pre-anaesthetic findings. Care must be taken to level the pelvis and relate movement to this fixed position. In many cases it will be found that there is no fixed deformity, but that movement is restricted under anaesthesia, compared to the opposite hip.

Demonstration of head shape

– Dye is injected into the hip joint under X-ray control using an anterolateral portal. Only 2-5 cc are required to outline the femoral head. Too much dye will obscure the view obtained.

– The shape of the femoral head is demonstrated anteroposteriorly, laterally and in the Billings position (20 degrees flexion, 10 degrees abduction, full external rotation). Deformity of the anterolateral segment of the femoral head in cartilage is best demonstrated by internal and external rotation of the leg in approximately 10-15 degrees of flexion and slight adduction.

Assessment of congruity

– The congruity of the joint is now observed using the image intensifier, as the hip is moved from adduction to abduction. Unstable movement will be first observed by rotating the leg in a few degrees of abduction. Typical hinge abduction may be noted as the leg is abducted, when the lateral aspect of the femoral head hinges on the cartilaginous or labral portion of the acetabulum.

Table V. – Clinical and radiological assessment.

	Doing well	Doing badly	Don't know
Clinical Factors			
Fixed deformity	No	Flexion/adduction	Flexion
Adduction	> 20°	> 5°	10°
Flexion with abduction	No	Yes	Yes
Radiological Factors			
Stage of disease	Any	Early	Any
Group	II, III, IV	II, III, IV	II, III, IV
Signs of "head at risk"	No	Yes	

Containment is contraindicated once healing has been established, unless congruity of the joint can be shown to be improved by position. Early disease in the older child demands separate and early arthrographic assessment as rapid deterioration in the shape of the femoral head may occur in these children *(fig 2)*. It must also be appreciated that continuing, intermittent discomfort is often present during the active phases of the disease in children who are simply being followed conservatively, without treatment. Recurrent acute symptoms or increasing discomfort may suggest deterioration. Parents must understand the natural history of the process through simple explanations and discussion [22].

The operations

With the above observations in mind, there are potentially three operations which can be considered in the surgical treatment of

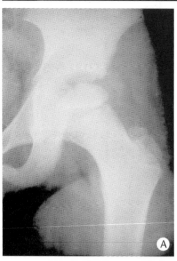

2 *Boy aged eight years who presented with a two-month history of right hip pain and limp. On examination, he localised his pain to the left thigh. There were 10 degrees of fixed flexion and no abduction. From the position of the fixed deformity, the hip flexed to 90 degrees and would adduct to 20 degrees.*
A. The AP radiograph shows the deformity of the femoral head with widening of the inferomedial joint space. There is narrowing of the ob-turator foramen.
B. The dynamic arthrogram shows that there is already early femoral head deformity and an increase in the medial joint space. The hip will centre in abduction.
C. The sequential radiographs 2 and 6 years following the lateral shelf acetabuloplasty show the remodelling of the femoral head that has oc-curred with time. The result is excellent and there is no alteration of the neck shaft angle.

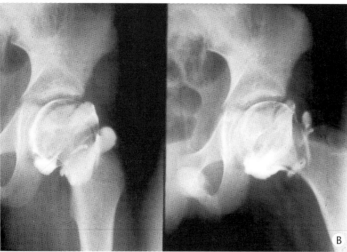

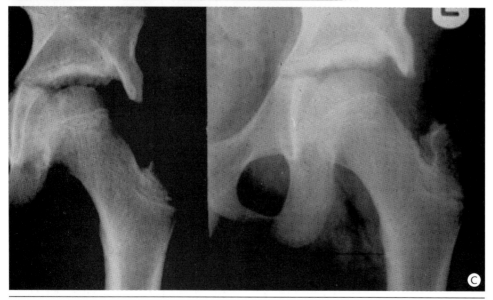

– The position of "best fit" or congruency is now assessed. In the majority of cases, this will be in the position of abduction + internal rotation for a "reducible subluxation" or containable hip and in adduction and flexion for the hip with hinge abduction. These positions identify the correction to be achieved at operation.

– Print-outs are taken to confirm the important observations of the investigation for the records.

LATERAL SHELF ACETABULOPLASTY [11, 23]

■ *Indications*

This is indicated if there is early presentation of a child over the age of 8 years, or in children between 5-8 years with "at risk" signs in Group II, III, IV disease in whom movement cannot be restored in the chosen position of realignment.

■ *Contraindications*

Lateral shelf acetabuloplasty is contraindicated in girls presenting over the age of 11 years with Group IV disease, and in children with unstable movement, with hingeing on a dynamic arthrogram.

■ *The operation*

Position

The patient is laid flat with a sandbag under the buttock.

Approach

– The incision is made below the iliac crest, passing below the anterior superior iliac spine. It then extends down in the line of the tensor fascia femoris.

– The interval between the tensor and sartorius muscles is developed and the lateral cutaneous nerve of the thigh is identified and mobilised.

– The tensor and gluteus medius muscles are elevated from the outer table of the ileum, which is exposed subperiosteally.

Dissection of the capsule and detachment of the rectus femoris

– The capsule is now cleared of fat and its overlying pericapsular fascia.

– The rectus femoris is dissected and its straight and reflected heads identified.

– The reflected head is detached from the straight head and mobilised on its proximal capsular attachment.

– The soft tissue between the capsule and the straight head of the rectus femoris is dissected so that bone can be placed anteriorly over the involved portion of the femoral head.

– At this stage the uncovered portion of the femoral head can be palpated as a lump. The object of the operation is to cover this "lump" with the lateral shelf of bone.

Acetabuloplasty

– A slot is now cut in the ileum just above the line of the capsular attachment and over the extent of the area for the acetabuloplasty *(fig 3)*. This usually extends to the proximal attachment of the rectus femoris. The direction of the slot is upwards and medial. It is just above the cartilage of the lateral acetabular epiphysis.

– Above this slot, a flap of bone based proximally is elevated from the outer table of the ileum.

– Corticocancellous bone is now obtained in strips from the outer table to provide enough bone to perform the acetabuloplasty.

– Strips of this bone sufficient to cover the uncovered portion of the femoral head or "lump" are now inserted into the pre-cut slot. This may be checked using an image intensifier.

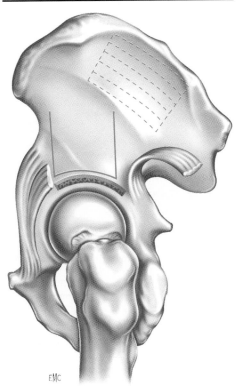

3 *A slot is cut in the ileum just above the line of the capsular attachment and over the extent of the area for the acetabuloplasty.*

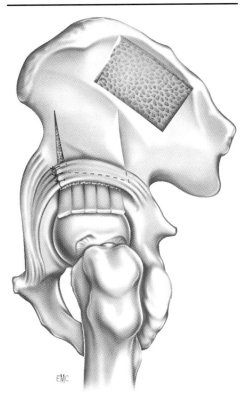

4 *Cancellous bone is packed under the elevated outer table.*

– Cancellous bone is now packed under the elevated outer table together with one or two strips of corticocancellous bone which are used to extend the outer table down to the lateral edge of the shelf of bone already inserted (*fig 4, 5*).

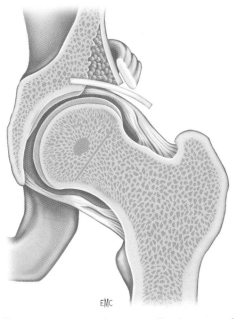

5 *One or two strips of corticocancellous bone are used to extend the outer table down to the lateral edge of the shelf of bone already inserted.*

– The rectus femoris is now reattached to the straight head, to help stabilise the graft that has been inserted.

Closure

The fasciae of the tensor fascia femoris and gluteus medius muscles are now reattached to the iliac crest.

If indicated, a suction drain is inserted between the graft and overlying muscles. The need for this is defined by the bleeding that has occurred.

The rest of the muscles are now repaired and the incision in the fascia lata closed.

A subcuticular stitch is inserted for skin closure.

Postoperative management

A check X-ray is taken to confirm that a shelf of satisfactory size has been inserted.

A 1 ½ spica is applied with the leg held in 15 degrees flexion, 15 degrees abduction and 15 degrees internal rotation.

The child is kept in hospital until his general condition is satisfactory. This is usually three to five days. For the first two days the child should be turned prone every four hours to allow the back of the plaster to dry.

The plaster cast is retained for a total period of nine weeks after which the child is readmitted for mobilisation. Physiotherapy and if possible hydrotherapy are required at this stage, but full weight-bearing may be permitted with the use of crutches.

The crutches are progressively discarded over a period of three to six weeks.

Routine follow-up is undertaken at 2, 5 and 8 months from operation. Follow-up at this point depends on progress. It can be on a six month basis once healing has established (*fig 2*).

FEMORAL OSTEOTOMY

Two types of femoral osteotomy can be performed during the course of the disease [6, 19]. Where containment is being or has been lost, a varus osteotomy is usually performed. In late disease, a valgus osteotomy is required to stabilise a hip with unstable movement and hinge abduction. It is essential that movement be restored in the chosen position of realignment when a varus osteotomy is performed. Failure to achieve this is often associated with poor results [7, 10].

■ *Indications*

Active stages

Groups II, III, IV with "head at risk" signs (doing badly) between the ages of 5 and 8 years and Group IV disease under the age of 5 years with "head at risk" signs with no central metaphyseal lesion.

Late stages

Pain with hinge abduction demonstrated on a dynamic arthrogram and persisting fixed deformity.

■ *Contraindications*

Femoral osteotomy is contraindicated when there is failure to restore movement in the chosen position for realignment.

Healing disease, unless congruity between the femoral head and acetabulum can be shown to be improved on a dynamic arthrogram.

■ *Position*

The child is laid flat for both a varus and valgus osteotomy with no sandbags under the buttocks.

■ *Approach*

– A standard approach is used for all osteotomies of the proximal femur.

– An incision is made on the lateral aspect of the thigh from the tip of the trochanter passing distally. The fascia lata is split in the line of the incision (*fig 6*).

– The vastus lateralis is identified and the distal overhang of the attachment of the gluteus medius muscle is released from the anterior aspect of the greater trochanter. Some bleeding is encountered, but better access to the anterior femur is obtained. An incision in the vastus lateralis is made in the line of its attachment to the femur, anteriorly and laterally (*fig 7*). Posteriorly, it extents down on the posterior margin of the attachment. Starting from the posterior corner, the muscle is elevated subperiosteally from the femur to expose both the anterior, lateral and posterior aspects of the bone. The muscle is retracted (*fig 8*).

– Using a periosteal elevator the anterior part of the neck is identified and a

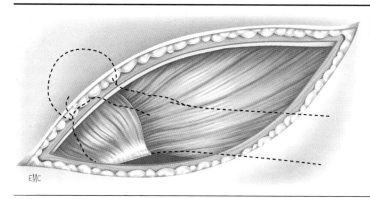

6 *The fascia lata is split in the line of the incision.*

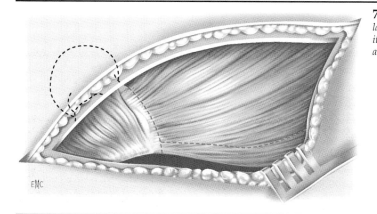

7 *An incision in the vastus lateralis is made in the line of its attachment to the femur, anteriorly and laterally.*

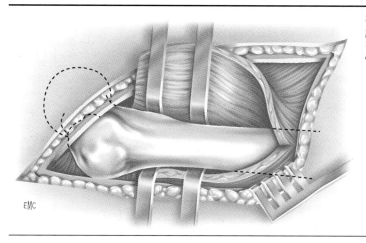

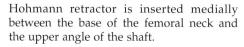

8 *The femur is now exposed subperiosteally, elevating the vastus lateralis medially.*

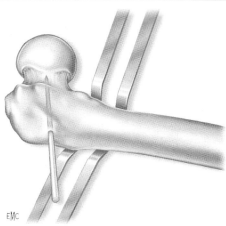

9 *A 2 mm Kirschner wire or small Steinmann pin is inserted through the flat lateral aspect of the femur just below the greater trochanteric growth plate up to the femoral neck under X-ray control.*

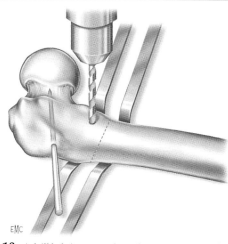

10 *A drill hole is now made on the anterior aspect of the upper femur. This will correspond to the second hole of a four hole femoral plate.*

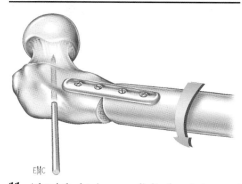

11 *A four hole plate is now applied to the anterior aspect of the upper shaft and the second screw inserted into the predrilled and tapped hole.*

Hohmann retractor is inserted medially between the base of the femoral neck and the upper angle of the shaft.

■ *Varus osteotomy*

– A standard lateral approach, as described above, is made to the proximal femur.

– The leg is placed in the position already established for realignment as the result of the dynamic arthrogram.

– A 2 mm Kirschner wire or small Steinmann pin is inserted under X-ray control through the flat lateral aspect of the femur just below the greater trochanteric growth plate up the femoral neck. It should be positioned parallel to the floor so that it can be used as a point of reference at the end of the operation *(fig 9)*.

– A drill hole is now made on the anterior aspect of the upper femur. This will correspond to the second hole of a four hole femoral plate. The drill hole is made at right angles to the floor. Its length is measured and tapped *(fig 10)*.

– A transverse osteotomy is now performed a few millimetres below the drill hole; this should be at right angles to the long access to the bone and to the floor.

– A subperiosteal dissection is now continued circumferentially distal to the shaft to allow correction of the rotation. The distal fragment is displaced medially by half its diameter and the leg twisted and realigned so that the patella points forward and the two legs are parallel. During this manoeuvre, the position of the proximal fragment should remain unchanged by holding the Kirschner wire.

– A four hole plate is now applied to the anterior aspect of the upper shaft and the second screw inserted into the predrilled and tapped hole. This screw should not be fully tightened *(fig 11)*.

– The two distal screws are now inserted into the plate. The drill should be positioned at right angles to the floor and the leg held so that the patella points directly anteriorly. Following this procedure the rotational element of the correction is now fixed.

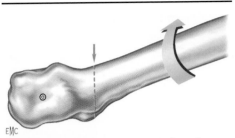

14 *The leg is now placed in the position for realignment which has already been established by the dynamic arthrogram. With the leg held in this position, an osteotomy is performed just below the Coventry screw.*

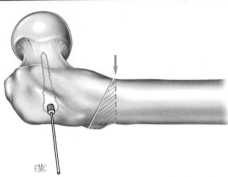

15 *A second osteotomy is performed at right angles to the long axis of the femur and the floor. The bony wedge is removed.*

– The leg is now placed in the position for realignment which has already been

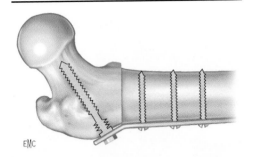

16 *The osteotomy is now closed and stabilised with an angled Coventry plate and screws.*

established by the dynamic arthrogram. With the leg held in this position, an osteotomy is performed just below the Coventry screw and at right angles to the patient and the floor *(fig 14)*. The leg is now returned to the neutral position with the patella pointing directly forward.

– A second osteotomy is performed at right angles to the long axis of the femur and the floor *(fig 15)*. The bony wedge is removed.

– The osteotomy is now closed and stabilised with an angled Coventry plate and screws. The angle of the plate must be adjusted to allow an accurate reduction of the osteotomy *(fig 16)*.

Closure

The vastus lateralis is repaired with a mattress suture, which reattaches its posterosuperior corner to its attachment. Other sutures are used to complete this repair.

The fascia lata is repaired. To ensure accurate closure, this should begin proximally and then continue distally.

The subcutaneous tissues are closed and the skin closed with a subcuticular suture.

After an X-ray has been taken to check that the position is satisfactory, a hip spica is applied.

Post operative course and mobilisation

The patient is placed on a Hamilton Russell type of traction.

Active movement is started on the day following operation. When the patient has regained active control of the leg, he is allowed to mobilise with limited weight-bearing on crutches. He is discharged home when safe on crutches.

The patient is reviewed at six weeks and thereafter at three month intervals for the first year. Once healing is established, follow-up can be at six month intervals.

References

[1] Banks MJ, Catterall A, Hashemi-Nejad A. Valgus extension osteotomy for hinge abduction in Perthes' disease. Results at maturity and factors influencing the radiological outcome. *J Bone Joint Surg Br* 2000 ; 82 : 548-554.

[2] Benson KD, Fixsen JA, Macnicol MF. Legg Calve Perthes disease. In : Children's orthopaedics and fractures. London : Churchill Livingstone, 1994 : 443-457

[3] Canario AT, Williams L, Wientroub S, Catterall A, Lloyd-Roberts GC. A controlled study of the results of femoral osteotomy in severe Perthes' disease. *J Bone Joint Surg Br* 1980 ; 62 : 438-440

[4] Catterall A. The natural history of Perthes' disease. *J Bone Joint Surg Br* 1971 ; 53 : 37-53

[5] Catterall A. Legg-Calve-Perthes syndrome. *Clin Orthop* 1981 ; 158 : 41-52

[6] Catterall A. The place of femoral osteotomy in the management of Legg-Calve-Perthes disease. *Hip* 1985 ; 24-27

[7] Catterall A. Adolescent hip pain after Perthes' disease. *Clin Orthop* 1986 ; 209 : 65-69

[8] Catterall A, Pringle J, Byers PD, Fulford GE, Kemp HB. Perthes''disease: is the epiphysial infarction complete? *J Bone Joint Surg Br* 1982 ; 64 : 276-281

[9] Catterall A, Pringle J, Byers PD, Fulford GE, Kemp HB, Dolman CL et al. A review of the morphology of Perthes' disease. *J Bone Joint Surg Br* 1982 ; 64 : 269-275

[10] Coates CJ, Paterson JM, Woods KR, Catterall A, Fixsen JA. Femoral osteotomy in Perthes' disease. Results at maturity. *J Bone Joint Surg Br* 1990 ; 72 : 581-585

[11] Daly K, Bruce C, Catterall A. Lateral shelf acetabuloplasty in Perthes' disease - A review at the end of growth. *J Bone Joint Surg Br* 1999 ; 81 : 380-384

[12] Grossbard GD. Hip pain during adolescence after Perthes' disease. *J Bone Joint Surg Br* 1981 ; 63 : 572-574

[13] Heikkinen E, Puranen J. Evaluation of femoral osteotomy in the treatment of Legg-Calve-Perthes disease. *Clin Orthop* 1980 ; 150 : 60-68

[14] Muirhead-Allwood W, Catterall A. The treatment of Perthes' disease. The results of a trial of management. *J Bone Joint Surg Br* 1982 ; 64 : 282-285

[15] Paterson DC, Leitch JM, Foster BK. Results of innominate osteotomy in the treatment of Legg-Calve-Perthes' disease. *Clin Orthop* 1991 ; 266 : 96-103

[16] Ponseti IV, Maynard JA, Weinstein SL, Ippolito EG, Pous JG. Legg-Calve-Perthes disease. Histochemical and ultrastructural observations of the epiphyseal cartilage and physis. *J Bone Joint Surg Am* 1983 ; 65 : 797-807

[17] Quain S, Catterall A. Hinge abduction of the hip. Diagnosis and treatment. *J Bone Joint Surg Br* 1986 ; 68 : 61-64

[18] Salter RB. The present status of surgical treatment for Legg-Perthes disease. *J Bone Joint Surg Am* 1984 ; 66 : 961-966

[19] Sponseller PD, Desai SS, Millis MB. Comparison of femoral and innominate osteotomies for the treatment of Legg-Calve-Perthes disease. *J Bone Joint Surg Am* 1988 ; 70 : 1131-1139

[20] Stulberg, SD, Cooperman DR, Wallensten R. The natural history of Legg-Calve-Perthes disease. *J Bone Joint Surg Am* 1981 ; 63 : 1095-1108

[21] Weinstein SL. Legg-Calve-Perthes disease: results of long-term follow-up. *Hip* 1985 ; 28-37

[22] Weinstein SL. Natural history and treatment outcomes of childhood hip disorders. *Clin Orthop* 1997 ; 344 : 227-242

[23] Willett K, Hudson I, Catterall A. Lateral shelf acetabuloplasty: an operation for older children with Perthes' disease. *J Pediatr Orthop* 1992 ; 12 : 563-568

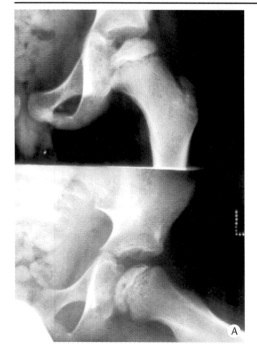

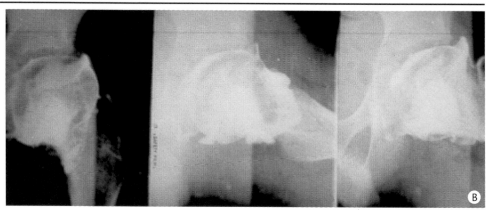

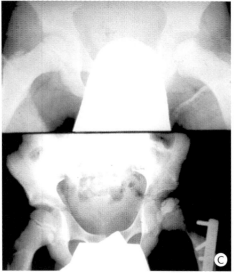

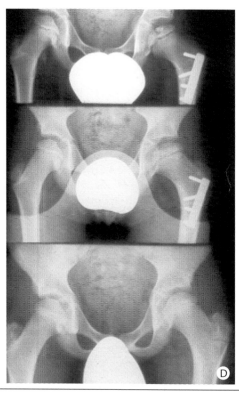

12 *Boy aged 6.5 years. There is a three-month hinge history of increasing pain and left sided limp. His walking distance is reduced. On examination the left leg lies 1.5 cm short, and there is a 10 degrees fixed flexion deformity. From the position of fixed deformity, the hip flexes to 90 degrees, but only abducts 50 degrees.*

A. AP radiograph of the pelvis and both hips. There is flattening of the femoral head and widening of the inferomedial joint space. The lateral radiograph shows Group III disease.

B. The dynamic arthrogram shows that there is already femoral head deformity with enlargement of the femoral head in cartilage. The overgrowth is mainly lateral. In abduction and in the frog position, the hip appears well seated and the overgrown portion of the femoral head lies within the acetabulum. It is therefore suitable for a realignment femoral osteotomy.

C. The radiograph at the top shows the appearance after two weeks in a broomstick plaster. The femoral head is now seated within the acetabulum in the same position as the arthrogram. After treatment by femoral osteotomy, the lower radiograph shows the position shortly after the plaster was removed.

D. The sequential radiographs at two, four and six years from operation. There is good remodelling of the femoral head and the varus which was induced by the operation has grown out as the condition has healed. The result in the long-term has been satisfactory.

– Holding the Kirschner wire in the predetermined position, a final adjustment is made to any varus or valgus correction and the second screw is tightened.

– The proximal screw of the four hole plate is now inserted and the Kirschner wire removed *(fig 11)*.

Closure

The vastus lateralis is repaired with a mattress suture which reattaches its posterosuperior corner to its attachment. Other sutures are used to complete this repair.

The fascia lata is repaired. To ensure accurate closure, this should be begun proximally and Perthen continue distally.

The subcutaneous tissues are closed and then the skin with a subcuticular suture.

After an X-ray has been taken to check that the position is satisfactory, a hip spica is applied.

Post operative treatment and mobilisation

The plaster is retained for six weeks.

At this point the patient is readmitted and the hip spica removed. Mobilisation is allowed with full weight-bearing with the use of crutches. The crutches are discarded progressively over the next four to six weeks, but may be needed for school.

The patient is reviewed at six weeks and thereafter at three month intervals for the first year. Once healing is established, follow-up can be at six month intervals *(fig 12)*.

■ *Valgus osteotomy* [1]

– A standard lateral approach is made to the proximal femur.

– The anterior aspect of the femoral neck and the angle between the inferior aspect of the femoral neck and the shaft are identified subperiosteally and a metal spike inserted to identify the position.

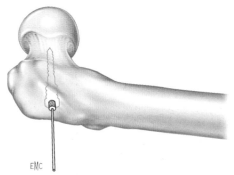

13 *A guide wire for a Coventry screw is inserted under X-ray control through the flat lateral surface of the femur, as close to the trochanteric growth plate as possible.*

– A guide wire for a Coventry screw is inserted under X-ray control through the flat lateral surface of the femur, as close to the trochanteric growth plate as possible. Its length is measured and a suitable Coventry screw inserted over it *(fig 13)*.

Slipped capital femoral epiphysis

H Carlioz
P Mary

Abstract. – Treatment of slipped capital femoral epiphysis is probably responsible for the serious early complications of the disease: osseous necrosis of the epiphysis and necrosis of cartilage. The danger lies in reduction of the displacement, whether as an emergency procedure for the acute situation or electively for the chronic form.
When there is only moderate displacement (up to 60°), treatment should therefore be limited to extra-articular screw fixation in situ.
When there is maximum, chronic displacement (90°), operative fixation using Dunn's operation is indicated as long as the junctional zone where slipping occurs—the former growth cartilage between the epiphysis and the femoral neck—is not ossified. If the junctional zone is already ossified, however, extra-articular osteotomy to reposition the upper extremity of the femur is an acceptable solution. This can only be done safely 6 to 12 months after closure of the junctional zone.
There is still no consensus as to the treatment of unstable, acute slipped epiphysis, for it is in this situation that early complications most frequently occur. Rather than emergency reduction of the displacement, our current preference is for cautious reduction in skin traction for one or two weeks, followed by extra-articular screw fixation to maintain the reduction thus obtained.
Prophylactic fixation of the unaffected contralateral capital femoral epiphysis, in our opinion, is an advisable precautionary measure. It is mandatory only when there is very extensive displacement on the affected side, i.e. more than 60°, which in itself increases the risk of early complications—osseous or cartilagenous necrosis—or the late complication of coxarthrosis.

© 2000, Editions Scientifiques et Médicales Elsevier SAS. All rights reserved.

Keywords: hip, children, femoral upper epiphysis, slipped capital femoral epiphysis, closed reduction, femoral head necrosis, femoral neck osteotomy, Dunn's operation, femoral neck osteotomy, pertrochanteric osteotomy, Kramer's operation.

Introduction

For each type of slipped capital femoral epiphysis (SCFE) – acute or chronic, major or minor displacement – there should be a logically corresponding treatment using well-defined techniques. This is the only way that the major risks of treatment, stiffening due to chondrolysis and osseous necrosis of the epiphysis, can be eliminated. Certain methods of treatment are particularly fertile grounds for such complications: attempts at forced orthopaedic reduction, immobilisation in plaster casts, and operations designed to reposition the epiphysis, whether intra-articular (femoral neck osteotomies) or extra-articular (intertrochanteric osteotomies).

Henri Carlioz, Chef de Service, Professor of Paediatric Orthopaedics and Reconstructive Surgery, University of Paris 6.
Pierre Mary, Assistant Chef de Clinique.
Hôpital Armand Trousseau, 26, avenue du docteur-Arnold-Netter, 75571 Paris, France.

Untreated SCFE, on the other hand, usually evolves without serious complications. Osseous necrosis of the epiphysis is almost always secondary to treatment. So too, probably, is stiffening due to chondrolysis (laminar coxitis).

We will deal first with the treatment of acute SCFE, then that of the chronic forms.

Acute slipped capital femoral epiphysis [2]

Sudden aggravation of the displacement can occur at any time, especially when the epiphysis has slipped by more than 30° or 40°. This results in pain and an absolute inability to move the leg. This is so-called "unstable" slipped epiphysis. When the child is seen shortly after SCFE of such sudden onset, an attempt to reduce the displacement should be made.

Two preliminary points are noteworthy:

– There is no definitive time interval, however approximate, after which repositioning of the epiphysis can no longer be carried out "orthopaedically". It is more important to consider inability to bear weight because of pain as proof that the epiphysis is unstable and that the sudden displacement is of recent onset.

– No attempt should be made to obtain perfect reduction, i.e. perfect positioning of the epiphysis in relation to the neck of the femur, which would signify a hyperre-duction endangering the epiphyseal blood supply. The epiphysis has already slipped by 20° to 40° when the acute displacement occurs. Reduction should do no more than return the epiphysis to that initial position.

CLOSED REDUCTION

In addition to a history of painful loss of use, certain signs on the hip radiograph allow assessment of the chances of reducing an acute SCFE:

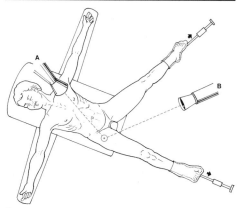

1 *Acute slipped capital femoral epiphysis (SCFE) on the right. Reduction of the displacement on an ortho-paedic table: traction in slight abduction without medial rotation. Direction of incident X-rays (image intensifier or 2 radiograph machines).*

– If the junctional zone where slipping occurs – the physis – is still open, the success of nonoperative reduction can reasonably be expected.

– If consolidation has begun and the physis is partly ossified, no such orthopaedic reduction can be expected, nor should it even be attempted.

Again, if the acute episode is not recent, and movement of the hip and weight-bearing are no longer painful, orthopaedic reduction should not be attempted. It is likely to end in failure and complications. In such cases, the radiological appearance is as described above, with partial or complete con-solidation of the displacement.

■ ***Closed reduction technique*** *(fig 1)*

The SCFE should be treated as an emergency. The less delay there is, the more easily the epiphysis can be repositioned. If reduction can only be carried out the next day, the child should be kept in bed, in longitudinal skin traction.

Closed reduction is attempted under general anaesthesia on an orthopaedic table. Two radiograph machines or an image intensifier should be available so as to provide anteroposterior and lateral views of the femoral neck.

No forcible manoeuvre should be undertaken to reduce the displacement. Manipulation should be limited to moderate, progressive traction in the neutral position, without flexion or rotation and in slight abduction. If reduction is not thus obtained within 5 or 10 minutes, traction is increased a little, but the radiological space between the epiphysis and the acetabulum should not increase, or should increase hardly at all. If a good reduction of the displacement is not obtained, there is a strong temptation to apply increased internal rotation and abduction. This should be resisted, and further attempts should be abandoned.

Indeed, even such a cautious approach may still be too brutal. If necrosis occurs, it is impossible to tell whether it is due to the

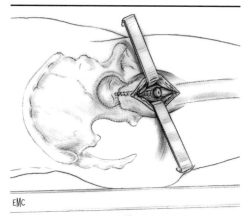

2 *Chronic or acute SCFE: extra-articular fixation. Lateral approach. Separation of vastus lateralis. Use of a single screw.*

suddenness of the slip, to immediate rupture of the medial femoral circumflex artery, or to manipulative treatment.

The procedure we have recently adopted, therefore, is as follows. On admission, the child is put to bed with both legs in skin traction. A radioisotope bone scan is requested. If the slipped epiphysis is very recent, traction alone will reduce it. The beginning of consolidation is allowed to take place over one or two weeks, after which the reduction is fixed with a screw. A further preoperative radioisotope bone scan and another scan several weeks later show whether the epiphysis is still viable or whether it is undergoing necrosis, and, if so, the point in time at which the ischemia occurred.

Reduction having been obtained, it must be maintained. Pelvis-to-foot plaster casts cause stiffening at the hip, and we never use them in the treatment of SCFE. The epiphysis therefore has to be fixed to the neck of the femur using a metallic internal fixation device, which in our case consists of a single calibre-7 screw.

Fixation by means of bone grafts, introduced by arthrotomy from the anterior aspect of the femoral neck towards the epiphysis, seems needlessly difficult to us. The ability of bone grafts to accelerate consolidation of the slip is hypothetical. Metallic internal fixation yields the same result with greater ease.

EXTRA-ARTICULAR SCREW FIXATION *(fig 2, 3, 4)*

The child is left on the orthopaedic table in the same position in which reduction of the slipped epiphysis has been obtained. The initially lateral approach is limited to 2 cm below the ridge for vastus lateralis. A narrow gap, created by separating the muscle fibres of vastus lateralis, is enough to allow 2 wires to be introduced, the best positioned of which will be used as a guide for the screw. The persistent displacement of the epiphysis necessitates a fairly anterior line of attack, at the junction of the anterior and lateral aspects of the trochanteric region.

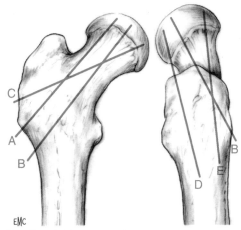

3 *Chronic SCFE.*
Ideal positioning of wires or screws: anteroposterior (A); lateral (B).
Imperfect positioning: anteroposterior (A and C); lateral (D and E).

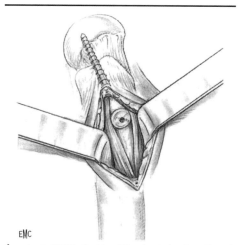

4 *Acute SCFE: fixation following reduction. Chronic SCFE: fixation in situ.*

The wire is directed upwards, inwards and backwards, so as to penetrate the epiphysis in its thickest, central part. If the wire is not ideally positioned but penetrates into the epiphysis nevertheless, it should be left in place for the moment, as it will be useful for preventing rotation of the epiphysis as the screw is tightened. A passage is prepared for the screw with an auger, using the best-placed wire as a guide. It is a good idea to "slip" the track for the screw within the femoral neck so as to obtain good tightening of the epiphysis to the neck. At no time should the articular cartilage be pierced, or the wire or screw allowed to enter the joint space, which would lead to stiffening as a result of necrosis of the cartilage. It is unnecessary for the screw to reach right into the periphery of the epiphysis, as its excellent hold in a centimetre or two of epiphyseal spongy bone will suffice. Both wires are withdrawn once the screw has been tightened. The screw should be directed quite far upwards, where the cortical bone gets thinner; if it is placed too low, in the thick part of the cortical bone, its entry hole will be at risk of subsequent fracture. We have never found it necessary to use two screws, which would probably not be without risk for the blood supply to the epiphysis.

The wound is closed, over a vacuum drain if necessary. Intermittent skin traction is set up. The patient is only permitted to bear weight 4 to 6 weeks later, when the junctional zone has closed. Meanwhile the hip is mobilised in bed, and walking with two elbow crutches allowed, without any weight-bearing on the affected leg until the time required for closure has elapsed.

If preventive fixation of the unaffected side is to be carried out, it can either be done immediately or a few days later.

The screws are removed only when the (radiological) translucency of the cartilage at the junction of epiphysis and femoral neck has disappeared.

OTHER METHODS OF FIXATION

Multiple wires provide fixation as solid as that obtained with a single screw, but their multiplicity increases the risk that the joint will be penetrated by one of them.

Chronic slipped capital femoral epiphysis

A number of preliminary remarks are necessary before describing operative techniques.

Correction of chronic displacement using a "closed" method, as described above for acute SCFE, should never be attempted.

A pelvis-to-foot plaster cast may prevent any progression of the displacement while closure of the growth cartilage is awaited, but such casts are uncomfortable and can also lead to stiffening. We never use them.

Osteotomy of the femoral neck is only rarely indicated, as it is difficult to perform and carries a risk of cartilage and bone necrosis. It should be considered only for cases with a maximum degree of displacement, close to 90°. The same restrictions apply to pertrochanteric osteotomy, which may be followed by stiffening due to necrosis of cartilage – although it is true that it involves no risk of bone necrosis.

Our policy, therefore, is to treat all cases of SCFE displaced by less than 60° with extra-articular screw fixation in situ. For greater displacement, we use either Dunn's operation, or pertrochanteric triple plane reorientation osteotomy. The choice between these two techniques principally depends on the state of the physis:

– If the physis has closed, we make do with a pertrochanteric osteotomy.

– If it is still open, Dunn's operation can be carried out, but so can pertrochanteric osteotomy, in which case the fixation material should cross the physis.

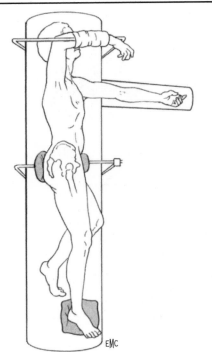

5 *Chronic SCFE. Position of the limb for anteroposterior view radiographs: no rotation, flexion or abduction.*

FIXATION IN SITU OF CHRONIC SCFE (DISPLACED BY 20° TO 60°)

The technique is the same as that described above. However, use of an orthopaedic table is not necessary; it is simpler to carry out the operation with the patient in lateral decubitus on an ordinary operating table. A single radiograph machine fixed in position, or an image intensifier set for horizontal use, allows anteroposterior and lateral views of the upper end of the femur to be obtained by repositioning of the limb (*fig 5, 6*).

The incision and approach are the same as those described for acute SCFE. It is possible to use only one wire, as there is no risk of rotating the epiphysis as the screw is turned. It is not necessary to "slip" the track of the screw within the femoral neck. If it has been decided to fix the good side preventively, this is done in the same operative program.

Weight-bearing on both sides is allowed from the second day onwards. No physiotherapy is necessary. Screws are only removed once any translucency of the growth cartilage has disappeared.

DUNN'S OPERATION [5, 11]

The purpose of this operation is to restore the normal orientation of the upper femoral epiphysis with regard to the femoral neck and acetabulum. Its originality lies in the fact that it safeguards the epiphyseal blood supply as much as is possible, thanks to the extensive lifting of periosteum which reduces tension on the posterior circumflex vessels, and also to the shortening and reshaping of the neck of the femur.

■ *Preliminary remarks*

In chronic SCFE, Dunn's operation should only be used when there is maximum

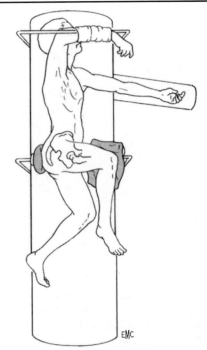

6 *Chronic SCFE. Position of the limb for lateral view radiographs: 90° flexion, 45° abduction, 10°- 20° medial rotation.*

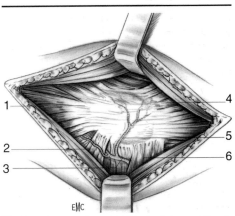

7 *Lateral approach to right hip. 1. gluteus medius; 2. piriformis; 3. medial circumflex femoral artery; 4. vastus lateralis; 5. trochanteric branch of medial circumflex femoral artery; 6. quadratus femoris.*

displacement of the epiphysis, and when no previous treatment has been attempted. In acute SCFE, Dunn's operation may be used following an (unsuccessful) attempt at closed reduction as described above. Should other treatments have been tried, it is inadvisable to resort to this difficult technique whose risks are increased by any previous interventions.

■ *Operative technique* (fig 7, 8, 9, 10, 11)

The patient is positioned in lateral decubitus. A straight, vertical skin incision is made, some 20 cm long, centred on the greater trochanter. The fascia lata and gluteus maximus are incised in the same line, and below them, the two edges of gluteus medius and the pelvitrochanteric muscles. The vastus lateralis is detached from its insertion ridge, from the anterior aspect of

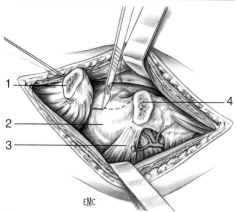

8 *Opening the joint capsule after section of the greater trochanter. 1. greater trochanter, raised; 2. joint capsule; 3. piriformis; 4. greater trochanter.*

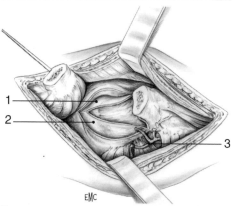

9 *Removal of periosteum from the femoral neck. 1. capsule and anterior periosteum; 2. posterior periosteum; 3. posterior circumflex artery.*

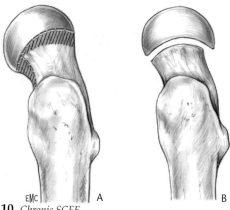

10 *Chronic SCFE.*
A. Posterior osteophyte (in gray). Bone resection (in rose).
B. The shortened and remodelled neck.

the greater trochanter, and over a distance of 2 or 3 cm from the diaphysis.

Identification of the circumflex vessels

At the posterior edge of the gluteus medius lies a branch of the medial circumflex femoral artery, which runs along it. Lower down lies another branch running to the lateral aspect of the greater trochanter.

The posterior circumflex artery itself lies behind the obturators and gemelli, and then plunges under the piriformis. It needs to be

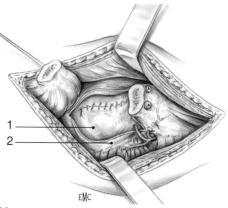

11 *Following fixation, the periosteum is replaced and closed (1). The capsule is shown still open (2).*

retracted away from the trochanter by turning it outside along with its accompanying fat tissue. It must be possible to reach the posterior edge of the greater trochanter without any risk of damaging the artery.

Section of the greater trochanter

Using a bone chisel, the greater trochanter is lifted up along with gluteus medius. The gluteus minimus often remains adherent to the capsule and must be detached from it separately.

Arthrotomy and removal of the periosteum from the femoral neck

The proximal aspect of the capsule is exposed anteriorly and incised in the axis of the femoral neck. The periosteum is incised at the anteroproximal edge of the femoral neck and then stripped of the whole of its periphery. Along with it, the insertion of the capsule is detached from the trochanter. However, at this stage of the operation, the periosteum is not detached from the posterior aspect of the femoral neck, being trapped between the neck and the slipped epiphysis. Only when the epiphysis has been separated from the femoral neck can the periosteum and the vascular bundle be easily stripped from the femoral neck.

Isolation of the epiphysis

With the help of a foam spatula, the plane in which the epiphysis has slipped is reconstituted little by little, starting at the anterior pole of the epiphysis, from inside outwards. It is now only held behind by the vessel-containing periosteum, which has been carefully stripped off the femoral neck. Immediately, the epiphysis spontaneously returns to its place within the acetabulum.

Cutting the neck of the femur

Economic resection of the metaphysis puts the femoral neck back into the right orientation and shortens it a little. The posterior osteophyte is chiselled away until the original cortical bone is reached.

Reduction and fixation

There should now be no difficulty in bringing the femoral neck back into line with the epiphysis by manipulating the

greater trochanter using Farabeuf's forceps. As soon as reduction seems easy, the femoral neck is dislocated again. Three wires are inserted into it, from the outside inwards, until they just reach its epiphyseal edge. They should be parallel with each other. The best-centred of the three will be used to guide the screw, while the other two will prevent the epiphysis from rotating while the screw is being turned. Reduction is resumed, the wires are pushed into the epiphysis, and anteroposterior and lateral radiographs are taken to check the quality of the reduction and the positioning of the wires. The best-placed wire is replaced with a screw and washer, to ensure good contact between femoral neck and epiphysis as the screw is tightened.

Closure

The periosteum and joint capsule are sutured, the greater trochanter is fixed in position with two screws, and the outer layers are closed over a vacuum drain.

Postoperative care

Skin traction makes immediate mobilisation possible. The child can start walking on the eighth day using elbow crutches, but weight-bearing on the operated side is only allowed once consolidation of the osteotomy has been radiologically confirmed.

PERTROCHANTERIC OSTEOTOMY
(fig 12, 13) [8, 9]

When SCFE is of maximum displacement, but Dunn's operation is not the chosen method of treatment—either on principle or because the junction cartilage is closed—pertrochanteric or subtrochanteric osteotomy can recentre the epiphysis in the acetabulum. This involves a combination of two basic repositionings of the cervico-epiphyseal segment, valgus and extension, together with medial rotation of the diaphysis. The rotation acts only on the position of the limb and not on the centring of the joint.

Preoperative calculation of each contributing element is difficult. We start by taking recentring views in maximum degrees of adduction, lateral rotation and extension. We generally end up with a position about 30° towards valgus and 30° to 40° towards extension. The diaphysis is rotated by whatever amount will balance lateral and medial rotation.

■ *Operative technique*

The fixation material to be used, a flange-plate or nail-plate, should be one that when put carefully in place will automatically ensure the required reorientation of the epiphysis after osteotomy.

Setting up

The patient is placed in the dorsal decubitus position on an ordinary operating table. It must be possible to take anteroposterior and lateral radiographs throughout the operation.

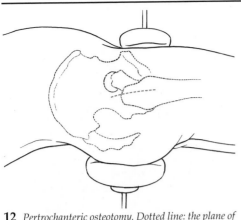

12 *Pertrochanteric osteotomy. Dotted line: the plane of the osteotomy. Positioning of the temporary 90° nail-plate. The flange is in flexion with regard to the diaphysis (2). Following osteotomy and exchange of nail, the plate, brought down against the diaphysis, will shift the epiphysis into extension. 1. gluteus medius.*

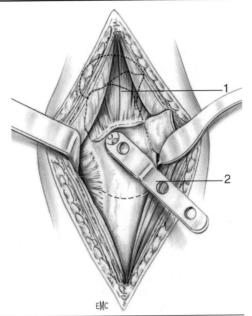

13 *Pertrochanteric osteotomy. Diagram of the positioning of the 90° nail.*
A. Anteroposterior view.
B. Lateral view.

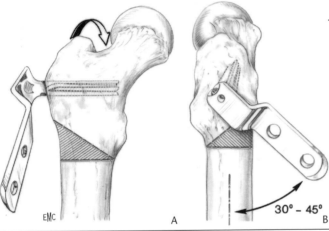

30° – 45°

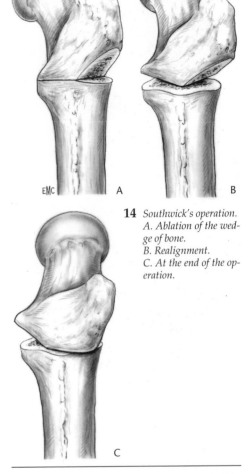

14 *Southwick's operation.*
A. Ablation of the wedge of bone.
B. Realignment.
C. At the end of the operation.

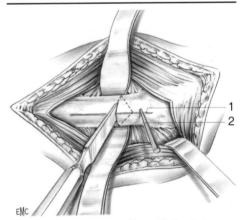

15 *Resection of the wedge of bone. The border between the anterior and posterior aspects of the femur is marked (1). A Chanz screw facilitates manipulation (2).*

Approach

The approach is a lateral one, as for any pertrochanteric osteotomy. The insertion of vastus lateralis is removed from the ridge of the trochanter and from several centimetres of the diaphysis.

Osteotomy

For the cervico-epiphyseal segment to be repositioned in valgus and extension with precision, a 90° nail-plate or flange-plate is used to start with. This allows the track of the final material within the femoral neck to be prepared, and it is the position of the plate that prepares for extension.

The nail or flange is introduced at a right angle to the axis of the diaphysis, and in line with the anteverted femoral neck. The flange is displaced anteriorly with regard to the diaphysis by an angle equal to the required degree of extension (30° to 40°, as we have explained). The plane in which osteotomy should be carried out is difficult to imagine. It can therefore be carried out in 2 stages to avoid any risk of the cut edges being in the wrong planes. The first cut is made horizontally, a centimetre lower than usual with regard to the hole for the nail.

This leaves room for a lateral cuneiform resection. Before these cuts in the bone are made, wires to pinpoint rotation are inserted on each side of the line.

The final material (110°, 120° or 130° according to the degree of valgus required) is put in place, before or after osteotomy, in its prepared track within the femoral neck. The plate is put in a position of flexion, which will put the femoral neck and epiphysis into extension when fixation is complete. Fixation is attained by holding the plate against the diaphysis using forceps and securing it in place with screws. Should excess muscular tension make it difficult to get the fixation material into place, it can be loosened by resecting a further 5 to 10 mm from the osteotomy. Lateral and medial rotation of the hip must be balanced, and it is therefore often necessary to rotate the diaphysis medially by 20° to 40° before completing the fixation.

The outer layers are closed over a vacuum drain.

Postoperative care

The limb is maintained in slight flexion at the hip and knee for 3 to 4 weeks. After this period, walking on crutches without weight-bearing on the side of the osteotomy is allowed.

SOUTHWICK'S PERTROCHANTERIC OSTEOTOMY TECHNIQUE
(fig 14, 15, 16, 17) [12, 13]

The following technique can be adapted to slipped epiphysis of 30° to 70°.

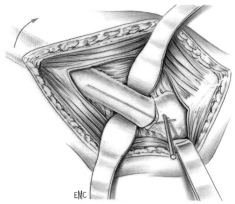

16 *Closure of the wedge in flexion, abduction and medial rotation.*

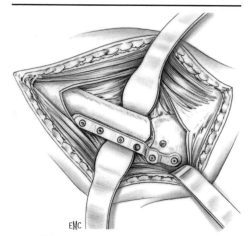

17 *Maintenance using internal fixation.*

■ *Operative technique*

The child is set up in the dorsal decubitus position. The approach is lateral, as for the technique just described.

A line marking the junction between the flat, anterior aspect, and the slightly convex, lateral aspect of the femur is cut with an osteotome. Another, transverse mark is then cut, perpendicular to the first, at the level of the smaller trochanter. A laterally-based 25° wedge of bone will be removed from the anterior aspect of the femur, and another 50° wedge from the lateral aspect. Both wedges share a base on the anterolateral border (marked). Their distal edges are in line and correspond to the transverse mark, and their third edges meet at a point on the anterolateral border. Each wedge of bone is resected within these marked-out edges. The two cut surfaces should be sufficiently flat to fit one another properly. A Chanz screw in the proximal fragment, parallel to its cut surface, makes it easier to manipulate. Osteotomy is then carried out at the level of the smaller trochanter.

The thigh is placed in an abducted and flexed position, bringing the resected surfaces of bone into contact, and opening up the lesser trochanter like a book with an elongating effect. The osteotomy is then maintained in position with an external fixation device or, preferably, by internal fixation using a flange or nail-plate.

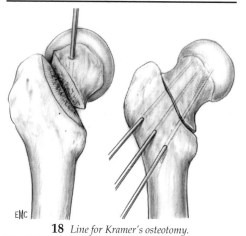

18 *Line for Kramer's osteotomy.*

Follow-up

Weight-bearing, at least partial, is allowed straight away. Fixation material is removed 12 to 24 months later.

Note: This technique is much used in English-speaking countries. In our opinion, however, neither the preoperative calculations nor the actual procedure are precise enough. In particular, it seems incorrect to consider rotation of the diaphysis to be a factor in reorientation of the epiphysis.

KRAMER'S BASE-OF-NECK OSTEOTOMY *(fig 18)* [1, 3, 7]

Anatomically halfway between Dunn's operation and the pertrochanteric osteotomies, Kramer's osteotomy is made at the base of the femoral neck; it is wedge-shaped with an anterior base.

■ *Operative technique*

The child is placed in dorsal decubitus on an orthopaedic table. The recommended anterolateral approach is a Watson-Jones. A T-shaped opening is made in the joint capsule and periosteum along the intertrochanteric line and down the anterior aspect of the femoral neck. The insertion of the vastus lateralis is removed from the lateral aspect of the femur.

The plane of the first osteotomy is distal, along the anterior intertrochanteric line and perpendicular to the axis of the femoral neck. It is chiselled, without ever going beyond the posterior cortical bone so as to avoid any risk of damaging the medial circumflex femoral artery. A large-bore retaining wire is then inserted into the proximal part of the femoral neck.

The line of the second osteotomy is inside the first, and is also perpendicular to the axis of the neck. The posterior convergence of the two planes removes an anteriorly based wedge. Three large-bore threaded wires are inserted into the trochanteric base of the femoral neck and directed towards the osteotomy. The leg is abducted and medially rotated to close the resected area as the weakened posterior cortical bone

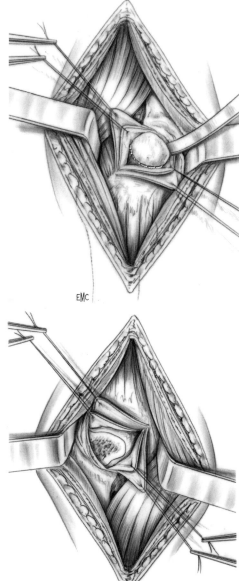

19 *Heyman's operation. After resection of the pathological outgrowth.*

undergoes greenstick bending. The wires are then pushed in as far as the epiphysis to maintain the correction that has thus been obtained. A vacuum drain is left in place in front of the closure of the joint.

Postoperative care

Weight-bearing is only allowed once consolidation of bone has occurred, i.e. about two months later.

HEYMAN'S OPERATION OR PHYSEAL REMODELLING *(fig 19)* [14]

Posterior slipping of the epiphysis tilts the anterior and medial part of the femoral neck forwards. In flexion, this projecting mass comes up against the anterior edge of the acetabulum and either limits mobility or else enters the acetabulum and scrapes the joint cartilage. Both possibilities are harmful, butfortunately the lump often gradually disappears. Indications for trimming it down with Heyman's operation are therefore rare. The operation can be used to complete the effect of a pertrochanteric osteotomy.

■ *Operative technique*

The patient is placed in dorsal decubitus. Hueter's approach is sufficient, as long as the common tendon of the rectus femoris is sectioned and turned downwards. The joint capsule is incised in the axis of the femoral neck. The slipped epiphysis is not visible, and the metaphysis constitutes an anterior projection whose blockage against, or penetration within, the acetabulum in flexion can be confirmed. It is resected as necessary, from outside inwards, with a curved chisel. At the end of the procedure, the anterior aspect of the femoral neck should be concave and should present no further obstacle. The insertion of the common tendon of the rectus femoris is reattached and the outer layers are closed over a vacuum drain.

Weight-bearing is permitted as of the following day.

Summary of indications for treatment

IN ACUTE SCFE:

1. either an attempt at gentle reduction, under general anaesthetic, using traction alone on an orthopaedic table, followed by maintenance of the result using extra-articular screw fixation;
2. or (our currently preferred option) continuous traction in bed for one or two weeks, followed by screw fixation.

IN CHRONIC SCFE:

1. screw fixation in situ for displacements up to 60°;
2. Dunn's operation for 90° displacements, when the epiphysis is still separated from the femoral neck by an unbroken radiological translucency;
3. triple effect pertrochanteric osteotomy for displacements of more than 60°, especially when translucency has disappeared;
4. Kramer's operation, with the same indications as pertrochanteric osteotomy.

When SCFE is unilateral, we always perform preventive screw fixation of the epiphysis on the contralateral side. This approach is not universally accepted, because of the risks involved in operating, small though they may be, and also because it is difficult to assess the risk of the problem becoming bilateral in terms of incidence. In our opinion, preventive fixation would seem mandatory, at the very least, when the future of the affected hip is uncertain, i.e. after acute SCFE or a major degree of displacement.

We have not described epiphyseal fixation in situ with bone grafts – Howorth's operation – as it seems to us more difficult than screw fixation without being more effective. Nor have we described the femoral neck osteotomies [4, 6, 10] – Compère's, Lagrange's and Muller's operations – as they seem less logical and more dangerous than Dunn's operation in terms of the blood supply to the epiphysis.

References

[1] Abraham E, Garst J, Barmada R. Treatment of moderate to severe slipped capital femoral epiphysis with extracapsular base-of-neck osteotomy. *J Pediatr Orthop* 1993 ; 13 : 294-302

[2] Aronsson DD, Loder RT. Treatment of the unstable slipped capital femoral epiphysis. *Clin Orthop* 1996 ; 322 : 99-110

[3] Barmada R, Bruch RF, Gimbel JS, Ray RD. Base of the neck extracapsular osteotomy for correction of deformity in slipped capital femoral epiphysis. *Clin Orthop* 1978 ; 132 : 98-101

[4] Derosa GP, Mullins RC, Kling TF Jr. Cuneiform osteotomy of the femoral neck in severe slipped capital femoral epiphysis. *Clin Orthop* 1996 ; 322 : 48-60

[5] Dunn DM. The treatment of adolescent slipping of the upper femoral epiphysis. *J Bone Joint Surg Br* 1964 ; 46 : 621-629

[6] Fish JB. Cuneiform osteotomy of the femoral neck in the treatment of slipped capital femoral epiphysis. A follow-up note. *J Bone Joint Surg Am* 1994 ; 76 : 46-59

[7] Kramer WG, Craig WA, Nicols SR. The compensating osteotomy for severe slipped femoral capital epiphysis. *J Bone Joint Surg Am* 1966 ; 48 : 1488

[8] Maussen JP, Rozing PM, Obermann WR. Intertrochanteric corrective osteotomy in slipped capital femoral epiphysis. A long-term follow-up study of 26 patients. *Clin Orthop* 1990 ; 259 : 100-110

[9] Merchan EC, Na CM, Munuera L. Intertrochanteric osteotomy for the treatment of chronic slipped capital femoral epiphysis. *Int Orthop* 1992 ; 16 : 133-135

[10] Nishiyama K, Sakamaki T, Ishii Y. Follow-up study of the subcapital wedge osteotomy for severe chronic slipped capital femoral epiphysis. *J Pediatr Orthop* 1989 ; 9 : 412-416

[11] Rey JC, Carlioz H. Épiphysiolyses à grand déplacement. Réduction sanglante par la technique de Dunn. *Rev Chir Orthop* 1975 ; 61 : 261-273

[12] Salvati EA, Robinson JH Jr, O'Down TJ. Southwick osteotomy for severe chronic slipped capital femoral epiphysis: results and complications. *J Bone Joint Surg Am* 1980 ; 62 : 561-570

[13] Southwick WO. Osteotomy through the lesser trochanter for slipped femoral capital epiphysis. *J Bone Joint Surg Am* 1967 ; 49 : 807-835

[14] Wong-Chung J, Strong ML. Physeal remodeling after internal fixation of slipped capital femoral epiphysis. *J Pediatr Orthop* 1991 ; 11 : 2-5

Hip deformity in cerebral palsy

JU Baumann†
R Brunner

Abstract. – Children with cerebral palsy develop skeletal deformities at the hip joint level due to alteration of forces acting on the growing bones. The increased femoral anteversion presenting with increased internal and decreased external rotation at the hip may require surgical correction, while valgus deformity is commonly overestimated on standard AP hip X-rays. The surgical technique and planning of the osteotomy are described in detail.

Hip dislocation is another common deformity, especially in severely handicapped children. The resulting pain and instability may impede the rehabilitation progress. The coxa valga et antetorta are combined with a channel-like deformation of the acetabulum, allowing the femoral head to slide out. The technique to repair this deformity is described. It combines a femoral and pelvic osteotomy, an open reduction, a capsulorrhaphy and an iliopsoas transfer.

To obtain a lasting correction, it is recommended that any bony surgery be postponed, if possible, to the age of 8 years or later. Earlier correction runs the danger of a recurrence of the skeletal deformation, due to the same abnormal forces acting during the growth period.

An adequate correction of the bony deformities at the hip joint facilitates rehabilitation of the patient by combining mobility with stability and freedom from pain. This enables any possible progress to be made in the individual patient and avoids destructive measures which interfere with function.

Keywords: hip, cerebral palsy, hip deformity, femoral osteotomies, periacetabular osteotomy.

Preface

Jürg U. Baumann dedicated his work to improving the living quality of handicapped people, especially patients with cerebral palsy. For his great experience and understanding care, he was loved by his patients and highly appreciated by his colleagues. In the midst of his work, he suddenly and unexpectedly died, leaving this chapter unfinished. This manuscript has been completed according to his principles and opinions by his former co-worker who is well acquainted with his treatment strategies and ideas.

Introduction

In children with cerebral palsy (CP), the musculoskeletal system is regularly normal at birth. The isolated defects in the organs of supraspinal motor control affect task-oriented sensory-motor functions. The subsequent aberrations in the temporo-spatial pattern of forces acting on the growing musculoskeletal system lead to a series of secondary deformations. Their rate of development depends on the speed of growth, their intensity, on the kind and severity of pathological movements, as well as on the loads on bones, muscles and ligamentous structures. These secondary deformities are particularly important around the hip joints.

The speed of growth is fastest during the first three years of life, but then slows down. It accelerates again before puberty, between 9 and 11 years of skeletal age in girls and from 11 to 13 years in boys. Deformities tend to be most severe in the presence of spasticity, less in prevalent dystonia with rigidity and in dyskinesia, such as athetosis.

Severe secondary skeletal deformities occur particularly in spastic tetraparesis with total body involvement (TBI). They can progress to neurogenic hip dislocation with typical femoral and pelvic changes, as well as scoliosis.

Neurogenic hip dislocation in children with CP is more incapacitating than "Developmental Hip Dysplasia" and subsequent hip dislocation. Spastic muscle hyperactivity and joint incongruence produce a vicious cycle of pain and instability, which increases the difficulties in sitting, standing and walking due the neuromuscular problems. However, children with CP are regularly born with normal hip joints. Their joints, which are usually well-formed, become deformed later and may finally dislocate, often between age 1 and 7 years [7]. Skeletal hip joint operations in CP children can be more than "salvage procedures", as they often result in almost normal hip joints [2]. With suitable care, the congruence of the joint surfaces can further improve during the remaining period of growth. The details of long-term postoperative management are highly important for the result in the adult, because the disorders of neuromuscular control persist and tend to produce recurrences or new and different deformities.

In clinical experience, particular danger for the integrity of the hip joints originates from the extensor spasticity in the trunk and lower extremities being stimulated and

Jürg U Baumann†, M.D.
R Brunner, M.D.
Paediatric Orthopaedic Department, Children's Hospital, Basle University, Basle, Switzerland.

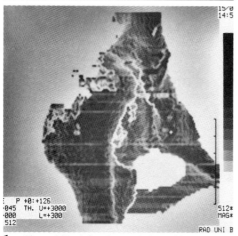

1 *Channel-like deformity in a dislocated hip joint. It is best seen in 3 dimensional reconstructions based on CT-scans.*

facilitated by excitement or weight-bearing, both sitting and standing. This leads to intensive spastic muscle contractions in all hip and knee extensors and adductors with co-contraction in antagonists such as the iliopsoas. This produces biomechanically harmful postures and movements in a position of extension, adduction and internal rotation of the thighs in relation to the pelvis and acetabulum.

The skeletal deformities at the hips observed in severe spastic CP consist of:

– Increased femoral anteversion (usually 50 to 80° of true anteversion).

– Increased femoral neck-shaft angle (usually 130 to 150° CCD).

– A channel-like defect due to compression of subchondral bone stock by the femoral head, mainly posterosupero-laterally in the acetabular roof *(fig 1)*.

In addition, the joint capsule is distended.

The deformities of femur and acetabulum are caused by the same factors of neuromuscular and biomechanical pathophysiology. The overwhelming intensity, duration and frequency of pathological muscle contractions and co-contractions lead to plastic deformation of both femur and acetabulum. Internal rotation, adduction and extension of the thigh lead to increased femoral anteversion and coxa valga, but the forces are strong enough to also produce compression damage by the femoral head to the posterosuperior aspect of the acetabulum, which extends into a gliding channel for the femoral head, facilitating hip dislocation *(fig 1)*. The skeletal deformations can be well repaired. The maintenance of the corrections is favoured by the end of skeletal growth, as well as by muscle tension-reducing postures.

It should be emphasised that increased femoral anteversion alone does not significantly alter the position of the femoral head and neck from normal in relation to the acetabulum in these children with their habitual internal rotation of the thighs.

During spontaneous movements and positions, their knees remain internally rotated by some 20° less than their measured anteversion. For assessment of joint congruity in function, the anteroposterior hip radiograph should be taken with corresponding internal rotation of the hip.

Operative indications

In a child aged 8 to 10 years with spastic diplegia, walking with internal rotation of 40 to 60°, the passive internal rotation at the extended hip joints is usually increased to 60, 70 or 80° with restriction of external rotation to around neutral. Hip radiographs, AP in neutral rotation (Dunn-Rippstein I) and an anteversion view, allow calculation of the true neck-shaft (CCD) angle and femoral anteversion (AT), as well as evaluation of the shape of the acetabulum. The CCD angle is only mildly increased in prevalent spasticity, but anteversion regularly measures 50 to 70°. In the "corrected position" of hip abduction by 20° and internal rotation by 50°, for example, the hip joint congruence is often normal. This is a clear indication for an isolated intertrochanteric femoral derotation–varus osteotomy, which should move the average functional axis for hip flexion-extension of the patient's hip joint obliquely into the frontal plane and thus help to restore a more normal gait pattern.

Femoral and pelvic joint reconstruction are indicated in the presence of severe subluxation with a lateralisation index of the femoral head of 50% or more, and when there is complete hip dislocation, even in the presence of severe multiple impairment, because this improves the quality of life, not only of the patient, but also of his caretakers, by facilitating long-term care. If the general health of the patient permits, it is possible at any age. Stable long-term results, however, have been observed in children aged 8 years or older [3]. In the presence of moderate subluxation, better long-term results and technical advantages are obtained by conservative treatment [1] up to age 8 or 9, i.e. to an optimal age for the success of this considerable surgery.

These interventions consist of a series of operative procedures, not all of them being necessary in every hip joint operated. If all are indicated in severe subluxation or complete dislocation, the single interventions must overlap or intersect as in a puzzle, and should be carried out in one operative session. Careful preoperative planning is essential for success.

The steps of orthopaedic surgical treatment for neurogenic hip sub- and dislocation in CP consist of:

1. Intertrochanteric femoral varus-derotation osteotomy with additional femoral shortening.

2. Open joint reduction.

3. Transposition and reinsertion of the trochanter minor with fractional lengthening of the iliopsoas. An anterolateral iliopsoas transfer (Mustard procedure modified) is valuable, but often unnecessary.

4. Acetabular reconstruction by a partial spherical acetabular osteotomy.

5. Capsular reefing.

Some femoral shortening always occurs in femoral derotation-varus osteotomy. This leads to relative elongation of the pelvi-femoral muscles including hip adductors. Whether additional aponeurotic muscle elongation of hip adductors and ischiocrural muscles is needed can be evaluated before femoral plate removal to permit combination of these interventions. Functional muscle training should immediately follow musculotendinous surgery.

Surgical procedures

ISOLATED FEMORAL DEROTATION VARUS OSTEOTOMY

■ *Indication*

Intertrochanteric femoral derotation-varus osteotomy alone

The procedure can bring particular benefit to children and young adults with the typical gait pattern of spastic diplegia or moderate tetraplegia with marked internal rotation of the thighs. The intervention can be seen not only under the aspect of rotation but also has an effect on the hip, knee and foot. By itself, it improves hip joint congruence in mild to moderate hip subluxation. It also reduces the dangers of treatment by exercise in standing and walking with externally rotated hip joints, irrespective of the presence of increased femoral torsion.

Girls should preferably be above age 8 and boys above age 10, optimally around skeletal age 11 in girls and 13 in boys. They should present with marked internal rotation gait and increased femoral anteversion of 45° or more, passive external rotation of the extended hip joint of 20° or less, and with congruent hip joints in the habitual position of internal rotation. The procedure with its important details, as described by M.E. Müller [4, 5, 6], has provided consistently reliable results with a minimal complication rate in CP patients. The surgical techniques described are based on materials recommended by the AO-ASIF Group (1992/2000). Intensive postoperative physiotherapy is needed for a year, in order to allow the control system to adjust to the restored anatomical situation and to overcome difficulties with equilibrium reactions while standing or walking. This must be made clear to patients and caretakers before the intervention.

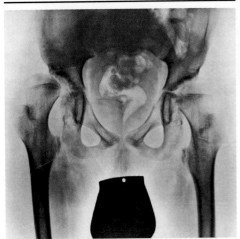

2 *Hip dislocation in standard AP view (same patient).*

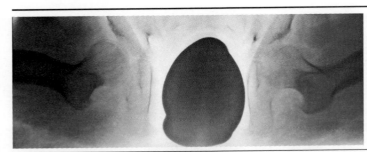

The treatment team should realise that in these persons with their habitual internal rotation of the femoral shaft, the transverse rotation of the femoral head and neck in relation to the pelvis and acetabulum remains nearly normal. Increased femoral anteversion is not a hip deformity. The femoral deformity, however, leads to internal rotation of the knee and often of the foot. The flexion-extension axis is rotated inward.

■ Contraindications

Surgical interventions which are useful for children near the end of skeletal growth frequently lead to recurrent skeletal deformation and to adverse neuromuscular compensations in younger children, aged 3-4 years, thus increasing the difficulties of long-term therapeutic management, including orthopaedic surgery. In spasticity, the true neck shaft angle is often almost normal. The damaging deformity of coxa valga is often not realised, but suggested by the radiographic projection in the presence of a marked increase of femoral anteversion on an image in the standard anatomic position of the extremity, which is abnormal for the patient.

■ Operative planning

– Gait documentation by video images, AP and lateral, or complete gait analysis is recommended for preoperative functional assessment and documentation.

– Radiographs for surgical planning: AP hip radiographs in neutral femoral rotation (Dunn-Rippstein I) and "anteversion view" (Dunn-Rippstein II), for measurement of the angles at the proximal end of femur (fig 2, 3). For surgical planning, an additional image in the corrected femoro-pelvic position, a posteroanterior (PA) view with anteversion fully corrected to 0 by internal rotation of the thighs, according to the amount of anteversion, as well as under abduction by the amount of planned correction of the neck-shaft-angle, is an essential help (fig 4).

– Graphic planning: copies of the AP and PA hip radiographs are made on transparent

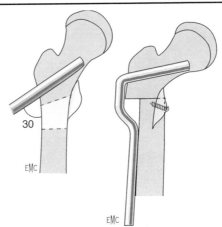

4 *Hip dislocation correction view (same patient).*

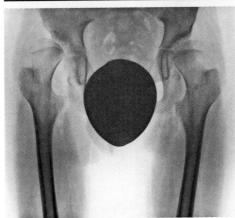

5 *Schematic drawing of the operation: the seating chisel is inserted at an angle of 180° - amount of varisation - angle of blade plate. The level of insertion of the seating chisel, of the osteotomy and the amount of shortening is determined.*
Operation on the right (28.10.98). Femur: CCD 145°, AT 40°.
Planned correction: Derotation, 20°; varisation 20°; shortening 15 mm; plate chosen: children 35 mm, 100°; open hip reduction, pelvic osteotomy; transposition of lesser trochanter (iliopsoas lengthening optional).

paper and the planned correction, including the chosen plate, are drawn in. This increases the safety and speed of the intervention, also reducing blood loss (fig 5).

■ Surgical procedure

The patient is placed on a radiolucent table with the pelvis inclined some 15° to the opposite side. The lower abdomen, pelvis and the entire leg are prepared and draped, thus preserving hip mobility.

Under general anaesthesia, a straight lateral incision is made from the tip of the greater

trochanter distally for 15-20 cm. The subcutaneous tissue and the fascia lata are divided in the same line. The interval between the anterior border of the gluteus medius and vastus lateralis is developed, and narrow Hohmann levers are inserted at the calcar femoris medially and laterally around the neck at the level of the tip of the greater trochanter. The vastus lateralis muscle is detached by an L-shaped incision along its proximal and posterolateral insertions to the femur. It is detached subperiosteally from the femur and reflected medially. The femoral neck is prepared on its anterosuperior aspect, avoiding the ascending branches of the medial and lateral circumflex arteries (fig 6). An incision in the upper anterior midline of the femoral neck opens the joint capsule. A Kirschner wire is positioned over the femoral neck; its tip is pushed into the base of the femoral head, indicating the direction of the neck. A second Kirschner wire is inserted into the greater trochanter in the plane of femoral anteversion and parallel to the planned angle of insertion of the plate.

The plate-seating instrument is now inserted immediately distal to the innominate tubercle with its epiphyseal cartilage of the greater trochanter, in the plane of the femoral neck and parallel to the guide wire in the greater trochanter, to a depth in accordance with the length of the blade plate planned for this patient. To avoid damage to the medial femoral circumflex artery and its branches supplying the femoral head posteriorly, the seating chisel must be inserted anteriorly in the femoral neck (fig 7).

Two cm distal to the guide blade, an intertrochanteric osteotomy is performed at a right angle to the axis of the femoral shaft, while the soft tissues including the medial femoral circumflex artery are carefully protected posteriorly by a wide Hohmann retractor.

In accordance with the planned varisation, a wedge cut off from the medial half of the shaft by a second osteotomy adds to the femoral shortening desired in these patients.

The plate-seating instrument is now extracted by gentle tapping and the blade plate is immediately inserted in exactly the same direction. The two femoral fragments are reduced by externally rotating the distal femur to a remaining anteversion-angle of the femoral neck, in relation to the axis of the knee joint, of 15 – 20°. The plate is

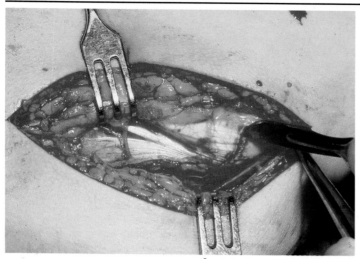
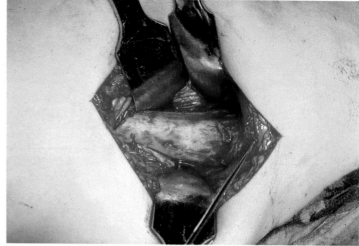

6 *Lateral approach to the femur after detachment of the vastus lateralis muscle.*

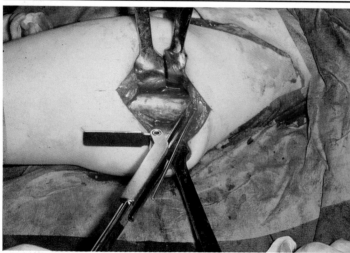

7 *Seating chisel in situ (guide wire shows planned angle of insertion).*

provisionally fixed by a Verbrugge compression clamp. Screws of correct length are inserted according to the AO technique to fix the plate to the femur and compress the osteotomy.

The wound is irrigated, inspected, treated for any remaining blood loss and supplied with deep suction drainage. The insertions of the vastus lateralis muscle are reattached by interrupted sutures. The wound is closed in layers.

■ Postoperative treatment

For pain control, the hip and knee joints are positioned in mild flexion and neutral rotation. No fixed immobilisation is used and non-weight-bearing treatment by gentle assisted active exercise is resumed the day after the operation.

The intradermal continuous suture is removed after 3 weeks. Wound compression by adhesive strips is advocated for 3 months and can be replaced by compression stockings to prevent hypertrophic scars. When recovery is uncomplicated, sitting in a wheelchair is resumed after 4 weeks, partial weight-bearing in a swimming pool after 4 weeks, and full weight-bearing following radiological control 6 weeks postoperatively.

Therapeutic exercise and gait training 2 to 3 times a week, as well as controlled home exercises, are advocated for one year.

■ Pitfalls and mistakes

The most dangerous complication of intertrochanteric osteotomy is avascular necrosis. It arises as a result of injury to the posterior retinacular vessels. During surgery, it may occur as a result of the reflection of the soft tissues from the posterior aspect of the intertrochanteric area, or by damage to the retinacular vessels due to faulty insertion of the seating chisel or plate, which may inadvertently enter the intertrochanteric fossa and cut the vessels.

Loss of position of the proximal femoral fragment can occur when the fixation is not sufficiently stable. This can happen if the blade breaks out of the fragment or if there is insufficient bone contact at the site of the osteosynthesis medially, leading to an insufficient medial buttress. Fixation can also be lost if the bridge of bone between the blade-plate and the osteotomy is too thin, because the blade may become loose or the bridge may break. In these instances, the situation can be saved by using the AO hook plate, gripping the trochanter major over its

top as far anteriorly as possible, thus avoiding damage to the retinacular vessels.

HIP JOINT RECONSTRUCTION, INCLUDING OPEN JOINT REDUCTION, INTERTROCHANTERIC DEROTATION VARUS AND SHORTENING OSTEOTOMY, ACETABULAR RECONSTRUCTION BY SPHERICAL PELVIC OSTEOTOMY

■ Indication

Neurogenic hip subluxation and complete dislocation

Optimal results are obtained in children with spastic tetraplegia including mixed types, with dystonia and dyskinetic components, at the age of 8-13 in girls and 10-15 in boys. Complete anatomical open joint reduction is facilitated in the presence of advanced subluxation or dislocation, because access to the primary acetabulum with the transverse acetabular ligament and the origin of the ligamentum teres is easier than in mild subluxation. Forceful dislocation of the femoral head must be avoided to protect its delicate circulation.

The patients complain most frequently of pain during exercise and while changing position, or inability to walk due partially to hip joint instability. Most patients have never before been able to walk even with support.

The goal of treatment is to permit standing and walking with support for transfer, freedom from pain and improved sitting posture, which also supports trunk and head control, as well as mobility of the upper extremities.

■ Contraindications

There are no absolute contraindications. A skeletal age of below 8 years is a relative contraindication because of danger of recurrence. After the end of growth, less perfect adaptation between an often deformed femoral head and the reconstructed acetabulum must be expected, with occasional mild pain in these non–ambulatory patients with their multiple impairments. Severe disorders of behaviour in adults requiring immediate postoperative mobilisation make total joint replacement a preferable alternative.

Detailed clinical and radiological evaluation, sometimes computed tomography with 3D-reconstruction and imaging, or additional separate modelling of the proximal femur and acetabulum, are prerequisites for regular success. Good functional results of skeletal reconstruction may be difficult to obtain following extensive previous soft tissue surgery, particularly adductor tenotomies. In children below age 4, age adapted procedures such as those recommended for developmental hip dysplasia should be used.

■ *Preoperative examination*

– Assessment of the passive range of motion of hip, knee and ankle joints, spine examination for neurogenic deformity, pelvic obliquity while sitting. General medical and neurologic examination to avoid surgical risks unacceptable for a planned reconstructive procedure.

– Radiography: Hip joints and proximal femur in neutral rotation of the thigh AP (Dunn-Rippstein I and Dunn-Rippstein II) as a basis for joint assessment and operative planning (*fig 2, 3*). The Dunn-Rippstein II view in 90° of hip flexion and 25° of abduction not only permits the calculation of the true neck-shaft and anteversion angles, but also provides an informative projection of the acetabulum in CP patients, with their regular hip flexion contractures tending to tilt the pelvis in the AP view.

– A preoperative CT with 3-dimensional optical reconstruction is very helpful to determine the direction of the acetabular elongation for optimal positioning of the patient and correction of the acetabular deformity.

■ *Operative procedure*

Preoperative planning

The planning of the varus-derotation-shortening osteotomy of the femur is based on a frontal radiograph with anteversion compensated by internal rotation (*fig 4*) in order to show the undistorted neck-shaft angle. A schematic drawing of the planned operative procedure is helpful to determine the amount of varus correction and femoral shaft shortening. The latter can be fine-tuned during the intervention (*fig 5*).

Access to the acetabular rim (first prepared by the anterolateral approach)

With the patient supine in 15 degrees of inclination toward the unaffected side, the skin on the involved side is prepared over the abdomen, the pelvis and the entire lower limb and draped, maintaining a freely mobile hip joint. The oblique skin incision

extends from 1 cm below the junction of the middle and posterior third of the iliac crest to 2 cm below the anterior superior iliac spine, continuing medially and distally to below the midline of the inguinal ligament. The subcutaneous tissue is divided. Over the iliac crest, the deep fascia and iliac apophysis are incised down to the bone. The fascia lata is opened from the anterior superior iliac spine distally, following the sartorius muscle. The lateral femoral cutaneous nerve is freed as it crosses the sartorius 2.5 cm distal to the anterior superior iliac spine from proximal medial to distal lateral, then protected by medial retraction. The groove between the tensor fascia lata muscle laterally and the sartorius and rectus femoris muscles medially is deepened by blunt dissection.

With a broad periosteal elevator, the lateral part of the iliac apophysis and the periosteum with the tensor fascia lata, gluteus medius and minimus muscles is stripped from the iliac wing down to the superior rim of the acetabulum anteriorly and the greater sciatic notch posteriorly.

The straight head of the rectus femoris originating from the anterior inferior iliac spine and the oblique head from the superior border of the acetabulum are dissected, marked by whip sutures, cut and reflected distally. The hip joint capsule is exposed superiorly, anteriorly and posteriorly by blunt and sharp removal of its fatty layer and the attaching fibres of the iliacus. The iliopsoas muscle can be elongated by 2-3 intramuscular transsections of its aponeurotic tendon as far proximal as possible. The wound is now packed with wet sponges and left open.

Femoral osteotomy

A straight lateral incision is made from the tip of the greater trochanter distally for 15-20 cm. The subcutaneous tissue and the fascia lata are divided in the same line. The interval between the anterior border of the gluteus medius and vastus lateralis is developed, and narrow Hohmann levers are inserted at the calcar femoris medially and laterally around the neck, at the level of the tip of the greater trochanter. The vastus lateralis is detached by an L-shaped incision along its proximal and posterolateral insertions to the femur. It is detached subperiostally from the femur and reflected medially. The femoral neck is prepared on its anterosuperior aspect, avoiding the ascending branch of the lateral circumflex artery which runs at the base of the greater trochanter. An incision in the upper anterior midline of the femoral neck opens the joint capsule. If there is marked hip subluxation, the available space allows the division of the transverse acetabular ligament and the acetabular insertion of ligamentum teres by this approach. A Kirschner wire is positioned over the femoral neck, and its tip is pushed into the base of the femoral head, indicating the direction of the neck. A

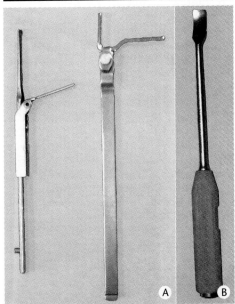

8 *Special instruments used for hip reconstruction.*
A. Seating chisel with AO hip blade plate.
B. Swan-neck chisel.

second Kirschner wire is inserted into the greater trochanter in the plane of femoral anteversion and parallel to the planned angle of insertion of the plate.

The seating chisel (*fig 8A*) is now inserted just distal to the innominate tubercle with its epiphyseal cartilage of the greater trochanter, in the plane of the femoral neck and parallel to the guide wire in the greater trochanter to a depth in accordance with the length of the blade plate chosen for this patient.

Two cm distal to the guide-plate, intertrochanteric osteotomy is performed at a right angle to the axis of the femoral shaft, while the soft tissues are protected posteriorly by a wide Hohmann retractor. The femoral shaft fragment is now shortened by the required amount obtained from the preoperative planning. If the minor trochanter is included, it is cut from the shaft by an oscillating saw, and a whip suture is attached to it and the psoas tendon. The femoral wound is inspected and treated for bleeding vessels, then packed with wet sponges.

Open hip reduction

Attention now returns to the anterolateral approach. A broad Hohmann lever is inserted into the greater sciatic notch and a small lever around the anterior inferior edge of the ilium. The capsule and synovium are incised parallel to the rim of the acetabulum at a distance of about 1 to 1.5 cm, the cut extending well anteriorly and posteriorly. At a right angle to it, a second incision completes the T-shaped approach. The free capsular edges are marked by whip sutures for later traction and reefing. The femoral head is inspected. Even severe damage to its cartilaginous surface and deformation by long-acting pressure are no impediment for the restoration and maintenance of a mobile hip joint with little or no pain in these patients. The ligamentum teres is cut at its insertion to the femoral head, then traced to its insertion at the acetabular notch and excised by one anterior and one posterior cut, thus avoiding injury to the acetabular branch of the obturator artery. It is essential to divide the transverse acetabular ligament, because it can effectively inhibit full reduction. The fibro-fatty tissue in the depth of the true acetabulum is excised.

The femoral head can now be reduced free of tension into an anatomical position in the acetabulum. This permits inspection and assessment of the location and depth of the deformation of the acetabular roof.

Spherical acetabular osteotomy

A cut around the acetabulum is made at a distance of some 8 mm from its rim, passing below the anterior inferior iliac spine and extending posteriorly to the cortex of the sciatic notch, by using a special spoon-shaped and spherical chisel of a diameter slightly greater than that of the acetabular surface (Swan-neck chisel, Synthes (fig 8B)). At the preferred age for the intervention, the depth of the osteotomy reaches some 2.5 cm. The osteochondral zone of the acetabular lip must not be damaged. The lamella of the acetabular roof must be thin enough to allow sufficient tilting of the anterior-superior rim downward and the posterior rim forward. The gap is filled with corticospongious bone grafts from the intertrochanteric varus-derotation-shortening osteotomy of the femur. It can be wedged in safely. No metallic fixation is used. Movement of the femoral head is now well centred.

Capsuloplasty is performed to reduce the large posterosuperior pocket. The capsule is pulled medially and closed by double-breasting sutures. Capsular material may be abundant enough to cover most of the inserted bone blocks at the acetabular rim. A gap may be left open anteromedially. The anterolateral wound is packed with wet sponges.

Femoral osteosynthesis

The plate-seating instrument is carefully extracted through the lateral approach to the femur by tapping and is exactly replaced by the blade-plate chosen before operation. The guide wire through the greater trochanter is left in place for checking the axis of the femoral neck. The surfaces of the femoral osteotomy are repositioned and adjusted to a remaining femoral anteversion of 20°; the plate is fixed provisionally by a Verbruge clamp. The amount of shortening is checked and if needed, an additional disk of bone can now be cut with a saw from the femoral shaft. The AO compression blade plate is fixed to the femoral shaft by compressing screws. The guide wire is removed and the vastus lateralis muscle sutured to its detached origins. A gliding screwhole is drilled through the trochanter minor with

its attached tendon of iliopsoas. It is then screwed to the proximal femoral fragment anteromedially. The fascia lata is closed over a deep suction drainage by interrupted sutures. The wound is closed in the routine manner.

Closure of anterior approach

In the ilioinguinal wound, the direct and oblique heads of the rectus are resutured to their origins with Z-lengthening. The detached lateral half of the iliac apophysis is carefully repositioned and sutured. The wound is closed in the routine manner. An anteroposterior hip radiograph is taken to control the reduction of the femoral head and the osteotomy. A hip spica cast is applied in 20-30° of flexion, 25-30° of abduction and neutral rotation with the knees flexed by 20-30° or more, according to the tightness of the ischiocrural muscles and to control transverse rotation of the leg.

■ *Postoperative treatment*

A hip spica cast including both legs and feet is applied immediately after surgery, holding the hips in slight internal rotation and abduction, and the hips and knees in slight flexion. The cast is removed after 3 weeks, together with the intradermal continuous suture. Non-weight-bearing treatment by gentle assisted active exercise is resumed. Four to five weeks after surgery, hip flexion usually allows sitting and adaptation of the seat, if necessary. As after femoral osteotomy alone, partial weight-bearing is possible after 4 weeks and full weight-bearing following radiological control 6 weeks postoperatively. Therapeutic exercise and gait training 2-3 times a week, as well as controlled home exercises, are advocated for one year, but rehabilitation, especially in walkers, can afford a much longer period.

■ *Results*

From 1978 to 1989, 52 patients underwent hip reconstructions. Five patients died during this period, 47 were evaluated at a follow-up in 1994. The age at surgery averaged 10.3 years (3.4 to 19.4 years), and the patients were seen 3.0 years postoperatively on average (0.5 to 10.9 years) and interviewed by a questionnaire 6.8 years (3.5 to 15.0 years) after surgery. In these patients, 64 hip joints were operated on. Fourteen hips had adductor and two had iliopsoas surgery, 7.4 years before to 3.2 years after the hip reconstruction. In 4 cases, a femoral varus derotation osteotomy preceded the hip reconstruction by 14.6 to 1.6 years, with recurrence of the femoral deformity. In one case, it was necessry to add a Chiari pelvic osteotomy after 1.6 years, and in another case, the reconstruction was redone after 1.5 years for re-subluxation.

At follow-up, 46 (72%) hip joints with a lateralisation index < 22% were graded well-centred, 15 (23%) with a lateralisation index

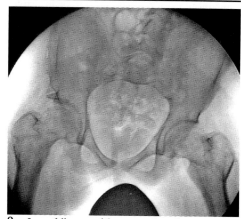

9   *2 year follow-up of the same patient shown preoperatively in figs. 1 to 4.*

between 22% and 50% were graded subluxed, while 3 (5%) had progressed to complete re-dislocation. While 32 patients suffered severe and/or continuous pain before surgery and only 15 had mild or no pain, pain was relieved in all, and 38 were pain free. None of the patients lost function, whereas 8 patients gained or re-gained transfer function and 4 patients even walked with an aid [3].

Fig. 9 shows the result 2 years after surgery of the same patient whose preoperative X-rays are shown in figures 1 to 4.

■ *Pitfalls and mistakes*

Redislocations of the hip joint are an imminent danger, as the neurological disease responsible for the dislocation cannot be cured. Hence, the hip joint needs to be stable in all directions before wound closure, and hip centring is mandatory.

Injury to the sciatic nerve is a complication common to all pelvic osteotomies, but seems to be of less importance with the procedure described above, as it never occurred in these patients.

Femoral head necrosis may result from cutting out of the seating chisel and the blade plate, if the circumflex vessels are damaged. They can also be affected if the T-shaped incision of the hip capsule is extended too far laterally. The marked osteoporosis in these patients requires adequate femoral shortening to avoid intra-articular pressure with flattening of the femoral head.

If the pelvic osteotomy is carried out too far from the acetabulum, bending down becomes difficult. The internal pelvic lamina may even fracture before the acetabulum becomes mobile. In this case, a second attempt after healing of the pelvis is recommended. If the osteotomy is too close, however, the acetabular surface will break. An intra-articular step needs to be avoided in this case.

Transposition of the iliopsoas muscle too far laterally (according to Mustard), tightening the anterolateral part of the capsule too much and pulling a capsular strip over the bone blocks inserted into the pelvic osteotomy may all result in an increased internal rotation of the hip which impedes rehabilitation and may even result in a posterior dislocation.

If the hip joint is centred and the femur is adequately shortened, hip abduction is usually regained. In case of insufficient abduction after femoral osteosynthesis, a mild adductor lengthening is recommended, which could, however, be postponed to the removal of metal, as at that time functional after-treatment is possible.

Pressure sores are the most frequent complication, especially in severely handicapped children who may be very lean and skinny. Enough padding with cotton wool is mandatory to avoid this annoying complication.

The strong forces of patients with spasticity and epileptic strokes require the use of strong implants. The fascia lata rubbing over the bulky metal, however, may produce pain shortly after the operation. Early metal removal will generally solve this problem.

References

[1] Baumann JU. Das therapeutische Angebot der orthopädischen Chirurgie bei Kindern mit zerebralen Bewegungsstörungen. In : Lohse-Busch H, Riedel M, Graf-Baumann T eds. Das therapeutische Angebot für das bewegungsgestörte Kinder. Springer-Verlag, 2001

[2] Baumann JU. Orthopaedic Surgery as a treatment procedure in cerebral palsy. In : Milivoj Velickovic Perat, Brian Neville ed. Cerebral palsy. Elsevier, 2001 (in print)

[3] Brunner R, Baumann JU. Long-term effects of intertrochanteric varus-derotation osteotomy on femur and acetabulum in spastic cerebral palsy: an 11- to 18-year follow-up study. *J Pediatr Orthop* 1997 ; 17 (5) : 585-591

[4] Müller ME. Die hüftnahen Femurosteotomien. 2. Aufl. mit Anhang: 12 Hüfteingriffe. Stuttgart : Thieme, 1971

[5] Müller ME, Allgöwer M, Schneider R, Willenegger H. Manual der Osteosynthese: AO-Technik. Berlin-Heidelberg : Springer-Verlag, 1977

[6] Müller ME, Allgöwer M, Schneider R, Willenegger H. Manual of Internal Fixation. Berlin-Heidelberg : Springer-Verlag, 1991

[7] Samilson R, Tsou P, Aamoth G, Green WM. Dislocation and subluxation of the hip in cerebral palsy. *J Bone Joint Surg (Am)* 1972 ; 54 : 8633-8687

Congenital proximal femoral deficiency

JA Fixsen
FP Monsell

Abstract. – *Congenital proximal femoral deficiency or congenital femoral deficiency (CFD) is a rare developmental disorder with a spectrum of presentations between femoral hypoplasia and virtual absence of the femur. The classification suggested by Gillespie in 1998 [5] is very useful for planning treatment. Patients in Gillespie Group A can be considered for limb reconstruction and lengthening. The majority of those in Gillespie Groups B and C require either rotationplasty and a prosthesis, or knee fusion combined with ankle disarticulation/Syme's or Boyd's amputation and a prosthesis. Some may be managed with a prosthesis alone. The surgical techniques are described with their indications, complications and post-operative management.*

Keywords: congenital femoral deficiency, proximal femoral deficiency, classification, limb reconstruction, lengthening, rotationplasty, knee fusion, ankle disarticulation, Syme's or Boyd's amputation.

Introduction

Proximal femoral deficiency may be congenital or acquired. Acquired deficiency may be secondary to trauma, tumour or infection, and its management is dealt with elsewhere in this work. Congenital longitudinal deficiency of the femur covers a broad spectrum, from minor hypoplasia to virtual absence of the femur. A number of classifications have been suggested. Aitken [1] at a symposium held in Washington in 1968, suggested the term proximal femoral focal deficiency (PFFD) which has become well established but concentrates on the more severe end of the spectrum. The classifications of Hamanishi [8] (1980) and Pappas [14] (1983) cover the whole range. However, as Aitken [1] pointed out, and later Sanpera and Sparkes [15] (1994), due to the characteristic delay in ossification seen in this condition, radiological groupings can change with time and radiological classification only becomes clearly established on serial X-rays over time.

In terms of clinical management, the classification suggested by Fixsen and

John A Fixsen, M.A. M.Chir, FRCS, West Barn, Clamoak Farm Banks, Weir Quay, Bere Alston Devon PL20 7BU, United Kingdom, formerly of The Department of Orthopaedic Surgery, Great Ormond Street Hospital for Children, Great Ormond Street, London WC1N 3JH, United Kingdom.
FP Monsell, MSc., FRCS (Orth.), Department of Orthopaedic Surgery, Great Ormond Street Hospital for Children NHS Trust, Great Ormond Street, London WC1N 3JH, United Kingdom.

Lloyd-Roberts [4] (1974) tries to distinguish between those patients in whom the relationship between the deficient femur and pelvis is inherently stable and those in whom it is not. Sanpera and Sparkes [15] confirmed that this classification was the most reliable for predicting outcome and Goddard et al [7] (1995) established that the X-ray taken at 12 – 15 months of age when the child was starting to stand and walk was easier to interpret and more reliable than that taken shortly after birth. Gillespie [5] (1998) in the report of a major symposium on "The Child with a Limb Deficiency" suggested a new clinical classification for planning treatment *(fig 1)*.

Gillespie classification of congenital femoral deficiency (1998)

Group A: The hip is stable and the proximal femur ossifies. If the femoral length is greater than 60% of the contralateral side, leg equalisation is possible. Coxa vara and retroversion of the femoral neck will have to be corrected. The knee is always to some degree dysplastic and unstable and is often valgus. Both these problems will have to be dealt with if lengthening is going to be successful *(fig 2A, 3A)*. If the femur is less than 60% of the length of the contralateral side, then some surgeons would recommend

a Van Nes rotationplasty, others prefer fusion of the knee and amputation through the ankle joint. Both are followed by prosthetic fitting.

Group B: Here the femoral length is less than 50% of the contralateral side and the hip is "unstable" as defined by Fixsen and Lloyd-Roberts [4]. The surgeon's aim is to maximise prosthetic function. Attempts to stabilise the upper end of the femur may be difficult, as reported by Goddard et al [7]. Fusion of the knee, as suggested by King [10] (1969), combined with through ankle disarticulation, Syme's or Boyd's amputuation can be very useful. Again, rotationplasty is an alternative in the presence of a satisfactory ankle joint *(fig 2B, 3B)*.

Group C: This is virtual absence of all except the most distal part of the femur. It is often associated with dysplasia of the hemipelvis and absence of any acetabular development. These patients require a prosthesis and, in the most deficient cases, retaining the foot may be beneficial to the prosthetist. Steel et al [17] (1987) suggested iliofemoral fusion for these patients, stabilising the femur on the pelvis, using the knee as a hip joint and either amputating the foot or performing a rotationplasty. Steel [16] reported good functional results in 22 patients at maturity in 1998 *(fig 2C, 3C)*.

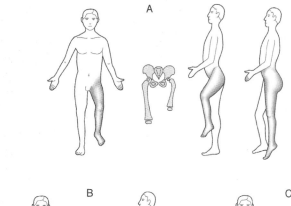

1 *Gillespie's clinical classification for planning treatment (adapted with permission from Gillespie R: Classification of Congenital Abnormalities of the Femur, in Herring JA, Birch JG eds. The Child with a Limb Deficiency. Rosemont, IL, American Academy of Orthopaedic Surgeons, 1998.*

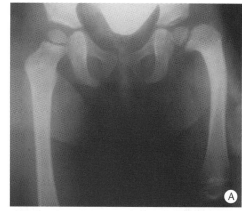

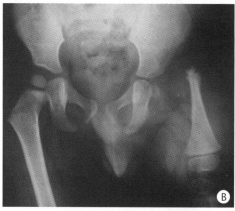

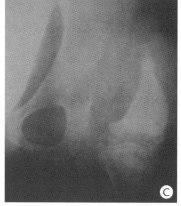

3 *Gillespie's classification: radiological features.*
  A. Type A.
  B. Type B.
  C. Type C.

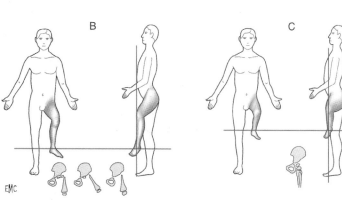
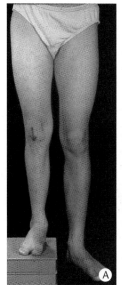
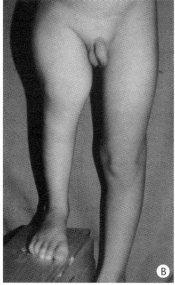
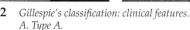

2 *Gillespie's classification: clinical features.*
  A. Type A.   *B. Type B.*
                        C. Type C.

Limb lengthening in congenital proximal femoral deficiency

The classification system described by Gillespie [5, 6] (1983, 1998) accounts for the extent of longitudinal deficiency, the morphology of the proximal femur and the stability of the hip. It is a straightforward system that defines those limbs in which surgical equalisation is a realistic option, and those that are more suitable for prosthetic reconstruction. The system described by Paley [12] (1998) approaches this condition in terms of surgical reconstruction and provides a classification that accommodates all degrees of deformity.

The indications for surgical reconstruction in Western Europe have broadened over the last twenty years, particularly since the introduction of the Ilizarov Method and the influence of the Association for the Study and Application of Methods of Ilizarov (ASAMI).

Whether surgical reconstruction should be applied to all degrees of deformity is a subject of continuing debate and is highlighted by these two classification systems.

The most appropriate treatment for an individual patient is governed by several competing factors. The available surgical expertise, the availability of suitable prostheses, and the wishes of the patient and family, which are in turn determined by the educational and cultural climate, all determine the optimum solution.

The goals of treatment must include optimum function, and surgical reconstruction must provide a limb that enables walking with a normal or near normal gait pattern. In our institution, we are fortunate to have access to excellent lower limb prosthetics, and this has influenced our approach to the management of more severe forms of congenital femoral deficiency, considered later in this chapter.

The management of a child with congenital femoral deficiency continues throughout childhood; it is essential to determine a strategy of management in infancy. With high definition antenatal ultrasonography, the diagnosis is often considered before birth. It is not usually possible to define the extent of the deformity until birth, and

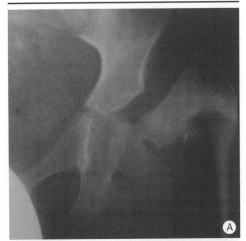

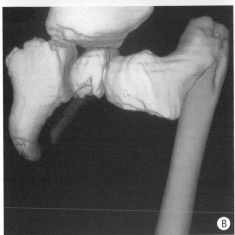

4 *Group A femur.*
A. Plain radiograph.
B. 3-D CT reconstruction. Note marked coxa vara and retroversion.

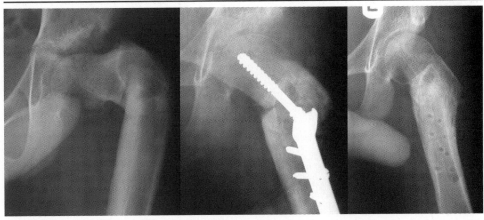

5 *Correction of coxa vara (fixation with Coventry lag screw and plate).*

management decisions are best delayed until a full examination can be performed. The morphology of the hip and proximal femur can be estimated between the ages of 1 and 2 years, using the radiological features described by Fixsen and Lloyd-Roberts [4] (1974), augmented by examination under anaesthesia and arthrography. The magnitude of the length discrepancy can also be estimated at this age, as the limbs develop in proportion until skeletal maturity.

A detailed management strategy must be formed during infancy, with a goal of limb equalisation at skeletal maturity. The Gillespie classification provides a basis and allows distinction, to be made in infancy, between those limbs suitable for surgical lengthening and those more suitable for prosthetic management. For the purpose of further discussion, this section will consider the surgical reconstruction of Group A, or hypoplastic femur, as defined by Gillespie [5] (1998).

The Group A femur is at least 60% the length of the contralateral femur and is usually associated with coxa vara and proximal femoral retroversion *(fig 4)*.

The acetabulum is often dysplastic and this predisposes to hip dislocation during lengthening.

As a precursor to lengthening, these anatomical abnormalities should be addressed using conventional osteotomies of the femur and pelvis.

Acetabular dysplasia (centre edge angle < 20°) predisposes the hip to dislocation during lengthening. This should be addressed with an inominate osteotomy directed to correct the predominant acetebular deficiency, which can be evaluated pre-operatively using 3-D CT, or visually at operation.

Anterolateral acetabular deficiency is addressed by a conventional Salter osteotomy. For posterior wall deficiency, a Dega's peri-acetabular osteotomy is performed. The proximal femoral deformity and subtrochanteric pseudarthrosis that is often present is corrected by an appropriate femoral osteotomy and secured with a Coventry lag screw and plate or similar device.

The anatomy of this region is often distorted and the normal tissue planes are absent, reflecting the field defect that is characteristic of this condition. It is often necessary to perform a radical soft tissue release before it is possible to correct the femoral deformity.

The fixation device is removed after the osteotomy has united, before lengthening proceeds. This allows fixation to the proximal femur without the risk of implant infection introduced via a pin site.

The lateral femoral condyle is often dysplastic, leading to a valgus knee deformity, which can be corrected as part of the femoral lengthening.

There is frequently an absence of the anterior cruciate ligament, which predisposes to posterior subluxation of the knee during lengthening. Following successful lengthening, the cruciate instability can limit function and may require reconstruction at skeletal maturity.

Proximal femoral osteotomy for severe coxa vara *(fig 5)*

INDICATIONS

The range of proximal femoral abnormality associated with this condition varies from subtle varus mal-alignment to complete absence of the proximal femur. There is no absolute indication for a stabilising or realignment procedure, and the following description is relevant to a progressive deformity with deteriorating gait, or as a precursor to femoral lengthening. The optimum age for stabilisation is controversial and depends on the overall management strategy. If surgical reconstruction is appropriate, the proximal correction is performed in early childhood. If the purpose of realignment is to improve prosthetic function, realignment may not be necessary until early adolescence. The choice of fixation device depends on the preference of the surgeon; the author favours a Coventry plate and screw in the younger child and an AO blade plate for the adolescent.

TECHNIQUE

The procedure is performed under general anaesthesia, with the patient placed supine on a radiolucent operating table. The limb is draped after skin preparation from the iliac crest to the knee, with a sandbag used to raise the buttock.

■ *Incision*

A direct lateral incision is made immediately proximal to the greater trochanter, along the line of the femur to the upper and middle third junction. As the dissection is deepened, the tissues usually appear abnormal and adherent. The anatomy of this region is often bizarre and reflects the field change that characterises this condition. The usual anatomical landmarks, including a well-defined fascia lata are often absent and the muscle layers may be indistinct. Dissection is continued to bone and the proximal femur is exposed subperiosteally; the periosteum is often thickened and the bone sclerotic.

The femoral neck is usually significantly retroverted and this must be appreciated when introducing a guide wire, irrespective of the fixation device. This relationship is clearly demonstrated in figure 4.

A guide wire is placed along the centre of the femoral neck and checked in two planes with an image intensifier. A Coventry initial reamer or AO seating chisel is introduced and two Kirschner wires are inserted to define the proximal and distal osteotomies at the inter-trochanteric level. These wires can be used to assess the rotational alignment; it is also useful to score the lateral femoral shaft with an osteotome.

The Coventry screw or blade plate is inserted and the osteotomies are performed using an oscillating saw, with copious saline irrigation.

The geometry of the osteotomy is determined by the extent of the deformity. The aim is to produce a neck shaft angle of 135° with a symmetrical range of internal and external rotation. The magnitude of the correction is determined by pre-operative clinical examination in addition to pre-operative computerised tomography (*fig 4*).

It is often necessary to perform a radical adductor release using a separate medial incision to facilitate full correction of the varus mal-alignment. It is essential to expose the proximal femoral shaft and release the linea aspera to achieve an adequate rotational correction.

The osteotomy is reduced onto the plate and secured with four screws in standard fashion.

The position of the implant and osteotomy are checked with an image intensifier and the wound closed in layers (*fig 5*).

POST-OPERATIVE MANAGEMENT

In the younger child, the osteotomy is protected in a plaster of Paris hip spica for a period of six weeks. In the older child with secure blade plate fixation, the initial management is with balanced traction for fourteen days. Toe touch weight-bearing is then permitted until the sixth post-operative week with a shoe lift or extension prosthesis. Full weight-bearing is allowed by the twelfth postoperative week, provided the radiographs demonstrate satisfactory progress.

COMPLICATIONS

The complications are not specific to this condition and include superficial and deep infection, implant failure leading to loss of position and delayed or non-union.

The most frequent specific complication involves recurrent deformity, and it may be necessary to repeat the procedure as growth progresses.

Modified Ilizarov technique for femoral lengthening

The following description is the authors' preferred method of lengthening in congenital femoral deficiency. This is a combination of the classic technique described by Ilizarov [9] (1992) and the techniques modified by Catagni and others [3] (1998). We describe the technique used to lengthen the femur and correct distal femoral valgus. The apparatus can be modified to address any three-dimensional deformity, but these techniques are beyond the scope of this chapter.

INDICATIONS

This procedure should be considered in Gillespie Group A patients in whom the predicted length discrepancy is between 20-40% of the uninvolved side. It is assumed that the hip and knee are intrinsically stable, or have been stabilised using the methods described above.

PLANNING

Clinical assessment of current length discrepancy, range of joint movements, joint stability and fixed joint deformity are essential for accurate pre-operative planning. The soft tissue dimensions of the thigh are measured to allow accurate fixator pre-construction.

Standard radiographs of the hip and knee are required to confirm the stability of the joints and estimate the extent of residual deformity. Long anteroposterior and lateral radiographs, which include the femur and tibia on one film, are required and are standardised with the patella centred forward and the pelvis leveled with blocks beneath the short limb.

The components of the deformity in the coronal and sagittal planes can be calculated using the methods popularised by Paley and colleagues [13] (1994), which allow accurate deformity correction in addition to lengthening.

The Ilizarov fixator is constructed before surgery; this simplifies and therefore shortens the surgical procedure. The basic construct involves a distal fixation segment composed of two complete rings. The proximal fixation segment is composed of an arch support and these are connected using a floating or force transmission ring.

The distal segment connects to the floating ring using four threaded rods, or clickers. The proximal arch connects to the floating ring using three oblique supports (*fig 6*). The device is constructed using the smallest ring that allows adequate soft tissue clearance; a circumferential clearance of one and one-half finger width is usually a good working compromise.

PROCEDURE

The procedure is performed under general anaesthesia, without neuromuscular blockade or non-steroidal anti-inflammatory medication. The patient is placed supine on a radiolucent operating table; the entire limb is draped after skin preparation from the toes to above the iliac crest. The ipsilateral buttock and flank are raised with a pillow or large sandbag to enhance access to the proximal femur and allow flexion of the hip and knee during wire and pin placement. An operating table with a detachable segment also allows satisfactory access to the leg, with the tibia supported on a Mayo table.

Using an image intensifier, a 1.8 mm reference wire is inserted in the distal femur, parallel to the joint line from lateral to medial, at the level of the distal metaphyseal flare. The fixator must be placed parallel to the mechanical axis of the femur to prevent medialisation of the knee during lengthening. The joint line is approximately perpendicular with the mechanical axis and therefore provides a good point of reference.

Careful attention to detail is required during wire placement to minimise subsequent pin site infection and allow maximum excursion of the knee and hip joints.

The knee is passively flexed and extended, and the skin over the lateral aspect of the distal femur is observed. There is a consistent area of skin that does not move during knee excursion and this is the optimum entry point for the wire. The knee is fully flexed before the wire penetrates the lateral quadriceps and this transfixes the muscle at its maximum length, preventing a tether that will restrict knee motion. The wire is inserted into the femur at its maximum diameter, avoiding high-speed insertion, which will generate intense heat, causing a ring sequestrum and early loosening. The wire can be cooled and sterilised and controlled using an alcohol soaked swab. The knee is fully extended and the wire advanced through the medial hamstring muscles using a mallet. Power insertion is to be avoided on the distant side to minimise the risk of damage to the neurovascular structures. At this point, the range of knee movement is checked, and any puckering or tethering of the skin is released with a scalpel.

A 5 mm half pin is inserted into the proximal femur at the level of the lesser trochanter. The image intensifier is used to insert this pin parallel to the line that joins the tip of the greater trochanter to the centre of the femoral head, provided the morphology of the proximal femur is normal. If there is a significant abnormality, the pin is inserted 7° to the anatomical axis of the femur, perpendicular to the mechanical axis.

The fixator is attached to the proximal pin and distal wire, ensuring that the femoral diaphysis is centred in the rings in the

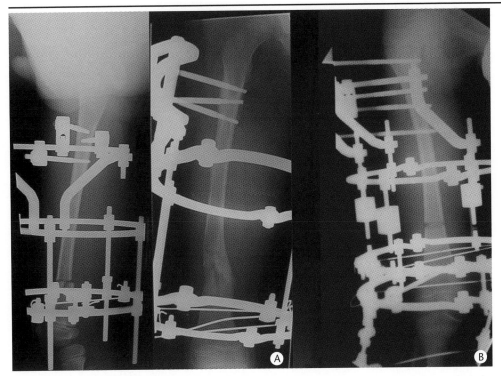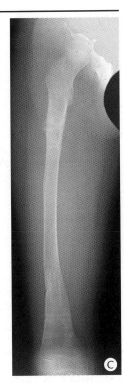

6 A. Ilizarov femoral lengthening.
B. AP radiograph during femoral lengthening. Note that the fixator crosses the knee to prevent posterior subluxation.
C. After lengthening and removal of the Ilizarov aparatus.

anteroposterior and mediolateral planes, with adequate soft tissue clearance. The fixator has now been positioned parallel to the mechanical axis of the femur, with the femur in the centre of the fixator.

The distal wire is tensioned to 110-130 Kg and the proximal pin is attached to the arch using a pin holder of suitable dimensions.

Distal fixation is secured using three further tensioned wires, placed with the maximum crossing angle that is possible without jeopardising the neurovascular structures. The technique of wire insertion described above is used for each subsequent wire.

Proximal fixation is completed using two further 5 mm half pins, inserted above and below the reference pin, with the maximum crossing angle that is allowed by the dimensions of the arch.

CORTICOTOMY

The method and site of division of the femur is also a controversial subject, with coherent arguments relating to differences in site and surgical technique. In general, there is agreement that the femur should be divided in the metaphyseal region using a low energy technique.

The authors favour a distal femoral metaphyseal osteotomy *(fig 6)* using the following technique. A 2 cm longitudinal incision is made in the mid lateral line. The iliotibial band is identified and dissected to its anterior and posterior extent and divided transversly under direct vision. The vastus lateralis muscle is defined and reflected anteriorly using a bone lever placed over the anterior surface of the femoral shaft. The

periosteum is identified and incised longitudinally. It is not necessary to strip the periosteum, as this will have a negative effect on bone formation. Using a sharp osteotome, the anterior and posterior corticies are divided completely, leaving the posteromedial corner undivided. The osteotome is rotated 45° in either direction, completing the osteotomy.

There is usually insufficient periosteum to allow satisfactory closure. The wound is closed in layers. The pin and wires are dressed with alcohol-soaked sponges and stoppers.

POST-OPERATIVE MANAGEMENT

The patient is encouraged to put 25% body weight through the limb as soon as comfort allows, graduating to full weight over a period of several weeks. Distraction commences after a latent period of 5 - 7 days, depending on the age of the patient, and continues at a rate of 0.25 mm every six hours until the target length has been achieved.

The patient attends follow-up on a regular basis, with radiographs to assess the quality of new bone formation. The rate of distraction may be altered to prevent premature consolidation or incomplete regenerate formation.

COMPLICATIONS

The nature of congenital limb deformity, with the associated field effect that involves all tissue types, creates substantial difficulties when surgical lengthening is undertaken. These techniques are associated

with an extremely high, but not necessarily prohibitive, complication rate. The knowledge that complication rates can approach 100% should not lead to a feeling of inevitability or complacency.

The detailed description of wire/pin insertion techniques, pin-site care and post-operative management is deliberate and leads to a substantial reduction of the frequency and severity of these complications.

Pin site infection is a common consequence of prolonged external fixation. Careful pin and wire insertion, wound care and post-operative pin-site care reduces, but does not abolish, this complication. Pain and erythema are usually the first signs of infection. The use of broad-spectrum antibiotics, in appropriate doses determined by body weight, is often effective. If resolution does not occur rapidly, hospital admission may become necessary, using parenteral antibiotics according to microbiological culture. The majority of infections will resolve if treated promptly, but it is occasionally necessary to remove the infected fixation and very rarely to abandon the procedure.

Pain is often associated with infection. Neurogenic pain may be associated with the lengthening process and may limit the rate of lengthening. Instability due to improper fixator construction or loosening must also be considered and appropriate adjustments made.

The quality of the new bone depends on a number of mechanical and biological factors. An excessive rate of distraction may lead to deficient regenerate whilst premature

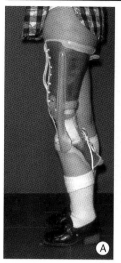 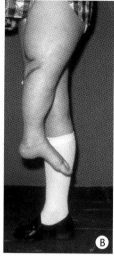

7 *Clinical appearance of a child after Van Nes rotationplasty with and without prosthesis.*

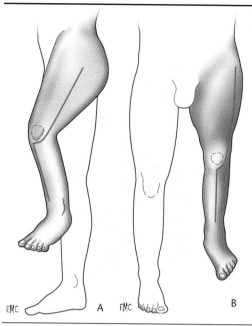

8 *S-shaped skin incision for rotationplasty. Lateral (A) and AP (B) views. The patella, which is commonly hypoplastic, is shown by a dotted line.*

consolidation is associated with slow distraction. Bone formation is monitored with frequent radiographs; in some centres ultrasound and CT are used. There is poor correlation between radiological and mechanical parameters and decisions are usually based on plain radiographs in two planes.

The optimum time for fixator removal is also difficult to predict in some cases. Premature removal is complicated by regenerate failure, with deformity or fracture.

The joint laxity that is commonly encountered in congenital femoral deficiency predisposes to joint subluxation and dislocation. This is an extremely grave occurrence and often leads to the procedure being abandoned. Careful pre-operative assessment, surgical reconstruction of the joints before lengthening, and aggressive physical therapy during lengthening are important to prevent this complication.

Rotationplasty in the management of congenital proximal femoral deficiency

Hip rotationplasty for the treatment of malignant tumours in adults is described by Professor Winkelmann in Section 6. Recently, a similar procedure has been described by Brown [2] (2001) in 3 cases of severe congenital femoral deficiency where the proximal portion of the deficient femur was excised, the leg rotated through 180° at the site of excision, and the remaining femur fused to the ilium. The knee is retained as a form of hip joint as it now lies at hip level, and the ankle, having been rotated through 180°, functions as a knee joint.

The so-called Van Nes rotationplasty for congenital defects of the femur, described by Van Nes [19] in 1950, subsequently reported by Kostuik et al [11] (1975), and

modified by Torode and Gillespie [18] (1983), is a somewhat different operation in which the hip is retained, the knee excised and rotation obtained through the excised knee and if necessary through a second rotation osteotomy of the tibia and fibula (*fig 7A, B, see also figure 10*).

The indications for rotationplasty in a child with congenital proximal femoral are as follows:

– unilateral involvement;

– the foot and ankle on the affected side should be relatively normal. Patients with significant ankle or foot deformity from associated severe fibular deficiency are not suitable;

– combined ankle and subtalar movements should be at least 50-60°;

– the degree of shortening of the leg should be such as to make any attempt at reconstruction by leg lengthening very arduous and hazardous, if not impossible.

Typically, these are the more severe forms of congenital femoral deficiency classified by Gillespie as Groups B and C and Aitken as Types C and D, in which the overall shortening is likely to be such that the foot is approximately at the level of the opposite knee. Some of the most severe cases in Gillespie group A (Aitken type A) may also be suitable for this procedure.

Psychological problems have been reported in some patients due to the abnormal appearance of the foot in the 180° rotated position. Careful counselling of the parents and child is necessary prior to operation. Preferably, they should meet and discuss the procedure with a patient who has already had it performed, so that they can appreciate the appearance of the limb and how it functions with a prosthesis. One of the problems in the growing child is that of spontaneous derotation with growth. Kostuik et al [11] in 1975 suggested that the

operation should not be done until the age of 12 years because of derotation problems. Using the modified technique of Torode and Gillespie [18], introduced in 1983, these problems seem to be much decreased, although they can still occur. Nowadays, surgeons would be prepared to operate as early as 2-3 years before the child starts school, and this may be helpful both from the psychological and the functional point of view.

TECHNIQUE

There are a number of variations of the technique described by Torode and Gillespie [18] in 1983.

■ **Position**

The patient is supine on a translucent operating table. The entire leg must be exposed from the iliac crest to the toes after skin preparation and draping. The opposite leg must be palpable under the drape to estimate accurately the level of the opposite knee.

■ **Incision**

An S-shaped incision is made starting proximal and lateral to the knee, crossing the knee anteriorly, and continuing distally along the subcutaneous border of the tibia as far as is necessary, depending on whether a mid tibial osteotomy is required to obtain the full 180° rotation after maximal rotation through the knee (*fig 8*).

■ **Procedure**

The skin flaps are elevated laterally and medially to expose the patellar tendon and the capsule of the knee. The patella is commonly hypoplastic and may be laterally displaced. On the lateral side, the common peroneal nerve (lateral popliteal nerve) is dissected out and protected. In patients with fibular deficiency, it may be abnormally placed and should be traced back to its origin from the sciatic nerve. The iliotibial band and the tendon of the biceps femoris can then be divided from their insertion on to the tibia and fibula if it is present. The lateral head of the gastrocnemius is detached from its origin on the posterior aspect of the lateral femoral condyle. The detached muscles and tendons should be marked for ease of identification following rotation of the lower part of the limb.

The popliteal neurovascular bundle is identified and carefully freed from the posterior aspect of the knee. The patellar tendon is then detached from the tibial tuberosity and turned proximally. The capsule of the knee is incised circumferentially and the knee joint, which is often grossly dysplastic with absent or deficient cruciates, is exposed and the cruciates, if necessary, divided. On the medial side, after detaching the sartorius from its tibial insertion so that it can be retracted out of the way, the insertion of the adductor magnus is carefully dissected out to the level of the femoral artery where it enters the adductor hiatus. The adductor magnus is divided to expose and free up the artery so that it may rotate anteriorly with the other popliteal vessels and nerves when the distal part of the limb is rotated at knee level *(fig 9)*.

The medial hamstrings and gracilis are detached from their origins on the tibia and the medial head of the gastrocnemius from the posterior aspect of the distal femur. Again, the tendons and muscles are marked. The popliteus is divided at the level of the knee.

The distal end of the femur is exposed and divided transversely with an oscillating saw above the epiphysial plate. The amount of femur removed depends on the amount of shortening required. The aim is to leave the ankle after rotation at the level of the opposite knee. The articular surface of the tibia is then removed via an osteotomy approximately 4-5 mm proximal to the proximal tibial epiphysial plate *(fig 10)*.

Having ensured that the popliteal vessels and nerve are free to rotate, the foot and lower leg are externally rotated, if possible through 180° *(fig 11)*.

Torode and Gillespie [18] suggested a second osteotomy at the level of the mid shaft of the tibia and that about 130-140° of the rotation should be gained at the knee, while the remaining rotation to 180° was gained in the tibia. Many authors, however, try to obtain all the rotation at the knee, particularly if significant shortening of the femur has been necessary. They advocate a second mid-tibial osteotomy (and fibular osteotomy if the fibula is present) only if there is evidence of vascular compromise, even after wide mobilisation of the neurovascular bundle at knee level.

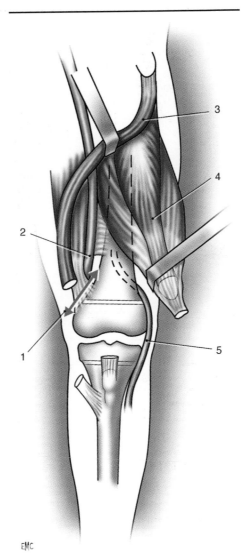

9 *Anterior exposure of the knee and line of division of adductor magnus insertion to allow the femoral artery to rotate anteriorly. 1. Line of division of adductor magnus insertion; 2. femoral artery entering the adductor hiatus; 3. sartorius released and retracted; 4. quadriceps released from tibial tubercle; 5. common peroneal nerve (note fibula is absent).*

■ *Fixation*

An intramedullary rod such as a Rush pin or stout Kirschner (K) wire is introduced retrograde into the femur and then distally into the tibia where it can be used to fix the tibial osteotomy if this has been necessary *(fig 12)*.

The final position of the rod is checked with the image intensifier. Provided the surgeon is happy that there is no vascular compromise, the rotation can be held by a single crossed K-wire at the level of the excised knee. If the surgeon is doubtful about the vascular status of the limb, then it is possible to control rotation with a hip spica which is not in a full 180° and to gain further rotation by serial changes of plaster. The skeletal muscles are reattached across the knee arthrodesis.

The incision is closed after careful haemostasis with suction drainage, depending on the surgeon's preference. The

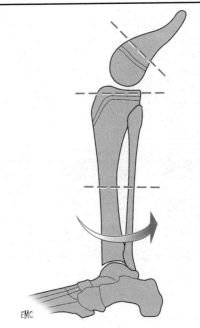

10 *Sites of osteotomies for rotationplasty at the knee and where necessary in the tibia.*
Note the position of the epiphyseal plates. The fibula is present and the foot dorsiflexes to neutral.

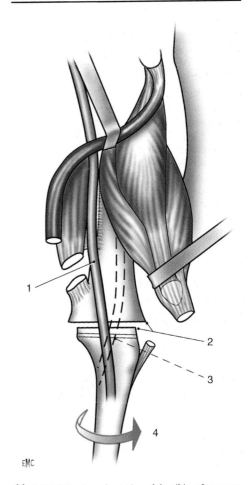

11 *140-180° external rotation of the tibia, after appropriate resection of distal femur and proximal tibia. Note the femoro-popliteal vessels free to rotate anteriorly and the common peroneal nerve posteriorly. 1. Femeropopliteal artery free to rotate anteriorly; 2. femur and tibia resected to appropriate level; 3. common peroneal nerve rotates posterioly; 4. tibia externally rotated 140-180°.*

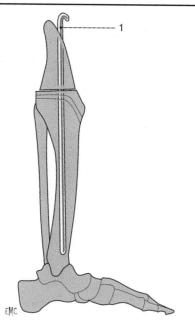

12 *The leg has rotated through 180° at the knee follow-ing osteotomy and excision of the knee. Note fixation with a rush nail (1). Rotation can be controlled by a crossed K-wire or spica. The fixed flexion at the knee can be corrected by knee excision.*

vascular status is again checked and a 1½ hip spica applied for 4-6 weeks.

POST-OPERATIVE CARE

Careful observation of the vascular status of the limb is maintained. When there is satisfactory soft tissue healing and bony union, usually at 4-6 weeks, the plaster can be removed and a modified below-knee prosthesis fitted. Physiotherapy is undertaken to regain movement and power at the hip and the ankle, which is now functioning as a knee.

COMPLICATIONS

Although this is a rare and major operation, when care is taken, excessive blood loss should be avoided. Vascular problems due to rotation of the vessels and nerves should also be avoided. Skin healing is usually satisfactory. The child usually adapts well to using the ankle as a knee, but it may be necessary to adjust the prosthesis both for alignment and fit of the socket several times in the first year to 18 months as the use of the ankle joint as a knee improves.

Arthrodesis of the knee combined with disarticu-lation through the ankle or Syme's or Boyd's amputation of the foot

INDICATIONS

This procedure should be considered in Gillespie group B and C patients where limb

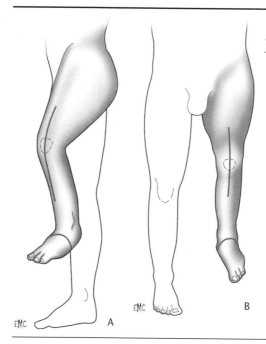

13 *AP and lateral views of the skin incisions. Note the generous skin flaps for disarticulation and the 3 ray foot.*

lengthening and reconstruction is not considered feasible. It should also be used in patients where the foot and ankle are unsatisfactory for rotationplasty and when the patient and parents find rotationplasty unacceptable.

AIM

The aim of the procedure is to provide a single stable strut at above knee level which can function satisfactorily with a modern above-knee prosthesis.

POSITION

The patient is supine, preferably on a translucent operating table, under general anaesthesia. The entire leg is draped after skin preparation from the toes to above the iliac crest. There is usually insufficient length of femur above the knee for a tourniquet to be used.

PROCEDURE

A longitudinal incision is made over the anterior aspect of the knee joint *(fig 13)*.

The soft tissues are elevated medially and laterally to expose the patella, the patella tendon and the capsule of the knee. The patella is often hypoplastic and abnormally placed and may even be absent. The interior of the knee is exposed by detaching the patella tendon and turning it upwards, dividing the capsule medially and laterally at the level of the joint line. The distal end of the femur and proximal end of the tibia are exposed subperiostally; the cruciate ligaments are frequently deficient or absent. The articular surfaces are removed with an oscillating saw *(fig 14)*.

It is often necessary to shorten the femoral fragment, both to correct a fixed flexion deformity at the knee and to remove the

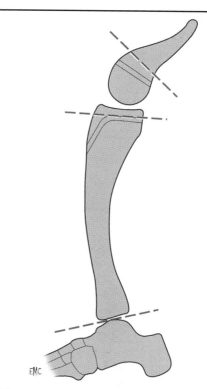

14 *Diagram showing sites for osteotomies at the knee and through-ankle disarticulation. Note the absent fibula, tarsal coalition and 3 ray foot.*

distal femoral epiphyseal plate in order to prevent overgrowth, as the aim of the operation is to position the amputation stump above the level of the opposite knee in order to allow room for the mechanism of the prosthetic knee which will be fitted. In younger patients, it is often not possible to accurately determine what the position will be at maturity, and so it is advisable to leave the stump rather long, until it is clear that growth will leave the stump at the correct level or a further adjustment of length is necessary. In younger patients, therefore, the proximal tibial epiphyseal plate is retained as it is in a rotationplasty.

FIXATION

An intramedullary rush pin or nail is introduced retrograde into the femur and then distally into the tibia to stabilise the arthrodesis *(fig 15)*. Rotation can be controlled either with staples across the arthrodesis or by crossed K-wires.

The surgeon can then proceed to ankle disarticulation or Syme's or Boyd's amputation. The techniques of these procedures are described elsewhere in this text. The technique in children is similar, although it is essential to use generous skin flaps and, if disarticulation is used, to anchor the heel flap over the end of the tibia with a K-wire for a period of six weeks *(fig 15)*.

CLOSURE AND AFTER-TREATMENT

After careful haemostasis, the wounds are closed with suction drainage. A hip spica is applied for 6 weeks or until bony union is obtained. When the spica is removed, the K-wire securing the heel pad, or the calcaneum if a Boyd's amputation has been performed, is removed.

COMPLICATIONS

Through joint amputations in children do not suffer from overgrowth. Similarly, one should not see problems with a Syme's or Boyd's amputation. It is important in the

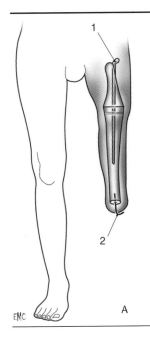
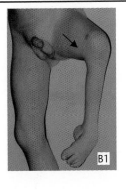
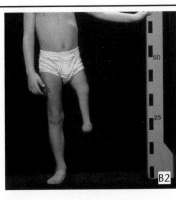

15 *A. Post disarticulation of the foot and excision of the knee. Note correction of the fixed flexion at the knee, rush nail internal fixation (1) and K-wire to secure the heel flap on the distal end of the tibia (2).*
B. Clinical photographs: pre-operative and following knee fusion and disarticulation through the ankle joint.

Boyd's amputation that the calcaneum be anchored vertically under the tibia and not allowed to drift posteriorly.

When this procedure is performed in young patients, as stated previously, it is advisable to leave the strut formed by the fused femur and tibia rather long, so that epiphyseodesis of the retained proximal tibial epiphyseal plate may be necessary later to adjust the length of the strut. This will allow adequate room for the fitting of a prosthetic knee within the prosthesis. In the authors' experience, patients manage extremely well with this type of treatment. They rarely develop problems with the stump, which may be slightly bulbous but this can be an advantage in prosthetic fitting. These patients are capable of taking part in the normal activities of life, including sporting activities, in their prosthesis.

References

[1] Aitken GT. Proximal femoral focal deficiency: definition, classification and management. In : Aitken GT ed. Proximal femoral focal deficiency: a congenital anomaly. Washington DC : National Academy of Sciences, 1969 : 1-22

[2] Brown KL. Resection rotationplasty, and femoro pelvic arthrodesis in severe congenital femoral deficiency. *J Bone Joint Surg Am* 2001 ; 83 : 78-85

[3] Catagni MA, Malzev V, Kirienko A. Advances in Ilizarov apparatus assembly. Fracture treatment, pseudarthroses, lengthening, deformity correction. Milan : Il Quadratino, 1998

[4] Fixsen JA, Lloyd-Roberts GC. The natural history and early treatment of proximal femoral dysplasia. *J Bone Joint Surg Br* 1974 ; 56 : 86-95

[5] Gillespie R. Classification of congenital abnormalities of the femur. In : Herring JA, Birch JG eds. The child with a limb deficiency. Rosemont: American Academy of Orthopaedic Surgeons, 1998 : 63-72

[6] Gillespie R, Torode IP. Classification and management of congenital abnormalities of the femur. *J Bone Joint Surg Br* 1983 ; 65 : 557-568

[7] Goddard NJ, Hashemi-Nejad A, Fixsen JA. The natural history and treatment of instability of the hip in proximal femoral focal deficiency. *J Pediatr Orthop B* 1995 ; 4 : 145-149

[8] Hamanishi C. Congenital short femur. *J Bone Joint Surg Br* 1980 ; 62 : 307-320

[9] Ilizarov GA. Transosseous osteosynthesis. Theoretical and clinical aspects of the regeneration and growth of tissue. Berlin : Springer-Verlag, 1992

[10] King RE. Some concepts of proximal femoral focal deficiency. In : Aitken GT ed. Proximal femoral focal deficiency: a congenital anomaly. Washington DC : National Academy of Sciences, 1969 : 23-49

[11] Kostuik JT, Gillespie R, Hall JE, Hubbard S. Van Nes rotation osteotomy for treatment of proximal femoral focal deficiency and congenital short femur. *J Bone Joint Surg Am* 1975 ; 57 : 1039-1046

[12] Paley D. Lengthening reconstruction surgery for congenital femoral deficiency. In : Herring JA, Birch JG eds. The child with a limb deficiency. Rosemont : American Academy of Orthopaedic Surgeons, 1998 : 113-132

[13] Paley D, Herzenberg JE, Tetsworth K, McKie J, Bhave A. Deformity planning for frontal and sagittal plane corrective osteotomies. *Orthop Clin North Am* 1994 ; 25 : 425-465

[14] Pappas AM. Congenital abnormalities of the femur and related lower extremity malformations. Classification and treatment. *J Pediatr Orthop* 1983 ; 3 : 45-60

[15] Sanpera I Jr, Sparkes LT. Proximal femoral focal deficiency: Does a radiologic classification exist? *J Pediatr Orthop* 1994 ; 14 : 34-38

[16] Steel HH. Iliofemoral fusion for proximal femoral focal deficiency. In : Herring JA, Birch JG eds. The child with a limb deficiency. Rosemont : American Academy of Orthopaedic Surgeons, 1998 : 99-102

[17] Steel HH, Lyn PS, Betz RR, Kalamchi A, Clancy M. Iliofemoral fusion for proximal femoral focal deficiency. *J Bone Joint Surg Am* 1987 ; 69 : 837-843

[18] Torode IP, Gillespie R. Rotationplasty of the lower limb for congenital defects of the femur. *J Bone Joint Surg Br* 1983 ; 65 : 569-573

[19] Van Nes CP. Rotationplasty for congenital defects of the femur. *J Bone Joint Surg Br* 1950 ; 32 : 12-16

Femoral neck lengthening osteotomy (FNLO)

EW Morscher
F Hefti
CC Hasler

Abstract. – The incidence of ischaemic necrosis in hip dysplasia depends on the method of treatment. It can go up to 20%. In more severe necroses with involvement of the metaphysis, a deformity of the proximal end of the femur develops which is characterised by coxa magna, short femoral neck and high-standing greater trochanter. Shortening of the femoral neck and proximal displacement of the greater trochanter cause a reduction of the leg length and insufficiency of the abductor muscles. Furthermore, the mechanical axis of the knee joint is lateralised with overload of the lateral knee compartment. With the first author's (E.M.) "Femoral Neck Lengthening Osteotomy" (FNLO) and simultaneous distal-lateral transfer of the greater trochanter, the normal anatomy and physiological functional conditions of the hip joint and the ipsilateral knee joint can be restored.

The operative procedure consists of six steps with three osteotomies. The femoral neck lengthening osteotomy is recommended in adolescents with the typical deformity after ischemic necrosis of the femoral head with closed epiphyseal lines. Severe degenerative changes of the hip joint are a contraindication for FNLO.

© 2000, Editions Scientifiques et Médicales Elsevier SAS. All rights reserved.

Keywords: hip, femoral neck lengthening osteotomy, hip dysplasia, avascular necrosis, proximal femur deficiency.

Introduction

Premature closure of the epiphyseal plate can follow congenital hip dysplasia, Perthes disease, trauma or septic arthritis of the hip. As a result, the proximal femur may develop a deformity. Classifications have been proposed for deformities of the proximal end of the femur after ischaemic necrosis of the femoral head, especially after treatment of developmental dysplasia of the hip joint [1, 4, 8, 10]. The most frequent deformity according to Specchiulli's classification (fig 1), where coxa magna, short neck and high-standing greater trochanter are combined with dysplasia of the acetabulum, is Type B3 which shows the worst prognosis concerning the development of osteoarthritis. A dysplasia of the acetabulum, therefore, must also be corrected to prevent osteoarthritis.

Closure of the epiphyseal plate predominantly occurs laterally, so that coxa valga develops as a rule. Coxa valga,

Erwin W Morscher, Professor, Felix Platter-Hospital, Burgfelderstr. 101, CH-4012 Basel, Switzerland.
Fritz Hefti, Professor.
Carol C Hasler, M.D.
Universitäts-Kinderspital beider Basel, Postfach, CH-4005 Basel, Switzerland.

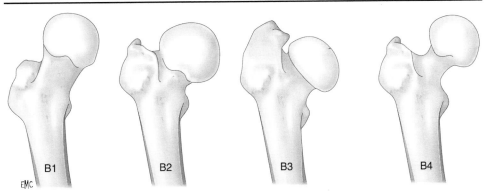

1 *Specchiulli's classification of deformation of the hip joint after avascular necrosis in development dysplasia. A) Partial, involving only the epiphysis, no alteration of the femoral neck; B) total, involving epiphysis and metaphysis. Four forms of B have been identified:*
B1: eventually resulting in coxa valga;
B2: eventually resulting in a short stubby neck, oval head and coxa magna;
B3: eventually resulting in coxa vara and severe acetabular dysplasia;
B4: eventually resulting in hypoplasia of the entire hip joint.

however, is not a contraindication to this operation since simultaneous varus correction is also possible [5, 9].

The "Femoral Neck Lengthening Osteotomy" (FNLO) aims to restore normal anatomy with restitution of the length of the femoral neck and the leg length, as well as improvement of the lever arm of the abductors (fig 2). The procedure includes three osteotomies parallel to a 130° or 120° blade plate. Lateralisation of the shaft effectively lengthens the femoral neck. Part of the overgrown greater trochanter is used to fill the gap above the lateralised shaft. The remaining trochanter is dislocated distally and fixed to the lateral side of the femur. This operation allows correction of limb shortening of 1 to 1.5 cm and improvement of the lever arm of the abductors. As a rule, this is followed by disappearance of, or at least amelioration of, a Trendelenburg-type gait.

All references to this article must include: Morscher EW, Hefti F and Hasler CC. Femoral neck lengthening osteotomy (FNLO). Editions Scientifiques et Médicales Elsevier SAS (Paris). All rights reserved. Surgical Techniques in Orthopaedics and Traumatology, 55-430-C-10, 2000, 4 p.

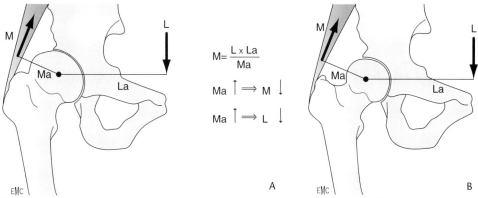

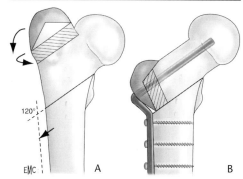

2 Rationale for the "Femoral Neck Lengthening Osteotomy". According to Pauwels' law [9] of weight bearing of the hip joint in the one leg stance phase, the equilibrium of the pelvis can be maintained only if the muscle force (M) is great enough to counteract the body weight (L).
  A. Since M x Ma = L x La (law of balance), a short femoral neck (Ma) increases the load of the hip joint and may lead to an insufficiency of the force of the abductor muscles (M) leading to a Trendelenburg limp.
  B. Under normal conditions, the lever arm of the body weight (La) is three times greater than the lever arm of the muscle force (Ma).

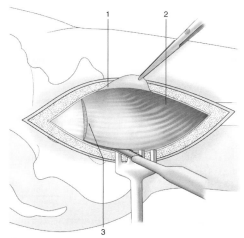

3 Femoral Neck Lengthening Osteotomy - FNLO.
  A. The typical deformity of the proximal femur after ischaemic necrosis of the femoral head. Schematic drawing of the FNLO with the course of the osteotomies, shortening and distal displacement of the greater trochanter and lateral displacement of the femoral diaphysis.
  B. Situation after FNLO, fragments fixed by an AO 120°-angulated plate.

This operation was first described by the first author (E.M.) in 1980 [7]. The results of the first 19 cases were published by Buess and Morscher in 1988 [2]. A similar osteotomy had already been described by Wagner in 1979 (the so-called "double-osteotomy") [11]. An almost identical operation was later published by Lascombes and Prevot in 1985 [6].

Surgical procedure

INDICATIONS

Indications include all conditions with shortening of the femoral neck, independent of their aetiology. This pattern of deformity is found particularly after congenital hip dislocation, Perthes disease or septic arthritis.

CONTRAINDICATIONS

– Open epiphyseal plates. As the osteotomies may cross the growth plate of the greater trochanter, the operation should not be performed in boys before the skeletal age of 15 years and in girls before the skeletal age of 13.5 years.

– Osteoarthritis of the hip joint.

PREOPERATIVE PLANNING

The FNLO is a technically demanding operation that requires precise preoperative planning. The osteotomies must be made at the right level exactly parallel to the blade of the plate.

The contours of the proximal femur are copied on translucent paper *(fig 3)*. The osteotomies are drawn at an angle of 130° or 120° to the shaft along with the blade plate. The length of the blade is measured. In doing this, the presumed lateralisation of the shaft must be taken into account. The blade should not penetrate into the femoral head.

ADDITIONAL PROCEDURES

■ *Pelvic osteotomy*

The hip joint should be well-contained and not subluxated. Insufficient coverage of the femoral head should be corrected with an osteotomy of the acetabulum (Chiari osteotomy, Bernese periacetabular osteotomy, etc.). Such an osteotomy can be combined with the femoral neck lengthening osteotomy, preferably in two stages, since the FNLO increases at least temporarily the pressure between the femoral head and the acetabulum.

■ *Varus/valgus angulation of the femoral neck*

In cases of lack of congruency of the joint space or limited mobility in adduction and/or abduction, bending films should be taken in order to decide whether a varisation or valgisation of the femoral neck should be undertaken in combination with its lengthening.

OPERATIVE TECHNIQUE

■ *Special instruments*

Three Hohmann retractors (2 with a sharp end, 1 blunt), K-wires in various sizes, AO-seating instrument for the blade with a measuring device for the angle, heavy hammer, slotted hammer, oscillating saw, 3.2 mm drill, bone holding forceps, 4-hole 130° or 120° blade plate, AO-cortical screws, bone clamp, cerclage (tension band) wires, AO wire tensioner.

■ *Positioning of the patient*

Supine position. The use of an extension table is recommended. An image intensifier should be available.

■ *Operative procedure*

The skin incision is made laterally on the thigh. It starts at the level of the tip of the greater trochanter and extends distally 12 to

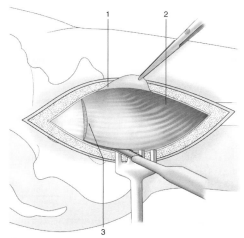

4 L-shaped incision and detachment of the vastus lateralis muscle at its origin. The incision and detachment of the vastus lateralis muscle follows the posterolateral insertion to the femur in a distal direction.

15 cm (depending on the thickness of the subcutaneous fatty tissue). The iliotibial tract is incised longitudinally.

The vastus lateralis muscle is then detached from its insertion in an L-shape *(fig 4)*.

The periosteum is incised and pushed distally with a periosteal elevator. The perforating vessels are dissected and ligated. Hohmann retractors are then inserted. A K-wire is positioned ventrally onto the femoral neck in order to gauge the anteversion angle. The tip of the wire should slightly penetrate into the femoral head. Another 1.6 mm K-wire is then drilled into the femoral neck parallel to the first wire, but with an angle of 50° to the shaft (when using the 130° plate). This wire should be placed simultaneously in the correct anteversion and direction of the blade of the plate as referenced by the first K-wire. A 3.2 mm drill is positioned at the insertion point of the blade. It is recommended to determine this starting point with the image intensifier. At the same time, the position of the K-wire can also be checked. Then, three holes are drilled with the 3.2 mm drill at the

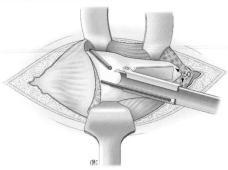

5 *The femur is exposed by three Hohmann retractors. The anteversion angle and the angle of the osteotomies (130° according to the angle of blade of the plate) is marked with a K-wire each. The seating chisel with angular device is inserted. The blade of the angular device must exactly follow the direction of the femur in order to avoid flexion or extension of the proximal fragment. The amount of lateralisation of the diaphyseal shaft must be taken into account when inserting the seating chisel into the femoral neck.*

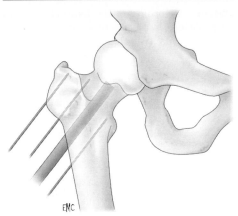

6 *The osteotomies and the position of the seating chisel (blade of the plate) are marked on the preoperative schematic planning. K-wires mark the course of the osteotomies running parallel to the seating chisel. This must be checked on the image intensifier.*

entry point of the seating chisel in order to facilitate the penetration of the edge of the seating chisel, preventing the disruptive effect of the instrument on cortical bone (fig 5). The blade of the seating chisel is now inserted using the angular device. The length of the blade within the bone is checked on the instrument. The blade of the seating chisel is inserted 5 mm longer than the calculated length of the blade of the plate. The amount of lateralisation must be taken into consideration when gauging this length (1.5 to 2 cm). Finally, the seating chisel is loosened with the slotted hammer, as it may be difficult to remove it after completion of the osteotomy.

The insertion of the vastus lateralis is split and the most distal part of the gluteus medius muscle is detached from the greater trochanter with a chisel. At the site of the planned osteotomies, K-wires are inserted parallel to the blade of the seating chisel. The insertion of the wires is guided by the image intensifier. The wires run the course of the osteotomies according to the preoperative planning (fig 6).

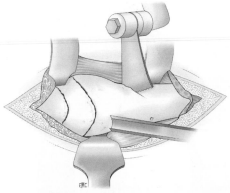

7 *The K-wires are removed. The osteotomies run parallel to the blade of the seating chisel at exactly a right angle to the frontal plane. The second osteotomy runs parallel to the first one and at the level of the upper circumference of the femoral neck. The greater trochanter is shortened. The cylindrical piece of bone between the two proximal osteotomies is harvested and used later on to fill the gap between the lateral "end" of the femoral neck and the fixation plate. The third osteotomy runs parallel to the first ones ending below the lower circumference of the femoral neck. To avoid penetration of the osteotomy into the femoral neck, the blade of the oscillating saw must be held in an anteroposterior direction (not from laterally to medially).*

The proximal osteotomy is carried out with the oscillating saw parallel to the blade of the seating chisel.

The second osteotomy is carried out parallel to the first one. A cylindrical piece of bone with a height of 1-1.5 cm is removed from the greater trochanter.

The third osteotomy is carried out distally to the blade of the seating chisel and parallel to it (fig 7). Care must be taken not to perform the osteotomy in too oblique a manner and not to penetrate into the femoral neck. The distance between this osteotomy and the blade of the seating chisel must be at least 2 cm to avoid a breakthrough of the plate later on.

Before replacing the seating chisel, the trochanteric fragment is perforated with the 4.5 mm drill three times to facilitate penetration of the blade of the blade plate. The blade of the selected 130° angled blade plate is now —with the resected trochanteric fragment— driven into the femoral neck after the seating chisel has been removed with the slotted hammer.

The blade must be inserted with the calculated length considering the amount of lateralisation of the femoral diaphysis. The shaft is then lateralised and provisionally fixed to the plate with a bone clamp. Careful control of the plate's position is mandatory. The first screw hole is drilled with the eccentric drill guide to compress the bony fragment. The arrow on the drill guide must point towards the osteotomy. Measurement of the length is followed by tapping and insertion of the first screw. The other drill holes are made with the neutral drill guide. Four full-length cortical screws are inserted for fixation of the plate (fig 8).

In the next step, the greater trochanter is lateralised and distalised. A thick (2 mm)

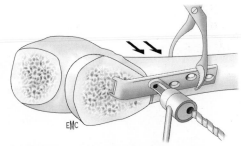

8 *Lateral displacement of the femoral shaft and provisional fixation of the plate by means of a bone clamp. The first drill hole is drilled eccentrically with the corresponding drill guide, the arrow pointing to the osteotomy, herewith compressing the osteotomy when inserting the first screw. The other drill holes are made with the neutral drill guide. The use of full threaded AO cortical screws is recommended.*

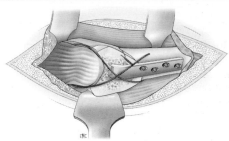

9 *The greater trochanter is distalised and fixed with cerclage wires to the distal diaphyseal fragment.*

cerclage wire is passed underneath the gluteus medius and minimus muscles running along the bony contour of the greater trochanter. A hole is drilled into the shaft of the femur and the wire is passed through it in a "figure eight" (fig 9).

Before closure of the wound, the vastus lateralis is reinserted. The posterior corner should be sutured with a U-shaped suture. The plate and the cerclage wire must be well-covered with muscle tissue. Three suction drains are inserted and the iliotibial tract is reapproximated. Skin closure and a compressive wound dressing complete the operative intervention.

Postoperative treatment

After surgery, the patient is in a supine position with the operated leg in abduction. He is allowed to discontinue bed rest on the first postoperative day and to ambulate with two crutches, non-weight-bearing on the operative side. After six weeks, the patient is controlled clinically and radiologically. If normal healing is evident, weight-bearing with 50% body weight is allowed. Full weight-bearing is permitted after nine to ten weeks.

Pitfalls and mistakes

Incorrect level of osteotomies: The level and direction of the most distal osteotomy in particular must be chosen correctly; otherwise there is the risk of splitting the femoral neck.

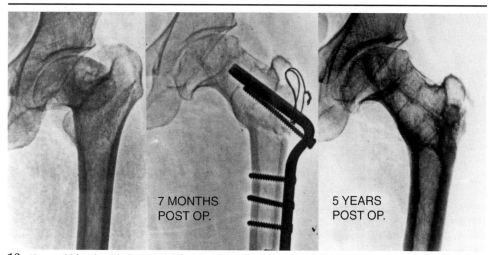

10 *40 year old female with the typical deformity after ischemic necrosis following treatment of a DDH of the left hip joint; 7 months after FNLO; after removal of the internal fixation material; 5 years postop.*

Inadequate fixation of the greater trochanter: As the greater trochanter is pulled down, significant traction must be applied to the gluteus muscles. Fixation, therefore, must be reliable. Care must be taken that the cerclage wire is in contact with the bone; otherwise the wire can cut through the insertion of the muscles and the greater trochanter looses its position.

Short blade length of the blade plate: Lateralisation of the shaft of the femur increases the lever arm of the femoral neck. Care must be taken that the blade of the blade plate penetrates the femoral neck far enough; otherwise the risk arises of the neck tilting into varus position.

Inadequate distance between blade of the blade plate and distal osteotomy: There must be a minimum distance of 2 cm between the blade of the plate and the distal osteotomy; otherwise break-out of the blade and, as a consequence, varus tilting of the neck will occur.

Results *(fig 10)*

Thirty-seven patients were assessed both clinically and radiologically with an average follow-up of 8 years (1 to 16 years). The average age at operation was 22 years (range 14 to 52 years); 14 were males and 23 females.

The leg length difference, of an average of 2.3 cm (0.0-6.0) preoperatively, was corrected by 1.3 cm (0.0-3.0). In 3 patients, the leg length remained unchanged. Normal gait was restored in 13 out of 14 patients with a preoperative "shortening limp". A Duchenne-Trendelenburg gait and/or positive Trendelenburg test —present in 30 cases preoperatively— became normal or was substantially improved in 21 cases. The FNLO did not influence the range of motion, except abduction, with an average improvement of 10°. Preoperatively, 5 out of 8 patients in the age group 30-49 years showed significant radiological signs and symptoms of osteoarthritis. Four of them required total hip replacement (THR) 1 to 9 years after surgery. One 62 year-old female patient still suffers from severe osteoarthritis 17 years after FNLO, but has refused THR. Twenty-four out of 32 patients without significant osteoarthritic changes who complained of muscular fatigue of their hip abductors with restriction of physical activities responded well to the operation. In the age group under 29 years, only one poor result was noted: a 16 year-old girl still walked on crutches two years after surgery due to persistent muscular insufficiency. Pre- and postoperative MDA-scoring could be figured out in 33 patients. Complaints about muscular fatigue were rated as pain. The overall score improved in 26 patients, remained the same in one patient, and deteriorated in 6 patients, amongst whom 5 patients developed osteoarthritic changes. Omitting these cases, the overall score improved on an average from 15.6 to 17 points (maximum 18 points). Regarding the MDA subgroups, gait (4.8 to 5.6 points) and pain (5.1 to 5.8 points) improved, whereas the score for range of motion showed only little improvement (5.4 to 5.6 points).

The following complications were noted: One nonunion of the greater trochanter after inadequate fixation with synthetic non-absorbable tension bands (Syntofil®) had to be revised, and healed uneventfully after tension band wiring. There was one transient peroneal nerve palsy due to inadequate postoperative positioning. One subcutaneous haematoma healed under conservative measures.

Indications

The femoral neck lengthening osteotomy aims to restore the normal anatomy and function of the hip joint. It should not be performed as long as the epiphyseal cartilage of the femoral neck and greater trochanter is open. The operation is also contraindicated in the case of osteoarthritis which is due to incongruency as a consequence of a dysplastic acetabulum and/or a deformity of the femoral head. In such cases, a pelvic osteotomy and/or valgus/varus osteotomy is indicated in addition.

References

[1] Bucholz RW, Ogden JA. Patterns of ischemic necrosis of the proximal femur in nonoperatively treated congenital hip disease. In : The Hip: Proceedings of the 6th open scientific meeting of the Hip Society. St Louis : CV Mosby, 1978 : 43-63

[2] Buess P, Morscher E. Die schenkelhalsverlängernde Osteotomie mit Distalisierung des Trochanter major bei Coxa vara. *Orthop Prax* 1988 ; 9 : 576-581

[3] Hasler CC, Morscher EW. Femoral neck lengthening osteotomy after ischemic necrosis of the upper femoral epiphysis. *J Pediatr Orthop* 1999 ; B8 : 271-275

[4] Kalamchi A, Macewen GD. Avascular necrosis following treatment of congenital dislocation of the hip. *J Bone Joint Surg Am* 1980 ; 62 : 876-888

[5] Keret D, Macewen GD. Growth disturbance of the proximal part of the femur after treatment of congenital dislocation of the hip. *J Bone Joint Surg Am* 1991 ; 73 : 410-423

[6] Lascombes P, Prevot J, Allouche A, Ligier JN, Metaizeau JP. L'ostéotomie d'allongement du col fémoral avec transposition du grand trochanter dans les coxa-vara acquises. *Rev Chir Orthop* 1985 ; 71 : 599-601

[7] Morscher E. Intertrochanteric osteotomy in osteoarthritis of the hip. In : The Hip: Proceedings of the 8th open scientific meeting of the Hip Society. St Louis : CV Mosby, 1980 : 24-46

[8] Ogden JA. Anatomic and histologic study of factors affecting development and evolution of avascular necrosis in congenital dislocation of the hip. In : The Hip: Proceedings of the 2nd open scientific meeting of the Hip Society. St Louis : CV Mosby, 1974 : 125-153

[9] Pauwels F. Biomechanical principles of varus/valgus intertrochanteric osteotomy (Pauwels I and II) in the treatment of the hip. In : Schatzker J ed. The Intertrochanteric Osteotomy. Berlin : Springer-Verlag, 1984 : 3-23

[10] Specchiulli F, Scialpi L, Solarino GJR, Laforgia R. Avascular necrosis in congenital dislocation of the hip: long-term results and proposed new classification. *Hip Int* 1995 ; 5 : 72-81

[11] Wagner H. Korrekturosteotomien am Bein. *Orthopäde* 1977 ; 6 : 145-177

Classification of total hip arthroplasties (THA)

J Witvoet

Abstract. – Before recommending a total hip replacement, it is vital that the surgeon appreciate the advantages and disadvantages of the different prostheses available. The actual choice of which model to use can be difficult given the number currently being manufactured. The aim of this chapter is not to review all these prostheses (more than 400 different designs), but to guide the surgeon by describing the advantages and disadvantages of the different materials used for each of the parts of the implant (socket, head and stem), the different bearing surfaces (metal or ceramic–polyethylene, ceramic–ceramic, metal–metal), the different methods of fixation of the prosthesis to bone (with or without cement), the different qualities of the surfaces and of their coating, and the qualities of osteointegration of those prostheses inserted without cement.

© 2001, Editions Scientifiques et Médicales Elsevier SAS. All rights reserved.

Keywords: hip, hip prosthesis, total hip arthroplasty (THA), classification, material, choices.

Introduction

Even if some surgeons always use the same type of prosthesis whatever the aetiology of the lesion, the age of the patient and his or her activities, it does seem reasonable to consider using different models, which often vary considerably in cost. For example, a stainless steel femoral component with a polyethylene (PE) cup (like that of Charnley [6]) costs four to five times less than one made of titanium with a rough stem covered with hydroxyapatite and articulating either with a metal-on-metal cup or a ceramic-on-ceramic cup. It is evident from the literature that a Charnley cemented prosthesis gives an excellent result in patients with a life expectancy of less than ten years; in this case there are no indications to use a more sophisticated implant.

In younger patients with a longer expectation of life, cemented prostheses with a metal or ceramic-on-polyethylene articulation deteriorate as a result of wear of the polyethylene, with osteolysis around the implant which leads to loosening. It is wise to use bearing surfaces with low coefficients of wear, such as metal-on-metal, ceramic-on-ceramic, or perhaps the newer polyethylenes.

It is essential that every new type of prosthesis suggested by manufacturers or others be not only tested in the laboratory, but also carefully studied with a clinical follow-up by appropriate experts before being released onto the market.

General properties [17, 21]

Total hip arthroplasty (THA) has been practised widely throughout the world since 1960. Before that, it had only been possible to replace a degenerate femoral head using a relatively simple prosthesis such as that of Judet or Moore. The first true total hip replacements were that of John Charnley, which had a metal femoral component and an acetabulum made of Teflon®, and that of Mackee-Farrar (fig 1), which had a metal-on-metal bearing (cobalt chrome alloy). Unfortunately, the early results of the Charnley metal-on-Teflon® were disastrous due to the rapid rate of wear of the Teflon® and to biological loosening. The results with the Mackee-Farrar were hardly better, as the occurrence of binding between the metallic surfaces led to early loosening from this mechanical cause. Charnley soon replaced the Teflon® with a high density polyethylene (HDP) of ultra high molecular structure in order to produce a Low Friction Arthroplasty (LFA), and this in fact is still the "gold standard". The original metal-on-metal prosthesis was soon abandoned.

In 1970, Pierre Boutin [3] devised a new bearing surface using alumina ceramic in order to reduce the amount of wear particles produced by metal-on-ultra high density polyethylene (UHDP) or metal-on-metal. Since 1990, new metal-on-metal bearings

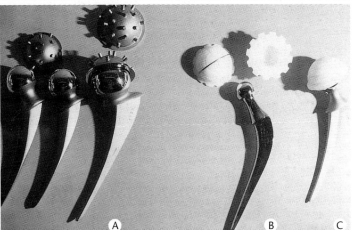

1 *The first total hip arthroplasties: McKee Farrar (A); Charnley (B); Charnley-Müller (C).*

Jacques Witvoet, M.D., Professor of Orthopaedic Surgery and Traumatology, Consultant, Orthopaedic Service, Hôpital Lariboisière, 75010 Paris, France.

All references to this article must include: Witvoet J. Classification of total hip arthroplasties (THA). Editions Scientifiques et Médicales Elsevier SAS (Paris). All rights reserved. Surgical Techniques in Orthopaedics and Traumatology, 55-430-D-10, 2001, 8 p.

have been developed which have an improved mechanical design and better wear characteristics than the original metal-on-metal prostheses.

Initially, acrylic cement was used for their fixation. In 1971, J. and R. Judet had the idea of not using acrylic cement to fix the two components, but to prepare the relevant surfaces to allow solid biological fixation by the in-growth of bone.

During the last 30 years, numerous types of prostheses have seen the light of day; some were used in many countries while the use of others remained more national or even regional. However, despite all the progress made, there is still no artificial hip prosthesis which can really replace the normal human joint.

The selection of which type to use depends on various criteria which include the material, the bearing surfaces and the method of fixation, as well as what is best for each individual patient and the specific training of the surgeon.

All complications and risks which can endanger life or jeopardise future function must now be reported to the relevant authorities established in all countries of Europe. All defects in design or manufacture which may result in fracture or excess wear must be reported by the surgeon. This means that he or she must be responsible for the selection of which prosthesis to implant, even if it is not of his or her design. All orthopaedic surgeons who perform total hip replacement must remain up-to-date with the current literature and regularly attend meetings of the specialist societies.

For several years in Europe, only prostheses bearing the mark "CE" have been acceptable; it is the surgeon's responsibility to ensure that only these are implanted. The characteristics of the selected prosthesis must be appreciated, including the material of manufacture, the type and any special preparation of the surfaces, the method of fixation, etc., as well as the renown of the manufacturer and the ISO 9002 label. Knowledge of any appropriate clinical trials of the specific prosthesis is also important, and will allow the surgeon to answer any questions posed by the patient.

Another problem arises when a total hip prosthesis has to be revised; this may involve the use of special instruments to remove a failed implant. It is essential that the surgeon be aware of the characteristics of the prosthesis, both when it is to be entirely replaced or when only one of the components must be exchanged. This is one of the reasons why the European Federation of National Associations of Orthopaedics and Traumatology (EFORT) has asked the European Hip Society to establish a European Hip Register.

A simple classification of total hip arthroplasties

As it is not my intention to list all the prostheses currently available on the European market, I have devised a simple classification which is easy to use, is based on each component of the prosthesis, the method of fixation, its modularity, and which stresses the advantages and disadvantages of each available model. References are quoted to allow further study of the current situation.

Components of a total hip arthroplasty

THE ACETABULAR COMPONENT

Available materials

Three materials are currently being used for the surface which receives the femoral head: ultra high molecular weight polyethylene (UHMWP), ceramics and metals.

• *Ultra high molecular weight polyethylene*

This is currently the most commonly used material for the bearing surface of the acetabular component. It must be of very high density with a molecular weight on the order of 2,500,000 to 4,000,000. The components are made either from a powder which is heated and then compressed in a mould, or from preformed cylinders or bars. The wear characteristics and resistance depend on the chemical composition, the molecular weight and the effects of sterilisation. As with all plastic materials, polyethylene (PE) is subject to deformation under pressure and to different types of wear (abrasion, adhesion corrosion or fatigue). Certain techniques have been used to try to improve the quality of PE (forging, chemical reticulation, heating or incorporation of carbon fibres), but as yet their value has not been proved.

The principal advantage of PE is its tribologic characteristics. It allows a sort of lubrication of the bearing surfaces which prevents binding and reduces wear. However, wear does exist in all load-bearing systems and occurs more on the less resistant surfaces (e.g. polyethylene against either metal or ceramic). Wear can result from abrasion, binding or fatigue. It depends on the materials used (50% less with ceramic than with metal heads), on the quality of the surface of the material, on the size of the head and on the life of the sterilisation. Sterilisation of the polyethylene by irradiation under normal air accelerates the oxidation process of the PE and increases the wear. There is less wear with metal heads of 22 mm than with those of 32 mm, as the bearing surface is smaller. This was Charnley's idea when he developed the Low Friction Arthroplasty (LFA) [6]. However, the penetration of the femoral head into the socket is more marked with 22 mm heads than with 32 mm heads, which can lead to impingement between the two components and to mechanical loosening. Heads of 28 mm seem a good compromise.

Another advantage of all PE acetabular components is the low modulus of elasticity (not so different from that of cortical bone), which does not modify the stress and strain on the pelvic bone.

The main disadvantage is the greater wear rate, of about 0.1 mm per year. This wear has two detrimental consequences. When the volume of wear particles exceeds the local possibility of resorption, osteolysis around the prosthesis appears due to proteolytic enzymes. Biological aseptic loosening is often the consequence of this osteolysis.

• *Ceramics*

There are two types of ceramics: alumina ceramic was first used by P. Boutin [24] in 1970 and zirconia ceramic appeared in 1989. Both use a powder of either alumina or zirconia heated to a high temperature. High quality control at every stage of manufacture and of every finished component is essential. The materials must fulfil very strict international standards: maximum purity (99.5% of aluminium oxide or zirconia), high density (>3.94 for alumina), very small grains (<3 microns for alumina and 0.1 micron for zirconia) and, above all, the homogeneous distribution of these grains. All these reasons explain why there are only a few ceramic manufacturers in the world and why the price is higher than that of plastics.

The principal quality of alumina ceramics is their stability and high degree of oxidation. This explains why the wear of alumina ceramics rarely produces inflammation reactions as described by Willer, Semlich, and Sedel. Their main fault is their fragility, which in the beginning resulted in fractures occurring in the femoral head (but not of the acetabular component) in about 3 to 7% of cases. The currently available alumina ceramics have a lower fracture rate of 0.02-0.04% (2-4 fractures per 10,000 prostheses).

Zirconia ceramic has the advantage of being more resistant to shock, compression and flexion, because it is a dispersoid ceramic where the propagation of fissures is more limited than in alumina ceramic. However, it is a less stable material than alumina ceramic, as during its manufacture it can pass from a stable monoclinical to an unstable tetragonal form which is less resistant to wear and breakage. This can be partially solved by adding yttrium oxide as a stabiliser.

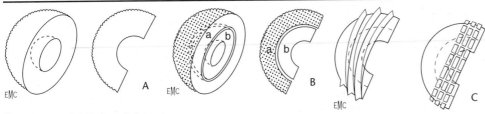

2 *Different models of acetabular cups:*
A. Monoblock (PE, metal, alumina).
B. Modular press-fit (a = roughened metallic cup; b = insert: PE, alumina).
C. Modular screw cup.

● *Metals*

The only metals currently used for the acetabular cup are the cobalt-chromium-molybdenum alloys (CCM) and titanium alloys. Stainless steel is used only for the femoral component. In evaluating metals, it is necessary to consider both those used for bearing surfaces and those used to form a rigid and strong backing of the cup.

McKee-Farrar and Ring used CCM alloy in their early prostheses. Unfortunately, at that time the quality of these CCM alloys was unsatisfactory; above all the quality of the surface of the head and the metal cup was unreliable. This resulted in a high proportion of loosening, either as a result of excessive friction at the bearing surfaces, from excessive wear, or from a combination of these two problems. In the last twelve years, improvement in the quality of the CCM alloys has allowed the production of smoother bearing surfaces and a much more accurate clearance between the head and the cup. One can only hope that these new metal-on-metal prostheses will not give the same poor results as their forebears. The advantage of a metal component is the absence of fracture. Yet, one unsolved problem remains: will the amount of chromium, cobalt and molybdenum ions circulating in the blood have deleterious effects? This risk would be increased if excessive wear occurs at the bearing surfaces. However, short term results seem to be very satisfactory.

■ *The different models of acetabular component* (fig 2)

There are two basic types of cup: monoblock or modular.

Monoblock acetabular cups *(fig 2A)*

These are produced in polyethylene, metal or ceramic.

Those made of **all polyethylene** must be cemented, as experience with these cups fixed directly to bone has been catastrophic after several years, due to excessive wear of the polyethylene at the convex outer surface. Morscher reinforced the polyethylene with a metal mesh; these components then did not require cement fixation nor did they suffer any significant thinning of the polyethylene [18].

All the models have some irregularities on their convex surface, so that the cup/cement interface can resist loosening produced by shear and stress forces. It is important that the polyethylene have a thickness of more that 8-9 mm so that the cup is not too supple and can therefore resist creep and wear.

As far as the **monoblock metallic cups** are concerned, some are made entirely of metal, while others have a sandwich form, i.e. metal-PE-metal. The PE in the sandwich acts as a shock absorber and spreads the forces acting on the bone. However, the creation of two interfaces (between the PE and the two layers of metal) with each material having a very different modulus of elasticity can create the risk of late failure.

Some **monoblock alumina ceramic cups** were originally fixed with the same cementing technique as used for PE cups. Unfortunately, the difference in the elasticity of the cement and of the ceramic cup produces significant stresses in the cement which can then lead to fracture or to separation of the cement from the ceramic cup.

Other non-cemented cups have been proposed: Mittelmaer's screw cups, Boutin's cup which has small knobs and Sedel's cup which uses press-fit. The results have not always been satisfactory, for it is rare if not impossible for the bone to grow into close contact with the ceramic. The relative high rate of loosening makes their use problematic.

Modular cups *(fig 2B, C)*

These consist of two parts: a metal-backed cup which fixes to the bone and accepts an inner cup made either of PE or ceramic.

The **metallic component** can be made either of titanium alloy or CCM alloy. Titanium alloy has a modulus of elasticity two times lower than that of CCM alloy and is better able to resist corrosion. Bone in-growth is easier than with the CCM alloy, but the titanium alloy is more susceptible to wear. To avoid migration of metallic cups, it is important that they have a rough surface which allows firm fixation to bone, encouraging a bone/metal interface which will resist movements resulting from the different elasticity of the bone and the metal cup. Metal cups with a smooth convex surface are no longer used. The roughened surface of the newer models can be produced by various techniques: sand blasting, coating the surface with microballs, or by using a porous mesh. To encourage

good in-growth of bone, many cups are now being covered with a calcium phosphate; the most often used is hydroxyapatite. Twelve years ago, the manufacture and the fixation of hydroxyapatite left much to be desired, due to difficulties in transforming it from a crystalline to an amorphous state, as well as to its poor fixation to the metal surface. Nowadays, these problems seem to have been resolved [5, 7, 8, 10, 11, 24]. The hydroxyapatite accelerates bone in-growth and, when the primary fixation is good, will produce a physical-chemical bond with the bone. This should completely obliterate the bone/cup interface (or the stem/bone interface) and prevent the penetration of particles of different materials resulting from joint wear. This should also decrease loosening due to any aseptic biological cause. The hydroxyapatite is very slowly absorbed, but will this too have long-term consequences? Only a good long-term study will supply the answer.

The exterior surface of the cup may be of various shapes. The majority are more or less hemispherical and have an equatorial diameter 1-2 mm greater than that of the polar diameter to ensure a good press-fit. Some cups have diameters identical to that of the cavity produced by an acetabular reamer, and are then fixed by five or six screws which produce compression between the component and the bone. However, this method of fixation will allow micro-movements between the screws and the cup, which can produce either metallic or polyethylene debris. These days, many cups are also being used that have either only two or no holes in the dome.

There are also various metallic rings which can be used with screws (such as the ZweiMüller); these too have a rough surface or may be covered with hydroxyapatite. Other cup designs include one or more slits (such as the Spotorno cup), which can improve both flexibility and fixation.

● *Insert*

The insert can be made of polyethylene or alumina ceramic. A PE cup must always have a thickness greater than 7-8 mm; otherwise, wear of the PE will result in a fracture of the insert after 3 to 4 years, and will often be associated with a massive osteolysis produced by metal-on-metal contact. An alumina ceramic insert should always be at least 4-5 mm thick to reduce the risk of fracture.

● *Fixation of the insert*

It is very important that the insert, whether ceramic or polyethylene, not move within the metal cup. The interior surface should be highly polished to decrease, in as far as possible, the production of wear debris. Various techniques for fixation are available when using PE, while inserts made of alumina ceramic are always fixed into the metal cup by inverse morse cone. It is important during surgery to ensure that good fixation and positioning of the inner ceramic has been achieved.

• *Cups with a mobile insert*

With the object of limiting wear and reducing the risk of dislocation, certain modular cups have a mobile PE insert. There is therefore a double mobility: between the metal cup and the PE insert, and also between the PE insert and the femoral head. This cup design reduces the risk of dislocation, but it is not certain whether its use decreases wear. The mobility of the insert on the metal may well increase the production of wear particles.

■ **Reinforcement of the acetabulum**

When there is a deficiency of bone in the acetabular region, it may be necessary to reinforce the iliac bone. Various devices and techniques have been devised, some in the shape of a ring are screwed to the internal wall of the acetabulum (Müller). Others have a inferior hook (such as the Kerboull cross or Gantz's ring) which is fixed to the superior margin of the obturator foramen. They have two advantages:

– they automatically centre the acetabular component in a good position,

– they prevent displacement of the reinforcement when combined with bone grafts.

Usually the cup is cemented into the reinforcing ring, but some are mechanically fixed (screws, a self-retaining fixation, or by other means) and this produces direct contact between the metal cup and its host bed.

FEMORAL COMPONENT

■ **Femoral stem**

The majority of prostheses (both monoblock and modular) consist of a femoral head which articulates with the acetabular component, and a femoral stem which occupies the medullary cavity of the femur. However, the stems of some femoral components are not designed to pass down the canal, but rather to follow the direction of the femoral neck (like a nail or a screw). In others, the head is attached to a femoral plate which is screwed onto the lateral cortex of the femoral diaphysis. These models are not being widely used, so it is difficult to determine their advantages and disadvantages.

The materials

Currently only metal femoral stems are being used, as other materials, such as reinforced carbon fibre, isoelastic plastic, glass fibre with or without composites, etc., have not yet been found reliable. Three metals are being used: austenitic stainless steel, CCM alloys and titanium alloys.

• *Austenitic special steels*

These are much more corrosion resistant than ferritic stainless steels. Steel 316 L is most commonly used. It contains 16-19% chromium which by oxidation creates a film of passivation (which resists corrosion) on the surface of the stem, 12-16% nickel which toughens the steel and reinforces the resistance to corrosion, and 2-4% molybdenum which prevents the formation of ferrite iron which itself reduces the resistance of the steel. It also contains 0.03% of carbon which eliminates contaminating elements derived from carbon intergranularity. The mechanical qualities of steel 316 L can further be enhanced by adding nitrogen using a heat treatment, by cold working, by casting in a vacuum.

• *CCM alloys*

The composition of these alloys (chrome, cobalt, molybdenum, nickel, tungsten, and carbon) depends on the individual manufacturers, but they can be considered in two major groups:

– those produced by a melting process following wax precision casting;

– those produced by forging (hot drop forging, usually by using a hydraulic press).

• *Titanium alloys*

Pure titanium cannot be used as it resists neither corrosion nor mechanical stresses. The commonly used titanium alloy contains 4% of vanadium and 6% of aluminium (Ti6A4V). Its modulus of elasticity (Young's modulus) is two times lower than that of steel or CCM alloys, and this helps to prevent stress-shielding particularly in the metaphyseal femoral cortex.

The disadvantage of titanium alloy is its lower resistance to wear, even if it has received a special surface treatment, than either steel or CCM alloys, but this inconvenience is decreased when the femoral stem has been well fixed, with or without cement. On the other hand, when the stem of the prosthesis has become loose, this will produce more metallic particles than arise from either steel or the CCM alloys, which can cause a significant soft tissue metallosis.

Surface of the femoral stem

Whatever material is used to make the femoral stem, the surface can be considered to be either smooth, mirror-like or roughened.

– **Smooth stemmed prostheses** are used only in conjunction with acrylic cement.

– **Rough stemmed prostheses** should never be used with cement. The rough surface can either be produced (as for the acetabular component) by using sand blasting, by the addition of microballs, or by a special technique (mesh, etc.).

The roughness of the surface encourages bone in-growth to ensure firm fixation, but certain conditions are essential if this is to occur:

– The most important is to ensure a good primary fixation of the stem in the diaphysis of the femoral canal. This depends on various factors, the most important of which is to use good operative technique. A really good bone/prosthesis contact must be achieved, so that the new bone formation arising from the cortex can reach the porous surface of the stem.

– The size of the pores should be between 50-300 μm.

– Biocompatability between the surfacing material on the stem and the bone is essential, and titanium alloy is the most effective.

The roughened surface can cover either a part (1/3, 2/3) or the whole length of the stem. The advantages of a proximal fixation (roughening of the proximal part of the stem) is that the maximum forces pass through this area, helping to improve the resistance of the bone to stress shielding. The other advantage is that it is easier to extract a firmly fixed prosthesis if for any reason this becomes indicated.

An as yet unproved disadvantage is the slight increase in the incidence of thigh pain compared to those patients with a totally roughened stem. This symptom may possibly arise from the distal unroughened end of the stem.

The advantages and disadvantages of a distal fixation (with entire stem roughening) are obviously the opposite of those with partial roughening: more stress shielding at the femoral metaphysis, less pain from the end of the stem, but more difficulty in extraction.

Use of a bioactive osteoconductor coating
[5, 7, 8, 10, 11, 24]

During the last twelve years, the work of Degroot, Geesing and Manley has encouraged the development of the use of calcium-phosphate materials such as hydroxyapatite (HA) coating, now being used more and more often. The HA is applied to the femoral stem by plasma spread. This accelerates bone in-growth both clinically and in the laboratory. Hydroxyapatite is an osteoconductor which guides and improves bone in-growth, but is not an osteo-inductor. Strict conditions apply to the use of HA. It must be a true hydroxyapatie, and not an inactive calcium-phosphate. The fixation of the HA to the support must be perfect to ensure that there is no gap between the HA and the roughened surface.

Other bioactive coatings can be used, such as a mixture of HA and tri-calcium-phosphate (TCP). TCP is absorbed faster than HA, but has a better osteoconductive activity.

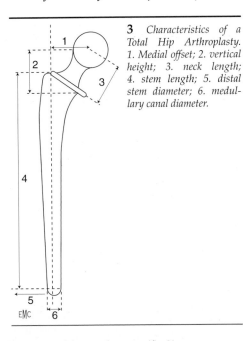

3 *Characteristics of a Total Hip Arthroplasty. 1. Medial offset; 2. vertical height; 3. neck length; 4. stem length; 5. distal stem diameter; 6. medullary canal diameter.*

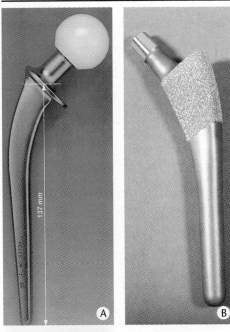

4 *Modular femoral stems.*
A. Cemented.
B. Porous coated.
C. Hydroyapatite coating.

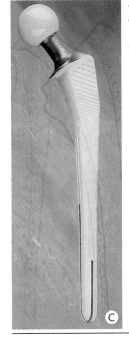

5 *Multiple modular femoral stems.*
A. Modular, head/neck and metaphysis/diaphysis.
B. Modular, head/neck, neck/metaphysis and metaphysis/diaphysis.

Designs of femoral stems *(fig 3)*

Femoral stems are not only characterised by the materials used and by their surfacing, but also by their specific design; this includes the shape, size, length, offset and anteversion, and the possible presence of a collar to bear on the calcar.

The design of cemented stems must help to reduce the strains exerted on the cement layer between the prosthesis and the bone, and in particular it should not have an acute angle. There are two types of stems used without cement fixation: those which fill as much as possible of the medullary cavity of the femur particularly at the metaphyseal level and are known as "anatomical press-fit"', and those which are straight and rectangular and which fix in the cortical bone at the level of its four angulations. The first have right and left stems, but the second type can be used for either side. Whatever the shape of the stem, it should be perfectly fixed in order to limit any micro-movement in three planes, which can occur at the bone/stem interface, particularly in the horizontal plane (in rotation).

Modular and monoblock stems

Femoral stems can be either monoblock, when the head and stem are made in the same mould or forged in one piece *(fig 4)*, or modular *(fig 5)* and therefore made in more than one part. Modularity is usually constructed at the head/neck junction, and the femoral head is fixed by a tight-fitting morse cone to the stem during the operation. The sides of the cone and its seating in the femoral head must correspond accurately so as to ensure perfect fixation. For this reason, it is forbidden to combine components made by different manufacturers.

Other parts of the stem can also be constructed in modular fashion, either with separate metaphyseal and diaphyseal components so that the prosthesis can be adapted to any shape of femoral canal, or at the junction of the metaphyseal portion and the neck, so as to be able to alter the offset and/or anteversion.

This modularity of the stem has several advantages:

– It is possible to adapt the stem to all femurs, whatever the shape of the femoral canal, the length of the neck, any deformity of the upper part of the femur whether primary or acquired, without the necessity of having available a large range of prostheses.

– It also allows a single part of the stem to be changed, for instance, in the case of a modular head inserted for a femoral neck fracture which can later easily be changed to a total hip replacement simply by changing the head and using the previously inserted stem.

However, there are several disadvantages. Galvanic corrosion can occur with or without wear between the two components if they are not a perfect fit. The mechanical strength of a modular stem is 10-20% less than that of a monoblock. Manufacture of the components must be very accurate as concerns the connecting parts of the two modules, and surgeons must take extra care during insertion to protect the junction, to clean both components thoroughly before they are fitted together, and, above all, to never use components made by different manufacturers.

Custom-made prostheses *(fig 6)*

Insertion of a total hip prosthesis can be approached by two routes. The most popular is to adapt the bones to a readily available prosthesis; this may involve the use of special instruments or the use of cement. The other method is to use a custom-made prosthesis designed and manufactured for a specific patient. This is more often necessary for the femoral component than for the cup. Appropriate CT scanning is necessary in the manufacture of these personalised components. A computer programme can control the actual manufacture by machine tools, producing a femoral stem designed to fit a specific femoral canal, its varus/valgus angles, and the offset of the neck. These specially-constructed stems are usually supplied with a rasp which is slightly smaller than the stem which is to be accurately inserted. The theoretical advantage of these custom-made stems, which do not require cement, is that they should be a perfect fit, allowing good bone in-growth and good transmission of stress between the component and the bone.

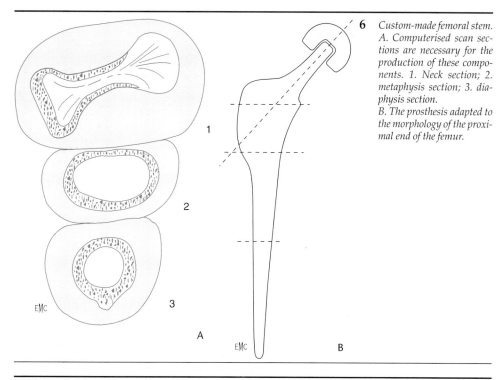

6 *Custom-made femoral stem.*
A. Computerised scan sections are necessary for the production of these components. 1. Neck section; 2. metaphysis section; 3. diaphysis section.
B. The prosthesis adapted to the morphology of the proximal end of the femur.

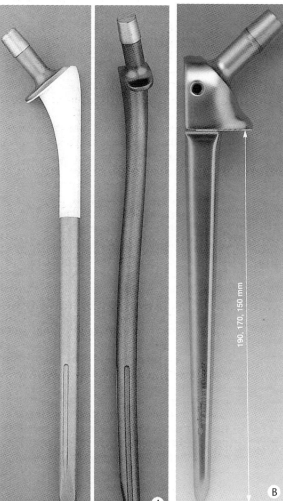

7 *Revision stem. These are longer than normal stems.*
A. Without cement and with or without HA.
B. Cemented.

The principal disadvantage is their very high cost. Even so, they have not yet been shown to have any real superiority over normally manufactured and readily available total hip prostheses.

Revision stems *(fig 7)*

It is often possible to use the same stem for both the primary operation and a revision, but on occasion the latter will require a prosthesis with a special stem. These are

usually longer so as to fill any bone defects and to bear on good quality cortical bone. Distal fixation of these long stems can be with cement (Wrobleski), by fitting tightly into the femur (Wagner), or by screws as used for interlocking intramedullary nails in the treatment of femoral shaft fractures. This latter will necessitate two or more holes in the distal part of the stem. They can be used when the shape and dimension of the medullary canal does not allow firm mechanical fixation.

■ **Femoral head**

This is the part of the femoral component which articulates with the acetabular cup.

Materials

The femoral head can be either metal or ceramic (alumina or zirconia), but whichever material is used it is essential that it be as smooth and polished as possible, and also perfectly spherical.

• *Metal heads*

Steel or CCM alloys are currently the only metals being used for femoral heads. Titanium is unsuitable, as friction against PE produces many wear particles which can produce a local tissue reaction. Some manufacturing techniques (ion implantation, ion nitriding) tend to stiffen the surface of titanium, but the long-term effects of these modifications is still awaited.

• *Ceramic heads*

Alumina ceramic heads have been used since 1970, and zirconia ceramic heads since 1988. The advantages and disadvantages of these two forms of ceramic have already been described, but the advantages of these materials over steel or CCM alloys are:

– greater resistance to wear resulting from friction, particularly in the case of three body wear.

– their smoother bearing surfaces which decrease the wear of the PE.

– better lubrication of the joint as they have a better coefficient of wetability (particularly alumina ceramic).

The disadvantage, particularly of alumina ceramic, is their fragility. A perfect fit between an alumina ceramic head and a metal stem is very important in order to reduce the risk of fracture.

Diameter of the head *(fig 8)*

The diameter of the head can vary considerably between prostheses; the most popular are those of 22, 24, 26, 28 and 32 mm.

Beside the problems of friction, which are considered in the next section, the diameter of the neck and the head is responsible for the amount of contact between the neck of the stem and the cup. This will be greater

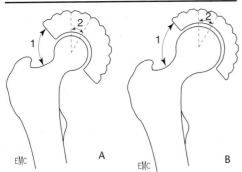

8 *Advantages and disadvantages of different diameters of femoral heads.*
A. 22 mm head. The advantages are greater thickness of the PE, low wear, low friction torque. The disadvantages are easier dislocation and small range of motion.
B. 32 mm head. The advantages are large range of motion, less risk of dislocation. The disadvantages are reduced thickness of PE, more wear, higher friction torque.

when there is a small difference between the width of the neck and the diameter of the head. A great difference will increase the range of movements and decrease contact between the femoral neck and the rim of the cup. It also will reduce the risks of PE wear (if the cup is of PE) or of the neck (if the cup is of metal or ceramic). By limiting contact between the neck and the cup, it will also lessen the mechanical stresses which can result in aseptic loosening.

Heads of 22 mm have a greater tendency to dislocate than those of 28 mm and especially those of 32 mm.

BEARING SURFACES

These provide another classification for total hip prostheses. The main surfaces in use are: metal-on-polyethylene, ceramic (alumina or zirconia)-on-polyethylene, alumina-on-alumina ceramic, and metal-on-metal.

■ *Metal- or ceramic-on-polyethylene bearing surfaces* [4, 9, 16, 27]

Metal-on-polyethylene can be either steel (very often 22.2 mm as in Charnley's prosthesis) or CCM alloys (very often with a diameter of 28 or 32 mm).

Although surfaces of 22 mm diameter decrease the amount of PE wear particles and help to maintain sufficient thickness of the PE in cups of small diameter, they have a greater risk of postoperative dislocation. Bearing surfaces of 32 mm produce more wear particles and decrease the thickness of the PE in cups of small size, but decrease the risk of dislocation.

Ceramic-on-PE decreases the production of wear particles when compared to metal-on-PE by about 50%.

However, the production of wear particles and the coefficient of friction does not depend only on the materials used, but also on the roughness and circularity of the bearing surfaces, the amount of play, the load, the type of movement (sliding and gliding) and the type of lubrication.

■ *Ceramic-on-ceramic bearing surfaces* [3, 19, 22, 25, 26]

Currently the only type being used is alumina-on-alumina ceramic. Zirconia-on-zirconia ceramic produces so much abrasion that it cannot be used. The use of alumina-on-zirconia ceramic seems to interest some surgeons, but this remains at an experimental stage.

There are three advantages for alumina-on-alumina ceramic (of 28 or 32 mm diameter):

– They have a low coefficient of friction which does not alter with time.

– Very little wear occurs (on condition that the alumina ceramic is of very good quality, that the clearance between the head and the cup is less than 10 mm, and that the operative technique is correct), and even so the particles of wear are completely inert and produce very little tissue reaction in contrast to that associated with PE-on-metal wear particles.

■ *Metal-on-metal bearing surfaces* [1, 2, 12, 15, 23]

The bearings used in the 1960s by McKee, Farrar, Ring and others were soon abandoned, as the cups often loosened due to the coefficient of friction between the two metal surfaces and the local osteolysis produced by metallic wear particles.

The fact that some of these prostheses have lasted twenty years has encouraged engineers and surgeons to study how to overcome the problems of friction. During the last twelve years, new metal-on-metal models have been used as a result of attempts to improve both the actual bearing surfaces and the sphericity of the contact surfaces. The advantages are the same as shown by the alumina-on-alumina ceramic except that the wear particles produce more reaction than those of alumina ceramic. However, any possible long-term allergic reactions of chromium and of cobalt are not yet known.

Fixation of total hip arthroplasties (fig 9)

Perfect fixation between bone and the prosthesis is vital to obtain a good result. This can be considered in three phases:

– **Primary fixation** (during the first 2 or 3 months after insertion) which depends basically on the surgical technique.

– **Secondary fixation** (during the first few years after insertion) which depends basically on the method of fixation used (with or without acrylic cement).

– **Tertiary fixation** (after 5-10 years) which depends on several factors: the quality and

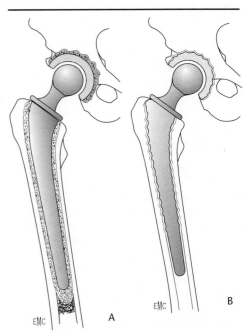

9 *Methods of fixation of total hip arthroplasties.*
A. Cemented prosthesis. Two interfaces: bone-cement and cement-stem.
B. Cementless prosthesis. One interface: bone-stem.

remodelling of the stress bone, the presence or absence of wear particles which can cause osteolysis, the quality of the materials used, and perhaps any peculiar reaction by the patient's tissues.

There are two currently available methods of fixation: the use of a acrylic cement (PMMA) or direct fixation with bone in-growth into any special applied surface coating of the components.

ADVANTAGES AND DISADVANTAGES OF FIXATION WITH ACRYLIC CEMENT

Any surgeon who uses acrylic cement should know its characteristics, as not all cements are identical. Its mechanical properties depend on its porosity and viscosity. There are two major types of cement: cement of standard viscosity which has good mechanical properties, but which penetrates very little into the roughened surface of bone, and cement of low viscosity which can be introduced under compression (syringe or cement gun) to improve penetration of the cement into the bone. The mechanical properties of low viscosity cement are not as good than those of normal viscosity cement.

The quality of the cement fixation depends largely on the surgical technique. The bone surface must be completely clean, free of any blood clot, fat or bone debris. Because the cement has only a mechanical fixation to the bone, it is important to conserve as much roughness as possible, especially of the floor of the acetabulum, and to save as much cancellous bone as possible in the metaphyseal region of the femur. Pressure insertion of cement is difficult to achieve for the acetabular component, but easy and recommended for the femur. The use of a special plug which blocks the femoral medullary canal distal to the tip of the stem improves compression of the cement and avoids inserting too much cement in this region.

There are two basic ways of inserting the femoral cement. The first, described by Harris, was devised to create a sheath of cement of at least 2 mm around the stem. This is aided by the use of a centraliser at the tip of the stem. While this gadget does keep the stem in a good position, there is some evidence that it may encourage local osteolysis. The second technique uses a prosthesis with the largest possible stem, with the aim of filling as much space as possible between it and the bone, especially at the metaphyseal region. This method has been shown to be beneficial with certain types of stems, as it reduces the risk of micro-fractures in the cement sheath which are likely to lead eventually to loosening.

The principal advantage of using cement is the excellence of the primary fixation, particularly of the femoral component, provided as previously emphasised that the correct technique has been used. It also improves the spread of load stresses in the bone as it increases the area of contact between the cemented prosthesis and bone.

There are two disadvantages with cement. Cardiopulmonary accidents have been reported at the time of cement introduction, although these are rare. The use of cement produces two interfaces, bone/cement and prosthesis/cement. As the modulus of elasticity are not the same for bone, cement and prosthesis, these materials will not have the same micro-movements at each interface.

Various theories have been proposed as to how these interface micro-movements may be limited. To limit movements between the cement and the prosthesis various suggestions have been made to improve adherence of the cement to the implant (roughened surfaces, pre-coating with cement or alumina ceramic, etc.).

It has been established that the results of inserting prostheses with roughened stems combined with cement are not as good as insertions using smooth stems with cement, and therefore must be abandoned.

ADVANTAGES AND DISADVANTAGES OF FIXATION WITHOUT CEMENT [13, 14, 18, 20]

To obtain good fixation when cement is not used, it is essential to obtain good bone in-growth to the prosthesis. Prostheses with smooth surfaces which were "jammed" into bone have now been abandoned; in the medium to long-term they were very likely to move.

Various conditions are necessary for good bone in-growth. The bone should be of good osteogenic property, the primary fixation must be perfect so as to limit micro-movement between the bone and the prosthesis, and the coating of the surface of the components must allow bone in-growth to occur. Not all of these criteria were respected with the original cementless prostheses, particularly in relation to the stem. This explains the relatively large number of failures with migration of the prosthesis and pain in the thigh some two years after insertion (10-20%). Improvement in the design and in the surface coating with the addition of hydroxyapatite produced

results comparable with those of cemented replacements. The number of symptomatic loosenings at 10 years is now on the order of 2-4%, but some pain in the hip can arise during the first 3-6 months after operation.

HYBRID PROSTHESES

For mechanical reasons it is easier to fix the acetabular than the femoral component without using cement. Some surgeons use different fixations for the cup and for the femoral component. Usually, the cup is fixed without cement, but the stem is cemented – these are considered to be hybrids.

Conclusions

There is a vary large range of available Total Hip Arthroplasties. Whichever is chosen, it is important that the surgeon be aware of the advantages and disadvantages of the implant he uses. Many patients now wish to know which prosthesis will be used and the respective merits of the different types. Even though some surgeons use only one type of prosthesis, it seems more logical (without creating problems of storage) to use different models according to the physiological age and life style of each patient, the quality of the bone stock available, the shape of the medullary canal, etc.

It also seems reasonable to use prostheses with low levels of friction and wear in patients who have a life expectancy of at least 10 years. On the other hand, for older patients it is sensible to use metal-on-plastic models, as their life expectancy and reduced activities will be less likely to produce loosening secondary to the production of wear particles.

References

[1] Amstutz H. Metal on metal hip prothesis: past performance and future directions. *Clin Orthop* 1996 ; 329 (suppl)

[2] August AC, Aldam CH, Pynsent PB. The MacKee Farrar hip arthroplasty. *J Bone Joint Surg Br* 1986 ; 68 : 520-527

[3] Boutin P, Christel P, Dorlot JM, Meunier A, De Roquancourt A, Blanquaert D et al. The use of dense alumina-alumina ceramic combination in total hip replacement. *J Biomed Mater Res* 1988 ; 22 : 1203-1232

[4] Callaghan JJ. Charnley total hip arthroplasty in patients less than fifty years old. A twenty to twenty five year follow-up note. *J Bone Joint Surg Am* 1998 ; 80 : 704-714

[5] Capello WN, D'Antonio JA, Feinberg JR, Manley MT. Hydroxyapatite coated total hip femoral components in patients less than fifty years old: clinical and radiographic results after five to eight years of follow-up. *J Bone Joint Surg Am* 1997 ; 79 : 1023-1029

[6] Charnley J. Low-friction arthroplasty of the hip. Berlin : Springer-Verbag, 1979

[7] D'Lima DD, Walker RH, Colwell CW Jr. Omnifit HA stem in total hip arthroplasty. A 2 to 5 year follow-up. *Clin Orthop* 1999 ; 363 : 163-169

[8] Epinette JA, Geesink RG. Hydroxyapatite et prothèses articulaires. In : Cahiers d'enseignement de la SOFCOT n° 50. Paris : Expansion scientifique française, 1985

[9] Garcia-Cimbrelo E, Diez-Vasquez V, Madero R, Munuera L. Progression of radiolucent lines adjacent to the acetabular component and factors influencing migration after Charnley low friction arthroplasty. *J Bone Joint Surg Am* 1997 ; 79 : 1313-1380

[10] Geesing RG. Eight years results of HA coated primary total hip replacement. *Acta Orthop Belg* 1997 ; 63 (suppl 10) : 72-75

[11] Geesing RG, Manley MT. Hydroxyapatite coatings in orthopaedic surgery. New York : Raven Press, 1993

[12] Jacobsson SA, Djerf D, Wahlström O. Comparative study between MacKee-Farrar and Charnley arthroplasty with long term follow-up period. *J Arthroplasty* 1990 ; 5 : 9-14

[13] Kelsey D. Design of the femoral component for cementless hip replacement. *Am J Orthop* 1997 ; 26 : 407-412

[14] Mont Ma, Maar DC, Krackow KA, Jacobs MA, Jones LC, Hungerford DS. Total hip replacement without cement for non-inflammation osteoarthritis in patients who are less than forty-five years old. *J Bone Joint Surg Am* 1993 ; 75 : 740-751

[15] MacKee GK, Watson-Farrar J. Replacement of arthritic hips by the MacKee-Farrar prosthesis. *J Bone Joint Surg Br* 1966 ; 48 : 245

[16] Madey SM, Callaghan JJ, Olejniczak JP, Goetz DD, Jonshon RC. Charnley total hip arthroplasty with use of improved techniques of cementing: the results after a minimum of fifteen years of follow-up. *J Bone Joint Surg Am* 1997 ; 79 : 53-64

[17] Malchay H, Herberts P. Prognostis of total hip replacement. Published by Department of Orthopaedics University of Göteborg, 1996

[18] Morscher E. The cementless fixation of hip endoprosthesis. Berlin : Springer Verlag, 1984

[19] Nizard RS, Sedel L, Christel P, Meunier A, Soudry H, Witvoet J. Ten year survivorship of cemented ceramic-ceramic total hip prosthesis. *Clin Orthop* 1992 ; 282 : 53-63

[20] Dowdy PA, Rorabeck CH, Bourne RB. Uncemented total hip arthroplasty in patients 50 years of age or younger. *J Arthroplasty* 1997 ; 12 : 853-862

[21] Paavolairen P, Slatis P, Hamalaimen M, Visuri T, Pulkkinen P. Long term results of total joint arthroplasty. Published by National Agency for Medecines, Helsinki, 1995

[22] Sedel L, Nizard RS, Kerboull L, Witvoet J. Alumina-alumina hip replacement in patients younger than 50 years old. *Clin Orthop* 1994 ; 298 : 175-183

[23] Streicher RM. Metal on metal articulation in total hip arthroplasty: the case for using metal on metal. *J Arthroplasty* 1998 ; 13 : 343

[24] Vidalain JP. HA coating. Ten years experience with the Corail system in primary THA, the Arthro group. *Acta Orthop Belg* 1997 ; 63 (suppl 10) : 93-95

[25] Willman T, Sedel L. Reliability and long term results of ceramics in orthopaedics. 4th International Ceramtec Symposium (March 1999). Stuttgart : G Thieme Verlag, 1999

[26] Winter M, Griss P, Scheller G, Moser Y. Ten to 14 years results of a ceramic hip prosthesis. *Clin Orthop* 1992 ; 282 : 73-80

[27] Wrobleski BM, Liney PD. Charnley low friction arthroplasty of the hip. Long term results. *Clin Orthop* 1993 ; 292 : 191-201

The Exeter cementing technique for the femur

M Fagan
G Gie
G Heyse-Moore
AJC Lee
RSM Ling
AJ Timperley

Abstract. – A technique for the use of acrylic bone cement for fixation of the femoral components of an artificial hip is described, based upon the fact that acrylic cement has no adhesive properties and obtains fixation purely by mechanical interlock with the endosteal bone of the femur. A "closed cavity" method is advocated, in which the distal femoral canal is occluded by a plug, the canal filled retrograde with cement dough, and the proximal opening of the canal then sealed to allow the cement dough to be pressurised to achieve penetration of the endosteal bone surface. Such pressurisation is continued up until the insertion of the femoral component.

Keywords: hip, cementing techniques, acrylic cement, total hip replacement, femoral component.

Introduction

In order to appreciate the basis for use of acrylic bone cement (self-curing polymethyl methacrylate (PMMA)) for fixation of the components of artificial joints, two fundamental facts must be understood. First, acrylic bone cement in its present form is not a glue and has no adhesive properties whatsoever. Second, the initial fixation of every skeletal implant, cemented or cementless, depends upon the establishment of a mechanical interlock [32] between that implant (cement being part of the implant) and the bone. On the strength and extent of that interlock depends the initial stability of the implant. Migration measurements have demonstrated that the "in-service" life of the implant depends substantially on its initial stability [14, 24]. Thus, the creation of the initial

Michael Fagan, Ph.D., Senior Lecturer.
Dept. of Engineering Design & Manufacture, University of Hull, Cottingham Rd, North Humberside HU6 7RX, United Kingdom.
Graham Gie, M.B., B.S., F.R.C.S., F.R.C.S. Ed. (Orth.), Consultant Orthopaedic Surgeon.
Princess Elizabeth Orthopaedic Centre, Barrack Rd, Exeter Devon, United Kingdom.
G Heyse-Moore, M.B., B.S., F.R.C.S., Emeritus Consultant Orthopaedic Surgeon.
James Paget Hospital, Great Yarmouth, Norfolk, NR31 6LA, United Kingdom.
AJC Lee, B.Sc., Ph.D., C.Eng., Honorary University Fellow.
School of Engineering & Computer Science, University of Exeter, Exeter Devon, United Kingdom.
RSM Ling, O.B.E., M.A., B.M.(Oxon), Hon.F.R.C.S. Ed., F.R.C.S., Honorary Consultant Orthopaedic Surgeon.
Princess Elizabeth Orthopaedic Centre, Barrack Rd, Exeter Devon, United Kingdom.
AJ Timperley, M.B., B.S., F.R.C.S. Ed., Consultant Orthopaedic Surgeon.
Princess Elizabeth Orthopaedic Centre, Barrack Rd, Exeter Devon, United Kingdom.

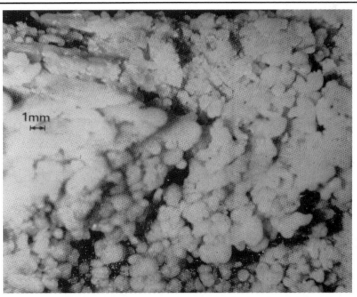

1 Photograph taken of the cement surface inside the upper third of the femur after the bone had been dissolved away in hydrochloric acid. The patient died of a ruptured aortic aneurysm 10 days following hip arthroplasty. The "'micro-interlock" that the cement has achieved with the endosteal bone of the femur is striking (reproduced with permission from Jefferiss CD, Lee AJC, Ling RSM. Thermal aspects of self-curing polymethylmethacrylate. J Bone Joint Surg [Br] 1975; 57-B: 511-18, Figure 9).

mechanical interlock is a vital step and is the sole responsibility of the operating surgeon. Cementing technique is concerned with the establishment of that interlock and, therefore, is an highly important part of the satisfactory use of cement in the clinical context of implant fixation. There is ample evidence that, in both man [5, 6, 20, 25, 30, 31, 36, 37, 50] and animals [10], living bone will form, without an intervening cellular layer, on the surface of the cement when the latter is associated with a "stable" implant – again

emphasising the importance of cementing technique in creating a durable implant-bone interface.

The unique property of acrylic cement in the dough state that allows it to function in the establishment of this initial mechanical interlock is its ability to take an incredibly accurate cast of any surface with which it comes into contact: polymerisation then "locks" that cast in place and so creates the mechanical interlock (fig 1). The establishment of the initial interlock between cement and bone requires penetration of bony spaces by cement dough.

When cement is used for the fixation of a component of an artificial joint, two interfaces are involved: the first between the cement and the bone, and the second between the cement and the implant. The latter is complex, controversial and outside the scope of this chapter that deals primarily with the former. Techniques for the establishment of the cement-bone interface can be divided broadly into two groups: one that might be termed the "traditional" or "old style" cementing technique and the other, that might be termed the "contemporary" cementing technique. The basic difference between them is that, with the former, the introduction of the cement dough into the bony cavity is performed simply by digital packing, following which its penetration into the bony interstices is primarily achieved by the insertion of the implant. With the latter, penetration of the dough into the bony spaces is achieved by closed cavity pressurisation techniques **before** the implant is inserted into the bone, any further extrusion of cement into the bone during implant insertion being, so to speak, a bonus.

Early development of the Exeter femoral cementing technique

Roughly speaking, penetration of cement dough into the bony spaces is directly proportional to the pressure applied to the dough and inversely proportional to its viscosity at the time of application of the pressure [40]. Therefore, not surprisingly, a number of authors have shown experimentally that by utilising a combination of a clean bone surface and the application under pressure of reduced viscosity cement dough, up to a four-fold increase in cement-bone interface shear strength can be achieved [16, 27, 28, 53]. Applying these experimental findings to the introduction of cement into the femur is the basis of the so-called "contemporary" cementing techniques.

The femoral cementing technique that evolved in Exeter in the late seventies and early eighties was based initially on two laboratory studies [16, 29]. The first of these dealt with the effect of a number of clinically relevant variables on the mechanical properties of acrylic cement. From this study came the recommendations that cement should always be physically constrained by bone and, as far as possible, should be loaded in compression. As far as the static strength of the cured resin was concerned, laminations, blood and tissue debris should be minimised in the cement dough.

In the second study [16], concerned purely with the cement-bone interface, it was shown that the strongest cancellous bone in shear in the femur is close to the

corticocancellous junctions, and that the improvements in cement-bone interface shear strength that could be achieved in vitro by pressurising low viscosity cement were increased when this strong cancellous bone was involved in the subsequent interlock.

In clinical practice, low-viscosity cement dough could not be handled or controlled digitally. This meant that the use of a cement gun was essential and that this was best employed to fill the canal retrograde, with cement above an occluding distal medullary plug [39, 43]. The plug, in conjunction with some form of proximal femoral seal that would fit round the gun spout, allowed a closed cavity to be created, into which the continued injection of cement dough would pressurise the medullary canal and force the dough into the endosteal bone of the femur.

The effects of different methods of cement and stem insertion on cement-bone interface pressures and on cement penetration into femoral bone have been studied in a number of laboratory models.

Laboratory models of femoral cementing

Both Markolf and Amstutz [39] and Oh and colleagues [43] demonstrated the major increases in peak cement-bone interface pressures that occurred during stem insertion just before the collar of the stem reached the cut surface of the femoral neck when the medullary canal was occluded distally by a plug. The main increase in pressure occurred distally in the canal, raising the possibility that the strength of the cement-bone interface distally might be greater than proximally. This, in fact, was subsequently confirmed by Reading et al [49]. Thus, the question of how to raise the cement-bone interface pressure in the proximal third of the femoral canal is important if significant proximal transmission of load into the femur is to be achieved clinically.

This issue was one of a number addressed in a laboratory study of femoral cementing that, to date, has only been reported [12] as part of a thesis submitted for the degree of Ph.D. in the Faculty of Engineering of the University of Exeter in 1984. Some important principles emerged from this work, some of which is reproduced here.

Two experimental models were employed. The first of these (*fig 2*) was a two-dimensional model of the medullary canal. The coronal section of a cadaveric femur was measured, reproduced in wood and sandwiched in 6 mm thick glass. Slots 1 mm in diameter and up to 20 mm deep were made on either side of the medullary canal. The penetration of cement into these long narrow slots was then measured to give the relative pressure distributions expected to occur during hip surgery. Two femoral stems

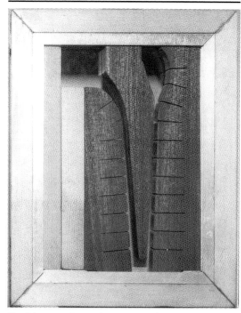

2 *The experimental apparatus showing the coronal section of a cadaveric femur reproduced in wood and sandwiched in 6 mm thick glass. The slots in the wood for measuring penetration are seen on the medial and lateral aspects of the canal. The penetration of cement into these long narrow slots was measured to give the relative pressure distributions occurring during surgery (reproduced with permission, first published in [12]).*

were produced from wood, modelling a tapered and a straight stem. For obvious reasons, regular PMMA bone cement could not be used in this model and an alternative model material was made from flour (40%), table salt (20%), water (35%) and paraffin oil (5%). By changing the nominal mix, a "cement" whose viscosity was similar to that of PMMA in its low and medium viscosity stages could be made. The viscosity of the "cement" was determined by measuring the flow through a nozzle calibrated for surgical Simplex P® bone cement. The model material could also be coloured and inserted into the model femur in layers to enable observation of the flow patterns during stem insertion. This apparatus allowed measurement of the relative pressure distribution down the femoral canal.

To determine the duration of the pressures experienced during the operation, tests were performed using a natural (cadaveric) femur with two pressure transducers (*fig 3*). Before any tests were performed with the two-dimensional model, it was necessary to confirm that the method gave reproducible results. This was achieved by inserting the tapered-stem model into the apparatus in 6 separate tests using material of the same viscosity and a plugged canal. These tests showed that the method did give reproducible results and could be used with confidence to make qualitative comparisons between different methods and devices (*fig 4*).

The models assumed that the canal was dry and clean. The advantage of this model is that it measures penetration of the cement which depends not only on pressure, but

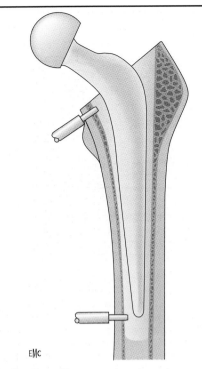

3 *Locations of the pressure transducers to measure the distal and proximal cement-bone interface pressures in a cadaveric femur.*

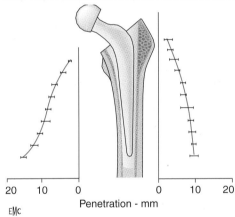

4 *The penetration and pressure distribution for an Exeter stem inserted into a plugged cavity showing the range of values recorded in six tests.*

also on the time for which the pressure is applied and the viscosity of the cement. Thus it is potentially a more valuable model than one where pressure alone is measured; for example, it is able to clarify the situation in which equal pressures are recorded for cements of different viscosities, i.e. it produces a greater penetration for a lower viscosity cement.

Only the graphic representations of the results are provided here. The raw data are, however, available from the authors for those who wish to see them.

The advantage of using a distal medullary plug is clearly demonstrated in Fig. 5. The findings are much as those in previous work [39, 43, 49]. The depth of cement penetration is presented for a tapered stem inserted into a plugged and unplugged canal. Without any distal restriction, the maximal penetration (and therefore

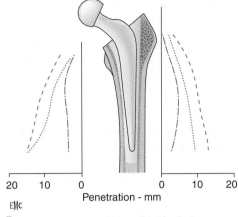

5 *The cement penetration recorded for the Exeter stem cemented into plugged and unplugged canals with and without a proximal restriction. (Unplugged canal: -.-. Plugged canal: ...... Plugged canal with proximal occlusion: - - - -).*

pressure) occurs near the centre of the stem. With a plug, the values are increased considerably, the greatest effect being recorded in the distal region, where rises of over 400% are observed; proximally the penetration remains low. Placing a proximal restriction on the opening of the femur during component insertion increases the penetrations throughout the canal, especially in the proximal region, although the values still do not approach those recorded distally (*fig 5*). The flow visualisation study showed that the main effect of the intramedullary plug was to reverse the flow of cement within the canal on stem insertion, i.e. with a plugged canal, stem insertion was associated with proximal flow of cement dough around the advancing stem. By contrast, in the absence of the plug, cement flow on stem insertion was distally directed down the medullary canal.

Therefore, to improve the proximal penetration, some form of pressurisation must be employed prior to stem insertion. The effectiveness of a femoral pressuriser is illustrated in Fig. 6 and compared to the pressure normally developed during the insertion of a tapered stem into a closed (i.e. distally plugged) cavity. The pressuriser

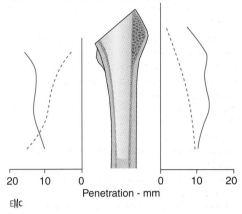

6 *The penetrations produced by the proximal pressurising device and by the insertion of the Exeter stem with a closed cavity. The main difference is in the proximal third of the canal. Stem insertion: ----. Femoral pressuriser ———.*

produces a constant pressure in the distal and central thirds of the canal, which increases to a maximum at the medial femoral neck. When compared to the distribution caused by stem insertion, the pressuriser performs favourably, particularly as it develops a high pressure proximally.

Finger packing of the cement was examined by direct measurement of the pressure induced in a complete femur. Fig. 7 compares the pressures developed in the proximal femur using either finger packing or a pressurising device. The finger packing produces transient pressure rises of up to 0.075 MPa (0.75 atm). Using the femoral pressuriser, peak values of 0.175 MPa are recorded with a steady base value of 0.1 MPa, i.e. the pressure is maintained through the period of pressurisation, and is evidently more effective than finger packing.

To investigate the effects of varying the viscosity of the cement, a range of model material was manufactured, equivalent to Simplex P™ between 2.5 to 7 minutes after the beginning of mixing. The variation of penetration with time at three sample positions on the medial and lateral faces is shown in Fig. 8 for the Exeter stem inserted into a closed cavity. On both medial and

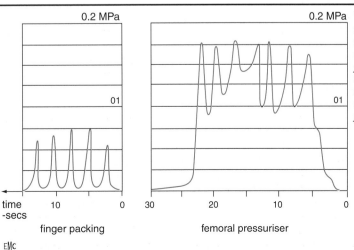

7 *A comparison of the interface pressure developed at the medial femoral neck when the cement is pressurised by finger packing (left) or a femoral pressuriser (right). Pressure is on the ordinate and time on the abscissa going from right to left.*

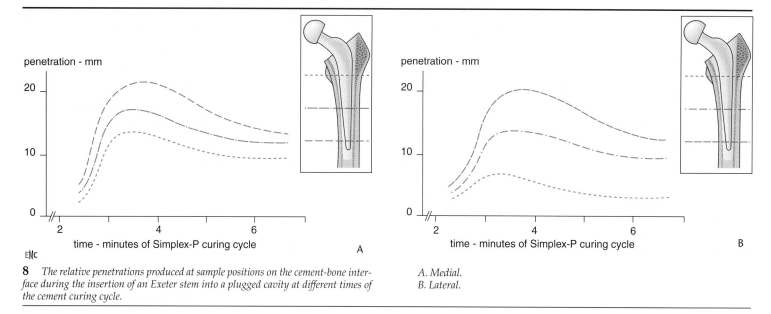

8 *The relative penetrations produced at sample positions on the cement-bone interface during the insertion of an Exeter stem into a plugged cavity at different times of the cement curing cycle.*

A. Medial.
B. Lateral.

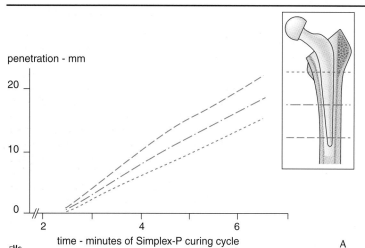
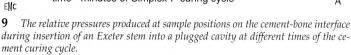
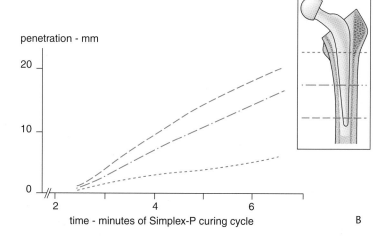

9 *The relative pressures produced at sample positions on the cement-bone interface during insertion of an Exeter stem into a plugged cavity at different times of the cement curing cycle.*

A. Medial.
B. Lateral.

lateral sides of the stem, maxima occur at 3 to 4 minutes, depending on the location within the canal. Insertion at this time, however, would leave the cement-bone interface vulnerable to the effects of bleeding. Since these graphs are derived for cements of different viscosities, the results do not immediately reflect the relative pressures. As expected, the magnitude of the penetration is proportional to the pressure developed during stem insertion and inversely proportional to the viscosity of the cement, i.e. penetration pressure/viscosity. Therefore, to compare the pressures generated when using different viscosities of cement, the product of penetration and viscosity must be used. Using this technique, the relative pressures developed at the sample positions have been calculated and presented in Fig. 9. The graphs show that the induced pressure increases almost linearly, as the viscosity of the cement increases. This is an highly important point clinically, i.e. the later the stem is inserted, the higher the interface pressures generated.

The experimental work cited here would seem to indicate a clear advantage to the use and pressurisation of cement dough in its low viscosity state. However, such recommendations made purely on the basis of in vitro experiments ignore the potentially damaging effects of bleeding from the exposed bone surfaces.

THE ADVERSE EFFECTS OF BLEEDING FROM THE BONE SURFACE

In 1981, one of the authors had employed the technique of pressurising cement dough in the low viscosity state onto a clean bone surface in a femoral revision arthoplasty, and whilst waiting for the cement to polymerise after the insertion of the stem, noted blood oozing out from the upper end of the cement-bone interface at the femoral neck. This observation immediately raised the question of the potentially damaging effects on the interface between cement dough and bone of bleeding from the bone. This matter was addressed in Exeter in two further

studies. Heyse-Moore et al [18] found that the bleeding pressure in the femoral canal during total hip replacement operations could be as high as 37 cm of water. In a series of 25 cases, the femoral canals in which bleeding was regarded by the surgeon as profuse were those in which the bleeding pressures were the highest. The extent to which such bleeding from the bone could compromise the cement-bone interface at surgery was then studied experimentally by Benjamin et al [1] who showed that bleeding pressures of 37 cm of water (the highest in vivo pressure recorded by Heyse-Moore) were capable of moving Simplex™ cement dough away from the bone up until 6 minutes after the beginning of mixing. These experiments made it clear that if relatively low viscosity dough (for example, Simplex™ at 3.5 minutes after the beginning of mixing) is put in to the femoral canal, pressurisation of that dough must be maintained at least until the viscosity of the dough is high enough on its own to provide tamponade. Utilising Simplex™, this would mean that pressure should be maintained until at least 6 minutes after the beginning of mixing. If it is not practicable to do this, then low or relatively low viscosity dough should never be used. Further confirmation of these findings was provided experimentally by Majkowski et al [34] in 1994, and the following year, Juliusson et al [23] showed in a clever clinical study that bone penetration (into the cancellous bone of the femoral head) by cement was increased by 100% when the circulation had been obliterated by cervical osteotomy.

The femoral cementing technique currently in use in Exeter

The implications of these experimental and clinical findings have been incorporated into the technique currently in use at the Princess Elizabeth Orthopaedic Centre.

MINIMISING BLEEDING FROM THE BONE

The anaesthetist plays an important part in achieving a dry field, which is so important for efficient and effective cementing. Epidural or spinal anaesthesia with or without a light general anaesthetic has many advantages [48, 51], not only from the standpoint of intra-operative bleeding [38].

CANAL PREPARATION

A trochanteric osteotomy is rarely used for exposure of the hip during hip arthroplasty at the Princess Elizabeth Orthopaedic Centre. Without it, the opening in the proximal end of the medullary canal is carried posterolaterally into the piriform fossa so as to allow the insertion of the taper pin reamer and rasps in the midline axis of the medullary canal. The use of appropriate rasps allows preservation of the strong cancellous bone in the femoral metaphysis, usually to within 2-4 mm of the corticocancellous junctions. The appropriate intramedullary plug is then introduced and should be a tight fit in the canal approximately 2 cm beyond the point at which the tip of the stem will eventually be sited. The fit of the proximal seal into the open proximal end of the canal is checked and, if needed, appropriate adjustments are made. The canal is very thoroughly washed with high volume, high pressure, pulsatile irrigation to clean the bone surface and remove fat. A sucker tube is inserted to just above the plug. The canal is then packed firmly with ribbon gauze soaked in 10 vols% hydrogen peroxide to assist in achieving haemostasis [17] .This also warms the bone surface slightly. Suction is maintained on the tube until the latter blocks during cement insertion.

CEMENT PREPARATION

Generally, Simplex RO™ cement with or without antibiotics is used. Mixing is carried out at approximately 1 Hz in a low vacuum to prevent the fumes from the monomer getting into the operating theatre. Full vacuum mixing is not employed nor are any other measures adopted to reduce porosity in the cement [33]. A double mix is employed except in very capacious femora that may require three mixes.

CEMENT INSERTION AND PRESSURISATION

The cement dough is poured into the cement gun barrel at between 1.5 and 2 minutes after the beginning of mixing (with an operating theatre temperature of 20° C). The ribbon gauze is removed from the canal and retrograde cement insertion is carried out under direct vision. The sucker tube is withdrawn as soon as it ceases to withdraw blood. Once the canal is filled, the spout of the gun is amputated level with the distal femoral seal and the latter is firmly impacted into the open end of the canal. Cement injection through the seal should initially be pulsatile [40] through repeated sharp pressure on the gun trigger. This process should be accompanied by the steady extrusion of fat and marrow through the proximal femoral cortex. Pressure is then maintained through the slow continued injection of cement until its viscosity is judged appropriate for stem insertion. This would never be before 6 minutes after the beginning of mixing in a primary intervention, depending on the theatre temperature, and is best judged by the feel of a bolus of cement retained in the surgeon's hand and kneaded in the fingers under the operating theatre light [11]. This is more reliable than using the clock.

If the seal cannot be made to fit the opening in the proximal femur satisfactorily so that adequate pressurisation with reduced viscosity dough cannot be achieved, the method described above should not be used. Instead, after canal preparation, the "suck down" method should be employed using a suction catheter with high viscosity dough and subsequent finger packing. This method requires a large bolus of dough to be kept over the mouth of the canal during suction, otherwise very large voids may be formed in the cement as air is sucked into the canal.

STEM INSERTION

The stem to be used is kept in a water bath at 60° C for a few minutes and then dried prior to insertion into the femoral canal. The aim of this is to accelerate polymerisation [9], on the basis that once the stem has reached its final position, the sooner polymerisation occurs, the better. There is evidence that heating the stem may also reduce porosities at the stem-cement interface [2], although this is less important when a stem with a polished surface is being used, as is invariably the case at the Princess Elizabeth Orthopaedic Centre.

Once the surgeon is satisfied that the viscosity of the cement has reached an appropriate state, the stem should be inserted accurately down the midline axis of the canal as far as varus/valgus is concerned, although with a straight stem, its point of entry into the cement should be near the posterior margin of the entry to the femoral canal at the cut surface of the femoral neck. Because of the double bow of the femur in the sagittal plane [8], this posterior entry reduces the chance of mantle deficiencies in the lower part of zone 8 [21] and the upper part of zone 9 [21]. Thus, centralisation of the stem at the level of the cut surface of the neck is positively contraindicated unless the level of neck section is extremely low.

Throughout the period of stem insertion, the exit from the canal medial to the stem should be occluded by the surgeon's thumb so as to maximise the cement-bone interface pressure in zone 7 (*fig 5*).

AFTER STEM INSERTION

Once the stem has reached its final position, the stem should not be in any way moved whilst the cement is polymerising. Any introducing instrument should be removed and, immediately thereafter, the "horse collar" seal is applied to the cut surface of the femoral neck around the stem and firm pressure maintained on the proximal cement until the latter has polymerised. This device prevents the cement-bone interface pressure in the upper end of the canal from falling below the highest bleeding pressures recorded by Heyes-Moore [18].

Discussion

The technique described above incorporates a number of the steps shown in the Swedish Hip Registry to have been associated with a significant improvement in survivorship with the end-point removal of the implant [35] and has also been associated with satisfactory outcomes in Exeter [54]. An interesting radiological comparison between the original Exeter polished stems [13], inserted with orthograde cement insertion through finger packing, and the current stems inserted with the technique described above [54] has demonstrated a five-fold reduction of diaphyseal hypertrophy in the latter by comparison with the former at the same length of follow-up. Since the stem geometries were substantially similar, it is tempting to suggest that this is a consequence of the far better proximal cement packing and pressurisation achieved with the current technique and that modifications of cementing technique, on their own, can affect load transmission from the stem through the cement and into bone.

The question of whether high or low viscosity cement should be used sometimes creates confusion. The time course of the viscosity changes through which cement dough passes from mixing to polymerisation varies between the different brands of cement. This affects the "working time" of the cement. From this standpoint, it is essential that the surgeon be familiar with the behaviour of the brand of cement that he is using and clear in his mind about exactly what he is trying to achieve. Whilst there are advantages to reduced viscosity as far as bone penetration is concerned, cement dough at this stage is vulnerable to bleeding from the bone surface and certainly cannot maintain the stability of the stem should the latter be inserted whilst the viscosity is still low. With certain cements (e.g. Zimmer LVC41™ [41], initially developed for use at the knee), the viscosity of the dough was initially very low and then increased rapidly as polymerisation approached. Such behaviour could create difficulties for the surgeon if he was unaware of the rapid viscosity changes; this is one of the reasons why the use of low viscosity cement has been associated with indifferent results in the Swedish Hip Registry [35]. Not all surgeons, however, shared this experience [4] and the issues are technical.

From the early days of the use of acrylic cement at the hip, there have been anxieties concerning fat embolisation and the central effects of absorbed monomer from the cement [19]. Whilst the evidence that absorbed monomer per se has any effect on the circulation peroperatively is poor [19], there can be no doubt that pulmonary fat embolisation does occur in association with femoral reaming and the insertion of both cementless [15, 26] and cemented [26] femoral components. Generally [26], though not always [44], its effects are minimal and transitory, and are maximal in very old and relatively unfit patients. Nevertheless, it is important for the anaesthetist and surgeon to take steps to minimise such changes. The anaesthetist should ensure that an arterial line and beat-to-beat measurements of mean arterial pressure are available in high risk patients so that prompt use of vasoconstrictors - inotropes is possible if needed. In all patients, he should be certain that the patient is normovolaemic at the time of insertion and pressurisation of cement. From the same standpoint, the most important step for the surgeon to take is to utilise high volume, high pressure, pulsatile lavage in the femoral canal before cement insertion [3, 7, 52]. Modifications to the cementing technique that are designed to reduce fat and marrow embolisation have been described [45, 46, 47] and may prove to be useful, but these involve measures that could also reduce cement-bone interface pressure and therefore may compromise fixation in the long term.

CONCLUSIONS

The basic principle underlying cementing technique in replacement arthroplasty of the hip is that cement in the dough state in the patient should always be kept under pressure and this must not be forgotten. Although some authors have placed the blame for indifferent results in cemented hip arthroplasty on what have been perceived as fundamental defects in cement as a material [22], Schmalzried and colleagues [50], from their postmortem studies, wrote: "Primary incompatibility and/or failure of the cement was not identified as a factor in either femoral or acetabular component loosening." This emphasises the overwhelming importance of the way cement is used in producing satisfactory clinical outcomes.

References

[1] Benjamin JB, Volz RG, Gie GA, Ling RS, Lee AJ. Cementing technique and the effects of bleeding. *J Bone Joint Surg Br* 1987 ; 69 : 620-624

[2] Bishop NE, Ferguson S, Tepic S. Porosity reduction in bone cement at the cement-stem interface. *J Bone Joint Surg Br* 1996 ; 78 : 349-356

[3] Byrick RJ, Bell RS, Kay JC, Waddell JP, Mullen J. High volume, high pressure pulsatile lavage during cemented hip arthoplasty. *J Bone Joint Surg Am* 1989 ; 71 : 1331-1336

[4] Carlsson AS, Nilsson JA, Blomgren G, Josefsson G, Lindberg LT, Onnerfalt R. Low- vs high-viscosity cement in hip arthroplasty. No radiographic difference in 226 arthrosis cases followed for 5 years. *Acta Orthop Scand* 1993 ; 64 : 257-262

[5] Charnley J. The reaction of bone to self-curing acrylic cement: a long-term histological study in man. *J Bone Joint Surg Br* 1970 ; 52 : 340-353

[6] Charnley J, Follacci FM, Hammond BT. The long-term reaction of bone to acrylic cement. *J Bone Joint Surg Br* 1968 ; 50 : 822-829

[7] Christie J, Robinson CM, Singer B, Ray DC, Byrick RJ, Mullen JB et al. Medullary lavage reduces embolic phenomena and cardiopulmonary changes during cemented hemiarthroplasty. *J Bone Joint Surg Br* 1995 ; 77 : 456-459

[8] Crawford RW, Psychoyios V, Murray DW, Gie GA, Ling RS. Incomplete cement mantles in the sagittal femoral plane: an anatomical explanation. *Acta Orthop Scand* 1999 ; 70 : 596-598

[9] Dall DM, Miles AW, Juby G. Accelerated polymerisation of bone cement using pre-heated implants. *Clin Orthop* 1986 ; 211 : 148-150

[10] Draenert K. Histomorphology of bone-to-cement interface: remodelling of the cortex and revascularisation of the medullary canal in animal experiments. In : The hip: Proceedings of the 9th open scientific meeting of the Hip Society. St Louis : CV Mosby, 1981

[11] Eni-Olotu DO, Nokes L, Rassoulian H, Goddard JR. The use of handheld cement sample as a guide to the setting of in situ cement mantle. *J Arthroplasty* 2001 ; 16 : 376-378

[12] Fagan MJ. A finite element analysis of femoral stem design in cemented total hip replacement. [thesis], University of Exeter, 1984

[13] Fowler J, Gie GA, Lee AJC, Ling RS. Experience with Exeter hip since 1970. *Orthop Clin North Am* 1988 ; 19 : 477-489

[14] Freeman MA, Plante-Bordeneuve P. Early migration and late aseptic failure of proximal femoral prostheses. [published erratum appears in *J Bone Joint Surg Br* 1994 Nov; 76 (6):999]. *J Bone Joint Surg Br* 1994 ; 76 : 432-438

[15] Gelinas JJ, Cherry R, Macdonald SJ. Fat embolism syndrome after cementless total hip arthroplasty. *J Arthroplasty* 2000 ; 15 : 809-813

[16] Halawa M, Lee AJ, Ling RS, Vangala SS. Shear strength of trabecular bone from the femur and some factors affecting the shear strength of the cement-bone interface. *Arch Orthop Trauma Surg* 1978 ; 92 : 19-27

[17] Hankin FM, Campbell SE, Goldstein SA, Matthews LS. Hydrogen peroxide as a topical haemostatic agent. *Clin Orthop* 1984 ; 186 : 244-248

[18] Heyse-Moore GH, Ling RS. Current cement techniques. In : Marti RK ed. Progress in cemented hip surgery and revision. Amsterdam : Excerpta Medica, 1982 : 71-86

[19] James ML. Anaesthetic and metabolic complications. In : Ling RS ed. Complications of total hip replacement. Edinburgh : Churchill Livingstone, 1984 : 1-17

[20] Jasty M, Maloney WJ, Bragdon CR, Haire T, Harris W. Histomorphological studies of the long-term skeletal responses to well fixed cemented femoral components. *J Bone Joint Surg Am* 1990 ; 72 : 1220-1229

[21] Johnston RC, Fitzgerald RH Jr, Harris WH, Poss R, Muller ME, Sledge CB. Clinical and radiographic evaluation of total hip replacement. *J Bone Joint Surg Am* 1990 ; 72 : 161-168

[22] Jones LC, Hungerford DS. Cement disease. *Clin Orthop* 1987 ; 181 : 92-99

[23] Juliusson R, Flivik G, Nilsson J, Ryd L, Onnerfalt R. Circulating blood diminishes cement penetration into cancellous bone. In vivo studies of 21 arthrotic femoral heads. *Acta orthop Scand* 1995 ; 66 : 234-238

[24] Karrholm J, Borssen B, Lowenhielm G, Snorrason F. Does early micromotion of femoral stem prostheses matter? *J Bone Joint Surg Br* 1994 ; 76 : 912-917

[25] Kawate K, Maloney W, Bragdon CR, Biggs SA, Jasty M, Harris WH. Importance of a thin cement mantle: autopsy studies of eight hips. *Clin Orthop* 1998 ; 355 : 70-76

[26] Kim Y, Oh S, Kim J. Incidence of fat embolism syndrome following cemented or cementless bilateral simultaneous and unilateral total hip arthroplasty. A randomised clinical trial. Transactions of the 47th annual meeting of the Orthopaedic Research Society, 2001 ; 26 : 1056

[27] Krause WR, Krug W, Miller J. Cement-bone interface: effect of cement technique and surface preparation. *Orthop Trans* 1980 ; 4 : 204

[28] Krause WR, Krug W, Miller J. Strength of the cement-bone interface. *Clin Orthop* 1982 ; 163 : 290-299

[29] Lee AJ, Ling RS, Vangala SS. Some clinically relevant variables affecting the mechanical behaviour of bone cement. *Arch Orthop Trauma Surg* 1978 ; 92 : 1-18

[30] Linder L, Carlsson A, Kindblom LG, Hansson HA. Histochemical and ultrastructural analysis of the tissue reaction to bone cement in man. *Acta Orthop Scand* 1984 ; 55 : 97

[31] Linder L, Hansson HA. Ultra-structural aspects of the interface between bone and cement in man. *J Bone Joint Surg Br* 1983 ; 65 : 646-649

[32] Ling RS. Observations on the fixation of implants to the bony skeleton. *Clin Orthop* 1986 ; 210 : 80-96

[33] Ling RS, Lee AJ. Porosity reduction in acrylic cement is clinically irrelevant. *Clin Orthop* 1998 ; 335 : 249-253

[34] Majkowski RS, Bannister GC, Miles AW. The effect of bleeding on the cement-bone interface. An experimental study. *Clin Orthop* 1994 ; 299 : 293-297

[35] Malchau H, Herberts P, Soderman P, Oden A. Prognosis of total hip replacements. Update and validation of results from the Swedish National Hip Arthroplasty Registry 1979-1998. Scientific exhibit at the 67th annual meeting of the American Academy of Orthopaedic Surgeons, Orlando, 2000

[36] Malcolm A. Pathology of low friction arthroplasties in autopsy specimens. In : Older MW ed. Implant bone interface. London : Springer- Verlag, 1990 : 77-82

[37] Maloney WJ, Jasty M, Burke DW, O'Connor DO, Zalenski EB, Bragdon C et al. Biomechanical and histologic investigation of cemented total hip arthroplasties: a study of autopsy retrieved femurs after 'in vivo' cycling. *Clin Orthop* 1989 ; 249 : 129-140

[38] Markel DC, Urquhart B, Derkowska I, Salvati EA, Sharrock NE. Effect of epidural analgesia on venous blood flow after hip arthroplasty. *Clin Orthop* 1997 ; 334 : 168-174

[39] Markolf KL, Amstutz HC. In-vitro measurements of bone-acrylic interface pressure during femoral component insertion. *Clin Orthop* 1976 ; 121 : 60-66

[40] Markolf KL, Amstutz HC. Penetration and flow of acrylic bone cement. *Clin Orthop* 1976 ; 121 : 99-102

[41] Miller J, Krause WR, Burke DL, Krug WH, Kelebay LC. Pressure penetration of low viscosity acrylic cement for improved fixation of arthroplasty components. *J Bone Joint Surg Br* 1982 ; 64 : 619

[42] Miller J, Krause WR, Krug WH, Kelebay LC. Low viscosity cement. *Orthop Trans* 1981 ; 5 : 532

[43] Oh I, Carlson CE, Tomford WW, Harris WH. Improved fixation of femoral component after total hip replacement using a methacrylate intramedullary plug. *J Bone Joint Surg Am* 1978 ; 60 : 608-613

[44] Ott MC, Meschia JF, Mackey DC, Brodersen MP, Burger C, Echols JD et al. Cerebral embolization presenting as delayed, severe obtundation in the postanesthesia care unit after total hip arthroplasty. *Mayo Clin Proc* 2000 ; 75 : 1209-1213

[45] Pitto RP, Hamer H, Fabiani R, Radespiel-Troeger M, Koessler MJ. Prophylaxis against fat and bone-marrow embolism during total hip arthroplasty reduces the incidence of postoperative deep-vein thrombosis. *J Bone Joint Surg Am* 2002 ; 84 : 39-48

[46] Pitto RP, Koessler MJ, Draenert K. Prophylaxis of fat and bone marrow embolism in cemented total hip arthroplasty. *Cl in Orthop* 1998 ; 355 : 25-34

[47] Pitto RP, Koessler MJ, Kuehle JW. Comparison of the fixation of the femoral component without cement and fixation with the use of a bone-vacuum cementing technique for the prevention of fat embolism during total hip arthroplasty. *J Bone Joint Surg Am* 1999 ; 81 : 831-843

[48] Ranawat CS, Beaver WB, Sharrock NE, Maynard MJ, Urquhart B, Schneider R. Effect of hypotensive epidural anaesthesia on acetabular cement-bone fixation in total hip arthroplasty. *J Bone Joint Surg Br* 1991 ; 73 : 779-782

[49] Reading AD, McCaskie AW, Barnes MR, Gregg PJ. A comparison of 2 modern femoral cementing techniques: analysis by cement-bone interface pressure measurements, computerised image analysis and static mechanical testing. *J Arthroplasty* 2000 ; 15 : 479-487

[50] Schmalzried TP, Maloney WJ, Jasty M, Kwong LM, Harris WH. Autopsy studies of the bone-cement interface in well-fixed cemented total hip arthroplasties. *J Arthroplasty* 1993 ; 8 : 179-188

[51] Sharrock NE, Salvati EA. Hypotensive epidural anaesthesia for total hip arthroplasty - a review. *Acta Orthop Scand* 1996 ; 67 : 91-107

[52] Sherman RP, Byrick RJ, Kay JC, Sullivan TR, Waddell J. The role of lavage in preventing hemodynamic and blood gas changes during cemented arthroplasty. *J Bone Joint Surg Am* 1983 ; 65 : 500-506

[53] Stone JJ, Rand JA, Chiu EK, Grabowski JJ, An KN. Cement viscosity affects the bone/cement interface in total hip arthroplasty. *J Orthop Res* 1996 ; 14 : 681-689

[54] Williams HD, Browne G, Gie GA, Ling RS, Timperley AJ, Wendover NA. The Exeter universal cemented femoral component at 8-12 years. A study of the first 325 cases. *J Bone Joint Surg Br* 2002 ; 84 : 324-334

Tribology of hip joint replacement

L Sedel

Abstract. – *The mechanisms of the artificial hip joint are presented, and the material characteristics and mechanical tests are summarised. The different friction systems on the market are identified: metal-on-polyethylene, metal-on-metal, alumina-on-alumina, zirconia-on-polyethylene. Other new materials such as improved polyethylene are only cited. Results of clinical studies and laboratory tests are presented. Tribology is of major concern in understanding why some materials are well tolerated over a long time period and others are not.*

Keywords: hip, total hip replacement, hip prosthesis, hip arthroplasty, biomaterials, polyethylene, alumina, metal-on-metal.

Introduction

Replacing a destroyed hip joint by a prosthesis has been a widely performed operation for more than 40 years. Although the surgical technique is now widely available, most patients are satisfied with the results, and the long-term outcome concerning the first designs is well known, many uncertainties still remain. These concern the long-term results in young or active patients, especially in terms of the basic science of this artificial system, such as: the mechanisms of friction and wear, material degradation leading to aseptic loosening of implants, debris formation, and their local and even general biological consequences, including bone remodelling in response to different local mechanical environments.

Tribology, or the science of friction, is one of the most difficult fields in mechanics. It can be summed up in two apparently simple aspects: sliding and wear. In fact, it concerns not only the chemical and physical characteristics of a material, but also fluid formation, geometrical configurations at a micro- or macroscopic level, stresses applied to the surfaces and the biomechanics of joint motion. As these materials are implanted in a living body, clearance and metabolism of wear debris are of concern. Will these debris degrade? Will they give rise to ionic particles? Will these particles or ions be

Laurent Sedel, Professeur des Universités, Chirurgien Chef de Service, Hôpital Lariboisière, 4, rue Ambroise-Paré, 75010 Paris, France.

stored or eliminated? In this limited format, it will be difficult to address all of these issues extensively.

Historical background

The first scientific approach to artificial joint lubrication is attributed to J. Charnley. His well-known pendulum experiments showed how the friction coefficient was a relevant factor in explaining acetabular loosening. He introduced the low friction concept with its two major innovations: the use of metal against polyethylene as a bearing surface and the small head (22.2 mm). He stated that polyethylene would wear but would not give rise to major problems, as he anticipated this linear wear to be in the range of 0.1 mm per year. This concept was widely accepted and eventually copied. However, several authors felt this system would give rise to some adverse effects. One of these was the risk of dislocation related to the small head; another was the amount of wear debris generated and not eliminated from the artificial joint environment. Willert in 1973 described the foreign body reaction that leads to loosening through a biological effect. Rose and Radin [54, 59, 60] described the mechanics of polyethylene degradation and ageing. Schmalzried [62, 63] in the early 1990s described the "effective joint space" where debris and fluids migrate around the prosthesis and cause bone osteolysis out of the joint space.

To prevent such problems, others worked on different friction systems, namely ceramic-on-polyethylene, ceramic-on-ceramic or, more recently, a come back of modified cobalt chromium on itself.

Parameters

As tribology is resumed by two concepts, sliding and wear, we will discuss the different parameters involved and how it is possible to study them [65].

FRICTION COEFFICIENT

When two materials slide on one another, a force is applied which is directly correlated to the nature of the materials by the equation $F\gamma = M$, where γ is the friction coefficient, F is the applied force and M the weight of the displaced material. This is true at a constant speed. To start the movement, it is necessary to exert an increased force which decreases as soon as the movement reaches a constant speed.

When a film is interposed, the problem is completely different as the friction then depends not only on the viscosity of the fluid, but also on its thickness and its speed of displacement. Each of these parameters will define what engineers call the friction system or the lubrication regimen, which includes boundary lubrication, fluid film, squeeze film, hydrodynamic and elastohydrodynamic lubrication systems. We will not discuss these different configurations, but present those parameters which play a major role and how it is possible to study them.

When surfaces are not flat but spherical, knowledge of the friction coefficient alone is not enough, as the frictional torque depends on the friction coefficient and also on the geometry of the contact. The smaller the contact area, the less the resistance to sliding.

It is therefore clear that many parameters have to be considered.

Some relate to hip biomechanics: the forces applied to the joint, surface in contact, speed, shock. Others are related to material characteristics: nature of the counterface, roughness, macrogeometry, ability or not to absorb water, contact surface. Yet others deal with the lubrication system: is there a fluid interposed? What is its thickness, its viscosity? Is there a third body interposed that could play a major role?

To answer all these questions, many approaches are required: material sciences and mechanical tests on the materials, using simulators, geometrical studies and stress analyses. Friction characteristics may be determined by simple or more sophisticated tests; in vivo studies use clinical and radiological measurements, and prostheses explanted after failure or from deceased patients may be analysed.

Three main fields are explored: biomechanics, material sciences, basic tribology. Consideration will be given to the results obtained using some of the surfaces as friction components in total hip replacement (THR).

BIOMECHANICS

Friction characteristics depend strongly on the load the joint has to sustain; other parameters such as surface contact, sliding speed and the number of cycles per day or year are of major concern.

Joint forces have been documented by many authors. Paul et al [56] indirectly measured these forces by using a force plate. The recorded force at the foot level was analysed and decomposed at each joint level in order to reach the value at the hip level. This type of calculation gave rise to large over-estimations of the real load applied. In vivo measurements were also performed: Rydell was the first to implant a prosthesis with a transducer. More recently, Hodge et al [29] and Bergmann et al [3, 4] used transducers in hip prostheses to directly measure pressure, applied load or generated heat. From these recent studies, it was found that applied load was 2 to 3 times body weight during walking. This load increased dramatically in some activities such as rising from a chair (6 times), running or jumping. Some very interesting results showed that the load decreased with muscle reinforcement due to rehabilitation. The movement characteristics of the hip are well known: walking generates a flexion angle of 20°, rotation of 5° and abduction-adduction of 5°. The heat generated during walking was also noted and this could play a role in the degradation of some plastic materials [4].

The mean number of steps per year is 1 to 2 million and, as measured by Wallbridge et al [72], there is a large decrease with age (4 times fewer steps for a 80 year-old person than for a 20 year-old one). Of course, there are large individual differences.

Other details may play a role but are little documented, for example, the shock absorption mechanism as related to the ground surface and type of shoe. Also, as demonstrated by E. Radin, individual parameters leading to different impedance characteristics may differ from one person to another. Individual behaviour can also play a major role, for example, the number of times a day a person gets up from a chair or starts walking. The number of steps he takes daily, walking distance, speed, stair climbing or descending, running – all these will modify the force and behaviour of each individually implanted material. It is probable that there may be some piston effect in the joint space. If this occurs, the wear profiles and lubrication will be greatly modified.

MATERIALS

Whatever the material used, some general considerations always apply.

■ *Contact area*

In a normal joint, the contact area increases as the load increases. This is related to surface adaptation and deformation of bone and cartilage under load and serves to maintain relatively identical pressures when load increases. When an artificial material is interposed, the initial surface area will be related to the matching sphericity and the clearance between the two components. This surface area will be directly influenced by the material's deformability. For a hard material, the initial sphericity will play a major role, while for two materials including one soft one, the deformability of the latter will play a major role. This explains why it is of major importance to achieve adequate initial clearance when the prosthesis is made of two hard materials such as ceramic-on-ceramic or in metal-on-metal. When there is a discrepancy between the two radii, Herz contact stresses will appear at the contact point with the risk of accelerated wear. These discrepancies may diminish in the long-term after a running-in period that can last for some millions of cycles.

■ *Surface geometry*

This is a relevant parameter that concerns many different aspects.

Microgeometry relates to roughness but also to the shape of surface irregularities. Roughness is measured by a special transducer that will give the value of Ra (mean height of irregularities). It does not measure the shape of these irregularities, sharp or smooth.

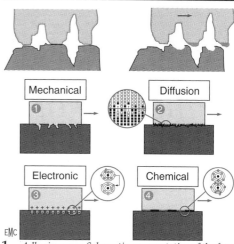

1 *Adhesive wear. Schematic representation of the four mechanisms of adhesive wear: mechanical, diffusion, electronic and chemical.*

SEM (scanning electron microscopy) examination of the surface reveals traces of machining, grain holes, porosity or any other irregularities.

By using **energy dispersive X-ray analysis (EDXA)**, it is possible to analyse the products found at the surface: for example the amount of carbide on a metallic surface.

Macrogeometry deals with the circularity of a prosthesis; this relates an equatorial plane section to a circle. Sphericity deals with circularities in all equatorial planes. These two parameters play a major role, especially if non-deformable materials such as metal or ceramics are used. The differences in radii between the two counterfaces or the clearance will be low. For an alumina ceramic, it must be around 50 μm; for two metallic surfaces, it must be a little larger to allow fluid to be interposed.

■ *Surface modification with time*

Many changes will occur under load and sliding. These changes are related to the cold flow of a plastic material, to wear with generation of debris, or to surface modification without debris formation. Some of these modifications, such as cold flow or running-in, can be considered part of the adaptation process, but some cause debris or severe surface deterioration that impair the system.

■ *Wear mechanisms* (fig 1, 2, 3)

The mechanisms by which pieces of material in contact with each other are released into the environment are defined as wear mechanisms and are not fully understood. They depend greatly on the characteristics of the material: its hardness, modulus of elasticity, rupture behaviour and corrosion products.

The four main mechanisms of wear behaviour are: adhesion, abrasion, fatigue and tribochemical causes. These mechanisms can occur simultaneously or successively.

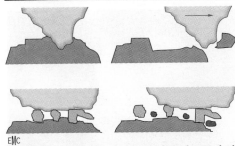

2 *Abrasive wear. The abrasion is dependent on both the roughness and the mechanical characteristics of the two materials. (Redrawn by permission from Sedel L. The tribology of hip replacement. Instructional Course Lecture, Journal of Bone and Joint Surgery 1997; 3 : page 7.)*

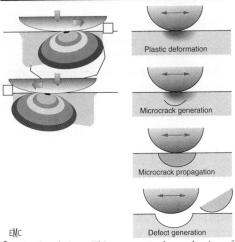

3 *Surface fatigue. This represents the mechanism of surface fatigue wear on alternative bearing. It occurs when hard material slides on soft material such as metal on polyethylene.*

Sensitivity to third body wear

When another material is interposed between the contact areas, it may give rise to increased wear. This phenomenon depends on the modulus of elasticity of the surfaces in contact. Softer materials are more sensitive than harder ones. The least sensitive material is alumina ceramic, while metal and plastic are more sensitive. Third bodies can also be cement or bone particulates, hydroxyapatite or metal. Harder materials will play a more destructive role than softer ones [10].

CHARACTERISTICS OF DIFFERENT BEARINGS IN USE

Different friction couples have been used. For some of them, very long-term experience in clinical use has enabled us to obtain a great deal of information. For other more recent couples, only partial knowledge is available. Information comes from many different sources; one of the most important is simulation.

■ *Mechanical simulation* (fig 4)

Two types of simulation are available:

Simple tribological studies: pin-on-disc or disc-on-disc machines. While many tests can

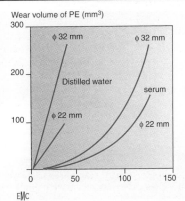

4 *Hip lubricant study with a metal-on-polyethylene couple with two different head sizes and two different lubricants. It can be seen that wear is strongly dependent on size but also on the type of lubricant used.*

be carried out at the same time, the conditions are very different from the physiological ones. These studies are relevant only for screening and to grossly separate good candidate materials from weak ones.

Hip simulator [13, 25, 49, 50, 51]: These relatively sophisticated machines are very useful. Different models are available where movements and load which are close to physiological values can be applied. To be able to understand the exact information these simulators provide, it is essential to have details about their design. Is the hip in a physiological position or is the socket displaced? Which lubricating fluid is used and what is its protein content? How is the fluid distributed? Is it a closed or an open circuit? What is the running speed? What is the applied load and what is the load cycle? How are the debris eliminated or are they kept in the sliding area? Is there a heat control system? These simulations often imply a very long and costly procedure.

After test completion, samples are examined, providing information on wear profiles, chemical changes in the material, debris type, volume, size and so on. However, these machine have some limitations. For example, if wear is measured by loss of component weight and if the material is hydrophilic, the results will be the sum of the two parameters: gain of weight from the adsorbed liquid and loss of weight from the debris generated.

■ *Biological simulation*

In vitro model: cell cultures are very useful for anticipating adverse reactions from particulates. Fibroblast cultures are the baseline [47], but for more accurate information it is better to use either osteoblast cultures or macrophages. Some teams [12, 26, 52] have used particulate-activated macrophages which revealed osteoclastic activity.

In vivo animal models are not very useful for studying sliding capacity, as their

biomechanics are far too different from those of humans. Animal experiments can only be run for a relatively short period of time. It is usually very hard to apply the results found in sheep or dogs to humans. Animal models are used mainly to test the biocompatibility of the sliding materials [30, 31, 33, 40], in bulk or particulate form. ISO standards define implantation procedures regarding sample size and shape, animal model, implantation period and histological studies. These studies are useful only for comparing one material to another [48, 52].

■ *Clinical trials*

Well conducted clinical trials are of course very useful; they must be prospective and study consecutive cases, examining many clinical and radiological details. It is essential to obtain excellent and reproducible X-rays in order to measure such parameters as migration, wear and bone modifications. Wear can be measured directly [35] when its magnitude allows it. However, for some materials such as ceramics or metal, wear cannot be measured on X-rays because it is under the sensibility level. It is also possible to quantify migration, and the incidence of radiolucent lines can provide indirect information about the amount of foreign body reaction. The occurrence of osteolytic areas must be recorded but this is usually in relation to wear of the sliding components. Calcar resorption is also a good marker of foreign body reaction.

X-rays can give more precise information about head/socket penetration. The use of stereophotogrammetry (RSA) requires beads to be implanted in the upper femoral extremity beforehand.

A great deal of information can be obtained after failures and revision surgery, but this does not provide information about the well-functioning prosthesis. A complete file is needed, including the reasons for revision and the time since adverse effects occurred (for example, socket tilting or head fracture). Samples must be retrieved so as not to create artefactual alteration of the materials. Samples should be sent to an engineering laboratory for tests: metal analysis, surface modifications, scratches, chemical modifications, polyethylene impregnation by particulates, or polyethylene modifications such as hardening of the surface [22].

Tissue samples can also be harvested for histological studies or quantification of inflammatory mediators (prostaglandin, growth factors, cytokines) [44, 45, 68]. Tissues can also be cultivated to quantify osteolytic activities. In the same tissues, particulates can be localised, quantified and identified, and this provides very valuable information about the respective role of each material in foreign body reaction processes [43, 48, 61] *(fig 5).*

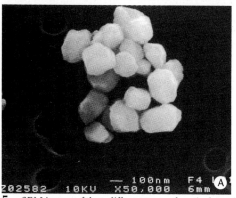
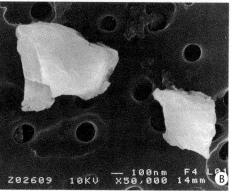
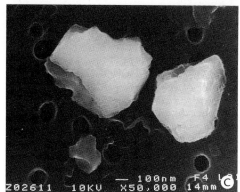

5 *SEM images of three different types of particulates. (Reproduced with permission from Lerounge S, Huk O, Yahia L'H and Sedel L. Characterization of in vivo wear debris from ceramic-ceramic total hip arthroplasties. Journal of Biomedical Materials Research, 1996 ; 32 : page 632. © 1996 John Wiley & Sons Inc.)*
A. *Zircon debris.*   B. *Titanium alloy debris.*   C. *Alumina ceramic debris.*

Results: different material couples

METAL-ON-POLYETHYLENE

Information is available from simulations and clinical studies which have been documented over many years. J. Charnley with his well-known pendulum demonstrated that metal-on-polyethylene with a small head size showed less friction than metal-on-metal components. He stated that both small head size and couple characteristics were responsible.

Metal-on-polyethylene experiences a very low friction coefficient (0.02), but is strongly dependent on the lubrication regimen, the roughness of the metallic counterface and the interposed fluid. It also depends on the temperature produced on contact.

In Boher's tribometric study [7], the friction coefficient ranged from 0.001 to 0.15. In a dry mode and in a pin-on-disc configuration, there are two successive changes:

– At first a thin film forms on the metallic surface by an adhesion mechanism. The sliding distance must be 500 km for this phenomenon to start and this distance diminishes if the load increases. Wear is in the order of $2.10^{-7}/mm^3/Nm$.

– In a second step, fatigue occurs. There is delamination of the superficial layer and transverse scratches appear. Wear is about $4.10^{-7}/mm^3/Nm$, and is now independent of the applied load.

If a lubricant is interposed, wear decreases so that twice the distance is necessary to observe identical abrasive wear. If the lubricant is associated with proteins, such as bovine serum or plasma, wear also decreases.

■ Effect of roughness

Wear is very sensitive to counterface roughness. Logically, it could be anticipated that increasing roughness increases wear. In fact, it is not so simple. There is an optimal roughness (Ra). If roughness is greater than this figure, wear increases by an abrasion phenomenon, and if roughness is less than this, wear increases by an adhesion mechanism. The optimal Ra for friction of a hard surface on polyethylene is 0.03 µm.

Polyethylene is very sensitive to any changes in the material or to any interposed material in the contact area. As regards material changes, the medical grade of polyethylene is ultrahigh molecular weight polyethylene (RCH1000). During its processing, voids or big masses of material organised as spherulites must be avoided as these can be the starting point for cracks leading to fatigue fractures. Recently, authors have pointed out the negative effects of oxidation on the long-term properties of polyethylene. This results in a layer of surface oxidation that will crack under load. This can be avoided by gamma irradiation in the absence of oxygen. Improved polyethylenes have been introduced. These improvements usually concern one aspect (for example, decrease of cold flow), but they can also increase debris generation or fatigue failures. Long-term evaluations in vivo are required to really know how these "improved polyethylenes" behave.

Any particles of bone, cement, or even hydroxyapatite will play an abrasive role. These three-body wear mechanisms may be responsible for early wear of polyethylene materials [10, 15].

■ Effect of temperature

During tests, the temperature rises in polyethylene while it is stable in metal. This rise in temperature can have adverse effects. Bergman and Rholmann [4] measured human temperature elevation during walking. This could play a role in the degradation process, especially if the hard material shows characteristics of poor heat dissipation.

■ Effect of the counterface material

The phenomena described above were observed for stainless steel or chromium cobalt counterfaces. For other materials, identical phenomena occur but are modified by the nature of the counterface.

For example, polyethylene against aluminum oxide provides a better sliding system. Abrasive wear and fatigue are also observed but at a sliding distance of 1000 to 4000 km and not at 500 km.

If the counterface is made of titanium alloy (TiAl6V4), there is an accelerated wear phenomenon. This is related to the regular destruction of the passivation layer of TiO_2 that is formed on the titanium alloy surface. This TiO_2 is detached and works as a third body increasing polyethylene and titanium alloy wear dramatically. This is not the case for the first million cycles if the titanium alloy has been previously treated by ion implantation. This ion implantation is effective only on the first microns of depth, leaving some uncertainties as to when this implanted layer will be destroyed by long-term use [16, 17].

■ Results from hip simulation

Many studies conducted on different types of hip simulators by MacKellop et al [49, 50, 51], Dumbleton et al [21] and Boher [7] provide very interesting results. Socket deformation includes both creep and wear and it is difficult to identify precisely which mechanism is predominant. Friction resistance is dependent on many parameters: increasing the head size increases the friction and equatorial contact also leads to increased friction. Micro X-rays of the polyethylene show macro-cracks due to abrasion and cracking of the surface under load. Micro-cracks are also initiated under the surface leading to large particulate release by a fatigue mechanism. The roughness of metallic heads made of stainless steel or cobalt chromium increased during the test. For alumina heads there was no change in roughness. Wear debris was measured by weighing released material, and showed 3 to 4 times more debris for metal-on-polyethylene friction than for alumina-on-polyethylene friction. Results concerning zirconia-on-polyethylene are controversial. Some simulation tests presented identical results for zirconia and alumina; others [69, 70] showed no improvement between cobalt chromium and zirconia, and still other described 40% to 60% reduction in polyethylene wear with zirconia [41]. Streicher [69, 70] looked at metal-on-metal systems and found this couple to be very sensitive to the size of the head diameter. With a diameter of 28 mm, the time the pendulum took to stop was the same as for metal-on-polyethylene. It was shorter for a 37 or a 32 mm head size. The annual wear rate of this combination is in the order of 2 to 5 μm per year. This is 200 times less than metal-on-polyethylene, but 2 to 10 times more than alumina-on-alumina. Metal-on-metal is very sensitive to the protein content of the lubricating fluid. In severe conditions with a high protein content and high loads, there can be some accelerated phenomena. The science of hip simulation is so well developed that some engineers are able to choose the test to suit one given material.

■ *In vivo studies*

These are the only reliable studies, as they give the true wear rate and in vivo behaviour of materials.

As polyethylene material has been in use for more than 30 years, a large amount of information on its long-term behaviour in humans is available. Socket deformation has been documented, measured and related to many parameters. This is due to a major contribution by Wroblewski et al [35, 76, 77] who analysed explanted sockets after loosening. Weightman et al [74, 75] presented studies showing that socket deformation was, in fact, more related to wear and associated with some apposition of detached particulates at the edge of the sliding area. Comparisons between explanted sockets and simulator tested sockets showed great similarities. These measurements introduced a bias: there was a strong correlation between loosening and wear but no arguments to assess which phenomenon occurred first.

Factors such as patient weight and time since implantation have not proved to be significant. The overall penetration rate per year is at its maximum at 2 or 3 years and then diminishes.

Other authors have quantified head penetration on X-rays. Larger heads result in more penetration. However, this increases dramatically if the head size reaches 35 mm in diameter. Mean penetration per year has been measured at 0.12 mm, but this may increase if head size increases, or decrease for alumina heads, even if penetration still remains around 0.08 mm per year. Many authors insist on the great individual variability of penetration rates over time. They all agree that a high penetration rate is related to an increased loosening rate.

Alumina-on-alumina couple

MECHANICAL CHARACTERISTICS

These mechanical characteristics concern fracture resistance, wear performance and ageing.

Alumina ceramic is a stiff, hard and brittle material, having a modulus of elasticity of 380 GPa, as compared with cobalt chromium (220 GPa), cortical bone (20 GPa) or bone cement (2 GPa). Standard alumina ceramics present a bending strength of more than 400 MPa and some good ceramics have a bending strength of 550 MPa.

Hardness is an important quality in terms of its resistance to wear. Alumina ceramic is harder than metal - in fact, it is one of the hardest materials after diamonds and carborandum according to the MOHR scale. This is why it is used as a cutting tool in industry.

■ *Fracture toughness*

The shock sensitivity or brittleness of alumina ceramic must be considered. Many people believe that brittle material will fracture under light impact loads resulting in catastrophic failure when the stress intensity factor (K1) reaches a critical value (K1c). This parameter is the fracture toughness of the material. It is determined by direct observation of a well-defined initial crack propagation under laboratory control. Alumina ceramic has a fracture toughness value of around 5 MPa(m) 1/2 which is lower than that of zirconia ceramic (9 MPa(m) 1/2). Thus, well-manufactured ceramic will sustain very high loads without breakage.

To avoid excessive internal stresses, the taper geometry of the head and stem must be accurate. This accuracy concerns not only the cone angle but also the cone circularity, roughness and linearity.

Laboratory tests to confirm the long-term behaviour of femoral ceramic heads include impact, fatigue and static strength tests. Cyclic testing is generally carried out for 10 or 20 million cycles with loads of 1.3 kN to 13.3 kN.

■ *Femoral head fractures*

Component fractures, and especially femoral head fractures, are one reason for failure of alumina-on-alumina total hip arthroplasty. The consequences of component fractures are one of the major limitations to the clinical application of alumina ceramic. Their frequency differs from one report to another: from 1/1200 to 10/130 [14]. We have already seen that fracture risk is dependent on alumina quality, the geometry of the sliding components and the applied load. Clinical cases of fracture are associated with small head diameter, poor quality alumina (especially large grain size up to 40 μm),

inborn stresses created during the material's production, less than ideal fitting of the male and female tapers, short term subluxation and reduction. Cement or bone fragments caught between the taper and ball do not appear to present any risk, which is different from other couple bearing surfaces including metal-on-metal. Since the early 1980s, improved manufacturing processes, taper design and quality control have resulted in a significant and general decrease of fracture risks. Moreover, heads with a diameter under 28 mm are no longer used in alumina-on-alumina prostheses. Due to these important improvements, it is difficult to estimate precisely from historical records the current risk of fracture. Out of more than 2000 hips, we have observed only one head fracture over the last ten years. With appropriate care taken during surgery, Clarke and Willmann [14] estimate that the risk of fracture may be reduced to below 1 in 2000 cases for a ten year period.

■ *Surface performance*

Alumina ceramic is an extremely interesting material as regards its wear resistance; this quality is related to its surface characteristics. It is possible to machine a very smooth surface with a Ra of 0.02 which is less than the best possible metallic surface finish.

Its wear properties are related to its ability to absorb water which is measured by the wettability or the angle of a drop of water on its surface. This is related to the hydrophilic character of its alumina surface and can also explain the excellent friction characteristics under load when the clearance is adequate and when the lubrication film fluid remains unchanged.

Many wear tests have been conducted. They were strongly dependent on the lubricant used; demineralised water gave worse results than did bovine serum.

The best results concerning friction coefficient and wear have been obtained with alumina-against-alumina. Boher [7] published experimental work on clearance and friction coefficients. It appeared that for alumina-against-alumina, the best clearance was from 10 to 50 μm. This was obtained by the Ceraver company using a special grinding process, but it required their selling the couple as a non-interchangeable unit. Since 1993, new manufacturing processes have allowed the provision of inter-changeable heads and sockets while retaining clearance.

Clinical measurements performed by J.M. Dorlot [19, 20] on retrieved specimens concluded that an alumina-on-alumina couple, under normal conditions and implanted for more than ten years, resulted in a yearly linear wear rate of 0.025 μm; this is around 4000 times less debris production than a metal-on-polyethylene couple. In some cases where the socket had tilted before retrieval or when the initial design or material were inadequate, some gross wear was documented, but this was during the 1970s [73]. Prudhommeaux [58] more recently compared alumina quality to wear in an ex vivo study; she found a strong correlation.

Metal-on-metal

Cobalt chromium-on-cobalt chromium, initially introduced by MacKee and Farrar, was abandoned because of its high friction coefficient and the relative toxicity of its wear particulates resulting in muscle necrosis and massive foreign body reactions. As some long-term implantations without any adverse effects were also documented, this concept was reintroduced 10 years ago. High-quality manufacturing has improved the sliding mechanism and adequate clearance has improved the lubrication mechanism. Surface performances have been improved by using forged Protasul-21WF® containing finely distributed carbides which increase surface hardness. Many laboratory tests are available on this new/old material. Retrieved material analysis has enabled the in vivo wear to be measured in the range of 10 μm per year. Preliminary clinical results are positive. Information from in vitro studies [11] or from retrieved long-term tissues suggests that biological reactions could be of concern if implanted in active and young patients. The measured in vivo

cobalt level in the blood also increases in patients with a metal-on-metal articulation, but nobody knows if this will have a deleterious effect. Few well-documented, long-term clinical studies are available at present, but preliminary studies are good. Some authors, such as Zweimuller, suspected some failures to be related to third body damage and have switched to alumina-on-alumina.

Zirconia ceramic-on-polyethylene

Zirconia ceramic has a better fracture toughness than alumina ceramics and is biocompatible in bulk form. It has a good tribological performance against polyethylene. The main interest of this product is the ability to produce a small size ceramic head with a low fracture risk. Some recent clinical results [1] have reported an increased loosening rate with zirconia ceramic-on-polyethylene compared to metal-on-polyethylene. This may be due to poor heat dissipation, instability of the material, or some other unknown reason. Zirconia-on-zirconia is not possible but it seems that zirconia-on-alumina can replace alumina-on-alumina with the added advantage of using a small head diameter. There are some upcoming studies with different mixtures of alumina and zirconia ceramics (A.Toni et al).

Others materials

The size of this chapter does not allow us to deal with other couples: titanium-implanted materials, polyethylene improved by irradiation, diamond and so on. It is possible that in the future some new material will provide a better answer to the remaining questions.

Conclusion

Tribology is a difficult field dealing with many different aspects; orthopaedic surgeons must understand that there is no simple answer to all these questions. Right now the best material as regards friction and low formation of wear debris is an alumina-on-alumina couple, provided an adequate system can be found to solve the problem of long-term bone/material fixation.
Tribology is one of the keys to long-term acceptance of joint prostheses, but it is not the only one: bone modelling, tissue biology and tolerance of degradation products are also concerned.

Acknowledgements – The author would like to thank Alain Meunier (researcher CNRS) who helped with some of the engineering aspects.

References

[1] Allain J, Lemouel S, Goutallier D, Voisin MC. Poor eight year survival of cemented zirconia-polyethylene total hip replacements. *J Bone Joint Surg Br* 1999; 81: 835-842

[2] Bely VA, Savkin VG, Sviridyonok A. Effect of structure on polymer friction, *Wear* 1971; 18: 11-18

[3] Bergmann G, Graichen F, Rohlmann A. In vivo measurement of temperature rise in a hip implant. Proceedings of the 37th Annual Meeting Orthopaedic Research Society, Anaheim, March 4-7 1991

[4] Bergmann G, Rohlmann A, Graichen F. Hip joint loading during going up and down stairs. Transactions of the first EORS meeting, Paris, Nov 1991

[5] Boehler M, Knahr K, Salzer M, Plenk H, Walter A, Schreiber V. Long-term results of uncemented alumina acetabular implants. *J Bone Joint Surg Br* 1994; 76: 53-59

[6] Boehler M, Schachinger W, Wolfi G, Krismer M, Mayr G, Salzer M. Do modular sockets with ceramic inlays migrate more? *J Bone Joint Surg Br* 1998; 80: 835-842

[7] Boher C. Simulation exprimentale du comportement tribologique des matériaux prothétiques de la hanche. [thèse], Toulouse, 1992

[8] Boutin P, Blanquaert D. Le frottement alumine-alumine en chirurgie de la hanche, 1205 arthroplasties totales. *Rev Chir Orthop* 1981; 67: 279-287

[9] Boutin P, Christel P, Dorlot JM, Meunier A, De Rocquancourt A, Sedel L et al. The use of dense alumina-alumina ceramic combination in total hip replacement. *J Biomed Mater Res* 1988; 22: 1203-1232

[10] Caravia L, Dowson D, Fischer J, Jobbins B. The influence of bone and bone cement debris on counterface roughness in sliding wear tests of ultra high molecular weight polyethylene on stainless steel. *Proc Inst Mech Eng* 1990; 204: 65-70

[11] Case CP, Langkamer VG, James C, Palmer MR, Kemp AJ, Heap PF et al. Widespread dissemination of metal debris from implants. *J Bone Joint Surg Br* 1994; 76: 701-712

[12] Catelas I, Huk O, Petit A, Zukor DJ, Marchand R, Yahia LH. Flow cytometric analysis of macrophage mouse response to ceramic and polyethylene particles: effects of size, concentration and composition. *J Biomed Mater Res* 1998; 41: 600-607

[13] Clarke IC, Gustafson A, Jung H, Fujisawa A. Hip-simulator ranking of polyethylene wear: comparisons between ceramic heads of different sizes. *Acta Orthop Scand* 1996; 67: 128-132

[14] Clarke IC, Willmann G. Structural ceramics in orthopaedics. In: Bone implant interface. St Louis: CV Mosby, 1994: 203-252

[15] Cooper JR, Dowson D, Fischer J, Jobbins B. Ceramic bearing surfaces in total artificial joints resistance to third body wear damage from bone cement particles. *J Med Eng Techn* 1991; 15: 63-67

[16] Davidson JA. Characteristics of metal and ceramic total hip bearing surfaces and their effect on long-term ultra high molecular weight polyethylene wear. *Clin Orthop* 1993; 294: 361-378

[17] Davidson JA, Poggie RA, Mishra AK. Abrasive wear of ceramic, metal and UHMWPE bearing surfaces from third-body bone, PMMA bone cement, and titanium debris. *Biomed Mater Eng* 1994; 4: 213-229

[18] Dayw H, Swanson SA, Freeman MA. Contact pressures in the loaded human cadaver hip. *J Bone Joint Surg Br* 1975; 57: 302-313

[19] Dorlot JM. Long-term effects of alumina components in total hip prostheses. *Clin Orthop* 1992; 282: 47-52

[20] Dorlot JM, Christel P, Meunier A. Wear analysis of retrieved alumina heads and sockets of hip prostheses. *J Biomed Mater Res Appl Biomater* 1989; 23: 299-310

[21] Dumbleton JH, Miller DA. A simulator for load bearing joints. *Wear* 1972; 20: 165-174

[22] Eyerer P, Ke YC. Property changes of UHMW polyethylene hip cup endoprostheses during implantation. *J Biomed Mater Res* 1994; 28: 1137-1151

[23] Frankel VH, Pugh JW. Biomechanics of the hip. In: Tronzo RF ed. Surgery of the hip joint. New York: Springer-Verlag, 1984: 115-131

[24] Fritsch EW, Gleitz M. Ceramic femoral head fractures in total hip arthroplaty. *Clin Orthop* 1996; 328: 129-136

[25] Galante JE, Rostoker W. Wear in total hip prostheses. *Acta Orthop Scand [suppl]* 1973; 145: 1-46

[26] Glant TT, Jacobs JJ, Molnar G, Shanbhag AS, Valyon M, Galante JE. Bone resorption activity of particulate-stimulated macrophages. *J Bone Miner Res* 1993; 8: 1071-1079

[27] Griss P, Heimke G. Five years experience with ceramic-metal-composite hip endoprostheses, part I. *Arch Orthop Trauma Surg* 1981; 98: 157-164

[28] Griss P, Von Andrian-Werburg H, Krempien B, Heimke G. Biological activity and histocompatibility of dense Al2O/MgO ceramic implants in rats. *J Biomed Mater Res Symp* 1973; 4: 453-462

[29] Hodge WA, Fuan RS, Carlson KL, Burgess RG, Harris WH, Mann RW. Contact pressures in the human hip joint measured in vivo. *Proc Natl Acad Sci USA* 1986; 83: 2875-2883

[30] Howie DW, Vernon-Roberts B. The synovial response to intra-articular cobalt chrome wear particles. *Clin Orthop* 1988; 232: 244-254

[31] Howie DW, Vernon-Roberts B, Oakeshott R, Manthey B. A rat model of resorption of bone at the cement-bone interface in the presence of PE wear particles. *J Bone Joint Surg Am* 1988; 70: 257-263

[32] Hummer CD 3ʳ, Rothman RH, Hozack WJ. Catastrophic failure of modular zirconia-ceramic femoral head components after total hip arthroplasty. *J Arthroplasty* 1995; 10: 848-850

[33] Hyanes DR, Rogers SD, Hay S, Pearcy MJ, Howie DW. The differences in toxicity and release of bone resorbing mediators induced by titanium and cobalt chromium alloy wear particles. *J Bone Joint Surg Am* 1993; 75: 825-834

[34] Isaac GH, Arkinson JR, Dowson D, Kennedy PD, Smith MR. The causes of femoral head roughing in explanted Charnley hip prostheses. *Eng Med* 1987; 16: 167-173

[35] Isaac GH, Hodgkinson JP, Wroblewski BM. A sinister bias in hip socket wear. Brief report. *J Bone Joint Surg Br* 1989; 71: 143-144

[36] Jenny JY, Boeri C, Tavan A, Schlemmer B. Résultats en fonction du couple de frottement. In: Pidhorz L, Sedel L éd. Symposium sur les prothèses totales de hanche avant 50 ans. *Revue de chirurgie orthopédique,* 1998; vol 84

[37] Kabo JM, Amstutz HC. Frictional torque in surface and conventional hip replacement. *J Bone Joint Surg Am* 1983; 65: 366-369

[38] Kawauchi K, Kuroki Y, Saito S, Ohgiya H, Sato S, Kondo S et al . Total hip endoprostheses with ceramic head and H. D. P. socket. Clinical wear rate. *Orthop Ceram Implants* 1984; 4: 253-257

[39] Kempf I, Semlith M. Massive wear of a steel ball head by ceramic fragments in the polyethylene acetabular cup after revision of a total hip prosthesis with fractured ceramic ball. *Arch Orthop Trauma Surg* 1990; 109: 284-287

[40] Kim KI, Chiba J, Rubash HE. In vivo and in vitro analysis of membranes from hip prostheses inserted without cement. *J Bone Joint Surg Am* 1994; 76: 172-180

[41] Kumar P, Oka M, Ikeuchi K, Shimizu K, Yamamuro T, Okumura H et al. Low wear rate of UHMWPE against zirconia ceramic (Y-PSZ) in comparison to alumina ceramic and SUS 316L Alloy. *J Biomed Mater Res* 1991; 25: 813-828

[42] LeMouel S, Allain J, Goutallier D. Analyse actuarielle à 10 ans d'une cohorte de 156 prothèses totales de hanche cimentées à couple de frottement alumine/polyethylene. *Rev Chir Orthop*1998; 84: 338-345

[43] Lee JM, Salvati EA, Betts F, Dicarlo EF, Doty SB, Bullough PG. Size of metallic and polyethylene debris particles in failed cemented total hip replacements. *J Bone Joint Surg Br* 1992; 74: 380-384

[44] Lerouge S, Huk O, Yahia LH, Sedel L. Characterization of in vivo wear debris from ceramic -ceramic total hip arthroplasties. *J Biomed Mater Res* 1996; 32: 627-633

[45] Lerouge S, Huk O, Yahia LH, Witvoet J, Sedel L. Ceramic-ceramic vs metal-polyethylene: a comparison of periprosthetic tissus from loosened total hip arthroplasties. *J Bone Joint Surg Br* 1997; 79: 135-139

[46] Livermore J, Ilstrup D, Morrey B. Effect of femoral head size on wear of the polyethylene acetabular component. *J Bone Joint Surg Am* 1990; 72: 518-528

[47] Maloney WJ, Smith L, Castro F, Schurman DJ. Fibroblast response to metallic debris in vitro enzyme induction, cell proliferation and toxicity. *J Bone Joint Surg Am* 1993; 75: 835-844

[48] Margevicius KJ, Bauer TW, McMahon JT, Brown SA, Merritt K. Isolation and characterisation of debris in membranes around total joint prostheses. *J Bone Joint Surg Am* 1994; 76: 1664-1675

[49] McKellop HA, Sarmiento A, Schwinn CP, Ebramzadeh E. In vivo wear of titanium alloy hip prostheses. *J Bone Joint Surg Am* 1990; 72: 512-517

[50] McKellop HM, Clarke IC, Marlkorf KL, Amstutz HC. Wear characteristics of UHMWPE: a method for accurately measuring extremely low rates. *J Biomed Mater Res* 1978; 12: 895-927

[51] McKellop HM, Clarke IC, Marlkorf KL, Amstutz HC. Friction and wear properties of polymer, metal and ceramic prosthetic joints materials evaluated on a multichannel screening device. *J Biomed Mater Res* 1981; 15: 619-653

[52] Murray DD, Rushton N. Mediators of bone resorption around implants. *Clin Orthop* 1992; 281: 295-304

[53] Nizard RS, Sedel L, Meunier A, Christel P, Soudry M, Witvoet J. Survival analysis of alumina-alumina total hip prosthesis: a 10 years follow-up study. *Clin Orthop* 1992; 282: 53-63

[54] Nusbaum HJ, Rose RM, Paul IL, Crugnola AM, Radin EL. Wear mechanisms for ultrahigh molecular weight polyethylene in the totalhip prostheses. *J Appl Polymer Sci*1979; 23: 777-789

[55] Oonishi H, Takayaka Y, Clarke I, Jung H. Comparative wear studies of 28-mm ceramic and stainless steel total hip joints over 2 to 7 year period. *J Long Term Effects Med Implants* 1992; 2: 37-47

[56] Paul JP. Bioengineering studies of forces transmitted by joints. Part2: Engineering analysis. In: Kenedi RM ed. Biomechanics and related bioengineering topics. Oxford: Pergamon Press 1965

[57] Plitz W, Hoss HU. Wear of alumina-ceramic hip-joints; some clinical and tribological aspects. In: Winter GD, Gibbons DF, Plenk H eds. Biomaterials1980. New York: John Wiley, 1982: 187-196

[58] Prudhommeaux F, Nevelos J, Doyle C, Meunier A, Sedel L. Analysis of wear behavior of alumina/alumina hip prosthesis after 10 years of implantation. In: Legeros RZ, Legeros JP eds. Bioceramics 11. Proceedings of the 11th international symposium on ceramics in medicine. New York: World Scientific Publishing, 1998

[59] Rose RM, Nusbaum HJ, Shneider H et al. On the true wear rate of ultra high-molecular-weight polyethylene in the total hip prosthesis. *J Bone joint Surg Am*1980; 62: 537-549

[60] Rose RM, Radin EL. Wear of polyethylene in the total hip prosthesis. *Clin Orthop* 1982; 170: 107-115

[61] Savio JA 3ʳᵈ, Overcamp LM, Black J. Size and shape of biomaterial wear debris. *Clin Mater* 1994; 15: 101-147

[62] Schmalzried TP. Light microscopic identification of high density polyethylene (HDP) wear debris using oil red- o staining. Transactions of the 38th Annual meeting of the ORS, Washington, February1992

[63] Schmalzried TP, Harris WH. Periprosthetic bone loss in total hip replacement:the role of high density polyethylene (HDP) wear debris and the concept of the effect joint space. Transactions of the 38th Annual meeting of the ORS Washington, February 1992

[64] Schuller HM, Marti RK. Ten-year socket wear in 66 arthroplasties. Ceramic versus metal heads. *Acta Orthop Scand* 1990; 61: 240-243

[65] Sedel L. Tribology of total hip replacement. In: Fulford P, Duparc J eds. Instructional course lecture. EFORT meeting, Barcelona, 1997

[66] Sedel L, Derethe P, Christel P. Mesure sur simulateur de l'amortissement d'une hanche normale et prothésée. *Rev Chir Orthop*1977; 63 (suppl 2): 100-107

[67] Sedel L, Kerboull L, Christel P, Meunier A, Witvoet J. Alumina on alumina in total hip replacement. Results in a serie of activepatients under fifty. *J Bone Joint Surg Br* 1990; 72: 658-663

[68] Sedel L, Simeon J, Meunier A, Villette JM, Launey SM. Prostaglandin E2 level in tissue surrounding aseptic failed total hips:effects of materials. *Arch Orthop Trauma Surg* 1992; 111: 255-258

[69] Streicher RM. Tribology of artificial joints. In: Endoprosthetics edited by E. Morsher

[70] Streicher RM, Semlitsch M, Schon R. Ceramic surfaces as wear partners for PE. In: Bonfield W, Hastings GW, Tanner KE eds, Bioceramics 4. Proceedings of the 4th International Symposium on Ceramics in Medicine, London, 1991: 9-16

[71] Sugano N, Nishii T, Nakata K, Mashura K, Takaoka K. Polyethylene sockets and alumina ceramic heads in cemented total hip arthroplasty. A ten year study. *J Bone Joint Surg Br* 1995; 77: 548-556

[72] Wallbridge N, Dowson D. The walking activity of patients with artificial hip joints. *EngMed* 1982; 11: 95-96

[73] Walter A, Plitz W. Wear of retrieved alumina-ceramic hip-joints. In: Vincenzini P ed. Ceramic in surgery. Amsterdam: Elsevier, 1983: 253-259

[74] Weightman BO, Paul IL, Rose RM. A comparative study of total hip replacement prosthesis. *J Biomech* 1973; 6: 299-311

[75] Weightman BO, Swanson SA, Isaac GH, Wroblewski BM. Polyethylene wear from retrieved acetabular cups. *J Bone Joint Surg Br* 1991; 73: 806-810

[76] Wroblewski BM. 15-21 year results of the Charnley low-friction arthroplasty. *Clin Orthop* 1986; 211: 30-35

[77] Wroblewski BM, Siney PD, Dowson D, Collins SN. prospective clinical joint simulator studies of a new total hip arthroplasty using alumina ceramic heads and cross-linked polyethylene cups. *J Bone Joint Surg Br* 1996; 78: 280-285

[78] Wu C, Rice RW, Johnson D, Platt BA. Grain size dependence of wear in ceramics. *Ceram Eng Sci Proc* 1985; 6: 995-1011

[79] Zichner LP, Lindenfeld T. In vivo wear of the slide combinations ceramic-polyethylene as opposed to metal-polyethylene*Orthopade* 1997; 26: 129-134

[80] Zichner LP, Willert HG. Comparison of alumina-polyethylene and metal -polyethylene in clinical trials. *Clin Orthop* 1992; 282: 86-94

Dislocations of total hip prostheses

D Huten
A Vidil
J Duparc

Abstract. – Instability, which occurs less often than loosening but more frequently than infection, is one of the complications which can spoil the result of a total hip replacement; an occurrence rate of about 2% is probably an underestimate. It can occur early or late after operation and result from trauma or malpositioning. The dislocation may be either posterior or anterior, and can happen once or be recurrent. Predisposing factors may be related to the condition of the bone and soft tissues, to the design of the prosthesis, to the surgical approach used, or to the postoperative follow-up. These causes may occur in various combinations, and this makes it difficult to investigate all the factors which may be responsible for instability.

An appropriate decision can only be taken after very careful assessment of the characteristics and causes of the instability. Severe malposition and nonunion of the greater trochanter are easily recognised, but often there is no obvious cause and one is reduced to hypothesising.

Conservative management is advised for a first and sometimes a second dislocation which do not have any obvious cause, and which often occur soon after operation. Recurring dislocations demand further surgery, which should be designed to correct any obvious cause which may be recognised either before or during the operation. The various available techniques are discussed and range from the simple fixation of an acetabular augment to the replacement of one or of both components of the prosthesis. These revisions weaken the peri-articular muscles and their success cannot be guaranteed. In practice, all these procedures have a significant rate of complications and of failure: 39% for Daly [13] *and 26% for Fraser* [19].

© 2000, Editions Scientifiques et Médicales Elsevier SAS. All rights reserved.

Keywords: hip, total hip replacement, dislocations, instability, conservative management, acetabular revision, femoral revision, long posterior wall (LPW) acetabular component, acetabular augmentation, constrained total hip prosthesis.

General principles [28]

When a total hip prosthesis gives problems of instability, it is always important to try to determine the characteristics and causes of the instability.

CHARACTERISTICS OF INSTABILITY

Instabilities should be classified according to type (subluxation or dislocation), when they occur (early, secondary, or late), the number of events, any specific reasons (trauma or malposition), and their direction (anterior or posterior).

■ *Type*

Subluxations can remain unrecognised for long periods and do not cause as severe problems as dislocations. Some patients learn to avoid the precipitating movement, but subluxations can progress to true dislocations.

■ *Timing*

Instability can appear soon after insertion of the prosthesis, as a secondary phenomenon, or as a later event.

Early dislocations (before 1 to 3, or even 12 months, according to different authors) are the most frequent. When there is no significant malposition or displacement of the greater trochanter, they can be considered as due to a lack of healing of the soft tissues, muscle hypotonia, loss of proprioception, and in some cases the presence of a deep haematoma. All of these can be followed by spontaneous resolution of the instability without further surgery.

Secondary dislocations occur when the patient recommences his normal activities, and are due to more extensive movements which follow the return of greater mobility, or sometimes to a traumatic incident.

Late dislocations, which appear by definition five years after operation, pose a special problem. They are especially likely to occur with prostheses which have a small head, with wear and deformation of the cup, distension of the capsule and weakness of the peri-articular muscles.

Early dislocations are more common than secondary, while late instability appears even less often.

■ *Number*

Recurrent dislocations are always alarming, and surgical treatment should be considered when the problem occurs sufficiently often to cause real inconvenience to the patient. These acute events always damage the soft tissues (rupture of soft tissue repairs with early dislocations, and distension of the pseudo-capsule with recurrent dislocations). They may damage the prosthetic components (deformation of the cup, scratching of the head), allow the interposition of foreign material (cerclage wires, fragments of broken screws), or dissociation of the individual components of

Denis Huten, M.D., Chairman.
A Vidil, M.D.,
Jacques Duparc, M.D., Honorary Chairman.
Chirurgie Orthopédique et Traumatologique, Hôpital Bichat, 46 rue Henri Huchard, 75877 Paris, France.

a modular prosthesis [4]. Most authors believe that a revision should be considered when there have been two or three dislocations.

▪ Predisposing factors

True traumatic dislocations of total hip prostheses do not occur very often and rarely require surgery. Conversely, dislocations due to certain positions of the patient frequently require surgery, especially if they follow relatively minor movements.

▪ Direction

Most dislocations are posterior because the hip is usually in flexion, adduction and medial rotation, but the direction can also relate to the original surgical approach. A posterior approach, which damages the posterior muscles, allows posterior dislocations. An anterior lateral approach, which damages the anterior muscles, allows anterior dislocations. The transtrochanteric approach avoids this hazard as it spares the muscles, but problems can arise when there is a nonunion of the osteotomy. The direction of any dislocation depends also on the orientation of the components, and this can explain instability in the opposite direction to that of the approach (excessive anteversion is likely to result in anterior dislocation even after a posterior approach). Multidirectional dislocations are rare and occur in patients with neurological problems, or who have a long history of prosthetic instability. The direction of the instability should be determined and is based on the movement which produces dislocation (flexion with internal rotation, or extension with external rotation), the position of the relevant leg, the lateral radiograph, and careful testing for the direction of instability after reduction. Sometimes, this remains unrecognised as a result of inadequate clinical or radiological examination, and this in turn can lead to errors in treatment.

CAUSES OF INSTABILITY [28]

There are two main mechanisms which can explain prosthetic dislocation (*fig 1*):

– Contact between the neck and the cup, bony structures or soft tissue structures, which provide a fulcrum which allows the prosthetic head to be leered out of the cup. This process is known as impingement or cam-effect and it can be incriminated with malpositioning (*fig 2*).

– Separation due to muscle weakness, which may be of several aetiologies (*fig 3*).

Management of dislocation is based on understanding the reasons causing dislocation to occur. The cause of instability is sometimes obvious from the malposition of the components, from muscle weakness produced either from a too-short or too-medial femur, nonunion of the trochanter, or

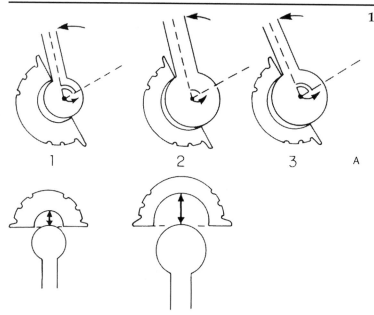

1 A. dislocation due to contact between the neck and the cup (cam effect). 1 and 2. The head/neck diameter ratio and the arc of motion are the same although the diameter of both heads differs; 3. The head diameter is the same as in 2 and neck diameter the same as in 1; the head/neck diameter ratio is larger than in 1 and 2.
B. Dislocation due to separation: large head sizes require greater displacement before the head dislocates.

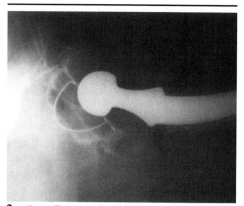

2 Cam effect: anterior dislocation due to contact between the neck and the posterior aspect of the cup during external rotation (too much anteversion of the cup).

paralysis. However, it is often impossible to be absolutely certain of a specific cause, and other factors may appear to be involved. This diversity of aetiological factors, which leads to associate procedures to improve stability, is characteristic of instability of total hip replacements.

▪ General condition of the patient

Old age is often associated with risk of falls, less ability to comply with dislocation precautions, and weak musculature which favours instability. It may also be a contraindication to extensive surgery.

Certain other general conditions produce a poor prognosis: poor compliance (alcoholism, psychiatric problems, old age), poor muscle control and contractures (central and peripheral neuropathies), and polyarthritis of the lower limbs.

The role of the aetiology of the original hip problem is more open to debate. Nevertheless, replacements made for cervical neck fractures have a high rate of dislocation [24], and this is probably related to advanced age and associated medical

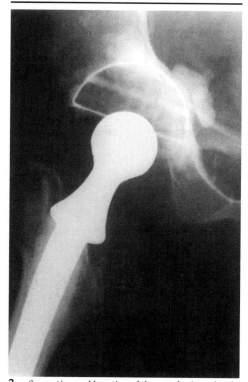

3 Separation: subluxation of the prosthesis under the effect of gravity in a paralysed hip and in spite of the re-establishment of correct leg length.

problems. Relatively high rates are associated with prosthetic replacement for avascular necrosis of the femoral head in young patients who are very active and who also frequently have a history of alcoholism.

An excessive degree of joint mobility, most often found in women, may also have a role.

▪ Local conditions

Previous surgery, particularly prosthetic, is a well-known cause of instability, largely as a result of damage to soft tissues. Repeated operations for loosening, and even more so for infection or for instability, also lead to a poor prognosis [48].

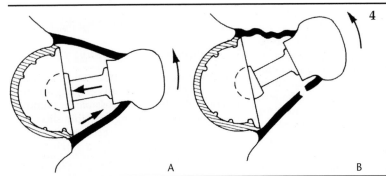

4 *A. Tension in the axis of healed (or intact) posterior transverse structures during internal rotation maintains good contact between the components.*
B. Lack of sound healing of these structures will allow increased rotation and cannot prevent dislocation.

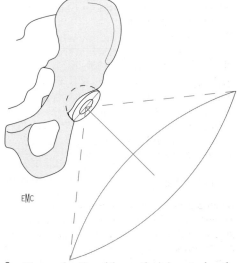

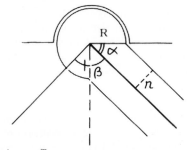

5 $\sin \alpha = r/R$.
The arc of prosthetic movement (angle β) = 180° - 2 α.
For r = 5 mm (neck of 10 mm) and R = 11.1 mm (head of 22.2 mm), the arc of motion is 126°.
For r = 5 mm (neck of 10 mm) and R = 14 mm (head of 28 mm), the arc of motion is 138°.

Approaches: The surgical approach used plays an essential role. Poor healing of the soft tissues which have been detached, or nonunion of a trochanteric osteotomy, can also explain the development of instability:

– the posterior approach weakens the posterior capsule and muscles, with a risk of posterior dislocation during the frequent movements of flexion-adduction-internal rotation *(fig 4)*.

– the various anterior lateral approaches in which the gluteus minimus and a part of the gluteus medius are detached predispose to anterior dislocation. They also run the risk of damaging the superior gluteal nerve.

– a transtrochanteric approach may result in nonunion of the osteotomy, which will result in a decrease of muscle power and a risk of dislocation, which is more important if the displacement of the trochanteric fragment is significant. Secondary fractures of the great trochanter have the same effect. Treatment is

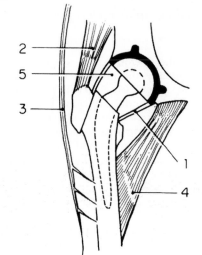

6 *A hip prosthesis. 1. Capsule; 2. gluteal muscles; 3. fascia lata; 4. adductors; 5. peri-prosthetic space.*

made more difficult if the fragment is small and displaced [47], or if the nonunion is old.

■ Type of prosthesis

The risk of dislocation is related to:

– A high neck/head diameter ratio, as this will decrease the range of possible movement and encourage dislocation by leverage between the neck and the edge of the cup *(fig 5)*. Heads with a skirt have the same deleterious effect as the large necks.

– A large head/neck angle, as this medialises the femur and thus decreases the moment arm of the gluteus medius.

– The presence of any large "dead space" between the capsule and the prosthetic head; this is often found with a large cup and a small head *(fig 6)*.

8 *The arc of motion of the prosthesis is centred on the axis of the cup. The risk of dislocation from neck-cup contact is greater when the arc of motion of the neck is not similar to the arc of motion of the normal hip.*

– A poor design of the cup: the extended cylindrical shape of the Charnley cup has been shown to prevent dislocation *(fig 7)*. Morscher has reduced his rate of dislocation by removing a 20° sector of the inferior part of the cup in order to avoid contact between the neck and the cup in extension and external rotation.

■ Postoperative complications

A deep infection is always a possibility and should be suspected from the clinical picture, and confirmed by blood tests (CRP) and aspiration, if any doubt still remains. Bone scanning is relatively non-specific. Some unstable prosthesis are also infected, especially after multiple revisions for instability. Infection encourages instability as a result of effusion formation and involvement of soft tissues. This requires specific treatment before any instability is dealt with.

■ Position of the components

Malposition of the cup is particularly likely to produce impingement. In fact, the axis of the range of movement of the femoral head is the axis of the cup, and dislocation is more likely if the axis of the cup does not match the axis of hip movement *(fig 8)*. If the cup is too vertical and in too much anteversion, dislocation will occur in an anterior direction, while a cup which is too-horizontal or retroverted will allow posterior dislocation [18]. Too-vertical cups may lead to lateral dislocation when the leg is adducted. However, it is difficult to give precise figures, particularly for anteversion, as this can vary according to which surgical approach is used. Increased anteversion is recommended by those who use a posterior approach because soft tissue restraint to internal rotation is less. Within limits, malposition of the femoral component seems to cause less trouble, and its correct

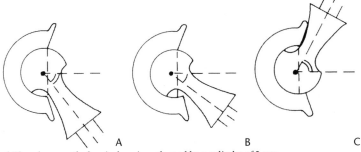

7 *A. Standard Charnley cup: the hemisphere is prolonged by a cylinder of 2 mm.*
B. Long posterior wall (LPW) Charnley cup: the posterior wall limits external rotation.
C. LPW Charnley cup: contact anteriorly of the components is the same as with a standard cup, but the posterior wall prevents posterior dislocation from occurring when the neck is in contact with the anterior rim of the cup.

orientation is easier to ensure during insertion. Lastly, malpositions of the cup and the stem are additive.

Shortening, resulting from malposition of either the femoral (excessive resection of the neck) or acetabular (too-high socket) component, will relax the soft tissues and lead to separation of both components. Shortening can be compensated for by lengthening the limb. Conversely, it is impossible to lengthen the limb in order to tighten the soft tissues, if the limb is either the same length or even longer than that of the opposite side. In this situation, it may be reasonable to shorten the longer limb if the discrepancy is unacceptable.

Dorr [14] describes three types of dislocations of increasing severity, and classifies them according to their cause:

– Type I: positional and without any obvious aetiology.

– Type II: resulting from an imbalance of the soft tissues, of which there are three causes (A: displacement of the greater trochanter, B: the cup is too high, C: excessive femoral resection). All the other abnormalities of the soft tissues are included in this type: ossifications, contractures, and spasticity.

– Type III: component malposition (A: acetabulum, B: femur).

In fact, there are usually several factors which may be responsible for a dislocation, and this classification does not cover all of the possibilities.

Preoperative assessment [28]

CLINICAL ASSESSMENT

Clinical assessment should include the age, associated medical problems (especially alcoholism, psychiatric and neuromuscular problems), the aetiology, the range of joint movement, and the length of the leg. It is also important to take into account the functional result of the arthroplasty, apart from the problem of dislocation. This means that it is more sensible to revise a prosthesis which is generally unsatisfactory, rather than one which is working well and only occasionally dislocates.

The type of prosthesis (manufacturer, design and size of each component) must be identified, and this can be difficult to do if the reports of the previous procedures on the hip are not available. It can occasionally be necessary to obtain special instruments to remove the prosthesis, or to obtain modular heads or acetabular liners to modify one component without interfering with its fixation. Decision may be difficult when a component is firmly fixed, but of an unsatisfactory design (too large a neck, too much neck-head valgus, etc.).

The surgical approach used for the index procedure will allow to inspect soft tissue lesions.

POSITION OF THE COMPONENTS

Examination should start with an assessment of any malposition, and this is done by appropriate imaging. However, it must be appreciated that there is no general agreement on what is the correct orientation, and therefore there is no precise definition of malposition. This is particularly true for anteversion of the cup, which should be 20-25° when using a posterior approach, and 5-10° with either an anterolateral or transtrochanteric exposure. This can be done by radiography and CT scan.

■ *Radiographic techniques*

Cup [1, 6, 39, 49]

During the operation, the surgeon should note carefully the position of the patient, paying particular attention to his longitudinal and transverse axes. Then, using a cup positioner and noting two anatomical landmarks (superior border of the obturator foramen and anterior rim of the bony acetabulum), the cup should be placed in the correct position of inclination and anteversion. However, unfortunately at this stage there is always the risk of a human misjudgement.

The "anatomical inclination" is the angle between the plane of the face of the cup and the horizontal plane. This angle is in the vertical plane which passes through the centre of the cup and perpendicular to the plane of its face. The angle of inclination measured on an anteroposterior radiograph is a projection of this angle in the coronal plane ("radiographic inclination").

The "anatomical anteversion" is the angle between the plane of the face of the cup and the sagittal plane. It is situated in the horizontal plane which passes through the centre of the cup and can therefore be measured directly by CT scan. The angle of anteversion measured on an anteroposterior radiograph or on a lateral view of the pelvis taken with the patient erect is the "radiographic anteversion". A reasonable idea of the degree of anteversion can also be gauged from a lateral radiograph of the hip, although this is not as accurate as the special measurements described above.

The relations between operative, radiographic and anatomical inclination and anteversion have been examined by Yao [49] and Murray [39], and the latter has produced tables which allow to convert anatomical orientation to radiographic or surgical orientation and vice versa. Nevertheless, it is not easy to make accurate measurements, and this does necessitate high quality radiographs (position of the pelvis, centring, tube/film distance), which can be difficult to obtain.

Femur

Methods for measuring femoral anterversion can also be used to study the position of the artificial hip and where they are subject to

the same errors. This applies to both the method of Dunlap and of Magilligan.

■ *Computed tomography*

The presence of pieces of metal complicated the first studies made by computed tomography, but it is possible to eliminate this problem by making very thin slices, and then to use these to reconstruct and to measure the anteversion both of the cup and of the femoral component.

Cup

CT scan can measure the anatomical anteversion. It can also reveal, in the region of the cup, ossifications of the soft tissues, osteophytes or extruded cement, which may produce a lever effect and hence instability.

Femur

CT scan is the most simple and most reliable technique for measuring anteversion of the femoral component. In practice, it is possible to superimpose the images of the femoral neck and the distal femoral epiphysis on the same cut, and thus measure directly the femoral anteversion using the axis of the femoral neck and a tangential line drawn between the posterior surface of the two condyles.

OTHER FACTORS WHICH MAY INFLUENCE THERAPY

– Wear of the cup, which above all is associated with late dislocations, incites to cup (or liner) exchange, provided that the patient has a reasonable expectation of life.

– A confirmed or potential loosening of one or more components will require appropriate revision.

– Significant bone weakness will complicate revision, as it allows the production of cortex perforations and will make fixation difficult.

– Associated infection will necessitate specific treatment (conservative, or more often prosthetic exchange either in one or two stages). This is sometimes only identified in the soft tissues during a revision operation, and will necessitate microbiological examination of joint fluid and histological examination of soft tissue.

Conservative treatment

A first dislocation should be treated conservatively unless there is an obvious cause which requires surgery. For obvious reasons, reduction should be performed as soon as possible. Other managements are still being discussed, but their aim is to encourage healing of the soft tissues around the prosthesis, improve muscle control and to protect the patient from further dislocation while these objectives are being reached. Their short-term success depends on the development of adequate "stiffness" of the hip, but further dislocation may occur if too much mobility reappears.

REDUCTION

The great majority of dislocations are reducible, sometimes even without anaesthesia. It is important to understand the direction in which the dislocation has occurred, and then to manipulate the joint in the reverse direction. It helps to have an assistant who is stabilising the pelvis, and manipulation should be gentle. After reduction, the stability or instability of the hip should be carefully assessed by testing for instability, but stopping just short of actual dislocation. The amplitude of these movements should be noted, and this will help to appreciate the degree of instability. Image intensification can be useful in difficult cases, and it may also be wise to perform the gentle manipulations with the patient on an orthopaedic table.

The dislocation has been found to be irreducible by manipulation in 4.5% of the cases of André [3], 6% of Woo [49], 13% of Courtois [11] and of Khan [31], and 18% of Dorr [14]. This irreducibility occurs particularly in dislocations which have either not been recognised or have presented late [17], or in the rare dislocations in which the capsule and muscles have been perforated in button-hole fashion by the femoral head [48]. In this situation, a fracture can be produced if too great a force is used. However, in 11 open reductions, Courtois [11] only once found a mechanical cause for the irreducibility, and this was an interposition of the gluteus minimus which perhaps may have resulted from attempts at closed reduction.

Certain specific complications have been reported:

– Interposition of soft tissues [3, 17], of fragments of cement [3], of cerclage wire or of broken screws. Whether obvious or only suspected from a widening of the joint space under anaesthesia, these problems will call for either open operation or arthroscopy [41], or a percutaneous manoeuvre (using pins or joint lavage) under radiographic control [3].

– The interposition of the psoas tendon behind the neck of the prosthesis can produce an anterior dislocation in extension [26].

– Complications related to the prosthesis have already been mentioned, and include separation of the components of a modular prosthesis. This will raise the suspicion of a design fault or of incorrect insertion technique.

The need to operate with little delay when a dislocation cannot be reduced, in the presence of interposition, when a modular prosthesis has come apart, or even in the presence of a haematoma will pose specific problems. The patient will not be prepared, and the risk of infection is increased if revision is performed as an emergency. Above all, the cause of the dislocation may not have become clear, and conditions may not be ideal for the use of appropriate imaging techniques. In this situation, it is necessary to depend on standard radiographs and the findings at operation, being prepared for every eventuality. Operating under these conditions may lead to poor results or the appearance of complications.

TRACTION-SUSPENSION

The goal of using traction is to immobilise the lower limb in a position which will allow sound healing of the soft tissues around the prosthesis and also to avoid, in the short term, the movement which dislocated the joint. Ideally, this should be for six weeks in order to allow really good healing, but from the literature it appears that it is difficult to maintain this immobilisation for longer than three weeks [3, 31]. Its major disadvantage is that three weeks in bed will predispose to all the usual problems, including pressure sores and muscle atrophy. In addition, there may be infection around the tibial pin, or from skin traction. However, there is no real evidence of the value of this treatment, which seems now to be being less and less used.

ORTHOSES

■ *Spica, braces*

An above-knee spica made from resin will control flexion and adduction while allowing walking, and this will help to maintain good muscle activity, but personal hygiene and skin protection require special attention. It can be replaced by a hip brace, which provides a less rigid immobilisation, but is likely to be better-tolerated. It provides 10 or 15° of abduction and has a flexion stop. It is removable, and this will facilitate personal hygiene, but will require close co-operation by the patient. The length of time this orthosis should be used seems to vary between three weeks [47], six weeks to three months [14], or even between six to nine months [7]. Six weeks seem to be a reasonable compromise. Although they are well-tolerated by young and active patients, they can be a heavy burden for those of more mature years. Most authors report good results with this technique: one recurrence out of 16 (Williams [45]), one out of 9 (Clayton [7]), two out of 12 (Dorr [14]). However, the period of follow-up in these series is often short or unknown. In Williams' series, 10 out of the 16 dislocations had been treated by open reduction before the immobilisation, and this influences his figures. In Woo's series of 331 dislocations, stabilisation was produced in two-thirds of the patients, but the hip had only been immobilised for three weeks [47].

It is also possible to use a long hip spica, but really only as a last resort.

■ *Knee splintage*

In posterior dislocations, immobilisation of the knee in extension will limit the range of hip flexion [14, 18], but the patient will be able to walk and to sit down. It is less efficient than a short double hip spica, as it does not immobilise the hip joint, but it is better tolerated by patients. Of course, knee splintage in extension may lead to stiffness of this joint, so the splint should be removable to allow regular exercise. Janecki [29] has shown the value of this treatment for dislocations of femoral prostheses inserted for fracture.

■ *Other splints*

A triangular splint (or a pillow) placed between the thighs will prevent adduction. An appropriate posterior splint immobilising the leg and the foot will maintain the hip in the desired rotation. However, these splints cannot be applied or removed by the patients themselves, as this would entail flexing the hip and this is contraindicated when there is posterior instability. They can only be used in patients who remain flat, and thus they may be applied either during rest periods or in patients confined to bed, for three weeks according to Wroblewki [48]. It seems reasonable to combine their use with a removable short double hip spica splint which is worn when the patient is out of bed and moving about.

■ *Physiotherapy*

This should be started as early as possible, but must also relate to any necessary immobiliation. It should include rehabilitation of the peri-articular muscles, largely using isometric techniques, help with walking when this is allowed, and maintenance of knee mobility, but must always avoid any movements which could produce a further dislocation or other instability.

It is always important to encourage the patient by not over-emphasising the problem of dislocation, and also to point out what movements and positions should be avoided.

This post-reduction management can be all that is required, or may be combined with a period of immobilisation. In fact, there is no general agreement on the role of conservative treatment, or of its efficiency. For right or for wrong, these treatments are less and less restricting.

■ *Results*

There is a very wide range of the reported rate of a further dislocation after treatment of the first dislocation: 17% [19], 22% [31], 26% [11], 35% [47], 42% [17], or even 61% [3]. Recurrent dislocation is more likely to occur after late dislocations [11, 31, 47], after closed reductions [11], or when there are factors which produce instability, such as after a revision arthroplasty, a trochanteric nonunion, or malposition. The divergence in the published series can be explained by their small size, the variety of cases, the different percentages of open reductions, and the variable mean follow-up.

Surgical treatment

It is important to realise that surgical management is the only possible treatment for some causes of dislocation (malposition, displacement of the greater trochanter). In other cases, surgery should be considered after a second or even third dislocation, particularly when these follow soon after the first dislocation.

Preoperative assessment does not always allow an exact diagnosis of the cause of the dislocation, so that one of the aims of operation is to try to elucidate any reasons for the instability.

The approach used often depends on the surgeon's preference, but there may not have been thorough healing of a previous approach, and thus this can easily be re-opened. Any trochanteric osteotomy should be performed early and not as a last resort to allow adequate exposure. If this is done at a later stage, it may aggravate soft tissue lesions. These should be recognised and dissection of the capsule and muscles designed to allow their adequate repair at the end of the operation.

Wound swabs should be taken for microbacterial examination, and the prosthesis is dislocated.

Any component loosening is noted. It is important to look for any zone of deformation of the cup resulting from repeated contact, and for any roughening of the articular surfaces. Under direct vision, the mechanism of the dislocation is sought and analysed. Sometimes, one or several causes may be found, but occasionally there will be little more than a suspicion.

PROSTHETIC REPLACEMENT

Malposition will necessitate revision of one or both components.

■ *Exchange of the cup*

Removal of the cup can be difficult and it is important not to damage bone. The new cup should be inserted in a correct position *(fig 9)*, and this means that the previous poor positioning must have been carefully analysed. It should be fixed in mechanically-acceptable conditions, and if necessary, the acetabulum will have to be reconstructed by a bone graft and reinforced by a metal implant. This reconstruction is also necessary when it is required to lower or lateralise the cup, as this re-positions the centre of the joint and increases the tension of the soft tissues. Reorientation of the cup is the most important part of the operation, and often is all that is required. However, the desire to avoid further dislocation raises other possibilities:

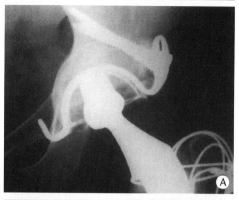
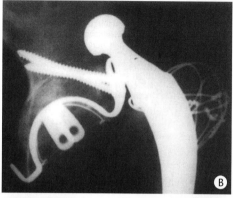
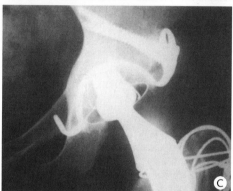

9 *A. Revision for loosening. Horizontal and a slightly anteverted cup.*
B. Posterior dislocation
C. No recurrence after exchange of the cup (more anteverted).

– the use of a cup which will accept a larger diameter femoral head than originally inserted (e.g. 28 mm instead of 22 mm), as long as this is possible with the design of the complete prosthesis, and the external diameter of the cup will accept an adequate thickness of polyethylene;

– the use of a long posterior wall cup (or elevated-rim liner), or the fixation of an augment screwed into place in order to prevent further dislocation.

■ *Exchange of the femoral component*

Malposition of the femoral component is less common, and the replacement of this component can be technically difficult. The extraction of a really well-fixed femoral stem, with or without cement, runs the risk of damaging bone. If there is a loss of bone substance, it may be necessary to use the

techniques designed for use with aseptic loosening in order to implant the new component under the best possible mechanical conditions. All these problems have encouraged some surgeons to propose a rotation femoral osteotomy when there is isolated retroversion [9]. The design of the new prosthesis should have corrected any design faults in the original model. In this respect, some surgeons like to use prostheses which increase the femoral offset without the need of lengthening the limb. The advantages of increasing femoral offset are reported to include an increased range of motion, better mechanical advantage for the abductors and decreased instability because of better soft tissue tension. However, these prostheses have the disadvantage of increasing varus forces which tend to tilt or loosen the components.

■ *Necessary action with the other component*

When one component has to be exchanged as a result of malposition, there are certain indications for changing the other component. These include real or potential loosening, wear or other alteration, or an imperfect design. In case of doubt, it is important to remember the difficulties which can be experienced in removal and in reimplantation.

As far as the cup is concerned, significant wear or the presence of adherent particles of cement or metal cannot be accepted. It is easier to change the liner of an uncemented cup than that of a cemented cup, but unfortunately, the adequate liner is not always still available. It is more debatable whether or not to change a cup when the cavity does not have the cylindrical shape suggested by Charnley, a modification which has established its place in preventing dislocation.

The femoral head often will be roughened and there may be linear marks. A modular prosthesis then has the advantage that the head can be changed without disturbing the stem. It will also allow to modify the length of the neck if the original head will accept this. The use of a more shallow head (and without any skirt) will lengthen the neck and tighten the soft tissues, and this can be beneficial, although it will also lengthen the limb by a few millimetres. More than 1 or 1.5 centimetre lengthening may not be well-accepted by the patient, particularly if he or she is not very tall. The ideal is to restore equal length to the legs, and if there is a preoperative increase in length, then a femoral head should be used which will have the effect of shortening the neck. However, this will relax the soft tissues, which may reduce stability. In this case, it is better either to accept (and encourage the patient to accept) this increase in length, or to advance the greater trochanter. This latter procedure should have been considered before surgery and the hip then approached using a transtrochanteric approach. A too-short or too-long neck which cannot be corrected by the use of a modular head may necessitate exchanging the stem. A large diameter neck will increase contacts between the components, and a prosthesis with a large neck-shaft angle which decreases the femoral offset is also likely to decrease stability. A modular head with a skirt should be replaced with a head without a skirt, as this modification increases the diameter of the neck and thus also increases contacts.

The idea is to eradicate all the factors which may give instability, and to restore a more normal architecture by using a more appropriately-designed prosthesis. This may necessitate exchanging both components. This will also hopefully produce a long-lasting good result. Published series suggest that the replacement of one or more components is the most successful treatment, whatever the aetiology: 69% of success for Daly [13], 76% for Fraser [19], 77% for André [3]. Nevertheless, an advanced age, poor local tissues, and the increased risk of complications of exchanges can lead to a compromise in management.

OPERATIONS INVOLVING THE GREATER TROCHANTER

■ *Treatment of a trochanteric nonunion*

Nonunion of the greater trochanter with displacement can be very difficult to correct surgically [10]. It is necessary to excise the fibrous tissue on the deep surface of the gluteal muscles in order to anatomically reduce the trochanter, and to expose two good bone surfaces. This reduction is often associated with an advancement in order to improve the tension of the buttock muscles. Various means of fixation have been suggested: wire cerclage, hooks and more recently cables, but they release metallic fragments which can migrate into the joint and increase polyethylene wear. A bone graft, preferably autologous, is useful. However, there is a significant failure rate, 3 out of 6 for André [3], and 7 out of 28 for Daly [13]. Courpied [10] had a 100% success rate with 19 nonunions treated with his bone hook, and occasionally a bone graft.

■ *Advancement of the greater trochanter*

Advancement of the trochanter increases tension in the gluteus medius and mimimus and increases their lever arm, as advancement also produces lateralisation as a result of the effect of the direction of the osteotomy. Kaplan [30] stabilised 16 out of 21 prostheses, and Ekelund [16] 17 out of 21, using this technique. Less favourable results have been reported by Daly [13] (10 failures out of 25 cases), and André [3] (2 failures out of 2 cases).

Besides the risk of failure, this procedure may also result in nonunion of the

trochanter, and this is in part due to the difficulty of obtaining adequate fixation, and to the poor bone surface contact. In turn, this may become another factor causing instability. Kaplan [30] reports six cases of nonunion, including two dislocations, and Ekelund [16] two cases including two dislocations.

Kaplan reports advancement of between 16 + and - 7 mm [30], and Ekelund 18 + and - 6 mm [16]. Too much advancement can cause problems, as it may be followed by secondary displacement and secondary laxity of the soft tissues resulting from distension of the muscle fibres [18, 48]. In addition, excess tension in the buttock muscles will tilt the pelvis, and the resulting hip abduction will produce apparent lengthening [15]. However, the apparent lengthening will often disappear spontaneously.

This risk, and the unreliability of trochanteric advancement, means that this technique should not be used in isolation. It is indicated when the instability results from laxity of the musculature resulting from medialisation of the femur without shortening. When there is a shortening, the responsible component (femoral or acetabular) must be repositioned so as to restore length, and thus muscle tension. It will also move the femur away from the pelvis. When there is also malposition of a prosthetic component, advancement of the greater trochanter seems to be inadequate [16, 30], although Kaplan reports no recurrence in three cases.

Trochanteric advancement is often combined with other procedures, notably revision of one or the other component [13, 37], and this is most often observed when a transtrochanteric approach has been used. However, in this situation it can be difficult the assess the value of the advancement.

ERADICATION OF SOURCES OF IMPINGEMENT

Any cause of impingement must be identified in all revisions for instability.

It is necessary to remove any protruding bone or cement around the cup as well as anterior (rarely posterior) hypertrophied or ossified soft tissues, as these can produce a dislocation [3, 11]. This procedure has in isolation had a variable effect, with success in 3 cases for André [3], but in only 5 out of 9 for Daly [13]. It is usually combined with other operations.

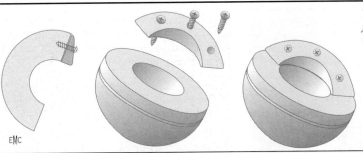

10 *Acetabular augment fixed with three screws onto the cup.*

Impingement arising between the greater trochanter and the iliopubic or ischial ramus in flexion with internal rotation result from cups which are too high, or from femurs which are too medial. These malpositions call for correction.

CUP AUGMENTATION

Olerud and Karlstrom [42] fashion a polyethylene segment from a cup of the same size, and then screw it onto the cup to be used. Using this technique has enabled them to stabilise 5 out of 6 prostheses, but in three patients the trochanter was also advanced, and in one the use of an anterior segment resulted in posterior dislocation. However, other surgeons have not been so successful with this technique. Bradbury [5] reports 3 failures in 16, Ekelund [16] 5 in 5, Graham [23] 3 in 3, Gie [21] 3 in 10, Gungor [27] 1 in 13, Meyryeis [35] 5 in 11, Mogensen [36] 0 in 2, Nicholas [40] 0 in 3, Watson [44] 1 in 2, and Williamson [46] 3 in 3. Combining all these series give a failure rate of 39% (25 in 74 patients), but as there was only a short follow-up, there remains a possibility of further failures.

These results are unsatisfactory. The majority of these poor results are due to a mechanical failure at the junction between the device and the cup (screw loosening or fracture), and this must reflect on the magnitude of the mechanical forces which can overcome the resistance of the device. Dislocation is in the opposite direction to that which occurred originally, as a result of contact between the neck and the device. Thus, it is important when treating a posterior instability not to place the device too low in order to avoid contact with the neck in extension and external rotation.

There are several types of augmentation (*fig 10*). They are about 5 mm thick and represent about a third to a half of the circumference. Some are designed to retain the head in the cup and some are not. Watson [44] suggests using 5 instead of 3 screws in order to ensure perfect contact between the augment and the cup, as well as the incorporation of a metal plate designed to prevent deformation of the augment. Caton et Vidil (unpublished) report stabilisation of 15 prostheses with a Watson's augment. Nicholas [40] has shown that it is the most efficient method of fixation, but also that it decreases the arc of movement and that it makes dislocation

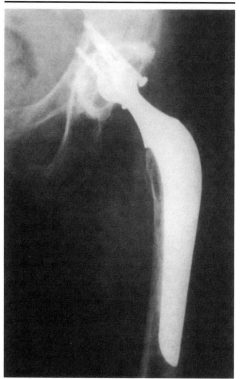

11 *Posterior dislocation without obvious malposition in an elderly patient. Stabilisation with acetabular augment and soft tissue repair.*

impossible, which can result in loosening of the cup due to excessive stresses.

The relative efficiency of acetabular augmentation, the risks of dislocation occurring on the opposite side, and loosening of the cup suggest that this technique should be reserved for older or relatively inactive patients *(fig 11)* who do not have an obvious malposition of their prosthesis [21, 44]. Meyrueis [35], using a retaining augment, has reduced his rate of dislocation from 5.1% to 2.5% in two successive series of primary prosthetic replacement, using a head of 28 mm and a posterior approach. The main purpose of the augment would be to stabilise the joint during the first three months after operation when early dislocation can occur, until there has been good healing of the local soft tissues and a good return of muscle tone. Using the same reasoning for revision operations, the main value of an augment would be to prevent a further dislocation after replacement of a malpositioned cup.

In any case, the use of augments should be limited because:

– they limit the arc of movement [40], and when screwed to the posterior rim of the cup, may predispose to anterior dislocation;

– mechanical stresses can loosen or break the screws [35] or detach the augment, and there is always the risk of a screw or fragment of a screw becoming jammed in the joint when a further dislocation is being reduced.

– the screws may scarify the head if there is a further dislocation, or during its reduction.

– insertion of the screws weakens the polyethylene, and there is a risk of contact between the head and the screw when the polyethylene becomes worn. This risk is greater with thinner cups used in short stature patients, or when the head is very large, or with uncemented cups.

– the risk of loosening may also be increased with the use of augments which retain the head [40].

SPECIAL CUPS

■ Long posterior wall cups, elevated-rim liners

Charnley in 1972 designed an asymmetrical "LPW" (Long Posterior Wall) cup in which the cavity is extended in its posterior half by a hemi-cylinder which reaches to the edge of the cup [38]. These cups, which are inserted in a lower position, produced in Charnley's hands a lowering of 0.6% in the rate of dislocation. This wall has the same theoretical effect as cup augmentation, but without the problems and failure which can be associated with screw fixation *(fig 7, 9)*. Murray [38] has criticised this cup because component contact occurs at 53° of forward movement and at 38° of posterior movement, while with a standard model cup, contact only occurs with 106° of movement. This allows greater contact between the neck and the cup in extension and external rotation. This has also been described by Krushell [32]. In addition, the moment of forces which tends to loosen a LPW cup and which results from contact with the femoral component is greater than with a standard cup. Finally, it does not produce more posterior stability than a standard cup inserted with 6° more anteversion.

The majority of uncemented cups can be used with an elevated-rim liner, whose orientation can be decided by the surgeon. The wall extends beyond the periphery of the metal cup and is therefore relatively unsupported. This may produce the same problems of contact between the neck and the posterior wall as in the Charnley's LPW cup, and produce the same stresses on the fixation when either subluxation or dislocation occurs, or during attempts at reduction. Cobb [8] has shown the value of a cup with a 10° posterior edge in preventing dislocations after primary replacements, and even more so with revisions, and whatever the surgical approach. However, he noted an increased percentage of anterior dislocations, which he attributed to contact occurring during extension and external rotation between the femoral component and the cup. In addition, he has stressed that wear and deformation of the wall occurs, as it is not supported by cement or metal, and that this may result in the production of wear particles. He recommends that these cups should only be used when there is a particularly high risk of dislocation, or with revision operations.

■ Constrained cups

The cavity of a constrained cup is more than a hemisphere and therefore their design includes a locking ring whose diameter is less than that of the femoral head ("captive head system"). The degree of retention therefore depends on the difference in the two diameters.

If the cup is made of one piece of material, this difference can only be of a certain degree, as otherwise it would be impossible to introduce the head into the cup. A satisfactory "clunk" should occur when the head is reduced ("snap-fit" cup). In the latest models of modular constrained cups [2, 34], the locking ring is fixed with screws to the uncemented cup, after the head has been reduced. It is also possible to transform a well-fixed standard cup to a constrained cup by using two polyethylene augments [42], but there is also the need to place several screws into the cup itself.

The degree of retention of a "snap-fit" cup is less at 37 °C than at room temperature, and it is probable that this reduces slowly as the polyethylene of the ring of retention wears and deforms. The efficiency of these cups seems to be limited by time, and this is revealed by a 1.3% rate of dislocation in the series of Lagrange [20]. Modular cementless constrained cups implants are more efficient but more constrained.

Both designs limit the arc of motion, as well as making the joint constrained. The use of these cups may therefore suggest the appearance of a higher rate of loosening. Moreover, a dislocation of a constrained cup usually needs an open reduction.

There are few reports of the use of constrained cups for recurrent dislocations. Anderson [2] had 6 failures out of 18 patients and Lombardi [34] 3 failures out of 31 patients when using the S-ROM modular design. It is difficult to be sure whether success results from the "captive head" system, or the reorientation of the cup, or both. In fact, the two effects are probably related, except when the metallic shell has been retained. The modes of failure of these implants are disengagement of the head from the liner (with pull-out of the locking ring), or disengagement of the liner from the metallic cup. One can also fear a separation of the head from the neck when using these cups with a modular femoral component.

These results suggest that these cups should only be used in elderly and inactive patients.

■ Angle-bore cup [48]

This cup simulates the anatomy of the normal acetabulum and thus the range of movements and stability of the normal hip. In the manufacture of the socket, the centre of the solid hemisphere is approached by the drill at a predetermined angle (less than 90°) to the face. This part having been completed, the socket is rotated backwards through 30° and the chamfer is cut anteriorly. This design gives more superior and posterior cover, but less anterior cover to the femoral head. It also leaves its lower pole uncovered and this allows more flexion, adduction and internal rotation.

The use of these cups has lowered the rate of dislocation after revision from 15% to 2% in Wroblewski's hands [48]. The posterior and superior part of the angle-bore cup is available as a separate piece. It can be fixed with two screws onto the socket face where the dislocation occurs and allows modification of a standard cup to an angle-bore cup.

■ ***Tripolar prostheses***

Bipolar prostheses provide stability, but they have been abandoned because they may be painful and migrate. Tripolar prostheses allow movement at two sites, as they have an unattached metal-backed polyethylene cup lying between the femoral head and the cup secured to the pelvis. The stability is obvious, the impingement is taken advantage of when the larger head diameter comes into function, and the range of motion is increased.

The "Lotus" hip [48] has a head of 22 mm seated in the free-moving central cup of 36 mm diameter which articulates with a cemented captive polyethylene cup. The range of movement possible is 125°. It is designed to be used when there is major instability due to the absence of the abductor muscles or a major replacement of the proximal end of the femur.

The Amstutz Prosthesis [25] is identical in its principles to the Lotus, and has a head of 26 or 28 mm seated in a central cup of 43 to 47 mm, which in turn fits into an uncemented non-captive cup. Goetz [22] reports a series of 56 prostheses of this type, cemented or not, with only 4% of new dislocations at 3 years, but 13% of loosening of the cup at 2 years.

Mobility at several interfaces raises the fear of a major production of polyethylene wear particles. Another problem arises from the very large exterior measurement of the cup, and this can limit the use of this prosthesis.

The Bousquet Prosthesis [33] has the same number of interfaces as the other two designs, but the exterior cup is metallic and fixed without cement. It articulates with a polyethylene cup which accepts heads of 22 or 28 mm. It can be used as a primary implant and has an almost total lack of dislocations (1 out of 1100 in Aubriot's series [33]), which supports its use for recurrent instability. The thin metallic uncemented cup allows the use of a standard size acetabular cup and is for this reason superior to the other tripolar prostheses already described. On the other hand, it is designed for implantation without cement, and this does limit the situations where it can be used. The standard model is fixed with one superior polar screw and two inferior metallic pegs. The models used for

revision have two or five small plates on their outer surface, which allow the use of several screws, and it can also be fixed with an inferior hook. A cemented model is currently being studied. Aubriot has reported good results in 13 recurrent dislocations [33], and this prosthesis seems to be particularly useful when there are soft tissue problems or an untreatable trochanteric nonunion. It is also useful in elderly patients with poor musculature, or in patients with neurological disorders.

SOFT TISSUE PROCEDURES

Some surgical approaches can cause significant damage to the soft tissues: poor healing of the capsule and short external rotator muscles in a posterior approach; poor healing (or palsy) of gluteus medius after an anterior lateral approach. However, it is often possible to mobilise these muscles and then reattach them. Some surgeons suggest posterior repair with a prosthetic reinforcement. It is also possible to obliterate the dead space which is created behind the cup by posterior dislocations. It is enough to freshen the surfaces of this dead space and to reinsert the soft tissues around the acetabulum by using screws with washers or anchors, using a technique similar to that described for the Bankart lesion in the shoulder. A distended pseudocapsule can be plicated [19, 37, 48]. It is also wise to suture the fascia lata with the leg in abduction, as this will have a tightening effect [19]. It is even better to fix it to the greater trochanter, as this will change the tensor into an abductor and will also limit rotation. These procedures are themselves not completely adequate, except possibly in an early dislocation without malposition, and where the soft tissues have not contracted and can be securely reattached. With late dislocations, they will be contracted and weak, and the muscles will have lost their ability to contract, and therefore they will not be able to help prevent further dislocation. In the worst situations, adequate restoration of the soft tissues cannot be attained, and the prognosis will be poor even if the prosthesis itself is in a good position. These soft tissue problems may reduce the possible surgical alternatives, and thus necessitate the use of a prosthesis with in-built stability.

POSTOPERATIVE PROTECTION

The high rate of failure calls for the provision of adequate protection to prevent early dislocation after revision. The soft tissues must be given adequate time to heal soundly. This takes between 6 to 12 weeks to occur, and therefore appropriate immobilisation is required during this period. The two principal movements which produce dislocation (flexion-adduction-internal rotation, and extension-external rotation) should be prevented, as well as movements which are likely to produce

dislocation as a result of the surgical approach used. This immobilisation does not prevent a good result with the return of useful hip movement. Walking, with if possible weight-bearing, should be encouraged as this improves muscle activity, and physiotherapy should also aid in muscle re-education (resisted exercises and work with pulleys). However, all this can be painful and runs the risk of redetaching muscles.

Certain precautions are necessary and these relate to the condition of the local tissues: traction-suspension, orthoses, etc. However, there are no relevant statistics available about the efficiency of these measures.

■ ***Removal of prostheses***

This is the ultimate salvage procedure after several revisions or with significant infection. Dorr reports 4 out of 17 cases [14], and Khan 12 out of 59 [31].

Results and indications

There is a very significant failure rate after revision surgery: 24% [19], 39% [13], 45% [3]. It is higher after surgery for recurrent dislocations than after a solitary dislocation or subluxation [13, 31], and perhaps this should encourage early revision. The chance of success depends on the identification and then the treatment of the exact cause of the instability [3, 13].

The most successful operation involves repositioning of one or both components; this must suggest that malposition is the principal cause of dislocation, and should always be very carefully considered and sought. However, there are other important considerations which have a role in ensuring a good result after exchange operations. These include increase of the range of motion (larger head on the same neck, removal of a skirted head, stem exchange for a smaller neck, etc.), increase of the femoral offset, or the use of a prosthesis with its own significant in-built stability (a cup with a cylindrical extension of its cavity, cup augmentation, etc.).

Firm fixation of a greater trochanter which is lying superiorly is necessary, and this procedure can produce stability if lack of fixation of the trochanter is the sole cause for the dislocation.

Eradication of cam effects and repair of soft tissues are essential parts of all revisions.

Other procedures only have a real chance of success when there is no significant malposition:

– advancement of the greater trochanter is indicated when there is an isolated medialisation, when the limb has to be shortened, and every time that a transtrochanteric approach is used for revision.

– the acetabular augmentation, which is a simple procedure, hardly seems indicated except in elderly and relatively inactive patients, provided there is good fixation. However, the insertion of screws into the polyethylene can be criticised. The use of posterior wall cups, which include an augment in their design, are perhaps preferable, but they necessitate changing the cup (or the liner). These two models have a risk of allowing dislocation in the opposite direction, of deformation and wear, and perhaps of loosening due to an increase of stresses onto the cup and to the liberation of wear particles. In addition, they only have a very moderate stabilising effect and are ineffective in case of malposition. Their principal function [8, 35] is to prevent further dislocation after correction of a malpositioned cup.

The multiplicity of causes of dislocation, as well as the difficulty in establishing the real reasons, lead to the association of stabilising techniques, but this makes it difficult to assess their individual value.

Other operations have to be considered in patients with specific problems, and should be kept in mind when considering failure of previous surgery, irreparable soft tissue damage, untreatable trochanteric nonunion or lack of patient co-operation (great age, alcohol abuse, neuropathies or psychiatric disorders). The value of constrained cups has not yet been established and some of their success can perhaps be attributed to better positioning of this component. We have no experience of the angle-bore cup. The Bousquet prosthesis seems to us to be better designed, but problems of cup fixation have yet to be solved.

Postoperative advice regarding prudence in resuming activities, and perhaps immobilisation, are important additional precautions.

Conclusion

Instability is relatively rare, but can produce considerable problems. There are numerous causes which make it difficult to elucidate exactly why there is instability, and also to decide on the best treatment. The main problems seem to relate to prosthetic malposition, and poor reconstruction of the normal anatomy of the hip, inadequate preoperative musculature and the presence of soft tissue lesions. Prevention is the best management and depends on appreciation of all the possible causes of instability. During revision for instability, it is important to use a prosthesis of appropriate design and to repair damaged soft tissues. In the most difficult situations, the tripolar prostheses seem to be promising a better future than constrained models, as these continue to be haunted by loosening and separation of the components.

References

[1] Ackland MK, Bourne WB, Uthoff HK. Anteversion of the acetabular cup. *J Bone Joint Surg Br* 1986 ; 68 : 409-413

[2] Anderson MJ, Murray WR, Skinner HB. Constrained acetabular components. *J Arthroplasty* 1994 ; 9 : 17-23

[3] André S, Feuilhade De Chauvin P, Tiberi T, Postel M. Luxations de prothèses totales de type Charnley modifiées Kerboull. *Rev Chir Orthop* 1983 ; 69 : 447-453

[4] Barrak RC, Burke DW, Cook SD, Skinner HD, Harris WH. Complications related to modularity of total hip components. *J Bone Joint Surg Br* 1993 ; 75 : 688-692

[5] Bradbury N, Milligan GF. Acetabular augmentation for dislocation of a prosthetic hip: a 3 (1-6) year follow-up of 16 patients. *Acta Orthop Scand* 1994 ; 65 : 424-426

[6] Chevrot A, Najman G, Nicolas B, Bicharzon P. Prothèses totales de hanche de type Charnley. Technique radiologique de mesure angulaire de la pièce cotyloïdienne (antéversion, inclinaison). *Rev Chir Orthop* 1983 ; 69 : 485-487

[7] Clayton ML, Thirupati RG. Dislocation following total hip arthroplasty. Management by special brace in selected patients. *Clin Orthop* 1983 ; 177 : 154-159

[8] Cobb TK, Morrey BF, Ilstrup DM. The elevated-rim acetabular liner in total hip arthroplasty: relationship to postoperative dislocation. *J Bone Joint Surg Am* 1996 ; 78 : 80-86

[9] Cohn BT, Krackow A. Femoral component retroversion treated by supracondylar rotational osteotomy. *Orthopaedics* 1987 ; 10 : 1057-1059

[10] Courpied JP, Postel M. Pseudarthroses trochantériennes après prothèse totale de hanche. *Rev Chir Orthop* 1986 ; 72 : 583-586

[11] Courtois B, Variel R, Le Saout J, Kerboul B, Lefèvre C. À propos de 87 luxations de prothèse totale de hanche. *Int Orthop* 1985 ; 9 : 189-193

[12] Coventry MB. Late dislocations in patients with Charnley THA. *J Bone Joint Surg Am* 1985 ; 67 : 832-841

[13] Daly PJ, Morrey BF. Operative correction of an unstable total hip arthroplasty. *J Bone Joint Surg Am* 1992 ; 74 : 1334-1343

[14] Dorr LD, Wolf AW, Chandler R, Conaty JP. Classification and treatment of dislocation of total hip arthroplasty. *Clin Orthop* 1983 ; 173 : 151-158

[15] Eftekahr NS. Dislocation and instability. In : Total hip arthroplasty. St Louis : CV Mosby, 1993 : 1505-1553

[16] Ekelund A. Trochanteric osteotomy for recurrent dislocation of total hip arthroplasty. *J Arthroplasty* 1993 ; 8 : 629-632

[17] Fackler CD, Poss R. Dislocation in total hip atrhoplasties. *Clin Orthop* 1980 ; 151 : 169-178

[18] Fontes D, Benoit J, Lortat-Jacob A, Didry R. La luxation des prothèses totales de hanche, modélisation mathématique. *Rev Chir Orthop* 1991 ; 77 : 151-162

[19] Fraser GA, Wroblewski BM. Revision of the low-friction arthroplasty for recurrent or irreducible dislocation. *J Bone Joint SurgBr* 1981 ; 63 : 552-555

[20] Gerard Y, Llagone B, Ameil M. Le caractère rétentif d'un cotyle prothétique est-il utile ou non ? *Rev Chir Orthop* 1989 ; 75 (suppl 1) : 123-124

[21] Gie A, Scott T, Ling RS. Cup augmentation for recurrent hip replacement dislocation. *J Bone Joint Surg Br* 1989 ; 71 : 338-344

[22] Goetz DD, Capello WN, Callaghan JJ, Brown TD, Johnston RC. Salvage of a recurrent dislocating total hip prosthesis with use of constrained acetabular component. *J Bone Joint Surg Am* 1998 ; 80 : 502-509

[23] Graham GP, Jenkins AIR, Mintowt-Czyz W. Recurrent dislocation following hip replacement: brief report. *J Bone Joint Surg Br* 1988 ; 70 : 675-680

[24] Gregory RJ, Gibson MJ, Moran CG. Dislocation after primary arthroplasty for subcapital fracture of the hip. Wide range of movement is a risk factor. *J Bone Joint Surg Br* 1991 ; 73 : 11-12

[25] Grigoris P, Grecula MJ, Amstutz HC. Tripolar hip replacement for recurrent prosthetic dislocation. *Clin Orthop* 1994 ; 304 : 148-155

[26] Grigoris P, Grecula MJ, Amstutz HC. Dislocation of a total hip arthroplasty caused by ilio-psoas tendon displacement. *Clin Orthop* 1994 ; 306 : 132-135

[27] Güngor T, Hallin G. Cup reinforcement for recurrent dislocation after hip replacement. *J Bone Joint Surg Br* 1990 ; 72 : 525

[28] Huten D. Luxations et subluxations des prothèses totales de hanche. In : Conférences d'enseignement de la SOFCOT. Paris : Expansion scientifique française, 1996 : 19-46

[29] Janecki CJ, Leve AR, Lai LK. The knee immobilizer as an aid in the prevention of postoperative endoprosthetic dislocations. *Clin Orthop* 1982 ; 168 : 83-85

[30] Kaplan SJ, Thomas WH, Poss R. Trochanteric advancement for recurrent dislocation after total hip arthroplasty. *J Arthroplasty* 1987 ; 2 : 119-124

[31] Khan MA, Brakenbury PH, Reynolds IS. Dislocation following total hip arthroplasty. *J Bone Joint Surg Br* 1981 ; 63 : 214-218

[32] Krushell RJ, Burke DW, Harris WH. Elevated-rim acetabular components. Effect on range of motion and stability in total hip arthroplasty. *J Arthroplasty* 1991 ; 6 (suppl) : S53-S58

[33] Leclerc S, El Blidi S, Aubriot JH. Traitement de la luxation récidivante de prothèse totale de hanche par le cotyle de Bousquet. *Rev Chir Orthop* 1995 ; 81 : 389-394

[34] Lombardi A, Mallory T, Kraus T, Vaughn B. Preliminary report of the S-ROM constraining acetabular insert: a retrospective clinical experience. *Orthopaedics* 1991 ; 14 : 297

[35] Meyrueis JP, Cazenave A. Prévention et traitement des luxations de prothèses totales de hanche par butée prothétique vissée. *Rev Chir Orthop* 1993 ; 79 (suppl II) : 157-158

[36] Mogensen B, Brynjoflur A, Arnason H, Jonsson GT. Socket wall addition for dislocating of total hip arthroplasty. *Acta Orthop Scand* 1986 ; 57 : 373-374

[37] Morrey BF. Dislocation. In : Joint replacement arthroplasty. New York : Churchill Livingstone, 1991 : 851-865

[38] Murray DW. Impingement and loosening of the long posterior wall acetabular implant. *J Bone Joint Surg Br* 1992 ; 74 : 377-384

[39] Murray DW. The definition and measurement of acetabular orientation. *J Bone Joint Surg Br* 1993 ; 75 : 228-232

[40] Nicholas RM, Orr JF, Mollan RA, Calderwood JW, Nixon JR, Watson P. Dislocation ot total hip replacement. A comparison study of standard long posterior wall and augmented acetabular components. *J Bone Joint Surg Br* 1990 ; 72 : 418-422

[41] Nordt W, Grangorra CE, Levy M, Habermann ET. Arthroscopic removal of entrapped debris following dislocation of a total hip arthroplasty. *Arthroscopy* 1987 ; 3 : 196

[42] Olerud S, Karlstrom G. Recurrent dislocation after THR: treatment by fixing an additional sector to the acetabular. *J Bone Joint Surg Br* 1985 ; 67 : 402-405

[43] Ries MD, Wiedel JD. Bipolar hip arthroplasty for recurrent dislocation after total hip arthroplasty. A report of three cases. *Clin Orthop* 1992 ; 278 : 121-127

[44] Watson P, Nixon JR, Mollan RB. A prosthesis augmentation device for the prevention of recurrent hip dislocation: a preliminary report. *Clin Orthop* 1991 ; 267 : 79-84

[45] Williams JF, Gottesman MJ, Mallory TH. Dislocations after total hip arthroplasty. Treatment with an above- knee hip spica cast. *Clin Orthop* 1982 ; 171 : 53-58

[46] Williamson JB, Galasko CS, Rowley DI. Failure of acetabular augmentation after hip arthroplasty: report of three cases. *Acta Orthop Scand* 1989 ; 60 : 676

[47] Woo RY, Morrey BF. Dislocations after total hip arthroplasty. *J Bone Joint Surg Am* 1982 ; 64 : 1295-1306

[48] Wroblewski BM. Dislocation. In : Revision surgery in total hip arthroplasty. London : Springer Verlag, 1990 : 29-46

[49] Yao L, Yao J, Gold H. Measurement of acetabular version on the axiolateral radiograph. *Clin Orthop* 1995 ; 316 : 106-111

Cement removal from the femoral cavity

B Bradnock

Abstract. – *The removal of cement from the femoral cavity can be a very difficult procedure to perform safely. As with any other surgical procedure, preoperative planning is essential to prevent complications during surgery. This planning should extend to obtaining adequate radiology and ensuring suitable instruments are available at the time of surgery. It is possible to remove cement using a variety of methods including hand instruments, ultrasound and osteotomies.*

© *2001, Editions Scientifiques et Médicales Elsevier SAS. All rights reserved.*

Keywords: hip, total hip arthoplasty, cement removal, hand instruments, extended trochanter osteotomy, high speed burrs, ultrasonic cement removal.

Introduction

As with any surgical procedure, it is important to carry out preoperative assessment and to plan the procedure in advance of the operation. Prior to removing cement from the femur it is necessary to carry out both AP and lateral X-rays of the femur and these should extend the full length of the cement mantle. From these X-rays it is possible to assess the curvature of the femur and to determine where it is weak or in fact broken or perforated from previous surgery. Due to the natural curvature of the femur, it is often necessary to remove bone from the lateral portion of the greater trochanter superiorly, to allow straight access to the medullary cavity. This can be planned preoperatively from the X-rays.

The planning should also involve the provision of any special equipment that may be required for removal of the prosthesis and cement.

It should be stressed at an early stage that it is preferable to remove the femoral prosthesis initially and leave the cement within the femur to act as an internal scaffolding to strengthen the femur while the hip is being revised on the acetabular side. Should the cement be removed from the femur first, it is possible to damage it, especially in cases of severe osteoporosis, during manipulation of the hip whilst operating on the acetabular side.

Cement removal can be performed using hand instruments, mechanical instruments and ultrasonic instruments. It is quite common for several methods of cement removal to be used during the operation.

Hand instruments

Removing cement using hand instruments without perforating or fracturing the femur is a very skillful art and many experienced surgeons are able to do this [5]. There is, however, a large learning curve and many fractures or perforations occur before the procedure can be carried out safely. Many surgeons use hand instruments to remove cement in the proximal third of the femur where visibility is good, especially if the bone is strong. However, in cases of severe osteolysis, when an osteotome is introduced into the cement mantle it makes it expand, and this expansion can cause a weak proximal femur to fracture. It is also very easy to fracture or splinter the femur while levering cement out of the femur using osteotomes. It is therefore preferable to remove the cement in the proximal femur without causing the cement mantle to expand. This can be carried out using ultrasonic techniques or by burring the cement.

Hand instruments can be used to move cement beyond the calcar (*fig 1*). It is essential to have good visibility and an intra-femoral light source or headlamp can be used to provide good illumination. Some surgeons find it necessary to use an image

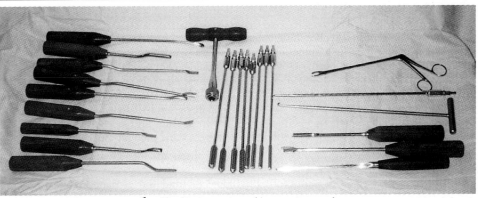

1 *Hand instruments used in cement removal.*

Brian Bradnock, BSc., MBCh.B., FRCS (Ed)., FRCS (Orth)., Consultant Orthopaedic Surgeon, St Albans City Hospital, St Albans, AL3 5PN Hertfordshire, United Kingdom.

intensifier during cement removal and, in selected cases, this may prove to be very beneficial.

If the bone stock is good and there is a fibrous membrane between the cement and the femur, the cement down to the region of the cement plug can usually be carefully removed using hand instruments.

It is recommended that the cement be removed in increments of 1-2 cm so that the outline of the internal surface of the femur can be well visualised. The plug poses a greater challenge to the surgeon armed with only hand instruments. The important questions to answer from the preoperative X-rays are whether or not the cement plug passes beyond the isthmus and whether or not the cement is wider distally. If the cement does not expand distally, it is possible to drill into the cement plug and tap into this with a threaded plug puller and gently remove the plug in a retrograde manner with some delicate hammer blows. However, if the plug widens distally this is contraindicated as the femur will expand and split when the plug is moved retrogradely.

If the cement expands distally, it is possible to drill through it centrally and ream out the cement incrementally but this is a formidable task and damage to the bone is highly likely.

Mechanical methods

The SEG-CES System® (Zimmer) has been used by some surgeons to remove cement from the femur.

This procedure involves removing the proximal cement to the level of the calcar using hand instruments. A Teflon®-coated threaded rod with nuts at 1 cm intervals is then cemented into the cement mantle (fig 2). Once this cement sets, the Teflon®-coated threaded rod is removed, leaving the well bonded cement and nuts at 1 cm intervals within the femur. It is then possible to thread a further instrument onto the nuts and, using a slap hammer, to remove the cement in 1 cm increments. This procedure is not without hazard.

Cases have been reported where the greater trochanter is avulsed, or the femur splits and in some cases it has not been possible to hammer out the cement leaving a bigger problem within the femur than at the beginning of the operation. When such a disaster occurs, it is necessary to do a femoral osteotomy to remove cement and nuts.

Extended trochanteric osteotomy [3, 6]

This procedure has been popularised by Paprosky and involves making numerous

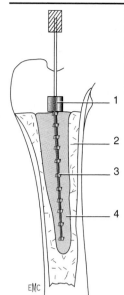

2 *The SEG-CES® system. If the distal plug of cement is well bonded, this system does not provide the solution. 1. Puller on slap hammer; 2. old cement; 3. nuts; 4. fresh cement.*

drill holes down the antero-lateral surface of the femur at a distance of 10-15 cm. The drill holes distally are then placed laterally, extending to the lateral margin of the femur, and are joined together using a sharp osteotome or a burr.

This produces a flap of bone which can then be elevated from the underlying cement using a fine osteotome. This has to be done carefully to avoid splitting the shaft of the femur. Once this has been folded over like opening a page of a book, the cement is clearly visible and can be removed using hand instruments. This does leave a problem with the cement plug, but because visualisation is excellent it is possible to remove the cement plug using hand instruments as described above, but without a huge risk of perforating the femur. Once the cement has been removed, it is necessary to apply tensioned cables around the femur to repair the defect; it is also advisable to use an uncemented hip replacement, as any attempt at pressurising cement will be flawed by cement leakage through the osteotomy sites.

High speed burrs

Several varieties of high speed burr are available commercially. These instruments are very effective at removing cement but they also remove bone when used in unskilled hands. They do not differentiate between bone and cement and in fact cut through bone preferentially.

One of the advantages of using high speed burrs is that they are "non-space-filling devices" and the cement mantle does not increase in dimension when burrs are used.

A disadvantage of burrs is that a lot of fine debris is produced both in the surrounding tissues and in the air and this can be a cause of contamination.

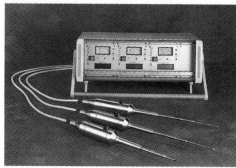

3 *OSCAR® (Orthosonics System for Cemented Arthroplasty Revision) is a computerised, automatic ultrasonic system.*

Ultrasonic cement removal

Many of the advantages outlined in the above methods are embodied in ultrasonic cement removal. This is also a "non-space-filling" type of cement removal. It is able to differentiate between cement and bone and is regarded as the optimal way of removing cement from the femur. Ultrasonic cement removal has improved dramatically over the last several years. A lot of the pioneering work has been done by Orthosonics in the development of the Orthosonics System for Cemented Arthroplasty Revision (OSCAR®) (fig 3). This equipment differs from its competitors in that it is computerised, produces more energy than other systems and is also very rapid at detecting cortical bone, resulting in less injury to bone when it is touched by an activated probe [2].

Ultrasound can liquify bone cement rapidly and this liquified cement can then be removed quickly [4]. Because cement is an excellent insulator, the conduction of heat from the liquid cement to the remaining cement is very slow and thermal injury to bone is consequently very small indeed.

Work carried out by Bhumbra [1] has shown that the temperature produced during cement setting is in fact greater than the temperature produced during cement removal using OSCAR®.

In the author's experience, it is simpler to remove the proximal cement using a groover; this is a flattened, spear-shaped, ultrasonic wave guide that is passed through the proximal mantle of the cement producing three longitudinal troughs (fig 4). These troughs are then interconnected by twisting the groover through 180° and cutting an internal circumferential groove in the cement. The proximal cement mantle can then be divided up into three thumb-sized fragments which can be removed simply using hand instruments. Care must be taken to avoid levering on delicate bone. The next portion of cement can then be removed using the back-scraper (fig 5). This involves removing cement in a retrograde manner and it is recommended this be performed in increments of 2-3 cm so that the bone/cement interface can be properly visualised.

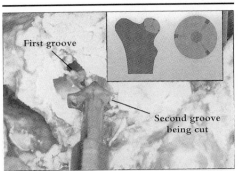

4 *The groover is used to remove proximal cement.*

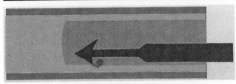

5 *The back scraper.*

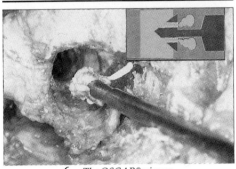

6 *The OSCAR® piercer.*

The plug of cement is the most challenging area of cement removal. However, with ultrasonic methods it is possible to liquify the solid plug of cement and remove it piecemeal with a piercer or ski-pole (fig 6). This device is conical-shaped with perforations. The cement liquifies within the beam of highly focussed ultrasonic energy, passes through the holes and then solidifies once it is out.

When the piercer is in contact with polythene, a resistance is met and it is necessary for the user to wait a few seconds before making progress through the polythene. This is because polythene absorbs more ultrasonic energy than polymethylmethacrylate. Should the tip of the piercer come into contact with bone, the OSCAR® will de-tune and produce an audible tone created by a change in the way the ultrasound is transmitting through the wave guide. When the wave guide is energised to cut through cement it expands in a longitudinal direction; however, when it touches bone it expands in a radial direction. The piercing device has a very small radius of curvature and should the audible tone be heard during cement removal, it is possible to simply rotate the hand set and find

another path through the cement. This equipment is so sensitive that if there is a lamination within the cement that is calcified, it will de-tune. Under these circumstances, it is a simple matter to insert a T-handled end-cutting reamer and scratch away on the surface of the cement, disloging the thin membrane of bone that is present. Cement removal can then progress normally. Once the plug has been pierced, the author's normal practice is to insert a back scraper and turn the plug into a C-shaped cylinder. It is then possible to hook a curette or ultrasonic probe distal to the plug and apply a retrograde force to remove the plug safely. If this remaining cement is well bonded the author advises removing the cement ultrasonically.

In some circumstances it may be preferable to leave some cement distally, if cementing in another stem, and use the remaining cement as a cement restrictor.

Following the removal of cement, it is recommended that a reamer or rasp be inserted into the femur to freshen up the internal surface. Some surgeons choose to perforate the plug of cement, pass a guide wire through the plug into the distal femur, and then ream the femur using flexible reamers. The author would caution against this practice because if the guide wire is not positioned centrally or the femur has a slight bow, it is possible to remove cement in a non-uniform pattern and severely compromise the thickness of the cortical wall by removing bone in preference to cement. During cement removal the femur should be washed out intermittently.

Special circumstances

REVISING FOR RECURRENT DISLOCATION DUE TO MAL-POSITIONING OF THE FEMORAL COMPONENT

Where there is no infection and a good cement/bone interface exists, it is preferable to remove cement from the femur and leave well-bonded cement. This can easily be performed using ultrasound. The cement/cement bond strength is several times stronger than the very best cement/bone bond strength and the cemented prosthesis can be cemented in safely.

In the author's experience, sticky cement adheres better than cement with a dough-like consistency, and it is advisable to insert the cement before it loses its sticky nature.

REVISING FOR INFECTION

Clearly when revising for infection, it is necessary to remove all foreign material and this can be a daunting task as the

cement/bone bond strength is well preserved. It is important under these circumstances to remove the cement with good illumination utilising a head lamp or a flexible light source. It may also be necessary to use an image intensifier to visualise the femur under X-ray. It should be stressed that any method of cement removal will leave spicules of cement in the canaliculi, and in the presence of good quality bone with well penetrated cement, it is advisable to ream the femur following cement removal and then utilise pulsed lavage to wash out the femur. By inserting the pulsed lavage distally into the femur and elevating it, fluid and debris can flow into the proximal femur during this procedure.

BROKEN STEM

The removal of broken stems can be difficult. With improvements in hip design and metals used, the problem is becoming rarer. It can be tackled in several ways: it is possible to drill into the metal, tap into it with a thread, and hammer the metal fragment out. It is also possible to use a thin ultrasonic probe to remove cement around the metal prosthetic stem and then using snipe-nosed mole wrenches to remove the broken fragment of stem. Should neither of these prove possible it would be advisable to make a window in the femur on the lateral surface and hit the metal stem with a tungsten carbide punch to dislodge it.

Conclusion

Hip revision surgery is becoming much more common and it is essential that revisions be done well, otherwise there will be an ever increasing number of re-revisions to be performed. Care must be taken to plan the operation preoperatively and to ensure that the necessary instruments are available at the time of procedure.

References

[1] Bhumbra B. Comparison of cement setting temperatures and ultrasonic cement removal temperatures. [thesis University College, London, 1996]

[2] Bradnock B, Young M. The removal of bone cement in cases of severe osteolysis. British Orthopaedic Association Spring Meeting, 1994

[3] Glassman AH, Engh CA, Bobyn JD. A technique of extensile exposure for total hip arthroplasty. *J Arthroplasty* 1987 ; 2 : 11-21

[4] Klapper RC, Caillouette JT, Callaghan JJ, Hozack WJ. Ultrasonic technology in revision joint arthroplasty. *Clin Orthop* 1992 ; 185 : 147-154

[5] Moreland JR. The removal of cement and cemented stems. Instructional Course Lecture. Presented at the Sixty-Sixth Annual Meeting of the American Academy of Orthopaedic Surgeons, Anaheim, California, February 8, 1999

[6] Younger TI, Bradford MS, Magnus RE, Paprovsky WG. Extended proximal femoral osteotomy. *J Arthroplasty* 1995 ; 10 : 329-338

The cementless total hip arthroplasty

G Scheller
L Jani

Abstract. – *Aseptic loosening of cemented total hip replacement (THR) in long term follow-ups has induced orthopaedic surgeons to develop implants for cementless biological fixation. The design, surface features and prerequisites of the surgical technique for osseointegration of cups and stems are discussed. After presentation of the preoperative planning, the surgical techniques using a threaded cup, a press-fit cup and a tapered stem are explained.*

Keywords: hip, arthroplasty, total hip replacement, cementless fixation, osseointegration, hydroxyapatite coating, press-fit, cementless femoral stem, cementless cup, threaded conical cup.

Introduction

Cemented total hip arthroplasties (THA) have been very successful in affording pain relief and improving function. However, the long term follow-ups of cemented Charnley PE-cups have shown between 11% and 25% loosening after 10 to 12 years [7, 15, 19]. The revision rate for failed cemented femoral stems using contemporary techniques is reported at around 5% at 10 years [8]. The results of cemented THA in younger patients are reported to be poorer. The reports show revision rates of up to 40% in mid-term results of some systems [1, 3, 4].

In the mid 1970s, the evident problems with cemented components in long-term follow-ups led many orthopaedic surgeons in Europe and the United States to develop implants for cementless fixation. Surface roughness, surface structures or porous coatings provided for direct bony ongrowth or ingrowth, and a biologic fixation of the implant by osseointegration.

Some of the early developments in the field of cementless THA also had high failure rates in the mid- and long-term results and were abandoned.

It became more and more evident that the amount of primary fixation and primary stability, the design of the stems, the geometry of the cups and the structure of the surface are more important and critical in cementless prostheses.

Gerhard Scheller, Privatdozent Dr. med.
Lutz Jani, Professor Dr. med.
Othopädische Universitätsklinik Mannheim, Theodor Kutzer, Ufer 1-3, D-68167 Mannheim, Germany.

Primary stability with micromotion under 50 µm at the bone/implant interface [16] is absolutely necessary for osseointegration and biological secondary fixation.

Surgical procedure

PREOPERATIVE PLANNING

The first step of preoperative planning is clinical examination of the patient. Leg length, range of motion, the presence of contractures and deformities should receive special attention.

The next step is radiographic analysis, requiring a minimum of two views. An AP view of the pelvis is necessary to estimate the leg length, to define the preoperative centre of rotation and the offset. The beam is centred over the pubis in the mid-line. The use of a magnification marker is useful. The dimensions of the proximal femur can be assessed more accurately from an AP view centred over the hip. The most popular lateral view of the hip is the Lauenstein lateral view, a modified frog-leg X-ray.

The general aims of preoperative planning are to restore the anatomic or premorbid centre of rotation and the femoral offset, and to equalise the leg length. The goals are to determine the correct centre of rotation and the size and position of the cup, the correct stem size and the optimal stem position as well as the neck length, if modular heads are used. Templates of the cup and the stem and a goniometer are necessary.

Drawing the following lines is helpful:

– A line across the roof of both acetabula.

– The tangent to both ischia, the interischial line.

– A line between both lesser trochanters.

The centre of rotation and the offset are determined at the contralateral, non-involved hip and measured in relation to Kohler's line and the inter-teardrop line. The centre of rotation of the operative side is found by symmetrically transferring this point from the opposite side.

Templating normally begins with the position and size of the acetabulum component.

The cup should be completely covered by bone and should fill the space between the teardrop and the superior-lateral rim of the acetabulum. The inclination should vary between 35° and 50° depending on the type of cup used. The correct size with respect to minimal resection of subchondral bone is chosen and the centre of rotation is marked.

Then, the femur is templated, referencing from the marked centre of rotation of the cup. The stem size and the stem position in relation to the anatomic landmarks of the greater and lesser trochanter are determined; the neck resection level and the neck length are defined (*fig 1*).

SURGICAL APPROACH

Different surgical approaches and variations in surgical techniques are used for the THA. The common variations are the postero-lateral approach with the patient in a lateral position and posterior dislocation of the hip, the anterolateral approach, as well as the lateral transgluteal approach modified according to Bauer with anterior dislocation

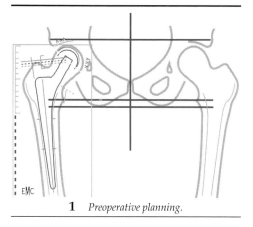

1   *Preoperative planning.*

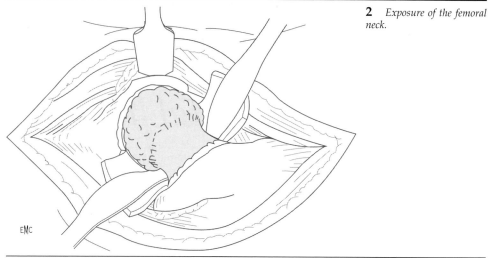

2   *Exposure of the femoral neck.*

of the hip. The joint capsule of the hip is prepared, exposed *(fig 2)* and resected. The osteotomy of the femoral neck is carried out according to the surgical procedure for the particular stem. The resected femoral head is removed and the acetabulum is exposed with special Hohmann levers *(fig 3)*.

CEMENTLESS CUP

Two different biomechanical concepts have gained wide acceptance in the last 10 years. On one hand, there are conical self-cutting threaded cups; on the other hand, there are hemispheric press-fit cups with different surface structures, which are normally slightly oversized for initial stability. The advantage of the threaded conical cups is a high initial stability. The advantage of the hemispheric press-fit cups is the minimal bone resection they require because their geometry respects the normal anatomy of the acetabulum.

Sometimes, the hemispheric cups come with additional fixation elements in relation to rotational and tilting movements, such as fins or cones or the possibility of using additional screws.

◼ *Threaded conical cups*

After exposing the acetabulum with Hohmann levers and excising the capsule, the osseous bed for the cup is prepared using the conical reamer, always starting with the smallest diameter. The axis of the reamer is positioned at an angle of 40° - 50° abduction and 10° - 20° anteversion *(fig 4)* with attention to the specific anatomic situation. The correct and exact orientation of the reamer is a prerequisite for accurate positioning of the conical implant. In contrast to hemispherical designs, there is no possibility of variation of the position between the conical reamer and the conical threaded cup. It is preferable to use a powered drive for this procedure. The optimal medialisation of the implant is achieved using the smallest reamer. The depth of reaming depends on the thickness of the acetabulum floor. Normally, the lamina interna is reached in the caudomedial section.

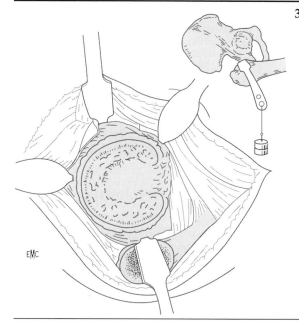

3   *Exposure of the acetabulum.*

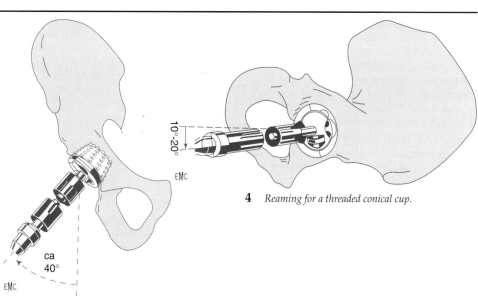

4   *Reaming for a threaded conical cup.*

Preparatory work using a chisel may be necessary when medialisation is difficult due to a hard acetabulum floor. It also may be useful to use the smallest hemispherical reamer as the first step. Otherwise, the conical reamer can deviate from its original, intended orientation and move into an area of softer bone.

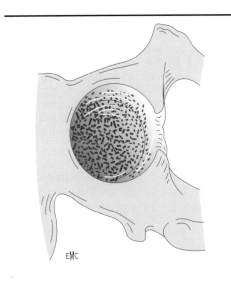

5   *Conical prepared acetabulum.*

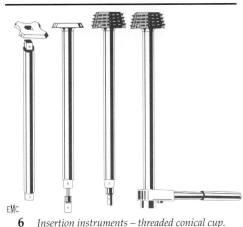

6   *Insertion instruments – threaded conical cup.*

Reaming is continued in 2 mm steps until the osseous acetabulum is accurately conical (*fig 5*). Interfering osteophytes should be removed. The dimension of the last reamer used indicates the size of the implant.

The conical cup is mounted on the insertion instrument. These instruments consist of a guiding shaft, a threaded rod for fixation of the cup, a ratchet and a pressure plate (*fig 6*).

The conical implant is placed in the acetabulum at the same angles as the reamers and centred by turning anti-clockwise. Then, the cup is screwed in, with the surgeon providing high axial load by leaning his body against the pressure plate.

After detaching the insertion instrument, the position and the distance to the osseous bottom can be checked through openings in the bottom of the implant.

Occasionally, the titanium cup cannot be screwed fully down to the floor of the reamed acetabulum. This is not disadvantageous for the functioning of the cup. It is possible to fill the gap with spongiosa. The outer edge of the implant should not rise up above the rim of the osseous bed too much or on greater parts of the circumference. Finally, the insert is mounted.

■ **Press-fit cups**

In the early 1980s, hemispherical cups, either all-polyethylene [14] or metal-backed [5, 6], were implanted with the same diameter as the last reamer.

The original surgical technique for the Harris-Galante Cup was called line-to-line reaming of the acetabulum. The implantation of the cup, equal in diameter to the last reamer, was followed by screw fixation. This "form-fit" or "exact-fit" led to the clinical observation of a high frequency of peripheral radiolucent lines in Zones I and III [11, 12, 17]

Mechanical tests showed that screws yield only a modest improvement in initial cup stability [2, 10] when using an oversized hemispherical implant. On the other hand, it became apparent that the use of fixation screws carries the risk of damaging neighbouring neurovascular structures [9, 20], that both screws and screw-holes could serve as a pathway for the migration of wear debris and that fretting may be a problem.

In 1985, Morscher introduced his press-fit cup into clinical use [13]. He defined "press-fit" as preload between bone and implant. The press fit cup by Morscher achieved this press-fit mechanism by flattening the hemisphere at the dome and using a cup size with an outer diameter larger than the corresponding reamer used last. Schmalzried [18] defined this mechanism to the American continent: "The cementless fixation of acetabular cups without screws relies on elastic distortion of the acetabulum and friction between bone and cup surface, optimally with good rim contact and high press-fitting."

Metal-backed fully-hemispherical cups and cups of less than a hemisphere are available. Sometimes the outer shape of the cup is basically spherical and the pole is flattened. The diameter of the implants is normally chosen 2 mm larger than the last hemispherical reamer, to generate equatorial tension to ensure good mechanical primary stability by over-sizing with respect to the reaming.

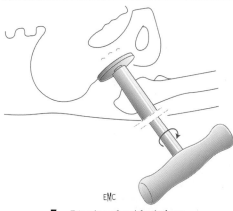

7   *Reaming a hemisherical cup.*

The operative technique will be described using the example of the press-fit cup by Morscher. After exposure, the acetabulum is reamed in 2 mm steps, starting with a reamer of at least 4 mm under the diameter of the removed head. The reaming under power is continued until all cartilage is removed and blood spots can be recognised at the subchondral bone (*fig 7*). A cup with the same nominal diameter as the last reamer, which includes an oversizing of 1.5 mm, is fitted onto a setting device. After the exact orientation is established (30° to the longitudinal axis of the patient and 10° anteversion (*fig 8*), the cup is temporarily fixed by light hammer blows, the position is checked, and then the cup is fully implanted using a heavy mallet (*fig 9*).

CEMENTLESS STEM

■ **Indications and contraindications**

Indications for cementless stems are primary and secondary osteoarthritis with respect to the bone quality. Parameters concerning the bone quality discussed here are sex, age and activity level of the patient. Radiographical parameters include classifications of osteoporosis and the relation between the diameter of the medullary canal and the cortical bone in the proximal femur.

Normally, younger patients with good bone quality should receive a cementless stem.

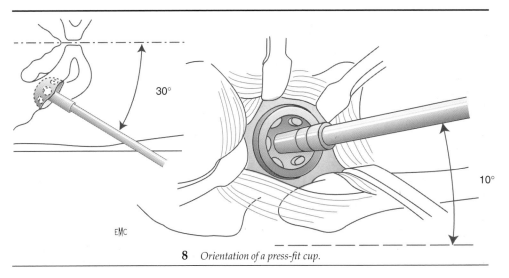

8   *Orientation of a press-fit cup.*

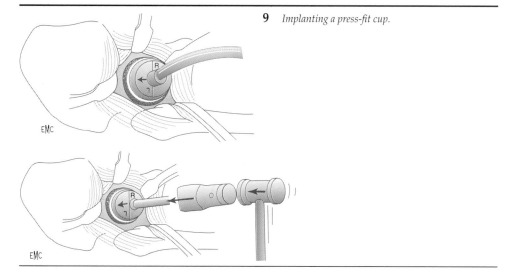

9 *Implanting a press-fit cup.*

Contraindications are severe osteoporosis and intraoperative complications in which primary stability could not be achieved for other reasons.

Design of cementless stems

Cementless hip implants are of two basic types: straight and anatomical stems.

Straight stems have symmetrical cross-sections. The dimensions of the cross-sections are variable. One type of straight stem is tapered with a proximal higher canal filling; the other type is parallel-sided with a smaller amount of proximal canal filling. One type fits both sides of the hip.

Anatomical stems correspond to the geometry of the femoral canal. Both a right and a left stem version are required, as the anteversion must be built into the cone segment of the prosthesis.

The aim of both types of stem is to achieve axial and rotational stability through their design, surface structure and sometimes special fixation elements such as grooves or ribs.

Custom-made femoral prostheses try to achieve a perfect fit between the individually-manufactured stem and the patient's cortical bone in the proximal femur. So far, published clinical data are not convincing. The costs and the reaming technique may be another problem. Some cementless stems have a porous-coated surface for bony ingrowth, whilst others can have a roughened surface for bony ongrowth.

Hydroxyapatite coatings on different surface structures are also available on the market. The osteo-conductive capacity should improve the early bonding between implant and the surrounding bone. The possibility of third-body wear due to hydroxyapatite particles is under discussion. The extent of porous or roughened surfaces is the subject of controversy, but there is no longer any doubt that surface structure should be circumferential at the proximal part of the stem. This feature provides a better barrier against the ingress of wear particles from

the articulation coupling. Supporters of a collared stem say that the collar avoids the penetration of wear particles into the femoral canal and that forces are transmitted directly to the medial cortex of the femur. Even if intra-operatively a perfect bone contact of the collar is achieved, resorption of the bone underneath the collar is quite often seen within the first year of bone remodelling.

Eight to twelve different sizes of stem are necessary to guarantee a perfect fit for the different sizes of the femur.

Surgical technique

The surgical technique described is for the CLS straight stem. The frontal and sagittal planes of the stem are conical; the anterior and posterior proximal surfaces are provided with parallel conical ribs. This "three-dimensional press-fit" design should provide initial mechanical, axial and rotational stability. Bony ongrowth on the roughened titanium alloy provides secondary fixation by osseointegration.

The proximal femur is exposed. Sometimes, a second exact osteotomy on the neck is necessary. The osteotomy is carried out parallel to the intertrochanteric line or as an

angled osteotomy. Because of the normal anteversion of the femoral neck, the stem can only be positioned in a correct axial direction if the osteotomy level on the medial side is no more then 10 mm above the superior margin of the lesser trochanter. The medullary cavity is opened by removing a trapezoidal segment of cancellous bone, reaching the tip of the greater trochanter by using a tuke saw or an osteotome.

Than an awl is introduced by rotating it into the medullary canal in the region of the resected tip of the greater trochanter (*fig 10*). The awl follows the longitudinal axis of the femur, orientates itself and gives a guideline for the positioning of the implant. If required, the canal must be widened laterally and posteriorly for this procedure.

The definite seating of the stem is prepared by using the sizing rasps, always beginning with the smallest one. The rasps should be introduced in the same place and direction as the awl to avoid a varus or valgus malposition. Rotational movements should also be avoided during the rasping procedure. The rasps are hammered into the marked depth with an antetorsion of about 10° (*fig 11*).

After the last rasp (referring to the preoperative planning) has been impacted, at least a 1 mm layer of compressed cancellous bone should remain between the rasp and the cortical bone, particularly in the medial section. After removing the last rasp, the medullary canal can be irrigated and the original implant impacted with a mallet to the preoperatively-determined depth (*fig 12*).

The position of the stem can be checked by measuring the distance from the shoulder of the prosthesis to the tip of the greater trochanter. The conical ribs of the stem should not make contact with the cortical bone at the level of the osteotomy. With direct cortical contact of the stem, further impaction could lead to a fissure or fracture of the proximal femur.

If a gap remains between the plane surfaces of the stem in the osteotomy level, we use

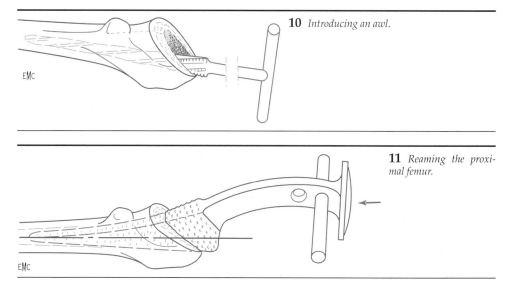

10 *Introducing an awl.*

11 *Reaming the proximal femur.*

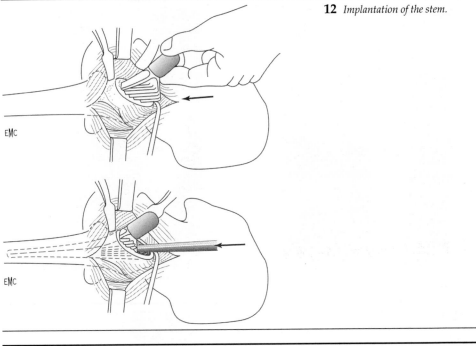

12 *Implantation of the stem.*

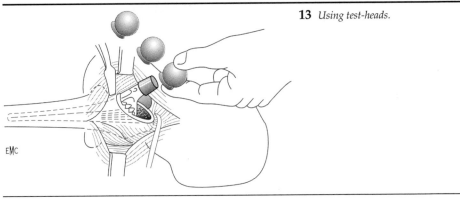

13 *Using test-heads.*

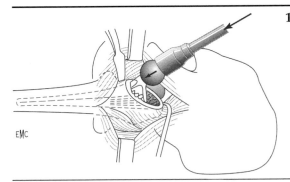

14 *Fixing the modular head.*

removed cancellous bone as proximal sealing and a barrier against wear particles from the wear coupling. A trial reduction with the planned test head and a stability check is performed (*fig 13*). Range of motion and muscular tension are checked. Then, the test head is removed and, after cleaning the cone, the definitive modular head is positioned and fixed with a gentle tap using a plastic-headed impactor (*fig 14*). Reduction and a function check follow, before drains are inserted and the wound is closed.

Special circumstances

PROTRUSIO ACETABULI

Acetabular protrusion is defined as a migration of the femoral head medially and superiorly towards the pelvic cavity beyond Kohler's line.

The primary form mainly occurs in relatively young women; both hips are involved. A combined varus deformity of the femoral neck is often found in association. The range of motion is reduced.

The age of the patients and the good results obtained with bone grafting of the defect favour the implantation of cementless cups when a THA is necessary. The intact peripheral rim is an ideal support for hemispherical press-fit cups.

The aim of the THA is to restore the centre of rotation of the hip by bringing it back to a more lateral and inferior position. The remaining cavity defect is grafted with particulate or morselised cancellous bone from the resected femoral head.

The restored centre of rotation and the CCD-ankle of the commonly-used stems cause a lengthening of the leg compared to the other hip. Careful planning and accurate information to the patient concerning this particular point are important. If available, a varus version of the stem may be helpful.

■ *Surgical technique*

The dislocation of the hip can be very difficult. A good exposure of the acetabulum with Hohmann levers and a total excision of the joint capsule is necessary. Often, it is helpful to carry out the osteotomy in situ, perhaps as a double osteotomy. It may also be helpful to carry out the exact osteotomy of the femoral neck after changing the position of the femur.

The medial wall of the acetabulum is usually thin or already partially penetrated. Medial reaming is not necessary. Soft tissue and cartilage in this area are removed with a curette.

The reaming starts with a spherical reamer; the diameter should be 4 mm less than the opening of the acetabulum. The reamer is introduced only to the level of the rim; reaming is continued in 2 mm steps. The oblong shape of the acetabulum requires careful reaming to create convergence of the acetabular rim. Pressure in the posterior direction avoids unnecessary reaming of the superior rim, thus causing a iatrogenic superior segmental defect. The bone graft is impacted by reverse reaming or by a trial cup. An oversizing of 2 (-4) mm is recommended for an initial press-fit of the cementless hemispherical cup.

Complications

After THA, as after any major surgical procedure, complications can occur. In principle, the same complications may occur after cemented or cementless THA. However, the occurrence of some problems is more frequent when cementless implants are used.

Haematoma formation out of the reamed bone surfaces seem to occur more frequently. At first glance heterotopic ossification may be a problem of cementless THA. However, there is no study published showing that increased bone debris in cementless THA induces more heterotopic ossifications. Patients at risk are men, and patients with ankylosing spondylitis, fused hip, hypertrophic osteoarthritis and Forestier's disease.

The danger of nerve injuries or vascular injuries may be slightly higher if cementless hemispherical cups are additionally fixed with screws. The penetration of the lamina interna of the acetabulum or of the ilium may be a risk for the passing nerves and vessels.

Acetabular fractures may occur during the implantation of oversized press-fit cups. These have no clinical significance if the initial stability of the cup can be achieved.

Intraoperative femoral fractures occur more often with cementless stems. The contact of the rasps or the implant with the cortical bone at the level of the osteotomy is normally the reason for these complications. Most of these fracture are small fissures from the calcar region to the lesser trochanter. It is hard to decide whether these fractures are stable. Therefore, the fracture line should be completely exposed to its distal end to avoid an underestimation of the fracture. We recommend cerclage wiring of all these cases.

In cementless THA, primary stability of the components is the indispensable prerequisite for osseointegration. The micromotion at the interface between implant bone must be below 50 μm to allow bony ongrowth or ingrowth of the structured surface. The surgeon should be fairly sure that the operative technique and implant design will guarantee the primary stability of every single implant.

Examples:

Morscher Press-fit Cup/CLS-stem *(fig 15)*.
MPF-Cup/CLS-stem *(fig 16)*.
Hofer/Imhoff-Cup/Zweymüller-stem *(fig 17)*.

Conclusions

The high revision rates and high rates of radiolucent lines for cemented PE cups seen in mid-term results, and even more in the long-term results, strengthen our opinion that today cementless cups should be the standard implant, even in older patients. Moreover, in terms of cost-effectiveness, the physiological age of an individual patient should be given more consideration than his chronological age.

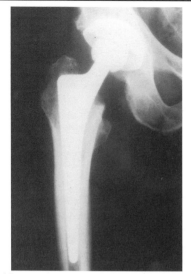

15 *Rö's: - Morscher-press-fit Cup/CLS-stem.*

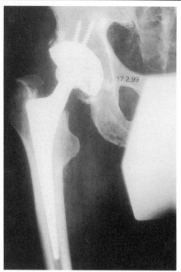

16 *MPF-Cup/CLS-stem.*

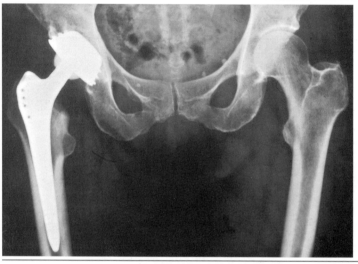

17 *Hofer/Imhoff-Cup/Zweymüller-stem.*

The hybrid version of THA is also strongly recommended for younger patients by some leading orthopaedic surgeons. In contrast, we recommend the use of proven cementless stem designs. Bone quality is the most important criterion for the implantation of cementless stems. Even in borderline cases – younger patients with osteoporosis, after inactivity or partial weight-bearing – we have regularly experienced a recovery of the bone quality after implantation of a cementless stem and a period of full weight-bearing.

References

[1] Chandler HP, Reineck FT, Wixon RL et al. Total hip replacement in patients younger than thirty years old: A five year follow-up-study. *J Bone Joint Surg Am* 1981 ; 63 : 1426-1434

[2] Clark HJ, Jinnah RH, Warden KE, Cox QG, Curtis MJ. Evaluation of acetabular stability in uncemented prostheses. *J Arthroplasty* 1991 ; 6 : 335-340

[3] Dorr LD, Luckett M, Contay JP. Total hip arthroplasties in patients younger than 45 years: A nine to ten year follow-up-study. *Clin Orthop* 1990 ; 260 : 215-219

[4] Dorr LD, Takei GR, Contay JP. Total hip arthroplasties in patients less than 45 years old. *J Bone Joint Surg Am* 1983 ; 65 : 474-479

[5] Harris WH. Advances in total hip arthroplasty. The metal-backed acetabular component. *Clin Orthop* 1984 ; 183 : 4-12

[6] Harris WH, Penenberg BL. Further follow-up on socket fixation using a metal-backed acetabular component for total hip replacement. A minimum ten-year follow-up. *J Bone Joint Surg Am* 1987 ; 69 : 1140-1143

[7] Hozack WJ, Rothman RH, Booth RE, Balderston RA, Cohn JC, Pickens GT. Survivorship analysis of 1041 Charnley total arthroplasties. *J Arthroplasty* 1990 ; 5 : 41-47

[8] Kavanagh BF, Dewitz MA, Ilstrup DM. Charnley total hip arthroplasty with cement: Fifteen-year results. *J Bone Joint Surg Am* 1989 ; 71 : 1496-1503

[9] Keating EM, Ritter MA, Faris PM. Structures at risk from medially placed acetabular screws. *J Bone Joint Surg Am* 1990 ; 72 : 509-511

[10] Kwong LM, O'Connor DO, Sedlack RC, Krushell RJ, Maloney WJ, Harris WH. A quantitative in vitro assessment of fit and screw fixation on the stability of a cementless hemispherical acetabular component. *J Arthroplasty* 1994 ; 9 : 163-170

[11] Lachiewicz PF, Anspach WE, Demasi R. A prospective study of 100 consecutive Harris-Galante porous total hip arthroplasties. *J Arthroplasty* 1992 ; 7 : 519-526

[12] Martell JM, Pierson RH, Jacobs JJ, Rosenberg AG, Maley M, Galante JO. Primary total hip reconstruction with a titanium fiber-coated prosthesis inserted without cement. *J Bone Joint Surg Am* 1993 ; 75 : 554-571

[13] Morscher E, Bern B, Jockers W, Schenk R. Rationale of a flexible Press-fit Cup in total hip replacement. 5-year follow-up in 280 procedures. *Clin Orthop* 1997 ; 341 : 42-50

[14] Morscher EW, Dick W, Kerner V. Cementless fixation of polyethylene acetabular component in total hip arthroplasty. *Arch Orthop Trauma Surg* 1982 ; 99 : 223-230

[15] Older J. Low-fiction arthroplasty of the hip: A 10-12-year follow-up-study. *Clin Orthop* 1986 ; 221 : 36-42

[16] Pilliar RM, Lee JM, Maniatopoulos C. Observations on the effect of movement on bone in growth into porous-surfaced implants. *Clin Orthop* 1986 ; 208 : 108-113

[17] Schmalzried TP, Harris WH. The Harris-Galante porous-coated acetabular component with screw fixation. *J Bone Joint Surg Am* 1992 ; 74 : 1130-1139

[18] Schmalzried TP, Wessinger SJ, Hill GE, Harris WH. The Harris-Galante porous acetabular component press-fit without screw fixation. *J Arthroplasty* 1994 ; 9 : 235-242

[19] Stauffer RN. Ten-year follow-up study of total hip replacement. *J Bone Joint Surg Am* 1982 ; 64 : 983-990

[20] Wasielewski RC, Kruger MP, Cooperstein LA, Rubash HE. Acetabular anatomy and transacetabular fixation of screws in total hip arthroplasty. *J Bone Joint Surg Am* 1990 ; 72 : 501-508

Total hip replacement in congenital hip disease

G Hartofilakidis
T Karachalios

Abstract. – *To improve communication, treatment planning and evaluation of results, we need a common classification to determine the different types of congenital hip disease in adults. The authors propose the use of the terms: dysplasia, low dislocation and high dislocation. Knowledge of the local anatomical abnormalities in these three types of congenital hip disease is very important. Total hip arthroplasty in all three types, especially in low and high dislocation, is a difficult operation and should be embarked upon only when there is an absolute indication. There are three major areas of difficulty: acetabular reconstruction, femoral canal preparation, and reduction of the components, especially in high dislocation, with overall improvement of leg length. The acetabular component must be placed in the area of the true acetabulum, mainly for mechanical reasons. In low and high dislocation, after reaming of the true acetabulum, if the remaining osseous cavity cannot accommodate a small cementless cup with at least 80% coverage of the implant, the cotyloplasty technique is recommended, rather than a bulk structural autogenous graft from the femoral head, to augment the superolateral aspect of the acetabular rim. In high dislocation, with the appropriate surgical technique and postoperative care, leg lengthening can exceed 5 cm without neurological complications.*

Keywords: hip, congenital dysplasia, CHD, arthroplasty, total hip replacement, low dislocation, high dislocation, acetabuloplasty, femoral reconstruction.

Introduction

Our early attempts to treat severe types of congenital hip disease (CHD) in adults by the use of total hip arthroplasty (THA) were frustrated by a lack of knowledge regarding the local anatomical abnormalities of these hips [3]. Later, following extended clinical and surgical experience treating these patients by THA, it became obvious that it was not feasible to compare the long-term results published in the international literature, due to the lack of a uniform terminology to describe the various types of the disease and the inclusion of dissimilar cases within the same series.

Terminology – Classification

TERMINOLOGY

The traditional term congenital dislocation of the hip (CDH), when used as a general

George Hartofilakidis, M.D., FACS, Professor Emeritus, Orthopaedic Department, University of Athens, 21 Photiou Patriarchou Street, 11471 Athens, Greece.
Theofilos Karachalios, M.D., Associate Professor Orthopaedic Department, University of Thessalia, 22 Papakiriazi Street, 41222 Larissa, Greece.

term to describe the wide spectrum of congenital hip malformations, is a misleading term and should be avoided [19]. Recently, the term developmental dysplasia of the hip has became more popular. However, this term is also indefinite and not representative of underlying pathology for all types of the disease. Therefore, the term congenital hip disease (CHD), as used by Wedge and Wasylenko is, in our opinion, more accurate as a general term, although it requires further classification [29].

CLASSIFICATION

Various systems of classification of CHD in adults are in use. Eftekhar recognised four types: dysplasia, intermediate dislocation, high dislocation and old, unreduced dislocation [6, 7]. The Crowe classification [4] is based on the degree of subluxation of the femoral head in relation to the acetabulum. Kerboull classified the deformity as anterior, intermediate and posterior [18]. In the present authors' classification [12, 14] three distinct types of CHD are recognised in adults: **dysplasia**, in which the femoral head articulates with the original acetabulum, despite the degree of subluxation (*fig 1*); **low dislocation**, in which the femoral head

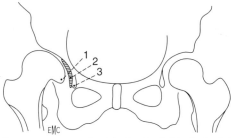

1 *Line drawing of a right dysplastic hip. 1. Capital drop; 2. the fossa covering osteophyte; 3. tear drop.*

articulates with a false acetabulum that partially covers the true acetabulum; and **high dislocation**, in which the femoral head migrates superiorly and posteriorly in relation to the hypoplastic true acetabulum and may articulate with the hollow in the iliac wing, which resembles a false acetabulum (*fig 2*).

Anatomy

ACETABULUM

Dysplastic hips present a gradually increasing deficiency of the superior

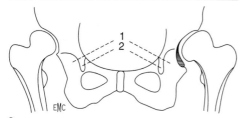

2 *Line drawing of a right high dislocation hip and a left low dislocation hip. 1. True acetablum; 2. tear drop.*

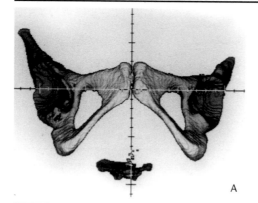

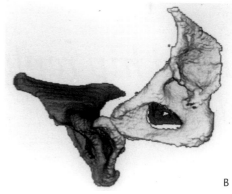

A

B

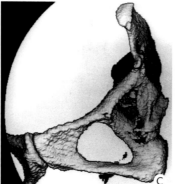

C

3 *The anatomy of the acetabulum in the three types of congenital hip disease in adults is shown in three-dimensional computerised tomography scans.*
A. Dysplasia (right hip). Left hip normal.
B. Low dislocation.
C. High dislocation.

segment, and a secondary shallowing due to the formation of an osteophyte that covers the acetabular fossa. In low dislocation, the inferior part of the false acetabulum is an osteophyte that begins at the level of the superior rim of the true acetabulum. The visible part of the true acetabulum has a narrow opening, anterior and posterior segmental deficiency and inadequate depth. In the majority of cases, there is also increased anteversion. In high dislocation, the true acetabulum is hypoplastic and triangular in shape. It has a segmental deficiency of its entire rim, a narrow opening, inadequate depth, and excessive anteversion *(fig 3A, B, C)*. The total iliac wing is hypoplastic, anteverted and the bone stock at the area of the acetabulum has an abnormal distribution, mainly located superoposteriorly.

FEMUR

In the dysplastic hip, the femoral head is initially spherical, but gradually becomes elliptical and elongated, due to the formation of marginal osteophytes. The femoral neck and the diaphysis are within the range of normal anatomy. In low dislocation, the femoral head, due also to the formation of marginal osteophytes, is often large and elliptical in shape. Occasionally, the femoral neck is anteverted and the diaphysis is narrow. In high dislocation, the femoral head is small and non-spherical. It either articulates with a false acetabulum or moves freely within the gluteal muscles. The femoral neck always shows increased anteversion and the lesser trochanter lies more anteriorly than normal. The diaphysis is hypoplastic with an extreme narrowing of the canal and with a thin cortex *(fig 4)*.

Indications for surgery

Total hip arthroplasty is a demanding operation in all three types of the disease, but especially in low and high dislocation. It should be performed only when there is a clear indication. Pain and/or severe functional impairment with limping, pelvic inclination, fixed flexion deformity of the hip, knee and spinal deformities are the main indications for operation. Limping alone is not an indication, especially in young active patients. According to the

authors' experience, patients with dysplastic hips present for total hip arthroplasty at an average age of 55 years, patients with low dislocation at an average of 51 years, and those with high dislocation at an average of 49 years when a false acetabulum is present, and at an average of 55 years when it is absent.

Preoperative planning

Templating of both the acetabulum and the femur is necessary. Acetabular components with a small outer diameter (e.g. 40-42 mm) and a small straight femoral prosthesis (CDH stems) are often used. In more complex cases, preoperative planning with a CT-scan or a 3D CT-scan is also necessary *(fig 3A, B, C)*.

Operative technique

Of the various approaches to the hip joint, the authors prefer the lateral approach recommended by Charnley. Trochanteric osteotomy is optional in the dysplastic hip, but strongly recommended for cases of low and high dislocation, to ensure better and safer exposure and reconstruction of both the acetabular and the femoral sides. The anatomic placement (true acetabulum) of the acetabular component is preferable, mainly for mechanical reasons [13, 14, 16]. In the case of inadequate bone stock at the level of the true acetabulum, the authors recommend performance of the cotyloplasty technique, which increases bone stock [14]. However, other surgeons suggest that if the bone stock

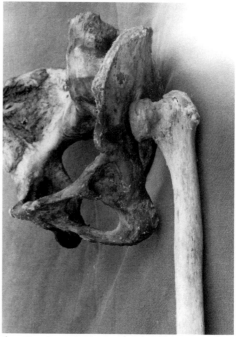

4 *The anatomy of the femur and the iliac wing in high dislocation is shown in a cadaver specimen.*

is better higher up, the cup should be placed superiorly but not laterally, and the anatomical position of the greater trochanter (lever arm of the abductor muscles) should be compensated for by a long neck femoral prosthesis [26].

SURGICAL APPROACH TO THE HIP

The patient is placed in a supine position. The skin incision, with the hip in 20° flexion and 20-30° adduction, starts approximately 3 cm proximally and posteriorly to the tip of the greater trochanter, and extends distally and anteriorly across the lateral aspect of the femur for approximately 20-30 cm. The fascia is incised in line with the skin incision and to the same extent. An initial Charnley retractor is then applied, keeping the edges of the fascia apart. The space between the anterior border of the gluteus medius and minimus is identified posteriorly, the tensor fascia lata is identified anteriorly, and a Hohmann retractor is applied, outside the capsule, around the junction of the greater trochanter and the neck of the femur, for better exposure of the front surface of the hip joint. The capsule is incised longitudinally at the middle of the neck and the Hohmann retractor is inserted into the capsule. Next, an osteotomy of the greater trochanter is performed, either with the use of a Gigli saw or with a wide, thin osteotome. Dislocation of the joint follows, adducting and carefully externally rotating the femur to avoid fracturing the shaft. A provisional osteotomy of the neck of the femur is performed at a level predetermined by the preoperative radiographs. The final adjustment is made during a trial reduction of the components. One of the most important instruments of the operation, Charnley's horizontal retractor, is then applied, holding apart the greater trochanter proximally and the femur distally, thus maximising the exposure.

RECONSTRUCTION OF THE ACETABULUM

In the **dysplastic hip**, the problem of superior bone deficiency is assessed with the use of acetabular trial components following the deepening process with the appropriate reamers. If at least 80% coverage of the periphery of the trial component can be obtained, a metal-backed cementless cup is implanted. If this is not feasible, an all-polyethylene cup fixed with cement is used. In this case, the cement mantle thickness in the area of the superior acetabular defect should exceed 10-15 mm *(fig 5A, B, C)*. In **low dislocation**, the true acetabulum has to be excavated underneath the inferior part of the false acetabulum. This is achieved by removing, with the use of a Lexer chisel, the osteophyte that covers the upper part of the true acetabulum. A complete absence of the upper wall of the true acetabulum may be noticed in most cases at this stage of the operation, and it should be developed during the reaming process *(fig 6)*. In **high dislocation**, the true acetabulum is identified by using the thickened and elongated joint capsule as a guide. Once the true acetabulum is located, two Hohmann retractors are inserted as markers of the most distal and anterior boundaries of the true acetabulum. One retractor is inserted at the acetabular notch, which corresponds to the superior margin of the obturator foramen. The second retractor is inserted anteriorly, taking great care to avoid

5   Reconstruction of the acetabulum in the displastic hip.
A. The preoperative appearance of the acetabulum.
B. Reconstruction by a metal-backed cementless cup. The arrow indicates the accepted uncovered part of the prosthesis.
C. Reconstruction by an all-polyethylene cemented cup. The arrow indicates the thick mantle of the cement at the upper part.

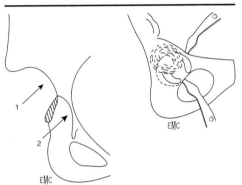

6   In low dislocation, the true acetabulum has to be excavated underneath the inferior part of the false acetabulum. 1. False acetabulum; 2. true acetabulum.

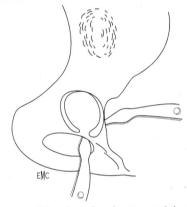

7   In high dislocation, when the true acetabelum is located, two Hohmann retractors are inserted, one at the distal end of the acetabular fossa and the second one engaging the anterior wall. The dotted lines indicate the direction of enlargement and deepening of the true acetabulum.

possibility of fracture, engaging the thin anterior wall into the inner wall of the pelvis at the junction of the ilium and the pubic ramus [6] *(fig 7)*. Once a wide exposure of the area of the true acetabulum has been achieved, the procedure follows the same steps in low and high dislocation. The hypoplastic true acetabulum is widened and deepened with small (38-40 mm) diameter reamers, directed superoposteriorly. Deepening is continued until the outer surface of the internal pelvic cortex is reached. After preparation of the true acetabulum, a press fit 40-42 mm cementless cup is inserted at an angle of 40-45° to the horizontal and with 10° anteversion, when the remaining osseous cavity can accommodate it with at least 80% coverage of the implant with bone. If this cannot be done, we suggest reconstruction of the acetabulum using an acetabuloplasty technique described and named cotyloplasty by K. Stamos [12-14].

COTYLOPLASTY TECHNIQUE

A controlled comminuted fracture of the entire paper-thin medial wall of the acetabulum is created using the Charnley deepening reamer or a Lexer chisel, or both *(fig 8A)*. The reamer is struck lightly with a hammer until the entire floor of the acetabulum fractures. Care must be taken not to perforate the internal layer of the periosteum.

A blind anchorage hole is then made with a Charnley starting drill in the roof of the acetabulum.

A large amount of autogenous cancellous morsellised (cut into small pieces) graft, taken from the femoral head and neck, is placed between the fragments of the acetabular floor and onto the periosteum of the fractured medial wall *(fig 8B)*. The graft

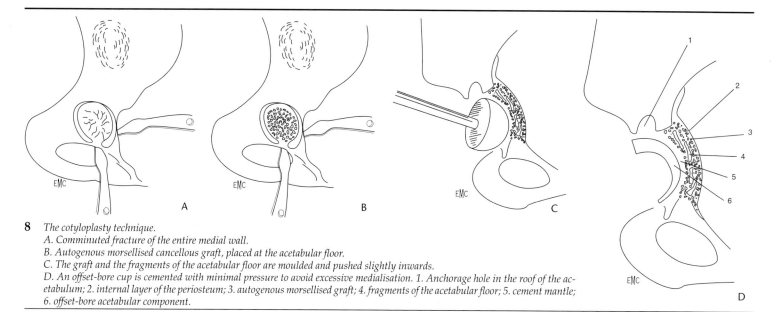

8 *The cotyloplasty technique.*
A. Comminuted fracture of the entire medial wall.
B. Autogenous morsellised cancellous graft, placed at the acetabular floor.
C. The graft and the fragments of the acetabular floor are moulded and pushed slightly inwards.
D. An offset-bore cup is cemented with minimal pressure to avoid excessive medialisation. 1. Anchorage hole in the roof of the acetabulum; 2. internal layer of the periosteum; 3. autogenous morsellised graft; 4. fragments of the acetabular floor; 5. cement mantle; 6. offset-bore acetabular component.

and the fragments of the acetabular floor are moulded and pushed slightly inwards with a hemispherical pusher or wrapped gauze, or both *(fig 8C)*.

The acetabular component, usually the offset-bore acetabular cup, fully covered [15], is then cemented at an angle of 40-45° to the horizontal and with 10° of anteversion, with minimal pressure being applied to avoid excessive medialisation *(fig 8D)*.

Dunn and Hess [5] proposed a similar technique, but with limited fragmentation of the medial wall, as well as reinforcement of the graft-cement interface with a wire mesh. The use of a bulk structural autogenous graft from the femoral head to augment the superolateral aspect of the acetabular rim was proposed initially by Harris [11], and the short-term clinical results were excellent. However, a high rate of failure reported after approximately twelve years [10, 21] raised doubts as to the efficacy of this technique, and those who still recommend it rely considerably less on the bulk graft than on the host bone for support of the acetabular component *(fig 9)*. The reason for such a high failure rate in this technique may be the complex pathological anatomy that we have described, and the abnormal distribution of stresses combined with the unfavourable long-term biological behaviour of structural grafts [9].

RECONSTRUCTION OF THE FEMUR

In dysplastic hips and in the majority of hips with low dislocation, the reconstruction of the femur is similar to that of conventional cases. Problems arise with the more hypoplastic types of low dislocation and in hips with high dislocation. The narrow canal is prepared with hand-operated reamers, since power reamers may cause a fracture or penetration of the thin cortex. A trial reduction of the components chosen, with the femoral component inserted at the

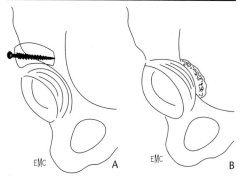

9 *The two techniques for reconstruction of the acetabulum.*
A. Use of a bulk structural graft to augment the superolateral aspect of the rim of the acetabulum.
B. The cotyloplasty technique. Complete coverage of the cup with controlled medialisation.

correct degree of anteversion (approximately 10°), is attempted after release of the psoas tendon and the small external rotators. If the reduction is not possible, additional shortening of the femur is performed with progressive resection of the femoral neck. Care is taken to keep the resection proximal to the lesser trochanter; otherwise the narrow diameter of the femoral canal, more distally, becomes a major problem. Shortening at the level of the neck of the femur is simple and uneventful, and thus we do not favour shortening of the femoral diaphysis, as suggested by others [22-25, 27]. The prosthesis is then inserted, using so-called modern cementing techniques. The surgeon must be prepared to use a straight, thin prosthesis leaving adequate space for a cement mantle of sufficient width. Special care must be taken to avoid inserting the stem with excess anteversion, or in a varus or valgus position. In agreement with other authors, we favour the use of cemented femoral prostheses. We consider that the principles and goals of cementless fixation of the stems (optimal canal fit and fill, initial implant stability and adequate bone

ingrowth) are not easily achievable in narrow femoral canals with such a thin cortex.

REATTACHMENT OF THE GREATER TROCHANTER

After the final reduction, reattachment of the greater trochanter is often difficult, and it may be necessary to release the gluteus medius and the remnants of the joint capsule. Fixation is achieved with the original «two wires» technique of Charnley [2].

AFTERCARE

It is recommended to use antibiotic prophylaxis for two days and anticoagulation in the form of newer low molecular heparins for 4 weeks. Two to three weeks of bed rest postoperatively, with an abduction pillow between the legs, is also recommended to allow better adjustment and balance of the soft tissues for most hypoplastic cases of low dislocation, as well as for cases of high dislocation. In cases of excessive lengthening, both the hip and knee joint should be kept in moderate flexion with the leg put on pillows to relieve tension on the femoral nerve (hip flexion) and on the sciatic nerve (knee flexion). The patient is instructed to start non-weight-bearing walking the third postoperative week, while full weight-bearing is usually permitted three to four months postoperatively.

Special cases

CONGENITAL HIP DISEASE WITH AN OLD SCHANZ SUBTROCHANTERIC FEMORAL OSTEOTOMY

The performance of a THA in the presence of an old femoral Schanz osteotomy is often indicated. When the underlying pathology is a low or high dislocation, THA can be

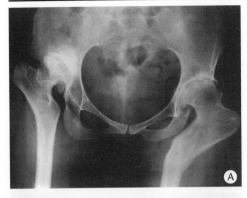
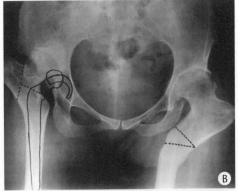
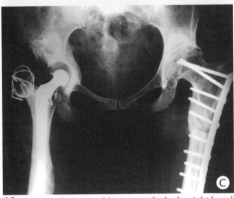
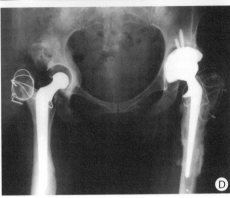

10 *A thirty-four year old woman who had a right low dislocation and a left dysplastic hip. Subtrochanteric Shanz osteotomies were performed when the patient was four year old.*
A. Preoperative anteroposterior radiograph of the pelvis.
B. Templating of both hips. A THA can be easily performed on the right hip, while on the left, a corrective osteotomy should first be performed.
C. Four years after a THA on the right side and one year after a corrective osteotomy on the left.
D. Anteroposterior radiograph of the pelvis at final follow-up (seven years following THA in the right hip and two years in the left hip). The intraoperative perforation of the right femur had no mid-term adverse effects.

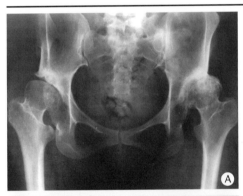
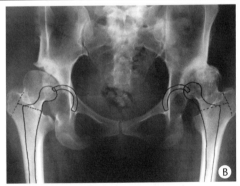
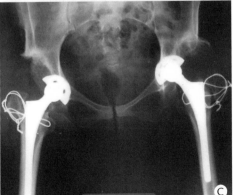

11 *A patient who had bilateral Chiari pelvic osteotomies at the age of three.*
A. Anteroposterior pelvic radiograph at the age of thirty-six. Both hips had developed low dislocation. The patient complained of severe pain and heavy limping.
B. Preoperative templating. It was planned to place both acetabular components at the level of the true acetabulae.
C. Two years following THA of both hips the radiological and clinical results were satisfactory.

performed in one stage. However, in a dysplastic hip, a two-stage operation is needed due to technical problems arising during the preparation of the femoral canal *(fig 10A, B, C, D)*.

CONGENITAL HIP DISEASE WITH AN OLD PELVIC CHIARI OSTEOTOMY

The performance of a THA in the presence of an old Chiari pelvic osteotomy may pose

technical difficulties when the osteotomy was performed in hips with subluxation *(fig 11A, B, C)*.

CONGENITAL HIP DISEASE WITH AN OLD ARTHRODESIS

Conversion of an old arthrodesis to THA is indicated when the hip is fused in unacceptable flexion, abduction or adduction. It is also indicated when the contralateral hip and the spine have developed osteoarthritic changes *(fig 12A, B, C)*.

Complications

Lower extremity nerve palsy, especially of the femoral and sciatic nerves, postoperative dislocation, femoral shaft fracture or perforation, and greater trochanter nonunion are the main complications encountered in total hip arthroplasty in patients with CHD. These complications are more frequent in low and high dislocation hips. Nerve damage can be avoided by cautious handling of the various instruments during the operation, especially the Hohmann retractors, and by the placement of both hip and knee in slight flexion after the operation for a few days. Postoperative dislocation can be minimised by proper orientation of the cup (inclination of 30-45° in the frontal plane and 10° of anteversion) and by 2 to 3 weeks of postoperative bed rest, for better soft tissue readjustment. Perforation of the femoral cortex is avoided by using hand-operated reamers, directed at the middle of the narrow femoral canal. Nonunion of the greater trochanter is a rather rare complication. Fibrous union is more frequent, but without any functional consequence.

Results

The results of THA in patients with CHD, published in various articles *(table I)*, are not easily comparable. The material is not homogenous since it includes various types of the disease [4, 8, 11, 20, 23, 28]. In the two homogenous series with completely dislocated hips, the most severe type of CHD that we are aware of has reported: a 25% failure rate in a group of 87 patients at an average follow-up of 10 years [17], and a 14.7% failure rate in a smaller group of 28 patients (34 hips) at an average follow-up of 9.4 years [1]. In the present authors' experience (1998) based on 84 hips in 67 patients, all with high dislocation who underwent THA during the years 1976-1994, 73 (87%) survived an average of 7.1 years (range, 2 to 20 years) postoperatively *(fig 13A, B)*. As a result of the operation, leg length increased by a mean of 3.5 cm (range, 1 to 7 cm). It has been suggested [8] that leg lengthening of more than 2 cm should be

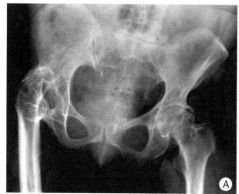
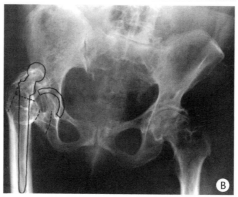
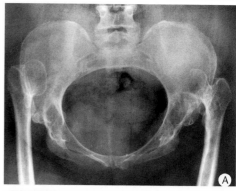
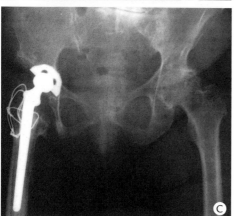
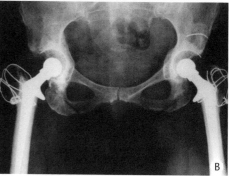

12 *A 61 year old woman who had a right high dislocation hip fused at the level of the false acetabulum at the age of 14. For fusion, an extra-articular Britain's ischiofemoral technique was used. The right hip had a 40° flexion and 30° adduction deformity. The left hip and both knees presented with severe arthritic changes.*
A. Anteroposterior radiograph of the pelvis.
B. Preoperative planning for THA. The dotted lines indicate the level of the osteotomies.
C. Two years following the conversion of the arthrodesis to THA. The ischiofemoral bar was resected and a 40 mm metal-backed acetabular component was placed at the level of the true acetabulum. A CDH cemented straight Charnley femoral component was implanted in the femur.

13 *Anteroposterior radiographs of the pelvis of a forty-seven year old woman who had bilateral high dislocation of the hip.*
A. Preoperative radiograph.
B. Nine years after bilateral total hip arthroplasty with offset-bore acetabular components inserted after cotyloplasty and Harris CDH stems. The length of the right lower limb increased from 71 to 75 cm and that of the left limb from 70 to 75 cm. The patient's height increased from 152 to 155 cm.

Table I. – Results of THA in patients with congenital hip disease.

Year	Authors	No of Hips	CHD type	Follow-up	Failure rate
1975	Tronzo et al	21	Cong. Subluxation and Dislocation	8m - 2yrs	9.5 %
1977	Harris et al	13	Trauma, cong. Dysplasia and cong. Dislocation	13m - 40m	7.7 %
1979	Crowe et al	31	Severe Dysplasia and Dislocation	2 - 6yrs	9.7 %
1991	Garvin et al	23	Severe Dysplasia and Dislocation	8 - 16.5yrs	26.0 %
1991	Kavanaugh et al	87	Complete Dislocation	5 - 16yrs	25.0 %
1993	Paavilainen et al	67	Severe Dysplasia and Dislocation	3 - 5yrs	44.8 %
1993	Anwar et al	34	Cong. Dislocation	5.6 - 14yrs	14.7 %
1995	Morscher	71	Dysplasia and Dislocation	1 - 9yrs	12.7 %
1998	Hartofilakidis et al	84	High Dislocation	2 - 20yrs	13.0 %

avoided, mainly because of the danger of neurological complications. However, in the 13 cases in our series where lengthening surpassed 5 cm (range, 5 to 7 cm), no neurological complications were observed. In the two cases of neurapraxia, the lengthening we achieved was 3 and 3.5 cm and both patients fully recovered. Therefore, the lengthening technique at the level of the neck of the femur may be considered safe.

Conclusion

A thorough understanding of anatomical abnormalities and the use of appropriate reconstruction techniques and implants make THA feasible in such complex cases of CHD. The three major areas of difficulty encountered, especially when a low or high dislocation hip is treated with total hip arthroplasty, are acetabular reconstruction, preparation of the femoral canal and reduction of the components. The complications are minimal and can be avoided with appropriate surgical techniques.

References

[1] Anwar MM, Sugano N, Masuhara K, Kadowaki T, Takaoka K, Ono K. Total hip arthroplasty in neglected congenital dislocation of the hip. *Clin Orthop* 1993 ; 295 : 127-134

[2] Charnley J. Low Friction Arthroplasy of the Hip. Theory and practice. Berlin : Spinger Verlag, 1979

[3] Charnley J, Feagin JA. Low friction arthroplasty in congenital subluxation of the hip. *Clin Orthop* 1973 ; 91 : 98-113

[4] Crowe JF, Mani VJ, Ranawat CS. Total hip replacement in congenital dislocation and dysplasia of the hip. *J Bone Joint Surg Am* 1979 ; 61 : 15-23

[5] Dunn HK, Hess WE. Total hip reconstruction in chronically dislocated hips. *J Bone Joint Surg Am* 1976 ; 58 : 835-845

[6] Eftekhar NS. Variations in technique and specific considerations. In : Eftekhar NS ed. Principles of Total Hip Arthroplasty. St Louis : CV Mosby, 1978 : 1-440

[7] Eftekhar NS. Congenital dysplasia and dislocation. In : Eftekhar NS ed. Total Hip Arthroplasty. St Louis : CV Mosby, 1993 : 1-925

[8] Garvin KL, Bowen MK, Salvati EA, Ranawat CS. Long-term results of total hip arthroplasty in congenital dislocation and dysplasia of the hip: a follow-up note. *J Bone Joint Surg Am* 1991 ; 73 : 1348-1354

[9] Goldberg VM, Stevenson S. The biology of bone grafts. *Semin Arthropl* 1993 ; 4 : 58-63

[10] Harris WH. Management of the deficient acetabulum using cementless fixation without bone grafting. *Orthop Clin North Am* 1993 ; 24 : 663-665

[11] Harris WH, Grothers O, Oh J. Total hip replacement and femoral head grafting for severe acetabular deficiency in adults. *J Bone Joint Surg Am* 1977 ; 59 : 752-759

[12] Hartofilakidis G, Stamos K, Ioannidis TT. Low friction arthroplasty for old untreated congenital dislocation of the hip. *J Bone Joint Surg Br* 1988 ; 70 : 182-186

[13] Hartofilakidis G, Stamos K, Karachalios TH. Treatment of high dislocation of the hip in adults with total hip arthroplasty. *J Bone Joint Surg Am* 1998 ; 80 : 510-517

[14] Hartofilakidis G, Stamos K, Karachalios TH, Ioannidis TT, Zacharakis N. Congenital hip disease in adult life. Classification of acetabular deficiencies and surgical management using acetabuloplasty (cotyloplasty) combined with total hip arthroplasty. *J Bone Joint Surg Am* 1996 ; 78 : 683-692

[15] Ioannidis TT, Zacharakis N, Magnissalis E, Eliades G, Hartofilakidis G. Long-term behavior of the Charnley offset-bore acetabular cup. *J Bone Joint Surg Br* 1998 ; 80 : 48-53

[16] Karachalios TH, Hartofilakidis G, Zacharakis N, Tsekoura M. A 12-18 year radiographic follow-up study of Charnley low friction arthroplasty. The role of the center of rotation. *Clin Orthop* 1993 ; 296 : 140-147

[17] Kavanaugh BF, Shaughnessey WF, Fitzgerald RH. Congenital dislocation of the hip. In : Morrey BF ed. Joint Replacement Arthroplasty. London : Churchill Livingstone, 1991 : 745-747

[18] Kerboull M. Arthroplastie totale de hanche sur luxation congénitale. *Encycl Méd Chir* (Elsevier, Paris), Techniques chirurgicales-Orthopedie-Traumatologie, 44-665-B, 1996

[19] Klisic PJ. Congenital dislocation of the hip. *J Bone Joint Surg Br* 1989 ; 71 : 136

[20] Morscher EW. Total hip replacement for osteoarthritis in congenital hip dysplasia. *Eur Instruct Course Lecture* 1995 ; 2 : 1-8

[21] Mulroy RD, Harris WH. Failure of acetabular autogenous grafts in total hip arthroplasty. Increasing incidence: a follow-up note. *J Bone Joint Surg Am* 1990 ; 72 : 1536-1540

[22] Paavilainen T, Hoika V, Paavilainen P. Cementless total arthroplasty for congenital dislocated or dysplastic hips. *Clin Orthop* 1993 ; 297 : 71-81

[23] Paavilainen T, Hoika V, Salonen KA. Cementless total replacement for severely dysplastic or dislocated hips. *J Bone Joint Surg Br* 1990 ; 72 : 205-211

[24] Pagnano WM, Hansen DA, Shaughnessy WF. Developmental hip dysplasia. In : Morrey BF ED Reconstructive Surgery of the Joints. New York : Churchill Livingstone, 1996 : 1013-1026

[25] Papagelopoulos PJ, Trousdale RT, Lewallen DG. Total hip arthroplasty with femoral osteotomy for proximal femoral deformity. *Clin Orthop* 1996 ; 332 : 151-162

[26] Russotti G, Harris W. Proximal placement of the acetabular component in total hip arthroplasty. *J Bone Joint Surg Am* 1991 ; 73 : 587-592

[27] Symeonidis PP, Pournaras J, Petsatodes G, Christoforides J, Hatzokos I, Pantazis E. Total hip arthroplasty in neglected congenital dislocation of the hip. *Clin Orthop* 1997 ; 341 : 55-61

[28] Tronzo RG, Okin EM. Anatomic restoration of congenital hip dysplasia in adulthood by total hip replacement. *Clin Orthop* 1975 ; 106 : 94-98

[29] Wedge JH, Wasylenko MJ. The natural history of congenital disease of the hip. *J Bone Joint Surg Br* 1979 ; 61 : 334-338

Total hip arthroplasty for ankylosed hips

M Kerboull
L Kerboull
M Hamadouche

Abstract. – Conversion of an ankylosed hip to total hip replacement may be technically difficult due to major local distortions. The simple wish to recover a mobile hip rarely leads to this procedure for a fused hip. It is more often motivated by its painful consequences on the lower back and ipsilateral knee, which are particularly marked in cases where the position of the hip is poor. To achieve a mobile and stable hip, two factors are essential: the hip abductor muscles must be in fair condition and the restoration of hip bio-mechanics must be anatomical, with a proper abductor lever arm ratio and correction of limb length discrepancy. Therefore, in order to carry out the conversion procedure properly, careful preoperative templating, using the contralateral normal hip as a reference, is mandatory. This will help to cope with the multiple technical difficulties, to determine the hip rotation centre and the abductor offset, and to select the femoral implant which will reduce the leg length discrepancy as well as possible. This conversion frequently leads to a pain-free and mobile hip, but normal gait and walking ability are less often achieved. However, even if there is a persistent limp, requiring a cane for distance walking, the patient always enjoys relief from back and knee pain, and especially being able to sit comfortably.

Keywords: hip, total hip arthroplasty, total hip replacement, ankylosis, arthrodesis.

Conversion of an ankylosed hip to a total hip replacement may be technically difficult, due to major local distortions related to many factors. It is necessary to take into consideration: the primary disease, the location and position of the fused hip, the way the ankylosis has been obtained, the duration of the ankylosis, and its consequences on periarticular muscles, body balance, the lower back and the ipsilateral knee.

Anatomical disorders due to ankylosis

The fused hip may be in the right place, but more often it is in a high position and sometimes in pelvic protrusion. Iliofemoral ankylosis resulting from extra-articular as well as intra-articular arthrodesis may be associated with iliotrochanteric or ischiofemoral bony bridges, intertrochanteric valgus osteotomy, and sometimes a femoral angulation due to a subtrochanteric osteotomy performed to correct the poor

Marcel Kerboull, M.D.
L Kerboull, M.D.
M Hamadouche, M.D.
Service de chirurgie orthopédique A, Hôpital Cochin, Pavillon Olier,
27, rue du Faubourg Saint-Jacques, 75674 Paris cedex 14, France.

position of the hip. The device used for arthrodesis fixation may still be in place. Its removal at the beginning of the procedure may be very difficult.

Periarticular muscles are always changed. In the best case, when ankylosis has resulted from simple cast immobilisation without any surgical procedure, they are all present and continuous, but they are atrophied, pale pink, extremely weak and flimsy due to long-standing inactivity. When ankylosis results from an arthrodesis, and sometimes after the failure of a first attempt or after the failure of a previous arthroplasty, not only are some muscles atrophied (especially the gluteus muscles), but some may also have been destroyed by surgery and replaced by fibrous tissue. The gluteus muscles may even be completely interrupted in two cases: when they have been totally destroyed or when they were not reattached to the greater trochanter.

The skin may have retained the marks of the primary disease and previous surgical procedures, such as scars of sinuses, depressed and adherent to bone, and multiple incision scars. Moreover, if the hip has fused in early childhood, ankylosis is frequently in a poor position, associated with a global hypotrophy of the lower limb, a real limb length discrepancy and a severe distortion of the ipsilateral knee with

epiphyseal growth troubles, varus or valgus deformity, chronic rotatory laxity and secondary degenerative changes.

Operative indications

Two complaints generally lead to mobilise a fused hip. It is rarely the simple wish to recover a mobile hip, but more often its painful consequences on the lower back and ipsilateral knee due to progressive arthritis [1, 2, 3, 5]. This process is all the more frequent when ankylosis is in a poor position and of long duration. Mobilisation of the hip is more justified in such cases and may achieve impressive functional improvement. Yet, the expected pain relief may be only partial if arthritic lesions are advanced, and if the hip remains stiff and becomes unstable after conversion. Even in this case, however, the patient always enjoys being able to sit comfortably. Nevertheless, to prevent disappointment on the part of the patient, it is advisable to try to anticipate the functional result of total hip replacement.

To achieve a mobile and stable hip, two factors are essential: the hip abductor muscles must be in fair condition and the restoration of hip bio-mechanics must be anatomical, with a proper abductor lever arm ratio and correction of limb length discrepancy [2, 5]. Assessment of the value of muscles around a long-standing fused hip is difficult. Electromyography has been demonstrated to be of little value; only careful and repeated digital palpation allows proper assessment of the anatomical and functional value of the muscles. Absence of scars means that all the muscles are present and continuous, even if they are atrophied and do not appear contractile at first examination. Six months later, after repeated isometric contraction exercises, their existence and activity can be felt. On the other hand, multiple previous operations with numerous skin scars, a bulky metallic device still in place, and a major anatomical distortion raise serious doubts as to the integrity and quality of the residual gluteus muscles. However, if most of the muscles are present and continuous, even though extremely thin, pale and fragile, and if the technical procedure has preserved them intact, they will gradually regain mass and strength. They will then be able to provide the hip with the correct functional stability, 3 to 12 months postoperatively. This stability will be achieved more rapidly if the artificial joint is reconstructed in an anatomical position and normal bio-mechanics are restored with a proper abductor moment arm [2, 5].

It is also difficult to anticipate the benefits that the lower back and knee will gain from the conversion. In general, there will be good knee improvement for a valgus knee beneath a hip ankylosed in abduction, for a varus knee beneath a hip ankylosed in adduction, for the patella beneath a hip in excessive flexion. However, for this to occur, the hip must become stable and its previous poor position must be totally corrected. In the absence of multiple and advanced arthritic lesions responsible for specific symptoms, the conversion may afford the lumbar spine great relief [1, 2, 3, 5]. This occurs when back pain is due to the over-stress of the lower back in hyperlordosis (ankylosis in excessive flexion). It also occurs when there is a frontal curve compensating pelvic obliquity, due to a hip fused in frontal malpositon. Even if stability of the hip is not perfect, the lumbar spine will be relieved from rotatory and sagittal stresses.

The functional improvement of the lumbar spine and knee afforded by the conversion of an ankylosed hip in the correct position to a total hip replacement may be of lesser value. Pain in a varus knee may even increase after arthroplasty, if the hip is unstable and has a positive Trendelenburg. As for the lumbar spine, pain relief may be partial if there is a definitive limp. At each step, the drop of the hip is compensated by a bend of the spine. Even if sagittal stresses decrease, the new frontal stresses may result in less relief of pain than expected from the hip mobilisation.

Therefore, relief of lower back and knee pain, the purpose of the operation, may not be obtained in every case. Careful consideration must be given before deciding to break ankylosis, as this decision may result in disappointment, especially if the ankylosis is in a correct position and surrounded by weak and changed muscles.

Preparation of the surgical procedure

Several X-rays and preoperative planning are required for the correct execution of the conversion. AP pelvic and hip views are usefully completed by an oblique obturator view that shows the greater trochanter, which is invisible on the AP view, and an oblique iliac view which opens the ischiofemoral space. It may show a bony bridge hidden on a AP view by superposition of femur and ischiatic bone (*fig 1*). A lateral view of the hip and femur is indispensable to assess the curve of the bone and show a major angulation unsuspected on the AP view. A large AP X-ray of the pelvis and lower limbs gives a precise idea of the general balance of the patient in the standing position, and also shows the global and segmentary lengths of the lower limbs and frontal deformity of the knees. With the patient in the standing position, X-rays of the lumbar spine (AP and lateral views, in spontaneous and extreme positions) show a possible lower back distortion and the possibilities of correction.

Templates of prosthesis components assist the pre-operative planning to determine the implantation position of the acetabular component, the osteotomy level and direction, and the type and implantation level of the femoral component.

The position of the socket is provided by superposition of the appropriate socket template (chosen according to the size of a healthy acetabulum) on the AP hip X-rays. To place the socket into the original acetabulum cavity, it should be leaned against the internal wall of the fovea, tilted at 45°, with its inferior margin at the tear drop level. In this anatomical position, the opening plane of the acetabular component determines the level of the osteotomy which will be done parallel to it, a few millimetres more laterally. The implantation level of the femoral component allows a proper estimation of the desirable lengthening of the limb based on the data obtained from X-rays of the lumbar spine, pelvis and lower limbs (*fig 2*).

Surgical procedure

Only the steps of total hip replacement on an ankylosed hip are described below [4].

1) The patient is placed in a **lateral decubitus position**, with the pelvis caught in a pelvic vice, the lower limb lying horizontally, knee slightly flexed, on two supports, one under the knee, the second under the foot.

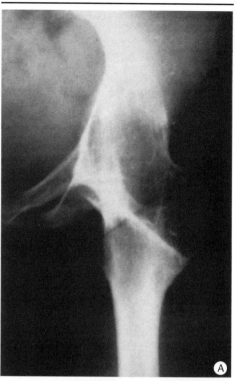
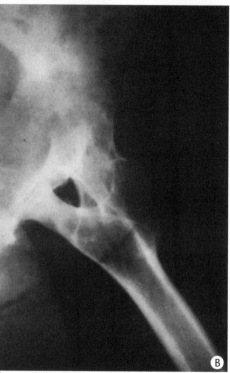

1 A. Ankylosis of the hip associated with an intertrochanteric valgus osteotomy.
B. The ischiofemoral bony bridge, hardly visible on the AP X-rays, clearly appears on the oblique iliac view.

2) The **skin incision** is lateral, centred on the greater trochanter, its inferior half straight and median, its superior half curved to the rear to follow the direction of the gluteus maximus fibres. Usually, there is a scar from a previous incision. It may be reused, and if necessary excised and lengthened, if it is not too far from the ideal site. After subcutaneous separation, the lateral approach is continued by incision of the fascia lata and discission of the gluteus

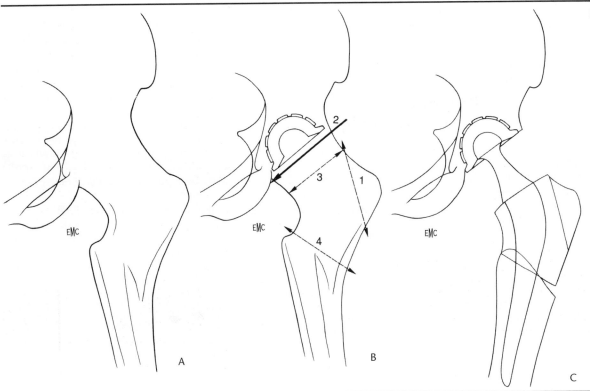

2 A. Ankylosis of the hip with a subtrochanteric femoral angulation.
B. Socket template in an anatomical position. The four femoral osteotomies: 1. Trochanteric osteotomy; 2. neck osteotomy; 3. base of femoral component implantation; 4. alignment osteotomy of the femur.
C. Anatomical result expected from a THR.

maximus fibres. They frequently adhere to the gluteus medius. This separation should be done with great care to avoid any muscular damage.

3) **Dissection of the trochanteric region.** Sometimes, dense fibrous scar tissue around the trochanter makes the dissection difficult and it is necessary to separate the anatomical elements with a scalpel. The shape and location of the trochanter itself may have been modified. Frequently, it is posterior, especially when the femur has an excessive anteversion or when the hip has fused in external rotation and anterior subluxation. It may sit astride the posterior part of the joint, as a pedicle graft, secured there with a pin or a screw. It may be located high, nonunited, hung on a contracted and fibrous gluteus medius, hiding the superior part of a cobra plate used to secure the femur to the iliac bone. It may be in a normal position, but drilled by 2 or 3 large screws (6 or 7 mm in diameter) of cobalt chrome alloy or stainless steel. Their removal is required before progressing and may prove difficult, even with the appropriate screw driver. Some cobalt chrome screws with a countersunk head and a slight linear print cannot be unscrewed and must be removed with a trephine. Sometimes, the trochanter is bare, if the gluteus medius has been destroyed by a previous operation or not reinserted on the trochanter. These are very annoying findings, because it may actually be impossible to restore a continuous muscular fan. It may even be necessary to stop the operation at this stage and give up the conversion to a total hip arthroplasty. Before osteotomising the trochanter, it is advisable to identify the anterior and posterior edges of the gluteus fan.

Frequently, dense sclerotic scar tissue includes the anterior edge of the gluteus medius and minimus, fascia lata and proximal insertions of the vastus lateralis. In this case, the different anatomical elements should be isolated and the space between the vastus lateralis and gluteus minimus opened. In the rear, the posterior edge of the trochanter, its posterosuperior corner and its muscular insertions must be identified, and the location of the sciatic nerve checked.

4) **Osteotomy of the trochanter.** This is usually done with a wide osteotome (20 mm). A plane section detaches a bony fragment on which are inserted all the gluteus and external rotator muscles except the quadratus femoris. This muscular fan is carefully elevated with a retractor and released from the capsule with a scalpel. Sometimes a bony iliotrochanteric bridge inside the muscles prevents its lifting. It is then necessary to isolate the insertion of the graft on the trochanter through the muscles and to cut it at this level with an osteotome. However, this risks damaging the trochanteric muscular insertions. After trochanteric osteotomy, it is also possible to cut the graft with a curved osteotome on its deep face; after reversing the trochanter and the muscles, the distal part of the graft is cut from the trochanter with an oscillating saw and the proximal part from the iliac wing with an osteotome *(fig 3)*.

5) **Exposure and section of the ankylosis.** Trochanter and muscular mass are kept elevated using 2 or 3 round-headed Steinmann pins. The articular capsule (which is sometimes thick, but more often thin but adherent to femoral head and neck) is removed. This excision widely exposes the fusion line between the femoral head and

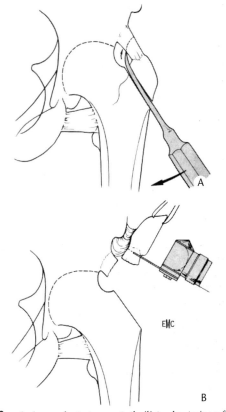

3 A. A curved osteotome cuts the iliotrochanteric graft through the trochanteric osteotomy focus.
B. After trochanter and muscle reversion, the bridge fragments are removed. Section with an oscillating saw of the trochanteric fragment close to its implantation.

the acetabulum. One should take care not to break the ankylosis at this level with convex and concave gouges, for this level is usually too high. This might result in digging a cavity which is too wide, not deep enough and too highly located. An acetabular

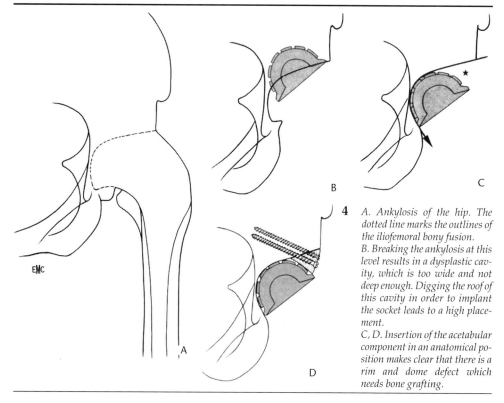

4 *A. Ankylosis of the hip. The dotted line marks the outlines of the iliofemoral bony fusion.*
B. Breaking the ankylosis at this level results in a dysplastic cavity, which is too wide and not deep enough. Digging the roof of this cavity in order to implant the socket leads to a high placement.
C, D. Insertion of the acetabular component in an anatomical position makes clear that there is a rim and dome defect which needs bone grafting.

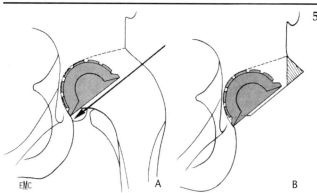

5 *The same case as figure 4.*
A. Socket template in anatomical position. The arrow indicates the level and direction of the osteotomy.
B. The acetabular bony cavity, in the right position, completely contains the socket. The superolateral excess bone is simply excised (hatched area).

of the socket should be tangent to the inferior margin of the acetabular fovea and the base of the iliopubic branch. This ensures that the socket faces 40-45° caudally and 15° anteriorly, whatever the position of the patient on the operating table. Then, the bone exceeding the opening plane of the socket is excised with a curved osteotome. After two anchoring holes have been bored into the pubic and ischiatic bones, the acetabular component is cemented. It is advisable not to weaken the roof of the cavity by boring a third hole. Sometimes the dome bone is so fragile that it needs to be strengthened with impacted bone fragments removed from the femoral head when preparing the cavity. In certain cases, it may be safer to rigidify this cavity by a metallic armature with an inferior hook inserted beneath the tear drop and a superior plate screwed to iliac bone. Some authors recommend the use of a cementless acetabular component.

7) Femoral preparation. This may be very simple. After marking the appropriate level of the neck section, based on the preoperative planning and a bony landmark, this section is carried out with an oscillating saw. Preparation of the femoral canal is started with a curette to obtain some cancellous fragments to be used to fill the medullary canal beneath the prosthesis tip, and finished with a cylindrical reamer so that the selected component will fit. The component is oriented at 10° anteversion, after a slight alteration of the cervical orifice if necessary.

Before cementing the femoral component, it is always necessary to check that reduction is possible, as well as that the trochanter can be put back into contact with its femoral base, as soon as limb lengthening due to arthroplasty reaches 2 centimetres. If the trochanter does not come into contact, even at 20° abduction, this might be because scar tissue at the deep side of the gluteus prevents it from being lowered. Excision of this fibrous tissue, associated with release of the lower part of the muscle from the iliac wing, allows 10 to 15 mm lengthening. If that is not enough, there is no other solution but femoral neck shortening. This shortening may also be imposed by the fact that it is impossible to reduce. The attempt to reduce should always be done by a direct push on the prosthesis with the limb in the adduction position, and not by traction on the limb. Indeed, traction on the limb tilts the pelvis and abducts the hip, which makes the reduction impossible if the hip is somewhat tight. After checking that reduction is possible and that the trochanter can be reattached with adequate bony contact, the metal wires for trochanter cerclage are run through a hole drilled in the lateral cortex. Bone cement is then introduced and the prosthesis inserted into the medullary canal. When the polymethyl methacrylate has completely set, the hip is reduced.

component implanted in such a cavity would be in a high position. If implanted in an anatomical position, there would be a superior acetabular defect of the dome and rim requiring bone grafting (fig 4). On the contrary, one should mark the place and orientation of the section plane on the femoral neck, as defined during peroperative planning (fig 5). However, before carrying out this section with an osteotome or an oscillating saw, the greatest care must be taken to protect the anterior and posterior soft tissues with two Hohmann retractors. One should also make sure that there is no ischiofemoral bony bridge. If there is, this graft is usually located beneath the quadratus femoris, which must be released from the femur to expose it. Then, the sciatic nerve being protected, the ischiofemoral bridge is cut with a curved osteotome (fig 6).

The section of the femoral neck is then performed with an osteotome or an ocillating saw (fig 7). Putting the lower limb in flexion, adduction and external rotation gives access to the inferior and medial part of the capsule (which is excised as well as the scar tissue) and to the obturator foramen. A Hohmann retractor slipped beneath its superior edge pushes the femur downwards and improves the view of the acetabulum, which is still filled with the femoral head united with iliac bone.

6) Preparation of the acetabular cavity. The first and main landmark is the superior edge of the obturator foramen. It is usually obscured with bone and fibrous tissue which should be carefully removed until the smooth cortical inferior margin of the acetabulum is exposed. When ankylosis has resulted from simple casting or extra-articular arthrodesis, the transverse acetabular ligament is present, marking the lower entrance of the acetabular fovea, and inside it are the remnants of the ligamentum teres and the fatty pad. From this landmark, which can always be identified, the acetabular cavity is progressively dug out with a gouge, rather than a reamer, until it has the adequate size for the selected acetabular component (fig 8). A trial socket is then introduced into this cavity with the proper orientation. If the cavity is prepared in an anatomical position, the opening plane

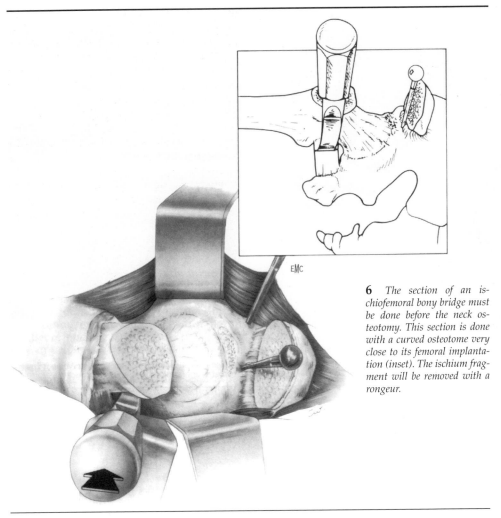

preparation of the bed of the prosthesis may be difficult. On the other hand, a three-dimensional angulation due to a previous subtrochanteric or diaphyseal osteotomy, carried out to correct a malposition of the fused hip, requires an alignment osteotomy. This is done at the tip of angulation according to the preoperative planning. It may be a simple or more complex transverse osteotomy. In any case, after the femoral stem has aligned proximal and distal fragments, the section must always be "touched up" to obtain accurate congruency and perfect bony contact. Cementing the femoral component (usually a long stem) assures strong fixation of this osteotomy, but it is advisable to surround the junction with autologous cancellous graft (from the femoral head) to hasten the bone fusion.

6 *The section of an is-chiofemoral bony bridge must be done before the neck os-teotomy. This section is done with a curved osteotome very close to its femoral implanta-tion (inset). The ischium frag-ment will be removed with a rongeur.*

8) Trochanter reattachment and closure.
After hip reduction, the lower limb rests on its supports, hip and knee in slight flexion. To restore the balance of the gluteus muscles, reattachment of the trochanter is done on a femur in the correct position if ankylosis was in the correct position; in other cases, it must be given a position opposite to the malposition of the fused hip (adduction for an abducted hip, abduction for an adducted hip, external rotation for a malposition in internal rotation, internal rotation for a malposition in external rotation). This sometimes leads to reattaching the trochanter elsewhere than its femoral bed, after preparation of a new bony laying.

After reinsertion of the vastus lateralis, the musculo-aponeurotic plane is closed over two suction drains, the subcutaneous cellular tissue and skin over a third. Then, a first dressing is applied, completed by a compression bandage spica.

Postoperative care

The patient lays free in his bed, knees slightly flexed and feet raised. The spica is removed on the first postoperative day and suction drains on the third. The patient gets up on the third day.

As soon as the operation is finished, the patient is encouraged to move foot and knee. The day after operation, passive manual mobilisation of the hip is started. On the third day, passive instrumental mobilisation is begun, using a simple installation made of a strap running under the knee, a cord, a grooved pulley and a handle. By traction on the handle, the patient slowly and painlessly moves his joint, gradually increasing its motion. Modern apparatuses for passive mobilisation may be used, but do not any better. Passive motion must be continued until active muscular contraction recovers enough strength to move the hip and take over from passive mobilisation.

The length of this phase of relative muscular impotence will depend on the patient and

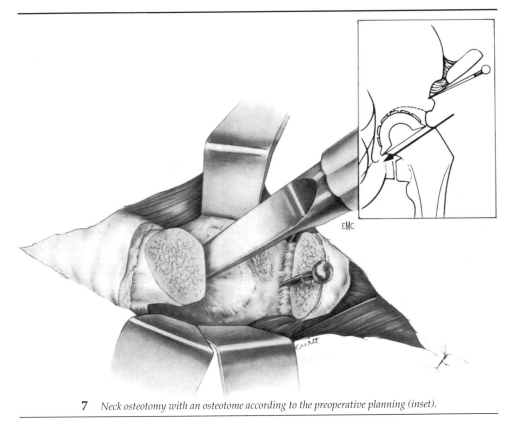

7 *Neck osteotomy with an osteotome according to the preoperative planning (inset).*

Femoral angulation due to a previous osteotomy can seriously complicate implantation of a femoral component.

However, if the osteotomy was intertrochan-teric, a new osteotomy is never necessary, even if a cortical graft crosses the callus, but

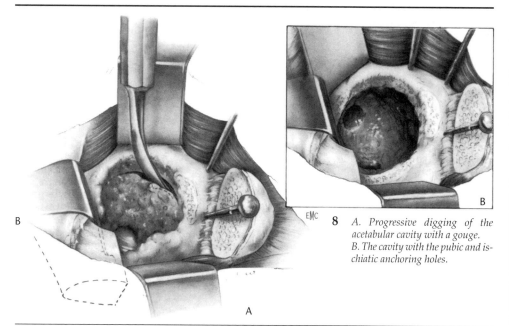

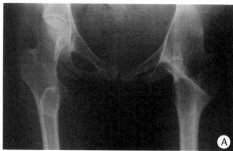

8 *A. Progressive digging of the acetabular cavity with a gouge. B. The cavity with the pubic and ischiatic anchoring holes.*

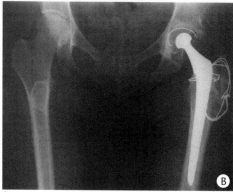

9 *The same case as figure 1. A. Before THR. B. Eight years postoperatively.*

the quality of the periarticular muscles (from a few days to 3 or 4 weeks). Recovery of motion is also variable. Usually patients easily and quickly recover 30° of frontal and rotational motion. Flexion motion may be harder to increase, especially when the hip was fused in a full extension position. The work of the physiotherapist and the patient must aim at increasing flexion. Numerous patients reach 90° at six weeks and finally will obtain 100° or 120°. Others will hardly reach 60°, without finding a satisfactory objective explanation for this stiffness in some cases.

Stability of the hip in a weight-bearing position improves gradually as abductor strength increases. Walking between two crutches with partial weight-bearing is allowed from the third day and continued until the sixth week when the trochanter has united. At this time, many patients are able to walk with a simple cane. The weight-bearing hip stability is rarely perfect before the fourth month. Some patients will take 6 to 8 months to walk without support and limping. Others will always need a cane due to a persistent limp (positive or negative Trendelenburg).

Medication is systematically used unless there is a specific contraindication. Prophylactic antibiotherapy starts with anaesthesia and continues for 3 or 4 days. In cases of tuberculosis sequelae, it is associated with specific antibiotherapy for 3 to 4 months. Anticoagulation therapy lasts 4 to 6 weeks. Anti-inflammatory treatment, using non-steroidal anti-inflammatory drugs, begins with the operation and continues 10 days. It seems to be of particular benefit for these patients; because it reduces pain and decreases the inflammatory reaction of early cicatrisation, it helps the patient to move the joint. Moreover, it substantially inhibits the development of heterotopic ossifications *(fig 9)*.

Results

The results of conversion of an ankylosed hip to total hip replacement according to this technique were evaluated in a series of 45 total hip arthroplasties in 45 patients, performed by one surgeon from 1969 to 1993 and reviewed with a mean follow-up of 8.5

years (5 to 20 years) [2]. Hip function was considered excellent or good for 91%. In 95% of the cases, the hips were pain-free and the mean arc of hip flexion was 88°. Fifty-one percent had normal gait and walking ability, whereas 35% had a slight limp but did not use a cane, and 13% had a marked limp and required a cane. The stability of the hip in the standing position was correlated with the state of the gluteus musculature assessed intra-operatively. The residual leg length discrepancy was an average 1.1 cm. Postoperatively, one operation was complicated by a transient peroneal nerve palsy, and one reactivation of tuberculosis occurred in a patient who had not had specific prophylaxis.

The main reports [1, 3, 5-7] published on long-term results of total hip arthroplasty on ankylosed hips are listed in table I and table II.

Table I. – Some long-term clinical results of total hip replacements for ankylosed hips.

Authors	Hips	Mean FU (yr)	Exc. + good clinical results %	Relief of back pain %	Relief of knee pain %	Walking no support %	Mean hip flexion	Residual leg length discrepancy (cm)
Hardinge et al [3]	112	8.2		80				2.4
Kilgus et al [5]	41	7	78	80	66	17	87	1.4
Reikeras et al [6]	55	7	63			21		
Stathy and Fitzgerald [7]	80	10.4	45			45		
Arlaud et al [1]	62	4.5		76	35	42	78	1.14

Table II. – The same reports. Complications and radiological results.

Authors	Hips	Complications	X-ray loose	Revisions
Hardinge et al [3]	112	2 infections, 11 nerve palsies	15	6
Kilgus et al [5]	41	3 infections, 2 dislocations, 1 nerve palsy	5	5
Reikeras et al [6]	55			7
Stathy and Fitzgerald [7]	80	9 infections, 1 dislocation	11	21
Arlaud et al [1]	62	2 infections, 4 dislocations, 3 femoral fractures; 6 heterotopic ossifications	3	9

References

[1] Arlaud JY, Legré G, Aubaniac JM. Arthroplastie de hanche après fusion osseuse. *Rev Chir Orthop* 1990 ; 76 : 411-419

[2] Hamadouche M, Kerboull L, Meunier L, Courpied JP, Kerboull M. Total hip arthroplasty for ankylosed hips. A five to twenty year follow-up study. *J Bone Joint Surg* 2000 (in press)

[3] Hardinge K, Murphy JC, Frenyo S. Conversion of hip fusion to Charnley low friction arthroplasty. *Clin Orthop* 1986 ; 211 : 173-179

[4] Kerboull M. Arthroplastie totale de hanche sur ankylose. *Encycl Méd Chir* (Éditions Scientifiques et Médicales Elsevier SAS, Paris), Techniques chirurgicales, Orthopédie, Traumatologie, 44-665-C, 1994 : 1-9

[5] Kilgus DJ, Amstutz HC, Wolgin MA, Dorey FJ. Joint replacement for ankylosed hips. *J Bone Joint Surg Am* 1990 ; 72 : 45-54

[6] Reikeras O, Bjerkreim L, Gundersson R. Total hip arthroplasty for arthrodesed hips: 5 to 13 year results. *J Arthroplasty* 1995 ; 10 : 529-531

[7] Stathy GM, Fitzgerard RJ. Total hip arthroplasty in the ankylosed hips. A ten-year follow-up. *J Bone Joint Surg Am* 1988 ; 70 : 963-966

Classification and treatment methods of acetabular deficiencies

EW Morscher
R Elke
B Berli

Abstract. – The management of acetabular deficiencies presents four major problems: replacement of the lost bone stock, restoration of the centre of rotation in the original acetabulum, stable fixation of the new acetabular cup and restoration of leg length.

The operative method selected for revision depends on the type of deficiency. Basically, we differentiate between two forms of deficiency and, therefore, two procedures: 1) cavity and rim supportive defects, and 2) segmental and rim non-supportive defects.

In cavity defects, the cortical acetabular rim is preserved and is thus supportive. In segmental deficiencies, the acetabular rim and the peripheral zones (1 and/or 3 according to DeLee and Charnley [6]) are non-supportive. Consequently, there must be substitution for their mechanical function as force-transmitting structures.

In Type 1 acetabular deficiencies (rim supportive cavity or cystic defect), a close peripheral contact of a cementless hemispherical press-fit cup can be achieved with a well-vascularised autochthonous pelvic bone. Morsellised homologous bone grafts should be used for filling of contained cysts only, and should not be exposed to weight-bearing.

In Type 2 non-contained and rim non-supportive acetabular deficiencies where segmental defects, large cavities and a non-spherical shape of the acetabulum do not allow firm fixation of a new cup by intrinsic press-fit, acetabular reinforcement rings (ARR) are recommended. The acetabulum is reconstructed with morsellised allografts which are impacted with a spherical (non-perforated) trial cup. These grafts must then be protected from loading with a reinforcement ring which is fixed to the original host bone of the pelvis by 3 - 5 ASIF (Association for the Study of Internal Fixation) cancellous screws. An all-polyethylene cup of corresponding size is then cemented into the support ring.

From 1988 to 1997 (10 years), 456 acetabular revisions have been performed at the Orthopaedic Department of the University of Basel, 255 with the author's "Press-Fit Cup". 201 acetabular deficiencies with segmental rim non-supportive defects have been provided with a Burch-Schneider or Ganz acetabular reinforcement ring. Of these 456 revisions, 26 had to be re-revised (5.7%): 19 for loosening of the stem (4.2%), and 7 for loosening of the socket (1.5%). Five were reinforcement rings (2.5%) and 2 were press-fit cups (0.8%), both for dislocation, none for aseptic re-loosening!

Keywords: hip, total hip replacement, revision, acetabular revision, acetabular deficiencies, press-fit cup, acetabular reinforcement ring.

Introduction

About 20% of all total hip replacements are for revision. The revision rate for isolated acetabular components is about 15% [14] to 18% [24].

The goal of an acetabular revision is to restore the "normal anatomy" which is disturbed by acetabular bone deficiencies. The management of acetabular deficiencies presents four major problems: replacement of the lost bone stock, restoration of the centre of rotation in the original acetabulum and the stable fixation of the new acetabular cup. With the restoration of the centre of rotation, the leg length discrepancy is, as a rule, corrected as well.

Classification of acetabular deficiencies

The operative method selected for revision depends on the type of deficiency. Several classifications have been proposed [4, 40]. A classification should be simple, allow preoperative planning and, therefore, serve as a guideline for operative treatment. Any classification is useful only if it aids the surgeon in the management of a given situation. The current generally used classification is that of the Hip Committee of the AAOS (American Academy of Orthopaedic Surgeons), which distinguishes five categories [4] (table I). Since load transmission occurs primarily in the cortical structures of the pelvic host bone, these are also the main supportive structures for the cup. Cortical, i.e. supportive, structures are the acetabular rim, the subchondral bone and the sclerotic bone surrounding the loose cup. From a practical point of view, we differentiate between two forms of deficiency and, therefore, two procedures only: Type 1 (contained, cavity deficiency) in which the acetabular rim is preserved and is thus supportive (AAOS category II), and Type 2 (non-contained, segmental

Erwin W Morscher, Prof.
Reinhard Elke, PD Dr.
Bernhard Berli, Dr. med.
Orthopaedic Department University of Basel, Felix Platter-Hospital, Burgfelderstr. 101, CH-4012 Basel, Switzerland.

Table I. – Classification of acetabular defi-ciencies (D'Antonio et al, 1989) [4]

Type I	Segmental deficiencies
	Peripheral
	Superior
	Anterior
	Posterior
	Central (medial wall absent)
Type II	Cavitary deficiencies
	Peripheral
	Superior
	Anterior
	Posterior
	Central (medial wall absent)
Type III	Combined deficiencies
Type IV	Pelvic discontinuity
Type V	Arthrodesis

Table II. – Practice-orientated classification of bone deficiencies in acetabular revision

| Type I | Contained, cavitary, rim supportive acetabular deficiency |
| Type II | Non-contained, segmental, rim non-supportive acetabular deficiency |

deficiency) in which the acetabular rim and the peripheralzones (zones 1 and/or 3 according to DeLee and Charnley [6]) are non-supportive (AAOS categories I, III and IV [34]) (table II).

Biomechanical principles of acetabular revision

RESTORATION OF THE CENTRE OF ROTATION

Apart from restoration of the deficient bone stock, anatomical placement of the acetabular component must be one of the main goals of acetabular revision. However, aseptic loosening with superior migration makes it difficult to obtain a close contact of the implant to the pelvic host bone while maintaining a normal anatomic hip centre of rotation. Due to the oval shape of the acetabulum, it is often not possible to enlarge it without damaging the anterior and posterior containment. Based on poor mid-term results with bulk allografts or cement filling of the defect, a more superior positioning of the cup ("high hip centre") has been proposed [20, 50, 52]. A smaller cup with an outer diameter of 46 mm or even less must then be used. In order to avoid too much shortening of the leg and insufficiency of the abductor muscles, the lost length should be substituted for by a long femoral neck or at least by a distal displacement of the greater trochanter. Under no circumstances should the cup (and therefore the hip centre) be located laterally, since this causes excessive overload of the hip joint with early failure [59]. All the same, the method of positioning the acetabulum superiorly remains controversial.

REPLACEMENT OF THE LOST BONE STOCK

Deficient bone stock, whether in primary arthroplasty (protrusio, dysplasia) or in revision surgery, can be restored by various means. Re-cementing the acetabular socket has revealed disappointing results. Re-revision rates of 30 to 50% after only 4 to 8 years have been reported [9, 11, 19, 36, 42, 43, 58, 61]. Therefore, there has been a strong tendency toward non-cemented revision during the last decade.

For acetabular defects showing the above-mentioned oval shape with the long axis in the craniocaudal direction (superolateral segmental and AAOS Type III combined cavity defect), special oblong components have been constructed [22]. Our concern about using oblong components is that the centre of rotation of the component and the centre of rotation of the articulation no longer correspond, so that damaging tilting moments in the implant-bone interface occur which could finally initiate loosening of the socket. However, favourable short-term results have been experienced with oblong sockets by Köster et al [22] and DeBoer et al [5]. Most surgeons prefer a biological reconstruction [4, 10, 32, 45, 47, 51, 54]. Various bone grafting techniques have been described for acetabular reconstruction. There is no doubt that, from a biological point of view, autologous grafts are superior to homologous grafts. However, since the amount of autologous graft is limited, for practical reasons the latter are used as a rule. Allografts are harvested from fresh-frozen femoral heads of patients undergoing primary total hip replacement. Since 1985, because of the risk of contamination by acquired immunodeficiency syndrome, the allografts have been sterilised in an autoclave before deep-freezing. Some surgeons prefer irradiation [47].

Large structural bone grafts reveal good early results [15]. A high failure rate in the mid-term, however, has been observed [23, 34] due to a collapse of the bulk grafts under load, because incorporation of large structural corticocancellous grafts remains incomplete even after a long period of time [17, 27, 34]. There is general agreement nowadays that solid grafts which cover more than 50% of the weight-bearing area of the cup should be avoided [12, 51, 52].

Cancellous, morsellised allografts can support neither an acetabular component [16, 39, 62, 63] nor a bipolar prosthesis [38] over time. Our own follow-up of 121 patients with 121 acetabular revisions, with an observation time of 8.6 years (6.7 - 11.2 years), showed good results if cystic defects were grafted. However, if large cavitaries and/or segmental defects were filled with bone grafts which were exposed to weight-bearing, slow but steady cup migration and progressive graft resorption over time was observed. The thicker the layer of morsellised bone grafts, the greater the resorption and the rate of migration. In other

words, there was a continuous resorption of the grafts under load with subsequent loosening in a high percentage of cases. The survivorship analysis indicated a revision rate of 40% after a period of 10 years [16]. Although these findings correlate well with the results obtained with other methods and data reported in the literature, they can by no means be rated as satisfactory. From this experience, we concluded that morsellised bone grafts that are loaded do not guarantee a permanent inert interface, and continuous resorption of the grafts takes place over time. Morsellised allografts, therefore, should be used for filling of contained cysts only, and should not be exposed to weight-bearing. On the other hand, grafts can be protected from excessive stress by an Acetabular Reinforcement Ring (ARR). Primary stability is obtained by using multiple screws. However, the main load transfer must still occur through cortical structures at the rim of the acetabulum. Zehntner and Ganz in 1994 could show that a reconstruction of the acetabulum with a Müller ARR can only be considered as adequate if an appropriately-sized ring has been in contact on the host pelvic bone cranially, posteriorly and inferomedially [63].

Grading systems as proposed by Moskal et al [33] may provide guidelines for treatment modalities and correspond well to our own concept of the management of acetabular bone deficiency:

– Grade I: Complete prosthetic host-bone contact, no bone graft required;

– Grade II: Incomplete prosthetic host-bone contact, prosthesis stable on host-bone, filler graft may be added;

– Grade III: Incomplete prosthetic host-bone contact, prosthesis is not stable in host-bone, structural bone graft required to stabilise the prosthesis or/and the use of ARR.

In Grades I and II, corresponding to contained, rim supportive acetabular deficiencies, the use of cementless acetabular components [53], preferably hemispherical, oversized cups [10, 33], is recommended.

In Grade III, we strongly recommend not to use structural bone grafts without a supporting ring if more than 50% of the weight-bearing surface of the graft must serve as a load transmitter [59]. A high rate of failure, i.e. collapse of structural acetabular allografts, has been described [17, 18, 34, 46, 52]. The greater the extent of coverage of the acetabular component by the graft, the greater the rate of late failure [17, 34, 47, 52] (table III).

In 1979, Slooff started to reconstruct acetabular deficiencies in revision surgery with impacted morsellised cancellous allografts from a bone bank, in combination with cement fixation of the new cup [51, 55]. This technique has become a standard procedure in acetabular revisions for many orthopaedic surgeons. In animal experiments, Schimmel et al (1998) [51] could

Table III. – Results of acetabular revision of non-cemented sockets against allograft [16, 17, 38, 40, 46]

Authors	Years	N	Obs'time	Result
Pollock (et al) [46]	1992	23	2 y	30 % re-revision
Hooten (et al) [17]	1994	27	46 months	12 (44 %) unstable
Paprosky (et al) [40]	1994	6	-	100 % failure rate
Herzog (et al) [16]	1994	121	8.6 y (6.7-11.2 y)	40 % re-revision
Papagelopoulos (et al) [38]	1995	81	3-8 y	53 % re-revision

show that cemented morsellised allografts have a high capacity to incorporate. Initial cup stability is adequate to provoke graft incorporation with decreasing stability after the incorporation process has been completed. Good early results have been published from clinical practice [51, 55, 56].

Operative guidelines

REMOVAL OF THE FAILED ACETABULAR COMPONENT

The joint is approached from the original incision and the newly-formed capsule is excised. The failed socket is removed. Sometimes, even a radiologically loose acetabular component may be found to be quite difficult to remove. Well-fixed cups may need to be removed because of infection or malposition.

To remove cemented sockets, the surrounding cement mantle is fractured with curved osteotomes and gouges. Anspach and Lachiewicz developed a pneumatic impact wrench that delivers repetitive shear loads to the implant/cement or implant/bone interface [2, 24].

Hemispheric, porous-coated, metal-backed cups can also be removed without greater damage to the surrounding bone with a double curved, swan neck-like osteotome. Where the cups are additionally fixed with screws, these screws must, of course, be removed beforehand.

Then, the acetabulum is cleaned of cement, and debridement of the fibrous tissue membrane is carried out with sharp curettes, forceps and reamers. The periprosthetic sclerotic zone is reamed until bleeding spots can be seen. However, excessive reaming which leads to damage of the anterior or posterior rim must be avoided. Curettage with debridement of inflammatory tissue of cysts and subsequent bone grafting is effective. There is no risk of recurrence of the osteolytic lesion [51].

ASSESSMENT OF THE ACETABULUM

Preoperative planning of an acetabular revision may be difficult or even impossible. Current radiographic descriptions of the defects are inadequate. Plain X-rays do not allow to distinguish exactly whether the acetabular defect is contained and rim supportive or not. Robertson et al, therefore, proposed to more accurately describe

remaining bone and improve surgical planning using 3D physical models based on CT data [48]. However, the ultimate assessment of bone loss and the definitive decision about the treatment method must be made intraoperatively, as a rule. In case of an intrapelvic dislocation of an acetabular component with concern about damage of the external iliac vessels, angiography is indicated. A retroperitoneal approach to extract the cup may be considered [8, 28].

With a (preferably perforated) trial cup of the same size as the last reamer, the surgeon must check whether the rim of the acetabulum is intact and supportive, and ready for a sufficient implant-bone contact of a press-fit cup at the periphery of the acetabulum.

MANAGEMENT OF CONTAINED RIM SUPPORTIVE DEFECTS

In Type 1 acetabular deficiencies (rim supportive cavity or cystic defect), a close peripheral contact of the cup to a well-vascularised autochthonous pelvic bone can be obtained. Cysts and cavities are filled with morsellised allografts and an oversized, hemispheric, porous-coated cup [29-31] is inserted and impacted (*fig 1*).

Stability of the new cup must be achieved by containment of the cup as fully as possible, and by secure fixation, preferably by intrinsic stability [10, 29, 31]. This method is currently the one most used for the majority of acetabular Type I revisions. A high success rate similar to primary arthroplasties can be achieved with these implants (*table IV*).

MANAGEMENT OF NON-CONTAINED RIM NON-SUPPORTIVE DEFICIENCY

In superolateral rim defects with a structural corticocancellous bone graft, the original anatomy and a non-cemented cup can be fixed. However, if more than 50% of the

1 *Revision of Type 1 contained, rim-supportive acetabular deficiency with press-fit cup.*
A. W.L., 68 year old female patient with "Girdlestone" situation after removal of the infected hip endoprosthesis due to septic loosening of the right hip arthroplasty.
B. X-ray after implantation of a noncemented press-fit cup into the contained rim supportive acetabulum and implantation of a non-cemented stem.
C. Complete radiological integration of the press-fit cup - result at 7 years.
D. 13 years after revision (17.11.98).

weight-bearing surface of the acetabular component is exposed to load transmission, this graft should be protected by an acetabular reinforcement ring.

Where segmental defects, large cavities and a non-spheric shape of the acetabulum do not allow firm fixation of a new cup by intrinsic press-fit, acetabular reinforcement rings according to Kerboull [21], Müller [41, 49], Burch-Schneider [13, 44] or Ganz [63] are preferable. The acetabulum is reconstructed with morsellised allografts which are impacted with a spherical (non-perforated) trial cup. These grafts must then be protected from loading with a reinforcement ring which is fixed to the original host bone of the pelvis by 3 to 5 ASIF cancellous screws.

With reinforcement rings (ARR) or antiprotrusio cages (APC), bone losses can be bridged, grafting and bone augmentation are allowed, and support is given to the new socket [13].

Cysts and the bottom of the acetabulum are filled with morsellised allografts, the segmental defects are reconstructed and then compressed with a trial cup or hemispheric

Table IV. – Results of acetabular revisions with hemispherical press-fit cups [7, 25, 26, 37, 39, 60]

Authors	Year	N	Type of Implant	Obs'time	Rate of Revision for Aseptic Loosening
Tanzer (et al) [60]	1992	140	Harris-Galante	2-6 y	1 %
Door (et al) [7]	1995	139	Anat. porous repl.	2-9.8 y (4.3 y)	1.4 %
Padgett (et al) [37]	1993	129	Harris Galante	3-7.5 y	0
Silverton (et al) [55]	1996	-	same group	6.5-11 y	0-4 % osteolysis
Paprosky (et al) [39]	1994	147	-	3-9 y	4 %
Lachiewicz (et al) [25]	1994	60	Harris Galante	2-8 y (5 y)	0
Lachiewicz (et al) [26]	1998	57	Harris Galante	5-12 y (7 y)	0
Present study	1998	255	"Press-Fit Cup"	0.5-10 y	0 (2 for dislocation)

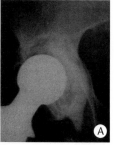
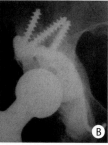

2   *Revision of a non-contained, rim non-supportive acetabular deficiency with allografts and Hooked Acetabular Reinforcement Ring (according to Ganz).*
   A. P.A., 60 year old female patient with aseptic loosening of a cemented all-polyethylene cup.
   B. 9 year result of a revision with morsellised allografts and Hooked Acetabular Reinforcement Ring.

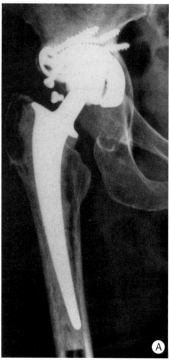
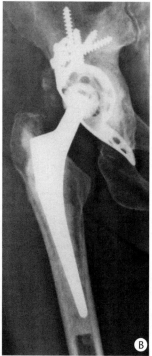
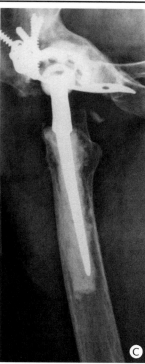

3   *Revision of non-contained, rim non-supportive acetabular deficiency with morsellised allografts and Burch-Schneider Acetabular Reinforcement Ring.*
   A. K. D., 60 year-old female patient with loosening and cranial migration of a screw fixated metal-backed acetabular socket.
   B. X-ray post-operatively a.p. The femoral stem has been revised by "cement-in-cement technique".
   C. Lateral view.

impactor. Even large segmental defects must not be reconstructed with structural corticocancellous grafts, since revascularisation of morsellised grafts is easier than with structural grafts, and the supporting ring protects the primary mechanically-weak morsellised graft well until it is revascularised and integrated.

The hook of the Kerboull reinforcement ring and Ganz reinforcement ring placed around the "tear drop" not only improves the stability of the ring but also brings the centre of rotation to its original location. With M.E. Müller's acetabular reinforcement ring, the anatomical centre of rotation could be restored, as well as with the Burch-Schneider anti-protrusio cage, in all but one of Gill and co-workers' 63 patients [13]. The hook can also bridge and fix pelvic discontinuities with minor bone deficiency. An all-polyethylene cup of corresponding size is then cemented (cement with or without antibiotics) into the supporting ring. Cement protruding through the holes of the reinforcement ring augments the stability of the graft-host bone supporting ring-cup construct (fig 2).

The Burch-Schneider anti-protrusio cage is placed with its inferior flange into a pre-cut slot of the ischium (fig 3). The larger superior flange is fixed with 6.5 mm cancellous screws to the lateral surface of the ilium. A best-possible fit with the acetabulum rim protects the screws from overload and subsequent fracture.

Postoperative management consists in immediate touch weight-bearing for 6 weeks followed by full weight-bearing, as a rule.

SALVAGE PROCEDURE

In cases of defects which cannot be reconstructed by any kind of method, or where the patient's general condition or severe recurrent infection does not allow a secure reconstruction, a Girdlestone excision arthroplasty or a "saddle prosthesis" [35] may be performed as a salvage procedure.

Discussion

The results of the various treatment modalities of acetabular deficiencies are listed in Tables *III*, *IV* and *V*. It is obvious that the reconstructions for contained, rim supportive defects with press-fit cups (oversized, porous-coated hemispherical cups) give the best results, comparable to those of primary arthroplasties. Revisions with reinforcement rings show — at least in the short term — satisfying results as well. However, the great variety of segmental and combined acetabular deficiencies make the predictability of this method more difficult. Furthermore, the risk of an infection or failure due to technical errors is higher in revisions with supporting rings.

An alternative to the above-described two methods of managing acetabular defects in revision is the method of "cemented impact allografting", which will be described by Slooff and co-workers in another chapter.

Table V. – *Results of acetabular revisions with reinforcement rings - with and without allografting, fixed by fully threaded 6.5 mm cancellous screws* [1, 3, 13, 41, 44, 49, 57, 63]

Author(s)	Year	Type of ARR	N	Obs'time, Re-loosening etc.	Re-revision
Aebi (et al) [1]	1989	Müller ARR	145	5.5-11 y (7.7)	0.7 %, 4.8 % infection
Rosson (et al) [49]	1992	Müller/Burch	31	5 y	7.5 % re-revision / asept.loosening
Berry (et al) [3]	1992	Müller ARR	42	5 y	12 % asept.loos, 12 % infection
Pascarel (et al) [41]	1993	Müller ARR	141	min. 5 y	2 re-rev. (1.4 %)
Zehntner (et al) [63]	1994	Müller ARR	27	5-10 y (7.2 y)	20 % re-rev. at 10 y
Peters (et al) [44]	1995	Burch-Schn.	25	33 months	0 re-revision, 14 % > 3 mm migr.
Starker (et al) [57]	1998	various types	174	5.6 y	6 (3.4 %) loosening
Gill (et al) [13]	1998	Burch-Schn.	63	8.5 y (5-18)	5 re-rev. (8 %)
Present study	1998	Ganz&B-Schn.	201	0.5-10 y	5 re-rev. (2.5 %)

References

[1] Aebi M, Richner L, Ganz R. Langzeitergebnisse der primären Hüfttotalprothese mit Acetabulumabstützring (ARR). *Orthopäde* 1989 ; 18 : 504-510

[2] Anspach WE, Lachiewicz PF. A new technique for removal of the total hip arthroplasty acetabular component. *Clin Orthop* 1991 ; 268 : 152-156

[3] Berry JD, Müller ME. Revision arthroplasty using an antiprotrusio cage for massive acetabular bone deficiency. *J Bone Joint Surg Br* 1992 ; 74 : 711-715

[4] D'Antonio JA, Capello WN, Borden LS, Bargar WL, Bierbaum BF, Boettcher WG et al. Classification and management of acetabular abnormalities in total hip arthroplasty. *Clin Orthop* 1989 ; 243 : 126-137

[5] DeBoer DK, Christie MJ. Reconstruction of the deficient acetabulum with an oblong prosthesis. 3- to 7-year results. *J Arthropl* 1998 ; 13 : 674-680

[6] DeLee JG, Charnley J. Radiological demarcation of cemented sockets in hip replacement. *Clin Orthop* 1976 ; 121 : 20-33

[7] Dorr LD, Wan Z. Ten years of experience with porous acetabular components for revision surgery. *Clin Orthop* 1995 ; 319 : 191-200

[8] Eftekhar NS, Nercessian O. Intrapelvic migration of total hip prostheses: Operative treatment. *J Bone Joint Surg Am* 1989 ; 71 : 1480-1486

[9] Ejsted R, Olsen NJ. Revision of failed total hip arthroplasty. *J Bone Joint Surg Br* 1987 ; 69 : 57-60

[10] Elke R, Morscher E. Klassifikation und Behandlung von Acetabulumdefekten. *Med Orthop Tech* 1997 ; 117 : 126-130

[11] Engelbrecht J, Weber FA, Sweet MB, Jakim I. Long term results of revision hip arthroplasty. *J Bone Joint Surg Br* 1990 ; 72 : 41-45

[12] Enneking WF, Mindell ER. Observations on massive retrieved human allografts. *J Bone Joint Surg Am* 1991 ; 73 : 1123-1142

[13] Gill TJ, Sledge JB, Müller ME. The Burch-Schneider anti protrusio cage in revision total hip arthroplasty. Indications, principles and long-term results. *J Bone Joint Surg Br* 1998 ; 80 : 946-953

[14] Harris WH. Modularity is unnecessary in primary femoral THA but has some advantages in primary acetabular THA. *J Arthropl* 1996 ; 11 : 334

[15] Harris WH, Crothers O, Oh I. Total hip replacement and femoral head bone grafting for severe acetabular deficiency in adults. *J Bone Joint Surg Am* 1977 ; 59 : 752-759

[16] Herzog R, Morscher E. Morselized homologous grafts in revision arthroplasty of the acetabulum. *Chir Organ Mov* 1994 ; 79 : 371-378

[17] Hooten JP Jr, Engh CA Jr, Engh CA. Failure of structural acetabular allografts in cementless revision hip arthroplasty. *J Bone Joint Surg Br* 1994 ; 76 : 419-422

[18] Jasty MJ, Harris WH. Total hip reconstruction using frozen femoral head allografts in patients with acetabular bone loss. *Orthop Clin North Am* 1987 ; 18 : 291-299

[19] Kavanagh BF, Ilstrup DM, Fitzgerald RH Jr. Revision total hip arthroplasty. *J Bone Joint Surg Am* 1985 ; 67 : 517-526

[20] Kelley SS. High hip center in revision arthroplasty. *J Arthropl* 1994 ; 9 : 503-510

[21] Kerboull M. Problems related to the acetabulum In : Postel M Kerboull M Evrard J Courpied JP eds. Total Hip Replacement. Berlin : Springer-Verlag, 1987 ; 84-90

[22] Köster G, Willert HG, Köhler HP, Döpkens K. An oblong revision cup for large acetabular defects. *J Arthropl* 1998 ; 13 : 559-569

[23] Kwong LM, Jasty M, Harris WH. High failure rate of bulk femoral head allografts in total hip acetabular reconstructions at 10 years. *J Arthropl* 1993 ; 8 : 341-346

[24] Lachiewicz PF, Anspach WE. Removal of a well fixed acetabular component. *J Bone Joint Surg Am* 1991 ; 73 : 1355-1356

[25] Lachiewicz PF, Hussamy OD. Revision of the acetabulum without cement with use of the Harris-Galante porouscoated implant. *J Bone Joint Surg Am* 1994 ; 76 : 1834-1839

[26] Lachiewicz PF, Poon ED, Hill C. Revision of a total hip arthroplasty with a Harris-Galante porous-coated acetabular component inserted without cement. *J Bone Joint Surg Am* 1998 ; 80 : 980-984

[27] Mankin HJ, Gebhardt MC, Jennings LC, Springfield DS, Tomford WW. Long-term results of allograft replacement in the management of bone tumours. *Clin Orthop* 1996 ; 324 : 86-97

[28] Masri BA, Masterson EL, Duncan CP. The classification and radiographic evaluation of bone loss in revision hip arthroplasty. *Orthop Clin* 1998 ; 29 : 219-227

[29] Morscher E. Current status of acetabular fixation in primary total hip arthroplasty. *Clin Orthop* 1992 ; 274 : 172-193

[30] Morscher E. Management of acetabular deficiency. *Orthopaedics* 1995 ; 18 : 859-862

[31] Morscher E, Berli B, Jockers W, Schenk R. Rationale of a flexible Press-fit Cup in total hip replacement. 5-year follow-up in 280 procedures. *Clin Orthop* 1997 ; 341 : 42-50

[32] Morscher E, Dick W, Seelig W. Revisions-Arthroplastik des Hüftgelenks mit autologer und homologer Spongiosa. *Orthopäde* 1989 ; 18 : 428-437

[33] Moskal JT, Danisa OA, Shaffrey CI. Isolated revision acetabuloplasty using a porous-coated cementless acetabular component without removal of a well-fixed femoral component. A 3- to 9-year follow-up study. *J Arthropl* 1997 ; 12 : 719-727

[34] Mulroy RD, Harris WH. Failure of acetabular autogenous grafts in total hip arthroplasty: Increasing incidence: a follow-up note. *J Bone Joint Surg Am* 1990 ; 72 : 1536-1540

[35] Nieder E, Elson RA, Engelbrecht E, Kasselt MR, Keller A, Steinbrink K. The saddle prosthesis for salvage of the destroyed acetabulum. *J Bone Joint Surg Br* 1990 ; 72 : 1014-1022

[36] Olivier H, Sanouiller JL. Reconstructions cotyloïdiennes par greffes spongieuses dans les révisions d'arthroplasties totales de hanche. *Rev Chir Orthop* 1991 ; 77 : 232-240

[37] Padgett DE, Kull L, Rosenberg A, Sumner DR, Galante JO. Revision of the acetabular component without cement after total hip arthroplasty: three to six year follow-up. *J Bone Joint Surg Am* 1993 ; 75 : 663-673

[38] Papagelopoulos PJ, Lewallen DG, Cabanela ME, McFarland EG, Wallrichs SL. Acetabular reconstruction using bipolar endoprostheses and bone grafting in patients with severe bone deficiency. *Clin Orthop* 1995 ; 314 : 170-184

[39] Paprosky WG, Magnus RE. Principles of bone grafting in revision total hip arthroplasty: acetabular technique. *Clin Orthop* 1994 ; 298 : 147-155

[40] Paprosky WG, Perona PG, Lawrence JM. Acetabular defect classification and surgical reconstruction in revision arthroplasty: a six year follow-up evaluation. *J Arthropl* 1994 ; 9 : 33-44

[41] Pascarel X, Liquois F, Chauveaux D, LeRebeller A, Honton JL. Utilisation des anneaux endocotyloidiens de Muller dans la chirurgie de révision des prothèses totales de hanche. À propos de 141 cas avec un recul minimum de 5 ans. *Rev Chir Orthop* 1993 ; 79 : 357-364

[42] Patterson M. Ring uncemented hip replacements, the results of revision. *J Bone Joint Surg Br* 1987 ; 69 : 374-380

[43] Pellici PM, Wilson PD Jr, Sledge CB, Salvati EA, Ranawat CS, Poss R, Callaghan J. Long-term results of revision total hip replacement. *J Bone Joint Surg Am* 1985 ; 67 : 513-516

[44] Peters CL, Curtain M, Samuelson KM. Acetabular revision with the Burch-Schneider antiprotrusio cage and cancellous allograft bone. *J Arthropl* 1995 ; 10 : 307-312

[45] Pitto RP, DiMuria GV, Hohmann D. Impaction grafting and acetabular reinforcement in revision hip replacement. *Int Orthop* 1998 ; 22 : 161-164

[46] Pollock FH, Whiteside LA. The fate of massive allografts in total hip acetabular revision surgery. *J Arthropl* 1992 ; 7 : 271-276

[47] Reikeraas O, Folleraas G, Winge JF. Allografting in uncemented acetabular revision. *Orthopaedics* 1998 ; 21 : 1191-1195

[48] Robertson DD, Sutherland CJ, Lopes T, Yuan J. Preoperative description of severe acetabular defects caused by failed total hip replacement. *J Comput Assist Tomogr* 1998 ; 22 : 444-449

[49] Rosson J, Schatzker J. The use of reinforcement rings to reconstruct deficient acetabula. *J Bone Joint Surg Br* 1992 ; 74 : 716-720

[50] Russotti GM, Harris WH. Proximal placement of the acetabular component in total hip arthroplasty. A long-term follow-up study. *J Arthropl* 1991 ; 73 : 587-593

[51] Schimmel JW, Buma P, Versleyen D, Huiskes R, Slooff TJJH. Acetabular reconstruction with impacted morselized cancellous allografts in cemented hip arthroplasty, a histological and biomechanical study on the goat. *J Arthropl* 1998 ; 13 : 438-448

[52] Schreurs BW, Slooff TJ, Buma P, Gardeniers JW, Huiskes R. Acetabular reconstruction with impacted morselized cancellous bone graft and cement. A 10- to 15-year follow-up of 60 revision arthroplasties. *J Bone Joint Surg Br* 1998 ; 80 : 391-395

[53] Schutzer SF, Harris WH. High placement of porous-coated acetabular component in complex total hip arthroplasty. *J Arthropl* 1994 ; 9 : 359-367

[54] Shinar AA, Harris WH. Bulk structural autogenous grafts and allografts for reconstruction of the acetabulum in total hip arthroplasty. Sixteen-year-average follow-up. *J Bone Joint Surg Am* 1997 ; 79 : 159-168

[55] Silverton CD, Rosenberg AG, Sheinkop MB, Kull LR, Galante JO. Revision total hip arthroplasty using a cementless acetabular component technique and results. *Clin Orthop* 1995 ; 319 : 201-208

[56] Slooff TJ, Huiskes R, VanHorn J, Lemmens JA. Bone grafting in total hip replacement for acetabular protrusion. *Acta Orthop Scand* 1984 ; 55 : 593-596

[57] Starker M, Kandziora F, Jager A, Kerschbaumer F. Pfannenrekonstruktion mit Pfannenstützschalen. *Orthopäde* 1998 ; 27 : 366-374

[58] Stillwell WT. Total hip revision, indications and surgical technique. *Orthopedics* 1982 ; 5 : 33-41

[59] Tanzer M. Role and results of the high hip center. *Orthop Clin North Am* 1998 ; 29 : 241-247

[60] Tanzer M, Drucker D, Jasty M, McDonald M, Harris WH. Revision of the acetabular component with an uncemented Harris-Galante porous-coated prosthesis. *J Bone Joint Surg Am* 1992 ; 74 : 987-994

[61] Wallenstein R, Olsson E. Rearthroplasty of the hip joint. *Acta Orthop Scand* 1982 ; 53 : 273-277

[62] Wilson MG, Nikpoor N, Alibadi P, Poss R, Weissman BN. The fate of acetabular allografts after bipolar revision arthroplasty of the hip. *J Bone Joint Surg Am* 1989 ; 71 : 1469-1479

[63] Zehntner MK, Ganz R. Midterm results (5. 5-10 years) of acetabular allograft reconstruction with the acetabular reinforcement ring during total hip revision. *J Arthropl* 1994 ; 9 : 469-479

Acetabular reconstruction with impacted bone grafting and cement

TJJH Slooff
BW Schreurs
JWM Gardeniers
P Buma

Abstract. – Aseptic loosening of an acetabular cup is often associated with extensive bone loss. This chapter describes a biological reconstruction technique with impacted allograft chips and cement in revision arthroplasty after failed total hip arthroplasty. With this technique, it is possible to replace the loss of bone and to repair normal hip mechanics in combination with a standard hip prosthesis, achieving a long-lasting stable reconstruction.
An overview is given of the essential issues concerned in bone grafting and, in particular, the use of morsellised allografts in combination with cement, as well as the rationale of the reconstruction method in acetabular revision arthroplasty. Subsequently, the chapter describes the surgical technique, the supporting scientific studies, and the clinical and radiographic results of the reconstruction.

Keywords: hip joint, total hip replacement, acetabular loosening, revision surgery, morsellised allograft, cemented acetabular component.

Introduction

The main problem in revision surgery of failed cemented and noncemented arthroplasties is the loss of bone stock, induced by the loosening process itself and by procedures to remove the prosthesis and cement. On the acetabular side, the loosening process often results in a combined cavitary-segmental defect (fig 1). The key problem in revision surgery is how to manage the periprosthetic bone loss. Although controversy still exists about the best treatment for bone stock deficiencies, this chapter presents an efficient biological method that uses tightly impacted morsellised cancellous allografts in direct contact with bone cement.

The treatment strategy for the acetabular reconstruction is aimed at:

– repair of hip mechanics by positioning the cup on the anatomic location, at the level of the transverse ligament;

– closing of the segmental defects to achieve a contained defect;

Tom JJH Slooff, M.D., Ph.D., Professor of Orthopaedics.
BW Schreurs, M.D., Ph.D., Orthopaedic Surgeon.
JWM Gardeniers, M.D., Ph.D., Orthopaedic Surgeon.
P Buma, Ph.D., Biologist.
Orthopaedic Department, University Hospital Sint Radboud, Nijmegen, P.O. Box 9101, 6500 HB Nijmegen, Netherlands.

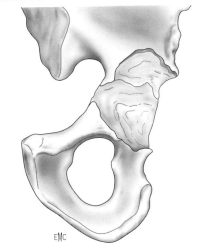

1 *Drawing after removal of the cup showing the central and peripheral segmental defects in combination with the cavitary defect.*

– replacement of the bone loss by filling the cavitary defect with allograft bone chips;

– restoration of stability by impacting the chips and the use of bone cement.

Background

Bone transplantation has a long history in medical practice. In the early years of surgical treatment, bone transplantation was not an accepted technique, but was rather considered an experimental approach with an unpredictable outcome. A major breakthrough came in 1947 when techniques were developed for preserving and storing allograft bone at minus 20°C [15]. Although it soon became clear that allografts would not be as successful as autogenous grafts, it became clinically possible to use allografts on a larger scale. During the 1960s, the clinical use of massive allografts became generally accepted to replace parts of the skeleton that had been lost through trauma or tumour. Another important clinical application of bone grafts began in the 1970s: the repair of osseous defects in association with primary and revision hip arthroplasty. Initial reports on acetabular reconstruction with, respectively, morsellised [6, 8] and structural bone grafts [4, 5] set the standard in this field. Regardless of the type of graft used, essential factors influencing the incorporation process are the stability of fixation of the graft, the amount of contact between host and graft, the load pattern within the graft, and the vascularity of the host bed. In addition, the size of the graft has also been found to play an important role in the graft incorporation process. Therefore, we make the distinction between "large fragment" and "small fragment" grafts. Large fragment grafts, such as massive cortical and corticocancellous structural grafts, incorporate incompletely, irregularly and slowly. The incorporation process is confined only to the outer few millimetres, leaving a more centrally-located core permanently necrotic [2, 13]. In time, this may cause failure of the graft due to microfracture and resorption. Impacted cancellous "small fragment" allografts allow rapid vascular invasion through the open structure and therefore enable a more rapid, complete and uniform incorporation without mechanical weakening. This is in accordance with our clinical and experimental observations. In animal experiments, incorporation of these impacted grafts was seen on both the acetabular and the femoral side [9, 10]. Incorporation was also observed in human biopsy specimens [1]. Since the late 1970s, the technique of impaction grafting combined with cement fixation of the prosthetic components has been our treatment of choice for restoring bone stock loss in primary deficiencies and in failed hip arthroplasties on the pelvic side [12]. Since the mid-1980s, the bone impaction grafting method has also been used on the femoral side [3].

Indications

The main indication for revision arthroplasty is the progressive loss of periprosthetic bone, followed by pain and physical disability in otherwise healthy patients. Surgery should be considered even before clinical symptoms appear. Radiographic signs of loosening often precede the clinical symptoms of failure. In our department, regular follow-up has been included since the 1970s in the standard postoperative protocol after primary total hip arthroplasty, to prevent extensive loss of bone (fig 2). When planning a revision arthroplasty, attention should be paid to assessing the diagnosis of loosening and establishing the cause of failure. A thorough physical examination should be followed by laboratory tests and good quality plain radiographs in three views: anteroposterior, axial, and abduction-external. These radiographs could be used to evaluate the severity of anatomic distortion, the location and the extent of bone lysis, the distribution of cement, and any acetabular or femoral deficiencies. It must be realised that the bone defects and the acetabular distortions in reality are much more serious than the preoperative radiographs suggest. Serial radiographs are mandatory to monitor changes in the position of the component, the cement and the bone stock over the course of time. If loosening is suspected, pre-revision management should include nuclear arthrography combined with an intra-articular needle biopsy and gamma-immunoglobulin scintigraphy to exclude infection as the cause of loosening.

Operative technique

Routinely, we use the posterolateral approach for cemented revision total hip arthroplasty with bone impaction grafting.

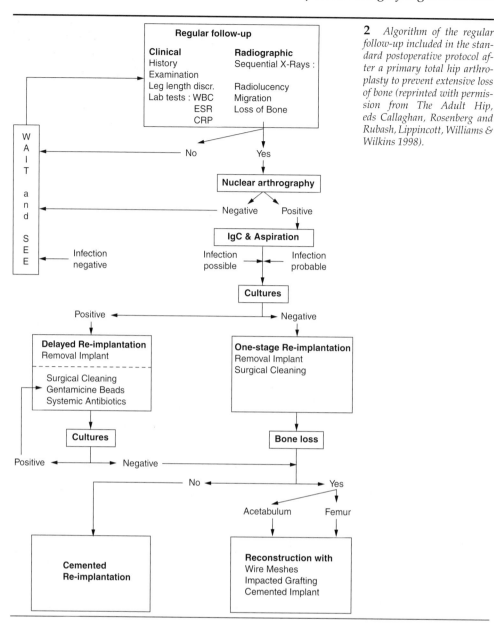

2 *Algorithm of the regular follow-up included in the standard postoperative protocol after a primary total hip arthroplasty to prevent extensive loss of bone (reprinted with permission from The Adult Hip, eds Callaghan, Rosenberg and Rubash, Lippincott, Williams & Wilkins 1998).*

This approach allows an extensive exposure of all aspects of the acetabulum and the proximal femur. In order to obtain access to the anterior aspect of the hip, the usual support on the anterior superior iliac spine cannot be used. We therefore recommend using a pubic symphysis pad next to the posterior pad. The contralateral leg is flexed 40 degrees in the hip and knee joint. The patient must be draped in such a manner that the incision can be extended to the region of the anterior superior iliac spine, if necessary. A trochanteric osteotomy is seldom indicated. Identification of the major landmarks and of the sciatic nerve is helpful to orientate the anatomy, which may be disturbed by scarring and distortions. These landmarks are: the tip of the greater trochanter, the minor trochanter, the tendinous part of the gluteus maximus and the lower border of the gluteus medius and minimus. Aspiration of the hip joint should be carried out at this stage to obtain fluid for gram staining. The proximal part of the femur is extensively exposed and mobilised before the hip is dislocated. A very wide exposure of the entire socket, by removing all scar tissue, is essential. A circumferential capsulotomy is performed and the iliopsoas tendon is divided. After removing the components and the cement, the fibrous interface is thoroughly removed from the irregular acetabular wall using sharp spoons and curettes. At least three biopsies are taken from this interfacial fibrous membrane for frozen sections and bacterial culture. After this sampling, systemic antibiotic therapy is started. Meticulous examination of the acetabular floor and wall is done to establish all defects that are present. Special care is devoted to locating the transverse ligament at the inferior side of the acetabulum (fig 3). From this level, the reconstruction will be built up in order to restore the hip mechanics. Placing a retractor at this level will be helpful. The combined medial and peripheral segmental and cavitary defects are evaluated. Flexible stainless steel meshes are trimmed (fig 4) and adapted to the defects using special scissors and clamps. At the periphery, these meshes are fixed with self-tapping screws at a minimum of three

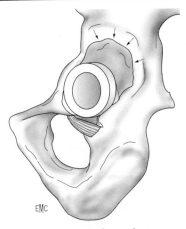

3 *Special care is given to locate the transverse ligament at the inferior side of the acetabulum to facilitate the reconstruction of the original centre of rotation. Arrows indicate the upper ridge of the segmental defect.*

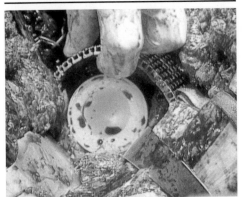

4 *With the trial cup positioned against the transverse ligament, the extent of the peripheral segmental bone stock loss can be demonstrated. Flexible stainless steel meshes are trimmed and adapted.*

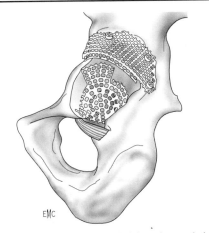

5 *After closing the segmental defects the acetabulum is contained and has become a cavitary defect.*

points to secure rigidity. The medial segmental defect is also covered with a metal mesh. After closing these segmental defects, the acetabulum is contained and has become a cavitary defect (fig 5). The sclerotic acetabular wall is subsequently "revitalised" with multiple small, superficial drill holes to enhance better surface contact and to facilitate vascular invasion into the graft.

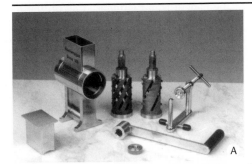 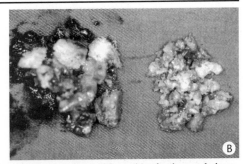

6 *A. A special bone mill was developed which can produce both large (1x1x1 cm) bone chips for the acetabular reconstructions as well as smaller chips for femoral impacted bone grafting.*
  B. On the left the larger and on the right the smaller bone chips.

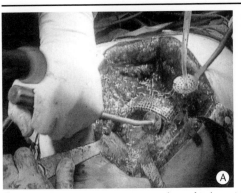 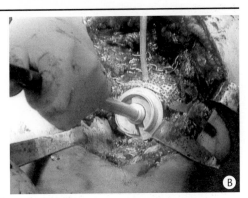

7 *A. Initially, smaller impactors can be used to impact the graft under the mesh.*
  B. Larger impactors are used to achieve stability by impacting the grafts using a metal hammer.

Preparation of the graft

Allografts from fresh-frozen femoral heads (hospital bone bank) are recommended. Autogenous cancellous chips may be mixed with the allograft if the surgeon wishes. The allograft is cleaned of soft tissues and divided into 4 parts. These will pass through a specially-developed bone mill providing substantially-sized chips, of about $1.0\,cm^3$ each (fig 6A, B). Alternatively, these grafts can also be prepared by hand with a rongeur. The more substantial size of the acetabular. chips is emphasized in contrast to the smaller size of the chips ($0.4\,cm^3$ each) used for femoral reconstruction. Bone slurry is not advisable because even after impaction its consistency is not stable. At least two femoral head allografts should be available for the reconstruction. In the heterogenous group of bone grafts, the morsellised fresh-frozen cancellous allografts are preferred. These chips incorporate rapidly and completely without mechanical weakening. To enhance stability between the chips, prerequisites for optimal results are: containment of the defect, tight impaction of the chips and the use of cement. The essential nature of these measures is confirmed by clinical follow-up of our patients [11] and by animal experiments [9].

Acetabular reconstruction

After rinsing, the acetabulum is packed tightly with chips. First, the small cavities

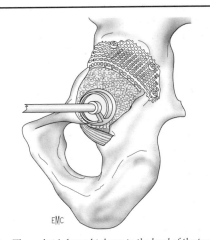

8 *The socket is brought down to the level of the transverse ligament.*

are filled, then subsequently the entire socket layer by layer. The use of the small and large impactors is indispensable to achieve stability within the graft (fig 7A, B). The last impactor used is 4 mm, which is oversized relative to the planned cup diameter so as to obtain a sufficient cement layer. Care is taken to reconstruct the anatomy of the hip by packing as much chip graft material as necessary until the socket is brought down to the level of the transverse ligament (fig 8). After impaction, the pre-existing enlarged acetabular diameter has been reduced to normal size (fig 9). During the preparation of the antibiotic-loaded cement, pressure on the graft is continued using the trial socket or the impactor. After insertion and pressurising the cement, the cup is placed and held in position with the pusher until

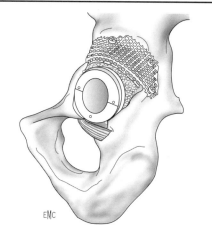

9   *After impaction, the pre-existing enlarged acetabular diameter has been reduced to normal size (diagram).*

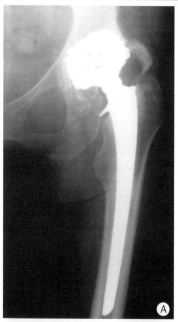

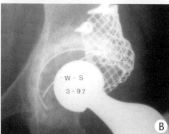

10   *A. Preoperative X-ray of a loosened implant. B. View of the same case after the acetabular reconstruction with a peripheral mesh (follow-up 3 years after operation).*

the cement is polymerised. Directly after the operation, and at regular intervals, X-rays of the reconstruction are made *(fig 10)*.

Postoperative care

Postoperative treatment includes oral anticoagulation therapy for 3 months and systemic antibiotics for 24 hours. Immediately after the operation, indomethacin is administered for 7 days to prevent heterotopic ossification. Mobilisation

of the patient is individualised according to the circumstances of the revision arthroplasty and based on the radiographic controls. A period of 2 to 6 weeks bed rest is required in cases of major acetabular reconstruction. Touch weight-bearing is maintained for 3 months, and weight-bearing is then gradually increased, changing to a single crutch, and then onto sticks and subsequently a single stick, as circumstances allow.

Results

The application of impacted morsellised allografts in cases with acetabular bone stock loss is attractive. However, only long-term follow-up studies can establish the true value of this technique. Therefore, we recently reviewed 56 patients (60 hips) with acetabular impacted bone grafts in cemented revision arthroplasty with a follow-up of 10 to 15 years (average 11.8 years) [11]. Five acetabular reconstructions were re-revised, due to two septic and three aseptic loosenings. After excluding the two cases with infection, this resulted in a survival rate of 94% at an average of nearly 12 years.

Prevention and management of complications

Generally, revision arthroplasties have a higher rate of complications as compared to primary total hip arthroplasty. This is because the surgery is more complex and time-consuming and is associated with higher blood losses. The patients are often elderly and many of these have age-related diseases. When a surgeon considers a revision or a re-revision arthroplasty, selection of the patient is a very important factor to prevent complications. In addition to the already mentioned age-related diseases, other factors require a thorough investigation prior to surgery. These factors are: pre-existing infection, preoperative assessment of the existing defects and bone loss, the availability of sufficient bone of good quality, all necessary instruments and implants to achieve initial stability of the reconstruction, and highly qualified and well prepared staff. In our material, five patients were re-revised. Of these, one was re-revised for recurrence of infection and one was infected, although antibiotic impregnated bone cement and systemic antibiotic treatment were routinely used. Three patients were re-revised because of aseptic mechanical loosening. Radiographic evaluation of the acetabular reconstructions suggested that a too-thin layer of chip allograft might be responsible for this failure. From clinical experience, we know that a thin graft layer, less than 0.5 cm thick,

will be pushed out of the acetabulum during pressurisation of the bone cement onto the graft. In fact, the remaining graft will be mixed with the cement and will subsequently become necrotic. In our opinion, the graft layer must have a substantial thickness, of at least 5 mm, to be stable. This is an essential part of ensuring the success of the surgical technique. It is therefore important to have sufficient graft available during surgery. In laboratory experiments, we observed a higher migration tendency in the grafted acetabulum in relation with the smaller size of the chips. Small sized chips (less than 0.4 x 0.4 x 0.4 centimetre each) behave like quicksand and, particularly at the acetabular side, result in instability of the reconstruction [14]. In other experiments, it was demonstrated that the mechanical behaviour of brittle materials such as bone substitutes is significantly different from impacted morsellised bone graft. In our opinion, these materials cannot replace morsellised bone grafts, and at this moment their use for this specific clinical application should be avoided. We emphasise that only fresh-frozen cancellous allografts must be used.

We also stress the fact that among all the factors determining the success or failure of a revision procedure, the expertise and the experience of the surgeon are probably the most important. Achieving initial stability of the reconstruction is essential to guarantee incorporation of the chip allograft and to prevent resorption of the graft and subsequent mechanical loosening of the component. The surgeon must have knowledge of the basic events of graft incorporation, of the necessity for correct preparation of the host bone and of the importance of using medium viscosity bone cement. On the basis of sound clinical experience and scientific data, the surgeon will select the standard components that fit this standardised surgical procedure, knowing that the geometry of these components influences the strain pattern in the cement and in the graft.

Dislocation of the components of the total hip is more frequently seen in revision arthroplasty. This is mainly due to increased muscular laxity, malposition of the components, impingement by heterotopic ossifications and neurological deficit. In most revision patients, atrophy of the gluteal muscles exists because of the deteriorating range of motion due to the painful and invaliding loosening process. During the reconstruction, if hip mechanics are not anatomically restored, the risk for dislocation will increase. Our technique is aimed at the restoration of the hip mechanics by placing the acetabular component at the level of the transverse ligament. The centre of the head of the femoral component must likewise be placed at the level of the tip of the greater trochanter. Before cementing the component, a trial reduction is recommended to test the muscular tension. We are very careful with exposing and incising the capsule during the revision procedure. We make a tendinous flap of the remnants of the rotators and the capsule that will stabilise the joint after reattachment to the crista trochanterica of the femur during closure of the wound. This is an adequate measure to prevent dislocation of the components of the total hip.

Another complication that may influence the outcome of the revision arthroplasty is the occurrence of heterotopic ossifications. From our research and clinical experience [7], we know that indomethacin successfully prevents the occurrence and recurrence of heterotopic ossifications. Immediately after the operation, prophylactic treatment with indomethacin is started and continued for seven days postoperatively. The effective dosage of 3 times 50 mg daily had no detrimental effect on the incorporation of the allograft used. Since the introduction of our reconstruction technique, the patients have been regularly followed-up, including critical evaluation of the serial radiographs. With all these measures, we try to prevent and to manage adequately the complications in revision arthroplasty.

References

[1] Buma P, Lamerigts N, Schreurs BW, Gardeniers JW, Versleyen D, Slooff TJ. Impacted graft incorporation after cemented acetabular revision: histological evaluation in 8 patients. *Acta Orthop Scand* 1996 ; 67 : 536-540

[2] Enneking WF, Mindell ER. Observations on massive retrieved human allografts. *J Bone Joint Surg Am* 1991 ; 73 : 1123-1142

[3] Gie GA, Linder L, Ling RS, Simon JP, Slooff TJ, Timperley AJ. Impacted cancellous allograft and cement for revision total hip arthroplasty. *J Bone Joint Surg Br* 1993 ; 75 : 14-21

[4] Gross AE, Lavoie MV, McDermott P, Marks P. The use of allograft bone in revision of total hip arthroplasty. *Clin Orthop* 1985 ; 197 : 115-123

[5] Harris WH. Allograft in total hip arthroplasty; In adults with severe acetabular deficiency including a surgical technique for bolting the graft to the ilium. *Clin Orthop* 1982 ; 162 : 150-164

[6] Hastings DE, Parker SM. Protrusio acetabuli in rheumatoid arthritis. *Clin Orthop* 1975 ; 108 : 76-83

[7] Hu HP, Slooff TJ, van Horn JR. Heterotopic ossifications following total hip arthroplasty: a review. *Acta Orthop Belg* 1991 ; 57 : 2-12

[8] McCollum DE, Nunley JA. Bone grafting in acetabular protrusio: A biologic buttress. In : Nelson CL ed. The Hip: Proceedings of the Sixth Open Scientific Meeting of the Hip Society, St Louis : CV Mosby, 1978 : 124-146

[9] Schimmel JW, Buma P, Huiskes R, Slooff TJ. Acetabular reconstruction with impacted morsellized cancellous allografts in cemented hip arthroplasty: a histological and biomechanical study on the goat. *J Arthroplasty* 1998 ; 13 : 438-448

[10] Schreurs BW, Buma P, Huiskes R, Slooff TJ. A technique for using impacted trabecular allografts in revision surgery with cemented stems. *Acta Orthop Scand* 1994 ; 65 : 267-273

[11] Schreurs BW, Slooff TJ, Buma P, Gardeniers JW, Huiskes R. Acetabular reconstruction with impacted morsellized cancellous bone graft and cement: A 10 to 15 year follow-up of 60 revision arthroplasties. *J Bone Joint Surg Br* 1998 ; 80 : 391-395

[12] Slooff TJ, Huiskes R, van Horn JR, Lemmens AJ. Bone grafting in total hip replacement for acetabular protrusion. *Acta Orthop Scand* 1984 ; 55 : 593-596

[13] Stevenson S, XiaoQing LI, Martin B. The fate of cancellous and cortical bone after transplantation of fresh and frozen tissue-antigen-matched and mismatched osteochondral allografts in dogs. *J Bone Joint Suirg Am* 1991 ; 73 : 1143-1156

[14] Van Unen JM, Verdonschot N, Schreurs BW, Huiskes R. The effect of morsellised bone graft size and operative technique on the initial stability of acetabular cups in revision surgery. 8th Meeting EORS, Amsterdam, May 4-7 1998

[15] Wilson PD. Experience with the use of refrigerated homogenous bone. *J Bone Joint Surg Br* 1951 ; 33 : 301-315

Acetabular revision with armature, allografts and cemented prosthesis

M Kerboull
L Kerboull

Abstract. – Among the numerous techniques used to restore a destroyed acetabulum, the one described in this chapter was developed 24 years ago in 1974. Since then, it has efficiently stood the test of time, even in the most severe cases of bone loss. Its goal is to reconstruct a bony cavity of normal size in an anatomic position into which a standard acetabular component is cemented. Bone reconstruction is composed of fragments of a frozen femoral head: a bulky piece carefully shaped to repair the damaged roof, slices to reconstruct or thicken medial, anterior and posterior walls, morselised cancellous bone to fill cavitary defects and gaps between structural grafts. This bony reconstruction is reinforced with a metallic hemispheric cross-shaped armature which is fastened to the bone by its inferior hook and superior screws. This device, which also serves as a guide for bone reconstruction, automatically provides the artificial hip with the right anatomical centre. It is stiff enough to secure a pelvic discontinuity, but because it is open, it remains flexible and does not change the elasticity of the iliac bone.

Keywords: hip, total hip arthroplasty, acetabular revision, bone allograft, acetabular loosening, reinforcement metallic armature, reconstruction of acetabular deficiencies.

Introduction

Total hip revision arthroplasty for mechanical loosening of an acetabular component raises numerous technical questions. The choice of approach, removal of prosthesis components, treatment of bone loss, type of revision prosthesis, cemented or cementless – these are the main and often controversial aspects of the procedure. Here, we will describe only revision with a cemented prosthesis after bone reconstruction of acetabular deficiencies with allografts and an acetabular reinforcement device.

Whatever the causes, mechanical or biological, total hip acetabular loosening results in bone loss which becomes more frequent and extensive after recurrent failures [14, 21, 22]. Bony deficiencies may be segmental, cavitary or combined. They may affect all the walls of the acetabular cavity and bring on a pelvic discontinuity of the most severe form [4, 21].

We have learned from experience, as have numerous other authors, that revision using an oversized socket or filling bone defects with cement leads to a new and sometimes early failure [12]. Therefore, repairing bone loss with bone is an absolute necessity. Yet, as an extensive reconstruction requires a great deal of bone, we must use allografts in most cases and often exclusively. In the early 1970s, a pelvic discontinuity associated with severe acetabular bone loss, as a complication of acetabular loosening of metal-on-metal prostheses, led us to design an implant able to solidly fix the fracture and to guide acetabular bone reconstruction [12]. This reinforced acetabular reconstruction has been our routine technique of acetabular loosening revision for 24 years. Its goal is to restore an anatomical state however extensive the bone defects. The efficiency and reliability of this technique have stood the test of time, even in the most severe cases of destruction.

This is just one possibility among others; numerous techniques of acetabular revision have been described. They can be classified into two categories, depending on whether a cemented or cementless acetabular component is used. Revision with a cementless component [5-7, 10, 11, 16] requires seeking host bone contact and leads to using extra-large sockets and placing them in a high position. This is not without mechanical disadvantages. Moreover, this technique cannot be used when there are extensive structural defects and especially when these are associated with a pelvic discontinuity.

Among reconstructions with allografts and cemented acetabular components, it is advisable to distinguish between reconstruction with impacted morselised allografts [2, 8, 15, 20] and the use of structural allografts [3, 9, 12, 17, 18] to repair segmental defects. The first technique is indicated in cavitary defects or in combined defects when it is possible to close segmental defects with metal meshes. The second is especially suitable to repair rim and dome defects. Both techniques are limited by the severity of bone destruction. When it is major and extensive, both cavitary and segmentary, the use of metallic armatures is required [1, 2, 12, 19]. There are different types of metallic armatures, with or without an inferior hook, with or without a superior iliac plate. Almost all are closed rings or hemisphere-shaped. As they are extremely rigid, they cannot become, mechanically speaking, an integral part of the bone, which remains elastic. They essentially support the acetabular component, but they do not reinforce bone reconstruction. That is a basic difference compared to the armature we use.

Allografts

Femoral heads resected during total hip arthroplasties are suitable for acetabular bone loss repair. Preparation, preservation and utilisation should be carried out within the framework of a bone tissue bank, of which the extremely strict operating rules have been established to prevent any risk of infection of the host by a transmissible pathogenic agent (bacterial or viral infection, neoplasia, nonconventional transmissible agent). Femoral heads are resected from selected donors and a sample is taken for bacteriological control to exclude per-operative infection. They are

Marcel Kerboull, M.D.
Luc Kerboull, M.D.
Service de Chirurgie Orthopédique A, Hôpital Cochin, Pavillon Ollier,
27, rue du Faubourg Saint-Jacques, 75674 Paris Cedex 14, France.

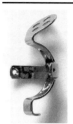

1 *Photograft of the acetabular armature.*

packed in the operating room in a threefold sterile and hermetically-sealed package, frozen at -80° and preserved at the same temperature. They are only used after "validation" when the results of tests on the donor and on the femoral head are negative. Residual soft tissues and cartilage are removed from the femoral head with an oscillating saw. Then, it is cut into fragments of varied sizes and shapes: a bulky piece to fill a large segmental and cavitary bone loss of the roof; slices which are more or less wide and thick to repair the walls; cancellous bone cubes or morselised fragments to fill minor cavitary defects or gaps between bigger pieces.

Metallic armature (fig 1)

The device used is a hemispheric cross with 4 arms made of stainless steel; it is intended to guide and reinforce the bone reconstruction of a destroyed acetabulum. Its shape results from the orthogonal crossing of 2 hemispheric plates. The vertical plate ends distally in a hook inserted under the inferior acetabular margin, and proximally in a rounded plate with 4 screw holes for iliac fixation. The horizontal plate is asymmetrical: the anterior arm is shorter than the posterior arm, which induces a 10° anteversion of the opening plane of the device. This device is available in two series (left and right) of 6 sizes for sockets from 37 to 53 mm in outside diameter. Three holes, one at the crossing of the plates and one at each end of the horizontal plate, allow the direct fixation of the graft to the plate with a 3.5 mm screw. Because of its shape and the inferior hook placed under the tear drop, this device automatically provides the artificial hip with the right anatomical position. It is stiff enough to assure a strong fixation of a pelvic discontinuity, but, because it is open, it remains flexible and does not disturb the elasticity of the acetabulum. It forms a single mechanical unit with the bony cavity which it reinforces, but it does not rigidify the acetabular component.

Technique of acetabular reconstruction

The goal of this reconstruction is to restore a bony cavity which is normal in size, which is in a correct anatomical position, and which has mechanical properties close to those of a normal acetabulum.

EXPOSURE, SOCKET REMOVAL AND CLEANING OF THE ACETABULAR CAVITY (fig 2)

A transtrochanteric approach is routinely used, but it is quite possible to carry out this reconstruction through a posterolateral approach.

The acetabular cavity is widely exposed using: distally, a hooked retractor in the obturator foramen, and proximally, 2 or 3 rounded head pins which keep the trochanter and gluteus muscles elevated, and two retractors, one posterior, one anterior. The removal of a loose socket, whether it is cemented or not, is not usually difficult if it is grossly loose. However, one must excise all the scar tissue (sometimes ossified), around the entire acetabular orifice in order to identify the periphery of the implant and the bony rim, before component extraction with a cup grasper. If the socket, though loose, is still fixed, the safest means of removing the acetabular component is to disrupt the cement-prosthesis interface. After removing some lateral cement with a narrow osteotome, a curved ostotome is introduced between the cement and the prosthesis and gradually insinuated around the acetabular component. Thus, the socket can be extracted without any damage to the bone of the acetabular bed. Removal of an intrapelvic component may be difficult and sometimes dangerous, but having to remove it through a retroperitoneal approach is exceptional. After widening, if necessary, the bony acetabular orifice, gentle working –combining traction, twisting and tilting– manages to progressively dislodge it without serious damage to the thin, weak walls of the bony cavity. Then, any cement fragments which are free or still adherent to bone are removed, and the bone is cleared with a cutting curette of the fibrous membrane which lines it and the granulomatosous tissue which fills cavitary defects. Finally, the cavity is washed with pulsatile irrigation. It is useless and not recommended to ream this cavity, to avoid weakening its flimsy walls.

CHOOSING THE SIZE OF ARMATURE

The reference is the size of a normal acetabulum. If there is a healthy hip, superposition of templates of acetabular components on the X-ray of the hip in a frontal view allows selection of the adequate size of device. When there is no reference, the

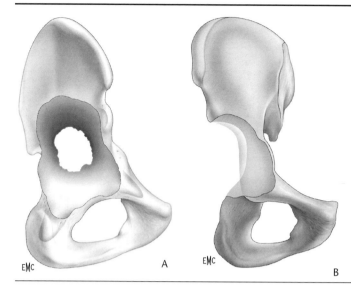

2 *Drawing of major acetabular destruction extended to the roof and the anterior, posterior and medial walls.*
A. Lateral view.
B. Frontal view.

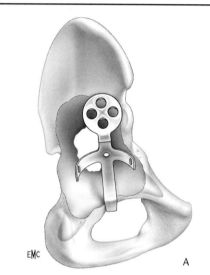

3 *Trial of acetabular armature in the acetabulum.*
A. The hook is inserted under the inferior acetabular margin near the ischium.
B. The armature is tilted at 45° and must not be more vertical, whether or not the superior blade comes into contact with the iliac bone.

size of the bony cavity in its inferior part must be taken into account, knowing that after bone reconstruction the anterior, posterior and medial walls must be at least 7 mm thick.

TRIAL OF THE DEVICE (fig 3)

After removal of fibrous or scar tissue, ossifications or osteophytes which hide it, the inferior margin of the acetabulum with its smooth cortical edge appears. Beneath it, a narrow curved periosteal elevator is introduced to make room for the hook inserted near the ischium. Then, the acetabular device is tilted at 45°. This movement should not tend to eject the hook from the tear drop. If it does, three possible causes must be explored: 1) The acetabular device is too large. Try a smaller one; 2) The inferior margin of the acetabulum is destroyed by a polyethylene granuloma. It should be repaired with an allograft fragment before inserting the hook; 3) The medial wall just above the tear drop is too thick. Thin it down with a rongeur or a gouge until the hook stays in the right position.

Then, one should check that the vertical branch of the device is located in a strictly frontal plane. When there is a defect, even slight, in the roof, the superior rounded blade does not come into contact with the bone. One must not place the device in a vertical position superior to 45° in order to bring the blade into contact with the bone; this would lead to ejection of the hook. The device should not be opened nor the blade bent to adapt them to the bone loss. On the contrary, the acetabular device should be used as a guide to evaluate the size and location of bony defects, as well as the shape and dimension of the allograft fragments needed to achieve bone reconstruction. Once this assessment is performed, the trial acetabular device is removed.

ROOF RECONSTRUCTION (SUPERIOR RIM AND DOME) *(fig 4)*

Unless there is a massive defect of the medial wall, bony reconstruction starts with reconstruction of the roof. Whenever possible, the superior bone loss is filled with a bulky fragment of a femoral head. It is carefully shaped with the trabeculae properly oriented, so that it can resist the pressure stresses in the bearing area. To give the defect a hemispherical shape, small cavities are filled with impacted cancellous bone and asperities are abraded. The graft is shaped so that its superior part, made convex, accurately fits the dome; its inferior part, made concave, matches the convexity of the device. The blade of the device lies on its lateral part, made of subchondral bone. Before flattening

4 *Roof reconstruction.*
A, B. A bulky fragment is shaped from a femoral head to fit rim and dome defect.
C. This fragment, embedded in the superior defect, is kept in place by the armature.
D. A slice from the femoral head slipped under the dome graft repairs the deficient medial wall.
E, F. Alternative possibilities of roof reconstruction with a single graft fragment (E), two superposed fragments (F).

this surface, it is advisable to put the armature in position to prevent an insufficient thickness of the graft. Several trials are sometimes needed to achieve a perfect fit of the graft to bone and armature. If the graft cannot be wedged into the dome defect, it can be screwed to the host bone. The device is again removed.

If superior bone loss is slight, it is sometimes enough to shape a small graft into an inverted L or give it a trapezoidal shape to augment the depth of the cavity and give the blade a

stable bed. If there is only a cavitary deficiency of the acetabulum, widening the cavity, but the superior rim is well-preserved, one may first screw the armature to iliac bone and then embed adequate slices of graft between the arms of the device and the walls of the cavity to thicken them *(fig 5)*.

MEDIAL WALL RECONSTRUCTION *(fig 6)*

In the majority of cases, bone loss is located in the middle part of the medial wall. A thick

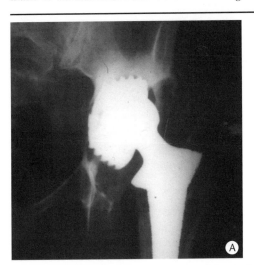
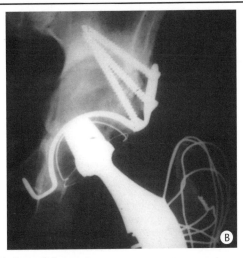
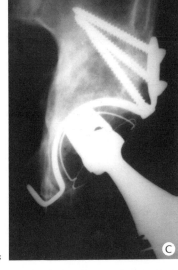

5 *Example of superior bone reconstruction with a single bulky graft fragment.*
A. Extensive acetabular bone loss associated with a pelvic discontinuity.
B. A large fragment from a femoral head cut to shape fills the superior defect. On this immediate postoperative X-ray, graft outlines and bone are clearly visible.
C. 18 months later, union between graft and native bone and the first steps of graft remodelling are obvious.

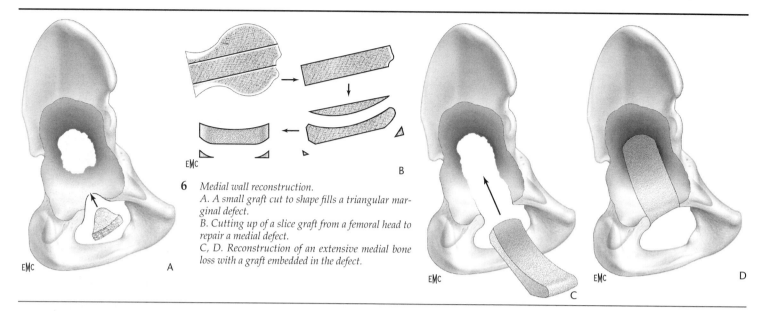

6 *Medial wall reconstruction.*
A. A small graft cut to shape fills a triangular marginal defect.
B. Cutting up of a slice graft from a femoral head to repair a medial defect.
C, D. Reconstruction of an extensive medial bone loss with a graft embedded in the defect.

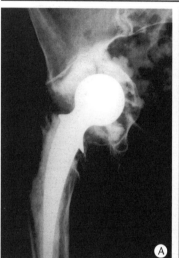
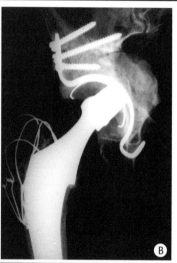
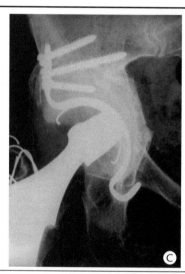

7 *Example of medial wall reconstruction.*
A. Acetabular medial deficiency.
B. The graft, which is too big, protudes into the pelvis on a postoperative X-ray.
C. At 10 years, graft remodelling and resorption of its intrapelvic part.

slice of femoral head is suitable to fill the defect after its edges have been bevelled and its exopelvic surface made concave to properly match the defect and the device. This slice must be thick enough (15 mm) so that it remains 7 mm thick after its shaping. It is not necessary to use a thicker graft, for the protrusive bone will progressively resorb. As for the endopelvic cavity –sometimes large– located beyond the graft, it will spontaneously disappear. In any case, it must not be filled with bone graft, which will certainly resorb and delay the collapse of the cavity.

If the inferior margin of the acetabulum is destroyed by a polyethylene granuloma, frequent in this location, it must be repaired to give the hook a grasp. A graft of adequate shape (rectangular, triangular or semicircular), thick enough to be wedged into the hook, suitably fills the defect.

If the destruction of the inferior margin extends far onto the medial wall, it is better, when a big femoral head is available, to repair the entire defect with one single slice, carefully shaped. The stability of the reconstruction will be stronger. It is also possible, by longitudinal cutting of a femoral

head and neck of normal size, to obtain a long and thick bony slice to fill an extensive defect.

If several fragments must be used, the stability of the medial reconstruction is rather poor. It may increase sufficiently when the armature is put into position. If it does not, the fragments may be fastened to the device with metal wires or a screw (*fig 7*).

FIXING OF THE ACETABULAR ARMATURE (*fig 8*)

After medial and superior reconstruction, we put the armature back in place, ensure that its position is correct, and test its stability with a punch introduced into the hole at the crossing of the arms. Then, the blade is secured to the iliac bone using 5 mm diameter screws. We begin with the lower hole, direct the screw upwards and to the rear towards the sacroiliac joint which it should not reach. Before fully tightening, we insert another screw in another hole (usually anterior) and partially screw it to stabilise the armature. Then we fully tighten the two screws in turn. The screws generally pass through the roof graft, and their path through the graft should be cleared so that tightening them forces the graft against the host bone. Tightening the

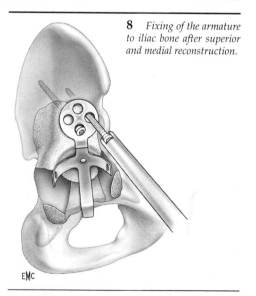

8 *Fixing of the armature to iliac bone after superior and medial reconstruction.*

lower screw puts the armature under tension, which is reflected by the hook tightening against the inferior margin of the acetabulum. If the hook is being ejected, this is because the upper graft is insufficiently thick. It is necessary to add a slice of bone of adequate thickness under the blade and resume tightening until the armature loses all

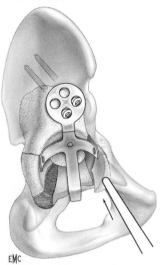

9 *Reconstruction of anterior and posterior wall by embedding sliced graft between the arms of the armature and remaining walls. Cancellous fragments are impacted in pubic and ischiatic cavitary defects and gaps between structural grafts.*

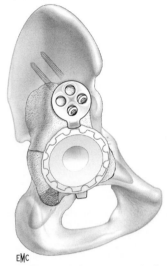

10 *Cementing of acetabular component in the repaired and reinforced bony cavity.*

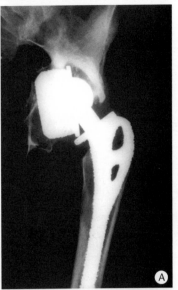

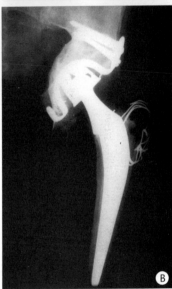

12 *A. Acetabular deficiency with a pelvic discontinuity. B. 17 years after revision. No resorption. Remodelling and incorporation of the graft.*

elasticity and forms a complete mechanical unit with the bone.

RECONSTRUCTION OF ANTERIOR AND POSTERIOR WALLS *(fig 9)*

This is achieved by embedding grafts that are cut to shape between the remaining wall and the horizontal branch of the armature. If necessary, these grafts may be screwed to the device, if embedding is impossible due to the complete destruction of the walls. This reconstruction is completed by packing cancellous bone into pubic and ischiatic cavitary defects and the gaps between the segmental grafts, in order to avoid any leak of cement between the grafts.

CEMENTING THE ACETABULAR COMPONENT *(fig 10)*

After cleaning the reconstructed and reinforced cavity with pulsatile lavage, we check that all the fragments are properly attached. If necessary, we remove any small free fragments and excise any bony projections with a rongeur. A trial cup is then introduced into the cavity to verify the match and accurate orientation. After final cleaning and drying, the corresponding acetabular component is cemented as usual.

Postoperative care

This type of acetabular reconstruction is strong enough to allow immediate and active mobilisation of the hip and partial weight-bearing with the help of two crutches as soon as the third postoperative day. The patient will keep the crutches for 2 or 3 months to progressively achieve full weight-bearing *(fig 11, 12)*.

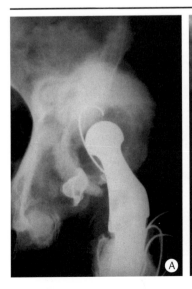

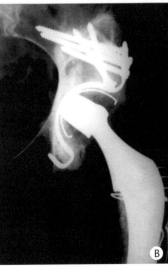

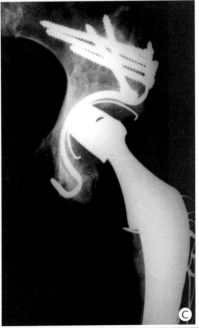

11 *A. Septic acetabular loosening associated with major roof destruction.*
B. One stage exchange revision. Bone reconstruction with allografts and acetabular armature. Postoperative X-ray.
C. 18 years later, infection has healed, the remodelled and incorporated allograft shows no signs of resorption.

References

[1] Bremant JJ. Renforcement métallique de l'acétabulum. In : Cahiers d'enseignement de la SOFCOT. Paris : Expansion scientifique française, 1990. 165-174

[2] Capello WN, Hellman EJ, Feinberg JR. Revision of the acetabular component. Use of cement. In : The adult hip. Philadelphia : Lippincott-Raven, 1998 : chap 89

[3] Chandler HP, Tigges RG. Structural grafting in acetabular recontruction. In : The adult hip. Philadelphia : Lippincott-Raven, 1998 : chap 88

[4] D'Antonio JA, Capello WN. Classification and management of acetabular abnormalities in total hip arthroplasty. *Clin Orthop* 1989 ; 243 : 126-137

[5] Emerson RH, Head WC, Berkhacich FM, Malinin TI. Non cemented acetabular revision arthroplasty using allograft bone. *Clin Orthop* 1989 ; 249 : 30-43

[6] Engh CA, Engh CA Jr. Cementless revision of failed total hip arthroplasty. Preoperative planning, surgical technique and postoperative rehabilitation. *Tech Orthop* 1993 ; 7 : 9-26

[7] Engh CA, Glassman AH, Griffin WL, Mayer JG. Results of cementless revision for failed cemented total hip arthroplasty. *Clin Orthop* 1988 ; 235 : 91-110

[8] Gie GA, Linder L, Ling RS. Impacted cancellous allografts and cement for revision total hip arthroplasty. *J Bone Joint Surg Br* 1993 ; 75 : 14-21

[9] Gross AE, Garbuz D, Morsi ES. Acetabular allografts for restoration of bone stock in revision arthroplasty of the hip. *Instr Course Lect* 1996 ; 45 : 135-142

[10] Harris WH. Management of the deficient acetabulum using cementless fixation without bone grafting. *Orthop Clin North Am* 1993 ; 24 : 663-665

[11] Harris WH, Krushall RJ, Galante JO. Results of the cementless revision of total hip arthroplasty using the Harris Galante prosthesis. *Clin Orthop* 1988 ; 235 : 120-126

[12] Kerboull M. Les réinterventions pour descellement aseptique des prothèses totales de hanche. La reconstruction du cotyle. In : Arthroplastie totale de hanche. Berlin : Springer-Verlag, 1985 : 89-96

[13] McCollum DE, Nunley JA. Bone grafting in total hip replacement for acetabular protrusion. *J Bone Joint Surg Am* 1980 ; 62 : 1065-1073

[14] Olivier H. Traitement des détériorations cotyloïdiennes aseptiques des prothèses totales de hanche. In : Cahier d'enseignement de la SOFCOT. Paris : Expansion scientifique française, 1995 : 23-34

[15] Olivier H, Sanouiller JL. Reconstructions cotyloïdiennes par greffes spongieuses dans les révisions d'arthroplasties totales de hanche. *Rev Chir Orthop* 1991 ; 77 : 232-240

[16] Padgett DE. Cementless acetabular reconstruction. In : The adult hip. Philadelphia : Lippincott-Raven, 1998 : chap 87

[17] Paprowski WG, Bradford MS, Jablonsky WS. Acetabular reconstruction with massive acetabular allografts. *Instr Course Lect* 1996 ; 45 : 149-159

[18] Paprowski WG, Magnus RM. Principles of bone grafting in revision total hip arthroplasty. Acetabular technique. *Clin Orthop* 1994 ; 298 : 147-155

[19] Pascarel X, Liquois F, Chauveaux D, LeRebeller A, Honton JL. L'utilisation des anneaux endocotyloïdiens de Muller dans la chirurgie de révision des prothèses totales de hanche. *Rev Chir Orthop* 1993 ; 79 : 357-364

[20] Sloof TJ, Buma P, Gardeniers JW, Schreurs BW, Schimmel JW, Huiskes R. Revision of the acetabular component: bone grafting. In : The adult hip. Philadelphia : Lippincott-Raven, 1998 : chap 90

[21] Vives P. Descellement aseptique des prothèses totales de hanche. *Rev Chir Orthop* 1989 ; 75 (suppl I) : 23-60

[22] Willert HG, Bertram H. Osteolysis in alloarthroplasty of the hip. *Clin Orthop* 1990 ; 238 : 108-121

Femoral revision with impaction cancellous allografting

GA Gie
RSM Ling
AJ Timperley

Abstract. – *For over more than a decade, impaction cancellous grafting associated with the use of acrylic bone cement, when properly applied to difficult revision situations associated with major bone stock loss, has proved to be a method capable of producing not only implant stability but also recovery of bone stock. It is, however, an operation whose success strongly depends on surgical technique. Implant stability using this technique is created by the operating surgeon on the operating table and requires a combination of adequate physical constraint for the graft and vigorous graft impaction, followed by accurate cementing and effective pressurisation of cement before implant insertion. Given these prerequisites, the present clinical evidence suggests that a surgeon can be optimistic with respect to the outcomes he can achieve for his patients, and such outcomes are likely to be maintained in the longer term.*

Keywords: hip, total hip replacement, revision total hip replacement femoral side, impaction grafting, femoral component loosening

Introduction

The orthopaedic surgeon involved in revision hip arthroplasty faces few greater challenges than that of a patient who has undergone multiple operations for femoral component loosening, associated with substantial loss of both cancellous and cortical bone stock in the femur. A method that not only produces a stable implant but also leads to restoration of bone stock is highly desirable, especially in young patients. Impaction cancellous grafting is one of the very few methods that can, when performed properly, achieve both these aims.

The method was initially applied to the reconstruction of the acetabulum, and was first reported by Slooff and his colleagues in 1984 [15]. At about that time, three patients at the Princess Elizabeth Orthopaedic Hospital in Exeter had undergone femoral impaction grafting with the use of a cementless stem for femoral component loosening with substantial loss of bone stock. Although symptomatic relief was initially good,

GA Gie, M.B., Ch.B., F.R.C.S. Ed., F.R.C.S. Ed. (Orth.), Consultant Orthopaedic Surgeon, Princess Elizabeth Orthopaedic Centre.
RSM Ling, O.B.E, M.A., B.M.(Oxon), F.R.C.S., Hon. F.R.C.S. Ed., Honorary Consultant Orthopaedic Surgeon, Princess Elizabeth Orthopaedic Centre.
AJ Timperley, M.B., Ch.B., F.R.C.S. Ed., Consultant Orthopaedic Surgeon, Princess Elizabeth Orthopaedic Centre, Barrack Rd., Exeter, Devon EX2 5DW, United Kingdom.

subsidence of the stems within the impacted graft was excessive. This experience, taken in conjunction with Slooff's success in combining impacted cancellous grafts and cement in the acetabulum, led to a trial of impaction grafting and cement in the femur at the Princess Elizabeth. The first case was carried out in May 1987 and the initial series was first reported in 1991 [14] and more fully in 1993 [6]. Since that time, the operation has become widely used. The initial enthusiasm for the procedure has been tempered by the fact that the complication rate has sometimes been reported as high [4, 10, 11, 13] and that it is strongly technique dependent [9, 17].

The achievement of implant stability in femoral impaction grafting depends on containment of the graft, impaction of the graft and the use of cement to immobilise the interface between cement and graft. Achieving stability in this procedure is a technical matter that requires exposure, time, trouble and experience.

Indications

In the original series of 56 hips reported in 1993 [6], the preoperative bone stock loss was mainly categorised as Endo-Klinik [5] grade II. There were 13 hips in grade III. Since that time, the generally satisfactory results

reported have been well-maintained and only one stem has been re-revised for aseptic loosening (at 8 years postimpaction grafting, in a case originally associated with an intraoperative femoral fracture that was unsoundly fixed) and none for femoral osteolysis. It therefore seemed reasonable to gradually extend the scope of the procedure and in the second series undertaken in Exeter, out of 102 hips, 46 were categorised as Endo-Klinik grade III and 3 as Endo-Klinik grade IV. With the further passage of time, increasing numbers of grade IV have been operated on using this method and recently, excellent results have been reported in severely damaged femora in the medium term [17]. As yet, there are no longer term results of the procedure applied to very severe problems of bone stock loss, and the limitations of the method are therefore not known at present. The longest follow-up in the original series now exceeds 12 years. Bearing these matters in mind, the indications can be simply stated as:

– Mechanical failure of cemented and cementless femoral stems, regardless of the length of the latter.

– Loss of proximal femoral bone stock with cortical defects and thinning as a consequence of instability, wear-induced osteolysis and possibly stress shielding.

All references to this article must include: Gie GA, Ling RSM and Timperley AJ. Femoral revision with impaction cancellous allografting. Editions Scientifiques et Médicales Elsevier SAS (Paris). All rights reserved. Surgical Techniques in Orthopaedics and Traumatology, 55-460-A-10, 2001, 6 p.

Preoperative planning

ESTABLISHMENT OF THE CAUSE OF SYMPTOMS

As a rule, the clinical history together with a careful study of serial radiographs are enough to be reasonably certain of the cause of the patient's symptoms. If there is doubt, however, an intra-articular injection of 10 ml of 2% lignocaine is a satisfactory method of clarifying the cause of pain. Furthermore, it gives the patient and the surgeon a good idea of the symptomatic relief that is likely to follow an effective revision procedure, a matter that is of assistance in coming to a decision about the need for revision surgery [3].

EXCLUSION OF INFECTION

This should be carried out along conventional lines. Sometimes, it is not possible confidently to exclude infection preoperatively. If the surgeon finds that there is evidence of infection after the hip has been exposed, the wisest way to proceed is to abandon the operation and wait for the bacteriological findings and antibiotic sensitivities.

ANALYSIS OF BONE DEFICIENCIES

In planning the operation, it is essential for the surgeon to have as much information as possible concerning the sites and extent of bone deficiencies in the femur. As a general rule, these are always more extensive than the plain X-ray appearances suggest. Many classifications of bone stock loss exist. The Endo-Klinik classification has been used in Exeter since 1987 [5]. A knowledge of the bone stock deficiencies helps the surgeon to plan the surgical approach to the femur so that he can provide adequate containment for the graft, using wire mesh fixed with cerclage where necessary. It also helps the surgeon to decide preoperatively whether a long stem or other supplementary fixation in the form of strut grafts or plating are required. In general, these should be used where there is significant structural weakness of the femoral shaft in the region where the tip of a standard length stem would be placed following revision. Without such supplementary fixation in these cases, there is a very real risk of postoperative femoral fracture.

TEMPLATING

Anteroposterior and lateral radiographs that extend beyond the most distal lytic area in the femur into normal diaphysis are essential, and allow the surgeon to decide the site in which the intramedullary plug should be placed. In general, this would be 2 cm beyond the most distal lytic area in the femur. Measuring the distance from the planned position of the plug to the tip of the greater trochanter enables the surgeon to place the plug with precision during the operation. The templates also allow the surgeon to estimate the size of the femoral component that may be required as well as the size of the proximal femoral impactor to be used to fashion the neomedullary canal in the impacted graft. However, a final decision on implant size is not wise until the operation is actually in progress.

Operative technique

There are now a number of different instrument systems available for femoral impaction grafting. Whatever system is chosen, the principles of the operation remain the same.

It is essential for the surgeon to create the circumstances under which the graft can be fully contained and vigorously impacted. This means that bone defects must be covered with wire mesh (fixed with cerclage) to reconstitute an intact femoral tube that will allow full containment of the graft. Without tight impaction and full containment of the graft, adequate stability cannot be obtained.

If infection is present, a two stage exchange is recommended. Once the infection has been overcome, a new prosthesis can be implanted with the impaction grafting technique at a second operation. Prophylactic antibiotics are always given intravenously but not until specimens for bacteriological culture have been obtained from the operative site.

The description of the technique of the operation that follows is based on the use of the X-Change III® instrumentation manufactured by Stryker Howmedica Osteonics.

EXPOSURE

Surgical exposure is according to the surgeon's preference but he must recognise that this operation cannot be performed correctly through an inadequate exposure. The upper end of the femur must be delivered into the wound to allow the proximal end of the canal to be opened into the greater trochanter, up to 1 cm lateral to the midline axis of the canal (depending on implant size). This requires free soft tissue release. Without this type of exposure, it is impossible for the new medullary canal to be correctly orientated, adequately impacted and properly cemented. In Exeter, the procedure is nearly always performed through a radical posterior approach that always includes a psoas tenotomy and section of the gluteus maximus tendon close to its femoral attachment. A conventional trochanteric osteotomy is rarely used because of the danger of possible loss of containment for the proximal and lateral part of the graft. However, an extended trochanteric osteotomy [18] is not open to this objection and may be a valuable addition to the exposure when there is substantial distal cement or a long ingrown stem to be removed. Obviously, the large trochanteric fragment following extended trochanteric osteotomy must be wired securely back to the femur before the impaction commences. This means that full exposure of the femur (adequate for the impaction) must be achieved before the extended trochanteric osteotomy is performed. If the femur is extensively manipulated while carrying out adequate exposure after such an osteotomy, there is an increased risk of fracturing the femur near the lower part of the osteotomy. After repair of an extended trochanteric osteotomy, implant stability following impaction grafting can be as good as is achieved in an intact femur [2].

REMOVAL OF THE OLD FEMORAL COMPONENT

If cortical integrity is tenuous, prophylactic wiring of the femur before removal of the old implant is wise. After removal of the old femoral component, all traces of cement, fibrous membrane, particulate debris and granulomatous material are cleaned from the femoral canal. Thorough lavage is important.

PREPARATION OF THE FEMORAL CANAL

Defects in the femoral canal should be made good with wire mesh that is secured by cerclage. Monofilament wire is advisable at the upper end of the femur to minimise the chance of debris production by fretting, should cables be used. The latter, however, should always be used to secure a mesh that has been employed for complete circumferential segmental deficits of the diaphysis. Using monofilament wire under these circumstances increases the chance of the distal femoral segment being driven out of the mesh during packing and impaction of the graft. Strut grafts may be needed to reinforce distal lytic defects. Before the cerclage is tightened to hold the strut, a layer of cancellous chips should be interposed between the strut and the femur. Where there has been significant loss of proximal medial bone stock, a proximal build-up with mesh may be needed but a decision on this is best postponed until the trial reduction is performed.

PREPARATION OF THE GRAFT

In Exeter, fresh frozen femoral heads constitute the main source of graft. All remnants of cartilage and soft tissue are removed from the femoral head which is placed in the bone mill; in these circumstances, the product of the milling contains some small cortical fragments. It may be advantageous to use purely cancellous bone but this means additional femoral heads may be needed. Irradiated

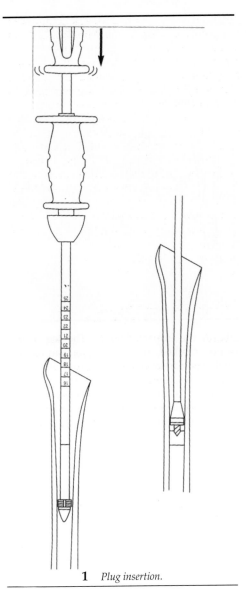

1   *Plug insertion.*

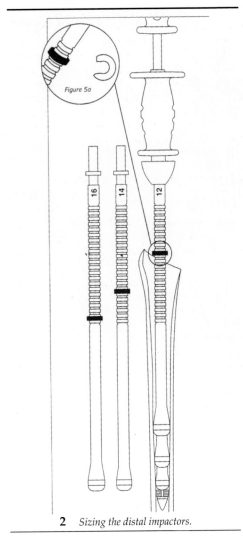

2   *Sizing the distal impactors.*

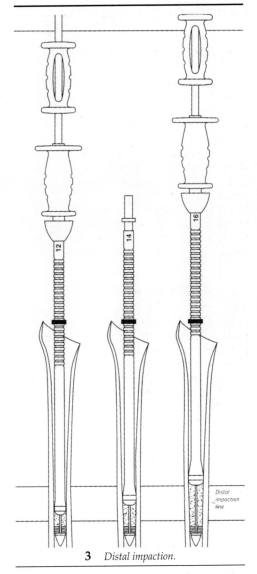

3   *Distal impaction.*

bone is used by many surgeons and there does not appear to be any convincing evidence to date that this is disadvantageous.

THE SIZE OF THE GRAFT CHIPS

This is important. Experimental studies have suggested that chips that are under 5 mm in diameter may be associated with compromised stability [16]. Bone mills should therefore be operated at low revolutions with the cutting blade at the largest aperture. Based on the principles of soil mechanics, there is evidence that the strongest impacted construct is achieved by the use of chips of variable size [1]. In Exeter, chips of approximately 10 mm in diameter are now routinely used for the proximal impaction of the femoral canal. Thorough washing and defatting of the graft is recommended by some surgeons [8], although it is possible this may reduce the viscoelastic behaviour of cement. This may be disadvantageous when femoral components of force-closed design [7] which function on the taper-slip principle are being used.

PLACEMENT OF THE PLUG

A tight fit of the intramedullary plug in the canal is essential. The plug is screwed on to the end of the guide wire and then driven down the canal to the predetermined depth using the plug introducer *(fig 1)*. If the proposed site for the plug is beyond the isthmus, it may be necessary to stabilise the plug temporarily by the use of one or two transfemoral Kirschner wires. If there is a soundly-fixed and non-infected plug of cement distally in an appropriate position, the guide wire may be drilled into the cement or the plug placed on top of the cement *(fig 1)*.

GRAFT IMPACTION

Before any graft is put into the femur, it is essential to try the proximal impactors down the canal over the guide wire in order to decide on the most appropriate size, starting with the one suggested by the templating. The largest size going easily down the canal to 1 cm beyond the level where the stem should be placed is the size to use. The surgeon should then ascertain how far down the canal each size of distal impactor will go before it is arrested by the endosteal wall of the femoral cavity. Each impactor should be slid over the guide wire and when it is stopped distally, the plastic cerclip should

be fixed to the impactor at the level of the greater trochanter *(fig 2)*. This provides an easily identifiable mark on each impactor that should never go beyond the tip of the greater trochanter during impaction. Unless this precaution is adopted, the surgeon may split the femur.

When packing the allograft chips into the canal, it helps to use the barrels of 20 ml syringes that have had their distal ends amputated. The chips are ejected from the syringe barrel into the open proximal end of the femoral canal and are then driven into the upper part of the canal with a large diameter, hand-held distal impactor and are impacted down on to the upper surface of the plug with the largest size of impactor that will pass down over the guide wire to the plug without catching on the bony wall of the canal. Impaction should not be unduly vigorous immediately above the plug, since this may drive it distally.

As soon as the surgeon has impacted to approximately 1 cm above the plug, he should then start vigorous impaction with the distal impactor *(fig 3)*. In between each set of blows of the sliding hammer on the impactor, the impactor should be withdrawn and more graft packed into the canal. Each

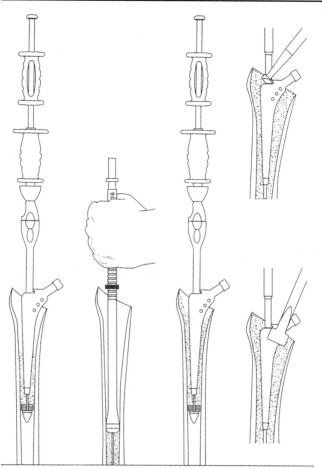

4   *The stages of proximal impaction.*

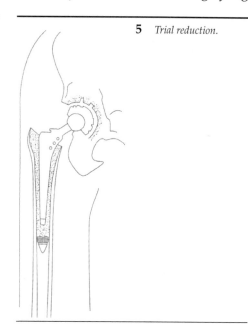

5   *Trial reduction.*

graft refill is packed proximally using a large diameter distal impactor and then vigorously impacted distally using the appropriate sized distal impactor. Once the graft has been impacted to the level of the distal impaction line using the distal impactor, the surgeon should change to using the proximal impactor or phantom (*fig 4*). The proximal impactor is driven firmly over the guide wire into the distally impacted graft. At this stage, the surgeon must recognise that the orientation of the proximal impactor or phantom is important because it controls the position of anteversion of the neomedullary canal.

After each pass of the proximal impactor, more graft material is introduced in the canal and is impacted using appropriate distal impactors held in the hand (*fig 4*) and not the slap hammer. The proximal impactor is then driven in again with vigorous blows of the sliding hammer. The proximal impactor should be so tightly impacted into the graft that it is impossible to withdraw it by hand. If it can be withdrawn by hand, the impaction is insufficiently tight. These steps are repeated until the femur is gradually filled and the neomedullary canal created.

Before the impaction reaches the top of the femur, it is wise to carry out a trial reduction (using the trial femoral heads on the phantom) to check on the final desired position of the stem and to decide on whether any proximal reconstruction of the

femur using mesh is needed. This is always required if there has been loss of proximal femoral bone stock to the extent that adequate proximal support for the stem cannot be achieved. If a proximal mesh is needed, it is best to apply the mesh whilst the proximal impactor is in place since it is then easy to ensure that sufficient space is left between the mesh and the impactor for an adequate amount of graft. Proximal mesh should never be placed so that it directly abuts on the stem. The trial reduction can usually be done with the guide wire still in place.

The importance of vigorous impaction of the graft around the upper end of the proximal impactor cannot be over-emphasised. Large chips are now used in the proximal end of the canal and vigorously hammered down round the proximal end of the proximal impactor using the small hand impactor and a hammer (*fig 4*).

At this stage, the proximal impactor should be absolutely stable in the neomedullary canal. If it is not, it is best to extract it and repack the canal more tightly. During impaction, any sudden reduction in the force needed to drive in the proximal impactor may mean that the femur has been fractured. Under such circumstances, the fracture line must be exposed and the fracture stabilised by appropriate means. The femur should then be repacked.

A trial reduction should then be repeated (*fig 5*) with the proximal impactor still in

situ in the impacted graft. The leg length can be checked, and the surgeon can make a final decision about the appropriate depth within the femur to which the proximal impactor is to be driven, to achieve the desired leg length. He should then withdraw the proximal impactor from the graft, using the sliding hammer in reverse for a distance of 2 cm, and then repack large chips into the upper end of the impacted graft around the proximal impactor, using the hand impactor and a hammer. The proximal impactor is then driven back into the impacted graft to the predetermined position to achieve the desired leg length. This final disimpaction, proximal packing, and reimpaction of the proximal impactor are important measures in achieving proximal stability.

INTRODUCTION AND PRESSURISATION OF CEMENT

When the guide wire has been removed, a suction catheter is passed down the guide wire cannula of the proximal impactor and suction applied to remove any blood that may have pooled at the distal end of the neomedullary canal. The catheter is left in place until immediately before cement insertion. Antibiotic-loaded cement is always used. Our preference is for the use of Simplex® cement. A double mix of cement should be available and loaded into the cement gun approximately 2 minutes after the beginning of mixing, with the operating theatre temperature at 20 C°. Vacuum mixing or centrifuging has not been used in Exeter. A narrow or tapered gun spout is essential for use with the cement gun to facilitate delivery of the cement into the distal part of the neomedullary canal (*fig 6*). Using a standard sized gun spout makes it very difficult to fill the distal canal properly and also risks compromising the graft on the canal wall. The femoral revision seal and backing plate should be passed over the gun spout up to the body of the cement gun before injection of cement is commenced.

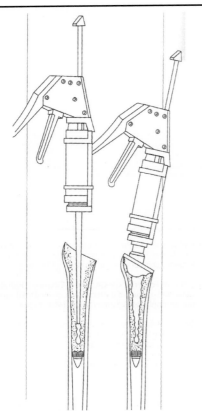

6   *Cement introduction and pressurisation.*

Retrograde injection of cement under direct vision is usually commenced 2 minutes after the beginning of mixing. The cement should be of relatively low viscosity, otherwise its adequate penetration of the graft cannot be achieved. Once the canal is filled with cement dough, the gun spout is cut off level with the distal end of the femoral revision seal and the seal is then impacted into the upper end of the neomedullary canal. The

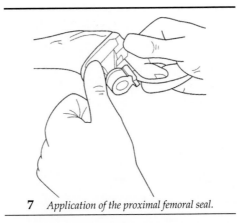

7   *Application of the proximal femoral seal.*

pressuriser seal and plate are then impacted into the opening at the upper end of the neomedullary canal and cement dough is steadily injected into the canal to generate the required pressure *(fig 6)*. Injection should continue until it is judged an appropriate time for the insertion of the stem. This is usually more than 5 minutes after the beginning of mixing. In general, stem insertion takes place a little earlier with impaction grafting than in primary interventions because with the former, the neomedullary canal has been "tailor-made" for the stem.

Once the stem has been inserted to the desired depth, the stem introducer is removed and the "horsecollar" proximal seal *(fig 7)* is placed around the upper end of the stem and held firmly in position with the backing plate until the cement has polymerised. The surgeon should place his thumb on the shoulder of the stem to make certain that it does not back out of the cement as polymerisation takes place.

The hip is then reduced and the range of movement checked. Any localised adjacent soft tissue or bony mass responsible for premature neck shaft impingement is removed. The wound is then closed in the usual way. Suction drainage is employed.

Postoperative care

Most patients are mobilised with elbow crutches (touch weight-bearing) on the second post-operative day. Two crutches are advised for twelve weeks, then one crutch, followed by two sticks, and then one stick so that full weight-bearing without any walking aids is achieved by six months. Patients who have undergone a very extensive acetabular reconstruction by impaction grafting as well as a femoral reconstruction are kept in bed for one week before mobilisation.

Conclusions

Femoral impaction grafting is a technique in evolution for which there are at present no long-term follow-up studies. Its true place in the armamentarium of the revision hip surgeon has therefore still to be established. There is no question that surgical technique is extremely important in achieving good results following this procedure, and herein lies perhaps its main drawback. However, it is equally true that no other procedure in this field is as capable of restoring bone stock in the femur as impaction grafting and for younger patients especially, this is a matter of major importance. So far, in our experience, the results have been maintained up to the medium term and we continue to remain guardedly optimistic for the future.

References ➤

References

[1] Brewster NT, Gillespie WJ, Howie CR, Madabhushi SP, Usmani AS, Fairbairn DR. Mechanical considerations in impaction bone-grafting. *J Bone Joint Surg Br* 1999 ; 81 : 118-124

[2] Chassin E, Silverton CD, Berzins A, Rosenberg A. Implant stability in revision total hip arthroplasty - allograft bone packing following extended femoral osteotomy. *J Arthroplasty* 1997 ; 12 : 863-868

[3] Crawford RW, Ellis AM, Gie GA, Ling RS. Intra-articular local anaesthesia for pain after hip arthroplasty. *J Bone Joint Surg Br* 1997 ; 79 : 796-800

[4] Eldridge JDJ, Smith EJ, Hubble MJ, Whitehouse SL, Learmonth ID. Massive early subsidence following femoral impaction grafting. *J Arthroplasty* 1997 ; 12 : 535-540

[5] Engelbrecht E, Heinert K. Klassification und Behandlungsrichtlinien von Knochensubstanzverlusten bei Revisionoperationen am Huftgelenl - mittlefristige Ergebnisse. In : Anonymous Primare und Revisionalloarthroplastik Hrsg - Endo-klinik. Berlin : Springer-Verlag, 1987 : 189-201

[6] Gie GA, Linder L, Ling RS, Simon JP, Slooff TJ, Timperley AJ. Impacted cancellous allografts and cement for revision total hip arthroplasty. *J Bone Joint Surg Br* 1993 ; 75 : 14-21

[7] Huiskes R, Verdonschot N, Nivbrant B. Migration, stem shape and surface finish. *Clin Orthop* 1998 ; 355 : 103-112

[8] Karrholm J, Hultmark P, Carlsson L, Malchau H. Subsidence of a non-polished stem in revisions of the hip using impaction allograft: evaluation with radiosteriometry and dual energy X-ray absorptiometry. *J Bone Joint Surg Br* 1999 ; 81 : 135-142

[9] Kuiper JH, Van Uem B, Nekkers GJ, Cheah K, Northmore-Ball M, Richardson JB. Early mechanical stability of impaction grafted prostheses correlates strongly with degree of impaction. Paper read at BATS/BORS/BSIG meeting, Oxford, 1998

[10] Masterson EL, Masri BA, Duncan CP. The cement mantle in the Exeter impaction allografting technique: a cause for concern. *J Arthroplasty* 1997 ; 12 : 759-764

[11] Mc Laren AC, Brown SG, Lucero EM. Early failure of impaction bone grafting for revision total hip replacement. Scientific Program of the Annual Meeting of the American Academy of Orthopaedic Surgeons, San Francisco, 1998

[12] Meding JB, Ritter MA, Keatinge EM, Faris PM. Impaction bone-grafting before insertion of a femoral stem with cement in revision total hip arthroplasty. A minimum two year follow-up study. *J Bone Joint Surg Am* 1997 ; 79 : 1827-1841

[13] Pekkarinen J, Ahlo A, Lepisto J, Ylikoski Y, Ylinen P, Paavilainen T. Impaction bone-grafting in revision hip surgery. *J Bone Joint Surg Br* 2000 ; 82 : 103-107

[14] Simon JP, Fowler JL, Gie GA, Ling R, Timperly J. Impaction cancellous grafting of the femur in cemented total hip revision arthroplasty. *J Bone Joint Surg Br* 1991 ; 73 (suppl 1) : 73

[15] Slooff TJ, Huiskes R, Van Horn J, Lemmens AJ. Bone-grafting in total hip replacement for acetabular protrusio. *Acta Orthop Scand* 1984 ; 55 : 593-596

[16] Smith EJ, Richardson JB, Learmonth ID, Evans GP, Nelson K, Lee R et al. The initial stability of femoral impaction grafting. *Hip Int* 1996 ; 6 : 166-172

[17] Van Biezen FC, ten Have BL, Verhaar JA. Impaction bone-grafting of severely defective femora in revision total hip surgery. *Acta Orthop Scand* 2000 ; 71 : 135-142

[18] Younger TI, Bradford MS, Magnus RE, Paprosky WG. Extended proximal femoral osteotomy. A new technique for femoral revision arthroplasty. *J Arthroplasty* 1995 ; 10 : 329-338

Revision total hip replacement: transfemoral approach and noncemented implantation

H Wagner
M Wagner

Abstract. – There are two problems to be solved in the surgical treatment of loosened total hip arthroplasties. The patient must be relieved of the pain caused by the loose implant by the insertion of a new and stably fixed prosthesis. Moreover, the loosening of the prosthesis is usually associated with bone resorption. This bone loss can be so advanced that implantation of a new prosthesis in the old bone bed is critical or impossible. Implantation of larger prostheses and filling the bone defect with cement only appears to solve the problem, because the defect will be even bigger when loosening occurs again. The femoral revision stem described here bridges over the damaged bone bed, leads to immediate exercise stability and allows early mobilisation of patients, who are usually elderly. At the same time, lively new bone formation can be observed, with filling of the bone defects. The transfemoral approach simplifies and speeds the revision, because the damaged former prosthetic bed is osteotomised and opened up to anchor a new femoral stem. Precise preoperative planning is essential in this procedure.

Keywords: hip, arthroplasty, revision arthroplasty, cementless implantation, transfemoral approach.

Introduction

Because of its spectacular success world-wide over the past decades, the total hip replacement is implanted very frequently, with ever-greater enthusiasm and in ever-younger patients. The most important late complication, after 15 to 20 years, is now proving to be aseptic loosening, which has been increasing from year to year.

The clinical problem with aseptic loosening is bone resorption in the prosthetic bed, which can progress so far that a considerable bone defect develops, making fixation of a new prosthesis in place of the old one increasingly difficult or even impossible.

At the early stage of loosening, when the bone is still of good quality, the prosthesis, cement and granulomatous tissue can be removed through the closed femur and a new prosthesis of equal length can be inserted. In recent years, noncemented prostheses have been increasingly used for revision, because revision with cement has considerable disadvantages in patients who still have a fairly long life expectancy. Because of the bone resorption associated with aseptic loosening, a larger bone cavity develops in the old prosthetic bed, and the inner surface of this cavity is smooth due to

Heinz Wagner, M.D., Professor.
Michael Wagner, M.D., PD.
Moorweg 1, D-90592 Schwarzenbruck/Nürnberg, Germany.

the bone resorption and the relative movement between implant and femur. When implanting a new prosthesis with cement, therefore, a larger cavity has to be filled with bone cement, which remains part of the foreign body. "The defect is still a defect" and it is not possible to make it smaller. Moreover, the stability of the cement fixation is considerably less than at the primary implantation, because the fine hollows on the inner surface of the bone defect are absent and the fine interdigitation between bone and cement does not take place. Revision with bone cement in a larger bone cavity therefore leads to a larger foreign body with less stable fixation, and thus to a shorter life-span of the prosthesis. At the next prosthetic loosening, the problem will be even more difficult. If noncemented titanium prostheses with a coarse-blasted surface are employed, new bone tissue can be formed by osseointegration, which leads to a reduction of the bone defect.

In the late stages of aseptic loosening, the bone defect is more advanced, and the shell of bone in the old prosthetic bed is thin and friable and no longer allows firm fixation of a new prosthesis in the old position. Prostheses with longer stems must be used, as they bridge the zone of the femoral defect and are fixed in healthy bone distal to the defect.

Indications for revision

The decision to revise the loosened hip replacement should not be delayed too long in a patient with a long life expectancy. One must not wait until increasing bone loss makes fixation of the new prosthesis quite difficult or until significantly larger implants must be used. In addition, unstable or broken prostheses have to be revised, as do infected prostheses. In the case of loosening with infection, it is necessary to consider whether the prosthesis should be removed initially with possible later reimplantation, or whether revision should be carried out at the same time. Many elderly patients manage well with a so-called resection hip after removal of the prosthesis without replacement. However, it is important that there be a stable proximal femur. A femoral shaft with a severe bone defect is ill-suited for a resection hip, due to a risk of fracture in the bone defect. A bilateral resection hip also cannot be considered, because this leads to such instability that the ability to walk is no longer guaranteed.

Femoral revision stem

A femoral prosthesis must always ensure proximal transmission of force, so that stress protection does not lead to bone atrophy in the proximal femoral segment. This also applies in principle to revision of the

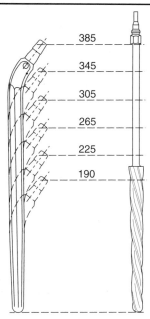

1   *Femoral revision stem in various lengths to fit the extent of the bone defect. There are markings on the reamer for the individual stem lengths.*

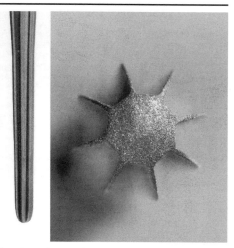

2   *Conical stem of the femoral revision stem of titanium-aluminium-niobium alloy with coarse-blasted surface. The stem has 8 longitudinal sharp conical ribs (right: cross section).*

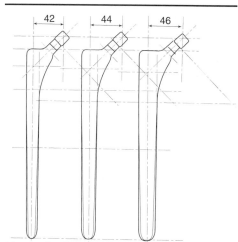

4   *Lateralisation variants of the femoral revision stem. Increasing offset of 42 - 46 mm with increasing stem diameter.*

prosthesis, though with modifications in cases in which the proximal femoral segment has lost its mechanical load-bearing capacity due to the bone resorption. In this case, the deficient stretch of bone must be bridged with a longer stem, and the stem must then be fixed distal to the defect in healthy bone – "as proximal as possible and as distal as necessary".

The femoral revision stem *(fig 1)* is designed for cementless fixation. Short stems are used when there is less bone loss and are fixed in the conically-reamed bone, utilising the old prosthetic bed. With extensive bone loss, long stems are fixed in healthy bone distal to the old prosthetic bed in the conically-reamed medullary cavity. The conical fixation distance should ideally be 10 cm, but at least 7 cm. The great strength of the cone connection ensures early mobilisation of the often elderly patients.

Revision stems in lengths from 190 mm to 385 mm are available to bridge bone defects in femurs of varying lengths *(fig 1)*. Diameters of 14 to 25 mm allow fitting to the diameter of the medullary cavity in each case.

The stem has a conical shape with a cone angle of 2° and is provided with 8 longitudinal and relatively sharp conical ribs, which cut into the bone during implantation, thus ensuring good stability, and especially great rotational stability *(fig 2)*. The stem is made from the titanium-aluminium-niobium alloy Protasul-100. The surface is coarse-blasted, which promotes the deposition of newly-formed bone tissue directly on the metal surface [4-6, 8].

The femur is reamed with conical reamers to obtain a close-fitting conical plug and socket connection with a large contact surface between the femur and prosthetic stem. Conical reaming of the bone is

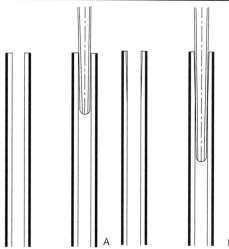

3   *A. The conical stem makes only point contact in a cylindrical medullary cavity.*
B. Stable conical fixation over a long area only occurs after conical widening of the medullary cavity.

essential for conical fixation of the stem. If a conical stem were to be driven into a cylindrical medullary cavity, mechanical resistance would arise naturally, which would have nothing to do with conical fixation. It would rather be an unstable point contact over a small area immediately at the entry site into the bone, which would also involve the risk of breaking the bone. On the other hand, if the medullary cavity is reamed conically, with only very little bone having to be removed when the cone angle is 2° *(fig 3)*, the conical stem penetrates further into the medullary cavity and achieves continuous stable contact with the bone over a long area.

The geometry of the stem, which is conical all around, allows spontaneous self-stabilisation of the prosthesis, even with the slightest sinking and even when there is bone resorption in the microscopic range. This phenomenon must not be mistaken for the clinically-important subsidence of the stem, when there is inadequate primary stability due to the selection of a stem with too small a diameter.

The neck of the prosthesis has the standard cone of 12/14 for the plug connection with the modular heads.

The shape of the revision prosthesis represents a compromise between the material strength and the anatomical circumstances, which has proven itself for many years. The proximal angulation of the prosthesis has a CCD angle of 145° with the thinner stem diameters. This diminishes as the stem diameter increases, i.e. when the prosthesis is of larger diameter, the lever arm for the pelvitrochanteric muscles becomes longer.

The steeper CCD angle with the thinner prosthetic stems has the advantage that a smaller torque is transmitted to the stem when standing up from the seated position and when climbing stairs, which allows smaller stem diameters to be used in slight patients, taking the material strength into account. With the transfemoral approach, there is also a spontaneous lengthening of the lever arm for the pelvitrochanteric muscles, in that the muscle pull leads to slight lateralisation of the greater trochanter.

Lateralisation stem

The standard model of the femoral revision stem has an offset of 36 mm. A lateralisation model is available for particularly broad varus hips, as are some primary stems, with an increasing offset of 40 – 50 mm as the stem diameter increases *(fig 4)*.

The stem of the revision prosthesis is straight and does not follow the physiological antecurvature of the femoral shaft. This has a number of crucial advantages: the straight stem allows conical reaming of the medullary cavity, facilitates implantation, allows unforced adjustment of the angle of anteversion and avoids the need to keep prostheses for the right and left sides, so that the number of implants does not have to be doubled. The straight stem makes modularity unnecessary, i.e.

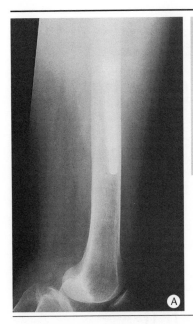

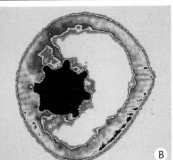

5 *A. The long straight stem runs distally from the femoral isthmus along the anterior cortex. The sharp ribs cut into the bone and stabilise the stem in the frontal plane.*
B. Cross section in computerized tomography.

assembling the prosthetic stem from several parts. This is important because modularity in long-term implants, especially in the case of small diameters, always comprises a mechanical weak point.

The most important advantage of the straight stem is apparent in cases in which long stems must be used because of the extent of the bone defect in the old prosthetic bed, which can extend far beyond the femoral isthmus. The conically-reamed bone channel in the medullary cavity for the revision stem should have a length ideally of 10 cm, but at least 7 cm. Depending on the thickness, the cortex usually only allows a bone cone 3 to 4 cm long distal to the femoral isthmus.

A straight prosthetic stem runs distally from this short bone cone along the anterior cortex because of the physiological antecurvature of the femoral shaft, when the sharp longitudinal ribs cut into the bone and contribute considerably to the stability of fixation in the frontal plane. The long straight stem thus has a two-fold fixation: the conical fit in the proximal area in the conically-reamed part of the medullary cavity, and a 3-point fixation in the distal area, when the stem becomes jammed between the proximal posterior and distal anterior cortex (*fig 5*).

A curved stem would follow the antecurvature of the femur after passing the relatively short bone cone and would not achieve firm contact with the anterior cortex.

However, the straight stem has the disadvantage that the tip of the stem can perforate the anterior cortex in the case of long stems with a length of more than 225 mm. Long stems can therefore only be implanted in association with a transfemoral approach where the antecurvature can be reduced at the transverse osteotomy. However, this is only of theoretical interest, because particularly long stems are used only when there is very extensive bone

damage, for which the transfemoral approach is appropriate anyway.

Preoperative planning

The most important function of the preoperative planning is selection of the correct stem length and the required stem diameter. The preoperative planning is very reliable with regard to the length, but is less precise with regard to the diameter of the stem, because the depth of penetration of the longitudinal ribs into the bone depends on the strength of the bone, which cannot be adequately assessed with certainty on the radiograph. It is therefore advisable to have the neighbouring stem diameters available during the operation and to make the definitive stem diameter selection according to the depth of penetration of the conical reamer.

The drawn plan enables the compensation of any leg shortening which has arisen due to the preceding prosthetic loosening, as well as the determination, if required, of the length of the transfemoral approach, taking into account the loss of bone in the old prosthetic bed.

The crucial usefulness of the preoperative planning is the fact that the individual steps of the operation and their sequence have been thought out before the operation and are recorded on the drawing. It is therefore unnecessary to start planning and "trying out" only after the operation has commenced. The planned operation can rather be carried out deliberately. This shortens the operating time and avoids surprises, because all of the details are familiar and recorded on the plan drawing. It is plausible that this results in an improvement in the quality of the operative procedure.

The basis for the preoperative planning consists of radiographs with a defined

degree of magnification. It has become established to use the average degree of magnification of 1.15:1. The planning templates are adapted to this.

To realise this degree of magnification, it is assumed that the hip joint lies 10 cm above the surface of the X-ray table. The distance from the table surface to the surface of the film is 5 cm and the distance from the focus of the X-ray tube to the film is 115 cm. In very obese patients, the bone can be higher above the table. In this case, either the distance from the tube to the film can be increased or a test body of defined length can be imaged at the height of the bone at the same time on the radiograph, from which the degree of magnification can be calculated.

Using the planning template which is placed on the radiograph, the suitable revision prosthesis is then selected: the length of the stem should be such that the accessory line for the centre of the head of the prosthesis touches the tip of the greater trochanter and the tip of the stem extends 10 cm (minimum 7 cm) distal to the old prosthetic bed into the intact medullary cavity. This establishes the required length of the stem and the desired lengthening of the femur, if there is any shortening present. Comparison with the radiograph of the opposite hip is required to ensure that both sides are of equal length. This can result in a variation in the height of the prosthetic head in relation to the greater trochanter.

The stem diameter required is determined with the planning template at the same time. This is a particularly important component of the preoperative planning, because this is where the most critical errors are made.

The accessory line for the midpoint of the head touches the tip of the greater trochanter, and the stem projects 10 cm (minimum 7 cm) distal to the old prosthetic bed into the intact medullary cavity. The stem diameter must be determined in this distal segment.

The outline of the planning template corresponds to the outline of the prosthesis. When a template is selected in which the outline for the prosthesis only has a close contact with the inner outline of the cortex, the stem diameter is too small, because it does not take into account the bone substance which is removed during conical reaming and the cutting of the longitudinal ribs into the bone. Such a prosthesis will not achieve adequate primary stability and will sink. When the correct diameter is selected, the outline of the prosthesis on the template will overlap the inner outline of the cortex by 1 mm on both sides (*fig 6*). During this procedure, in the case of very hard bone, it can rarely happen that the prosthesis does not penetrate sufficiently deeply into the medullary cavity during insertion. This does not cause any problems, because the prosthesis can be withdrawn and the medullary cavity can be widened slightly with the conical reamer. The opposite

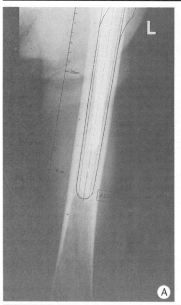
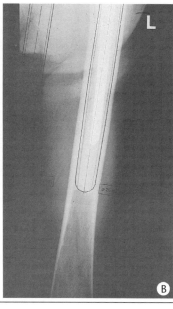

6 *Selection of prosthetic size with the planning template on the radiograph.*

A. The outline of the planning template touches the outline of the cortex. The diameter of this stem is too small, and the prosthesis will sink.

B. When the stem diameter is correct, the outline of the planning template overlaps the outline of the cortex by 1 mm on both sides.

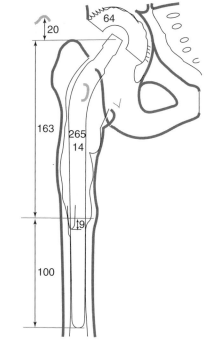

7 *The result of the planning is entered on the plan drawing. The lengths and the implant diameter are entered and can be read during the operation.*

situation is much more unpleasant, that is, when the selected stem diameter is too thin and the prosthesis sinks in too far from the start. A new and thicker implant must then be taken from its sterile packaging, which increases costs unnecessarily.

The most common mistake made during the preoperative planning, and consequently during implantation, is selection of a stem which is too thin and too long. With the correct stem diameter, fixation over a length of 10 cm is fully adequate.

The outline of the ilium including the acetabulum and planned cup implant are first drawn on the plan drawing, and the centre of the articulation is marked. The preoperative position of the femur is also entered by marking the tip of the greater trochanter (or another reference point) to check the intended length or correction of length.

The planning template is then placed under this drawing of the outline, with the selected revision stem in slight physiological adduction, so that the centre of the head on the template lies under the previously marked centre of the cup implant. The outline of the prosthesis is then traced from the template onto the outline drawing.

The outline drawing, which now contains the ilium, the cup implant and the outline of the revision stem, is now placed on the radiograph. By moving it appropriately, the stem can be brought into the centre of the medullary cavity. At the tip of the greater trochanter (or another previously-selected reference point), the leg length or lengthening can be checked against the preoperative marking.

The outer and inner outlines of the femur are then drawn in. The tip of the loosened prosthesis and the distal tip of the old cement mantle should also be entered for orientation during the operation.

The size of the stem and the important length measurements are now entered on

the plan drawing: the depth of the tip of the loosened stem, depth of the old cement mantle, depth of the tip of the intended revision stem and site of the transverse osteotomy, if a transfemoral approach is planned. The distal limit of the transverse osteotomy in the transfemoral approach is generally placed at the distal end of the bone defect. It is often necessary to deviate from this rule in the case of broken prosthetic stems or particularly long cement plugs. All lengths are determined with the ruler on the template, which takes into account the magnification factor of the radiograph of 1.15:1 *(fig 7).*

All of these measurements must be made from a reliable reference point which can also be found easily during the operation. The tip of the greater trochanter is nearly always used; it can be found at operation and marked with a Steinmann nail.

When there is very severe loss of bone, it can happen that the tip of the trochanter cannot be used as a reference point. In that case, another, or possibly several, reliable reference points must be chosen, e.g. a prominent bone edge, cerclage wires around the bone or screws and, in particularly difficult cases, the lateral epicondyle or even the lateral knee joint line.

When using the transfemoral approach, the greater trochanter is split longitudinally. In the second phase of the operation, the tip of the trochanter is then no longer suitable as a reference point. The required measurements during the operation, especially the depth of penetration of the stem, can be made from the transverse osteotomy, the position of which is defined precisely on the plan drawing.

Radiographs of the femur in two planes extending 15 cm distal to the tip of the stem of the loosened prosthesis are required for the preoperative planning – not only to show the implant correctly, but also to assess the "physiological" antecurvature which can show great individual variability in the

patients and can cause unpleasant surprises during the operation when it is not identified beforehand.

Correct orientation is likewise required for revision of the prosthetic cup. A view of the pelvis shows the relation to the opposite hip. The centre of rotation of the affected joint can be determined from this, if findings are physiological in the opposite hip. Köhler's teardrop figure permits orientation when the hip disease is bilateral, as is frequently the case. Wherever possible, the original centre of rotation of the hip joint and the centre of the prosthetic cup should coincide.

Prosthetic heads of different diameter have been used for total hip replacement. If only one component is to be changed, it is necessary to clarify what size head was implanted. The diameter can be measured with planning radiographs with 15% magnification. However, it should be noted that there are prosthetic systems having head diameters of 26 mm or 33 mm.

A total hip replacement or revision without preoperative planning is an "unplanned" operation.

Operative technique

The most important and difficult operative problem in revision after aseptic or septic loosening of a hip prosthesis is stable fixation of a new prosthesis in the damaged bone of the old bed. The stability of the new stem must be good enough that the patient can be mobilised again at once after the revision operation. The operative procedure must be guided by the extent of the bone damage.

Even if opening of the femur is not necessary, it is beneficial to carry out these measures through the posterior approach with the patient in the lateral position. If an unexpected situation occurs at operation, e.g. a fissure or fracture of the bone, or firmly attached cement cannot be removed, it is easy to extend the approach distally without significant damage to the muscles. There is also significantly less venous bleeding when the patient is in the lateral position.

Transfemoral approach

For the transfemoral approach, the patient is placed on his/her side and fixed with supports. The fascia lata and gluteus maximus muscles are split in the direction of their fibres, and the femoral shaft is exposed along the linea aspera. The transfemoral approach is limited distally by a semicircular transverse osteotomy. The level of this osteotomy is determined by the preoperative planning. A Steinmann pin is inserted in the tip of the trochanter, and the distance distally according to the preoperative planning is measured and marked. The soft tissues are released from the femur only at this site.

For the anterior and posterior limits of the transverse osteotomy, two drill holes are made with a 3.2 mm drill, one hole on the linea aspera and the other about 120° anterior to this. The width of the bone lid is determined by the gap between the drill holes. The femur is split along the linea aspera with a flat chisel as far as the innominate tubercle. The osteotomy extends further anteriorly towards the tip of the greater trochanter, so that a sufficiently strong dorsal strip of bone of the greater trochanter is preserved for the subsequent suture (*fig 8*). The tendon of gluteus medius can be split longitudinally over a distance of 3-4 cm, but should not be divided any further because of the risk of injuring the superior gluteal nerve. The oscillating saw should not be used, as otherwise cement particles can be spread in the wound; in any case, the bone is so thin that only a few chisel blows are needed. The anterior border of the bone lid is made with a few stab osteotomies, using a narrow flat chisel which is passed bluntly through the fibres of the vastus lateralis muscle. The bone lid is opened carefully along the linea aspera with chisels and fragment spreaders. When the cortex is very thin and pliable, the stab osteotomies referred to above can also be made at this point through the medullary cavity. The bone lid can then be raised with the vastus lateralis muscle attached which is important for the blood supply of the bone lid. The stem now lies free and can be removed. Cement particles and large granulomas are cleared out.

In order to minimise blood loss, the granulation tissue which is firmly attached

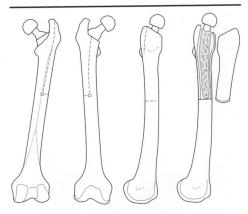

8 *Principle of the transfemoral approach.*
A. Posterior drill hole on the linea aspera for the posterior limit of the semicircular transverse osteotomy. The longitudinal osteotomy to open the bone lid runs along the linea aspera.
B. Anterior drill hole to mark the anterior limit of the transverse osteotomy. Multiple stab osteotomies run cranially from this hole for the regular anterior limit of the bone lid.
C. The longitudinal osteotomy inclines slightly anteriorly above the innominate tubercle.
D. Opening the bone lid with exposure of the stem with its cement mantle.

to the bone shell should be removed only after the cup implant has been exchanged. After exchanging the cup through the transfemoral approach, the femoral medullary cavity is prepared for the revision stem. It is important that precise preoperative planning has been carried out and that the surgeon follow this at operation. The tip of the trochanter is usually no longer suitable as an intra-operative orientation point after removal of the bone lid, but with planning drawings all the measurements can be made from the transverse osteotomy, the position of which is known from the planning.

The femoral medullary cavity is widened with the conical reamers until firm frictional resistance to reaming can be felt. The transverse osteotomy is now the reference point and the required depth of penetration must be measured from the distance between the transverse osteotomy and the marking on the reamer.

A frequent problem in the fixation of noncemented femoral stems when bone is atrophic consists of fractures or fissures of the femur. In the literature, this complication is described in over 25% of cases [1]. In a revision procedure, at which there is further weakening of the cortex due to osteolysis and removal of the stem and bone cement, the risk of femoral fissures must be noted particularly [1, 2].

In order to prevent this unpleasant complication or to allow stable implantation even with a longitudinal fissure, it is often necessary to place a cerclage distal to the transverse osteotomy. The cerclage technique is particularly important in this situation. Thin cerclage wires which are tightened with two flat-nosed pliers can often not withstand the torques and forces which occur, and they

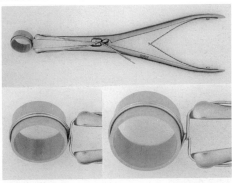

9 *Double cerclage with pliers. The two wire ends are threaded at the tips of the arms and are then placed in the clamping device on the pliers lock. When the pliers are opened only a little, the wire ends are locked. When it is opened further, great tension can then be placed on the cerclage. The cerclage is secured with a simple turn of the pliers while maintaining the tension (below right). [Manufacturer: Sulzer Orthopedics]*

loosen or break. Fragments of the cerclage can get into the articulation and produce considerable three-body wear or possibly lead to corrosion due to contact with the implant.

In an experimental arrangement with a standardised model, it was demonstrated that the stability of a cerclage is considerably influenced by the wire size and operative technique [10]. Cerclages with wire sizes of under 1.2 mm diameter are not a match for the forces and torques which occur with a femoral stem. A cerclage should therefore always be placed using a steel wire with a diameter of 1.5 mm. Double encirclement of the femur proved to be superior to single encirclement in the in vitro experiments referred to above. Wires of greater diameter are difficult to handle at operation. Furthermore, a double cerclage should be placed with a special tightening instrument (*fig 9*). With these instruments, the cerclage is not tightened by twisting the wire, but tightening of the wire and securing the cerclage by twisting are performed separately from one another. The wire twist thus cannot break when the cerclage is tightened, which is often observed when flat-nosed pliers are used. The necessity for the cerclage depends on the strength of the bone. If in doubt, a cerclage should always be placed, but meticulous care is necessary to ensure that the wire does not touch the stem.

After preparing the bone, the femoral revision stem is then pushed into the conically-widened medullary cavity. It is driven in with a few hammer blows only until it has become just secure enough for it to be loosened again easily in case correction of rotation is necessary.

If no leg lengthening is planned, the distance between the transverse osteotomy and the tip of the trochanter corresponds to the distance between the transverse osteotomy and the marking on the reamer. That is, the marking for the centre of the head of the selected prosthesis is at the original level of

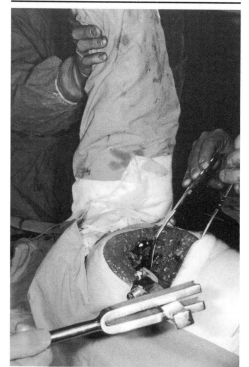

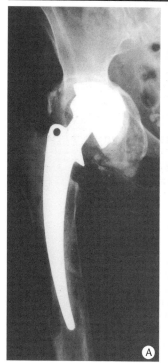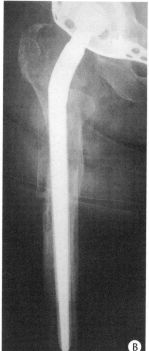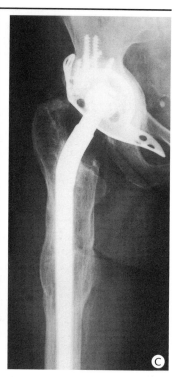

10 *Checking the angle of anteversion when implanting the femoral revision stem. The illustration shows a left hip using the transfemoral approach with the patient in the lateral position. The slotted hammer has been placed onto the impactor. The direction of the slotted hammer is checked against the long axis of the lower leg which is flexed to a right angle. If the slotted hammer is turned anti-clockwise, the angle of anteversion becomes greater (vice versa for the right hip).*

11 *Lively new bone formation after the transfemoral approach.*
A. Loosening and subsidence of the femoral stem with severe bone loss and paper-thin cortex in a 67-year old woman.
B. 2 weeks after the transfemoral approach.
C. 2 years and 7 months after the transfemoral approach with complete bone filling of the defects.

the tip of the trochanter. The same applies to the depth of penetration of the stem.

The revision stem is hammered in with the impactor, using steady hammer blows and checking the angle of anteversion. Anteversion is adjusted and checked against the lower leg, which is flexed to a right angle (fig 10). If the knee ligaments are lax, this check may not be sufficiently reliable. It is therefore useful to also carry out a trial reduction and to check the stability of the joint. This should be done as soon as the stem has become sufficiently secure in the bone after a few hammer blows, and not only after the final firm fixation, because loosening of the implant to correct rotation can be very troublesome. Trial reduction is carried out with a manipulation head which is shorter than the definitively planned prosthetic head. When correct anteversion has been established, following re-dislocation, the definitive fixation of the stem takes place with steady firm hammer blows. With each hammer blow, the stem penetrates a bit further into the medullary cavity until firm fixation has been achieved; this can be recognised from the fact that while continuing hammer blows with equal intensity, the stem no longer penetrates any further into the medullary cavity. A change in the sound can also be heard regularly at this point. After a further trial reduction with the manipulation heads, the final prosthetic head is put on and the hip is reduced.

After reduction, soft tissue tension is now checked: with longitudinal traction on the extended leg using approximately 10 kg, the joint should open about 2-8 mm cranially. If the opening is more than 10 mm, a longer head should be used. The wound is then closed. The pseudomembranes are removed from the inner surfaces of the bone shell and the osteotomised shells of the transfemoral approach are replaced. If the physiological leg length was restored, the bone lid of the transfemoral approach is usually adequately replaced by stretching the gluteus medius and vastus lateralis. Additional cerclages of either wire or strong absorbable sutures are required only when the soft tissues are hypotonic.

After repositioning, the bone lid of the transfemoral approach often has a tendency to remain on the anterior surface of the stem and must be repositioned on the lateral surface, while avoiding a diastasis at the transverse osteotomy. When the muscles are atrophic, the anterior part of the greater trochanter together with the bone lid can, in rare cases, remain too far cranial and must then be held in the correct position with a tension band wire running between the tip of the trochanter and the diaphysis distal to the transverse osteotomy. It must also be ensured in this situation that the wire does not touch the stem.

If autologous bone chips have been obtained during the preparation, these should be placed laterally beside the bone lid. New bone formation is generally so lively that there is no indication for the use of frozen bone bank chips between the bone shells

and the implant. If, on the other hand, there are still bone defects on the lateral surface of the femur, these should be filled with fine bone chips. Bone defects on the medial surface of the femur do not require any special attention, because spontaneous ossification starts rapidly at this site [3, 5, 8, 11].

Stabilisation of the transfemoral approach is basically achieved with strong sutures between the two parts of the divided greater trochanter. Consolidation is problem-free, because the bone and the soft tissues were split in the direction of the tensile forces.

Septic stem loosening

Many loosened prostheses are also infected, but detection of bacteria does not succeed in every case. If infected arthroplasties are to be revised, very careful debridement is essential. The complete prosthesis, all of the bone cement, all necrotic tissue and the inflamed granulation tissue must be removed. The organism should be identified by preoperative hip joint aspiration. Antibiotics must be given peri- and postoperatively according to the sensitivity. We have found intraoperative irrigation and subsequent continuous instillation with the antiseptic Lavasept™ (hexamethylene biguanide and polyethylene glycol in 0.1% solution) very useful [7, 9]. Even when revising infected loosened prostheses, it has become apparent that when these principles are followed, there is rapid restoration of the damaged bone bed. However, if the infection is not brought under control, osseointe-gration does not take place, so that the noncemented stem can be removed easily after consolidation of the transfemoral approach.

Results

The described technique with the femoral revision stem has been used since 1986. In all cases, there has been rapid new bone formation *(fig 11)* in the damaged bone bed [3]. Histological investigations [4] have shown that the bone grows first on the ribs of the conical stem. Complications were observed infrequently, and the severity of the initial findings should be taken into account. The most important complication is subsidence of the femoral stem with insufficient primary stability. This leads to shortening of the leg and relaxation of the muscles surrounding the hip, which can lead to a tendency to dislocation. In these cases, either the diameter of the stem was too thin or the stem was not hammered in with the requisite force. Proximal bone atrophy, such as often occurs with long cemented stems, was not observed in any case. Periarticular ossification is no more common after the transfemoral approach than after other approaches.

Complications

In 150 revisions using the femoral revision stem:
Secondary subsidence of the stem: 9
Thigh pain: 5
Dislocation of the prosthesis: 3
Pulmonary embolism: 3
Reinfection: 2
Fatal complications: 0

Discussion

Loosening of implants is associated with loss of bone. The problem can be solved in the long term only by restoring the damaged bone. With the described technique of the transfemoral approach, a rapid restoration of the bone bed can be achieved without the use of foreign bone. At the same time, the revision is simplified; the stem is fixed in stable bone, and the removal of the old stem along with granulation tissue and cement residues takes place rapidly. The high primary stability permits early mobilisation. It should be noted that elderly patients cannot observe partial load-bearing anyway, which makes reliable stable fixation of the stem especially necessary. Precise preoperative planning is indispensable for this technique.

References

[1] Burke DW, Bragdon CR, O'Connor DO, Jasty M, Haire T, Harris WH. Dynamic measurement of interface mechanics in vivo and the effect of micromotion on bone ingrowth into a porous surface device under controlled loads in vivo. *Trans Orthop Res Soc* 1991 ; 37 : 215-218

[2] Herzwurm PJ, Walsh J, Pettine KA, Ebert FR. Prophylactic cerclage: a method of preventing femur fracture in uncemented total hip. *Arthroplasty Orthop* 1992 ; 15 : 143-146

[3] Kolstad K, Adalberth G, Mallmin H, Milbrink J, Sahlstedt B. The Wagner revision stem for severe osteolysis. *Acta Orthop Scand* 1996 ; 67 : 541-544

[4] Schenk RK, Wehrli U. Zur Reaktion des Knochens auf eine zementfreie SL-Femur-Revisionsprothese. Histologische Befunde an einem fünfeinhalb Monate postoperationem gewonnenen Autopsiepräparat. *Orthopäde* 1989 ; 18 : 454-462

[5] Wagner H. Revisionsprothese für das Hüftgelenk. *Orthopäde* 1989 ; 18 : 438-453

[6] Wagner H. Revision of femoral stem with important loss of bone stock. In : Postgraduate Lectures n° 1. EFORT. Paris : Masson, 1993 : 64-74

[7] Wagner H, Wagner M. Infizierte Hüftgelenkprothesen - Gesichtspunkte für den einzeitigen und zweizeitigen Prothesenwechsel. *Orthopäde* 1995 ; 24 : 314-318

[8] Wagner H, Wagner M. Konische Schaftverankerung zementfreier Hüftprothesen - Primärimplantation und Prothesenwechsel. In : Morscher EW ed. Endoprothetik. Berlin : Springer-Verlag, 1995 : 278-288

[9] Wagner M. Lokale Antisepsis bei infizierten Hüfttotalendoprothesen. *Orthopäde* 1995 ; 24 : 319-325

[10] Wagner M, Knorr-Held F, Hohmann D. Measuring stability of wire cerclage in femoral fractures when performing total hip replacement. In vitro study on a standardized bone model. *Arch Orthop Trauma* 1996 ; 114 : 32-37

[11] Weill D, Scarlat M. La prothèse fémorale de révision de Wagner : à propos d'une série personnelle de 40 implantations. *Ann Orthop Ouest* 1995 ; 27 : 105-108

Revision of failed femoral prostheses: transfemoral approach and cementless distally-locked stem

C Picault
P Vives

Abstract. – In very severe failures of femoral prostheses with notable bone damage, a cementless stem stabilised by distal locking with screws in the healthy femoral diaphysis is implanted with the use of an anatomical transfemoral approach which lifts one or more pedicled femoral flaps. The good clinical and radiological results of this technique are reproducible, as demonstrated in a multicentre study of 183 cases with a 1 to 11 year follow-up. Revascularisation and restoration of the bone stock are obtained. Definitive stability of the stem in the metaphyseal region is achieved in more than 80% of these very severe cases. This technique is time- and blood-saving when precisely performed. The durability of the results is due to the new living bone spontaneously produced by the callus of consolidation of the longitudinal femoral osteotomies, as well as to the rebuilding of normal biomechanical constraints in the upper femur. In case of failure of definitive metapyseal stability, this type of stem is easily removed and replaced by a new one, cemented or cementless, which can be reimplanted in a perfectly rebuilt femur.

Keywords: hip, total hip replacement, femoral component failure, transfemoral approach, cementless implantation, distal locking of stem.

Introduction

Revisions for femoral implant failures have become more and more frequent, and more and more difficult to treat. Following successive operations, the problem of bone stock loss is worrying. The operative difficulties of removing the failed implant and of completely cleaning the femoral cavity create complex situations. The implantation and stability of a new implant are progressively more uncertain in a deformed femoral cavity with a weakened cortical bone.

A conventional intracanalar approach, or a unique longitudinal femorotomy (using unilateral cortex splitting) to simply enlarge the canal, is commonly used in simple cases of loosening without bone damage.

In very severe failures of femoral implants, an anatomical transfemoral approach with the implantation of a cementless stem distally locked in the healthy distal diaphysis is the technique suggested. The revision of the implant as well as the rebuilding of both the bone stock and the anatomical shape of the femur may become a standardised and reproducible technique.

Charles Picault, M.D, Clinique Saint Charles, 69001 Lyon, France.
Pierre Vives, M.D., Centre Hospitalier Universitaire, 80054 Amiens, France.

The "transfemoral approach technique" [4, 7] begins with an anatomical elevation of pedicled vascularised femoral flaps and finishes with a careful architectural rebuilding of the femoral shape. In addition, the possibility of a complete cleaning of the bone cavities and the consolidation of femoral flaps represents a biological technique. The distal locking with screws of a relatively small-sized stem must be considered as a temporary vertical stabilisation, the target being to obtain proximal osteo-integration of the stem. A distal wedging (or jamming) technique which uses a press-fit into the diaphyseal canal is not recommended: stress shielding or by-passing the normal biomechanical loading triggers proximal bone atrophy. With the transfermoral approach technique, the long-term risks of distal wedging are eliminated, as well as the very difficult removal of a distally blocked stem. Bone grafting is unnecessary, because the bone defect is filled by the active bone of the callus of consolidation of the femoral flaps.

Operative technique

PREOPERATIVE REQUIREMENTS

A precise preoperative plan (using templates) *(fig 1)* must be carefully

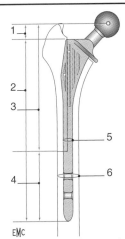

1 *Preoperative planning. The metaphyseal damage and the diaphyseal diameter in the locking area dictate the choice of stem size. The length of the femoral flap is calculated taking into consideration both the femoral lesions and the distal security zone required for safe locking (at least 60 mm for two screws). 1. neck length + 15 mm; 2. stem length; 3. flap length; 4. length of penetration of the tip of the stem; 5. stem diameter; 6. screw length.*

elaborated and strictly followed, based on the mensurations resulting from radiological magnification. The goals are to remove the failed stem and reimplant a new one, with preservation of the remaining bone stock and biomechanical rebuilding resulting from intense revascularisation of the femur following consolidation of the femoral flaps. The lateral position is recommended. A posterior approach is the most efficient way of obtaining a wide and safe exposure of the femur and the acetabulum.

Two procedures can be undertaken, according to local difficulties: in the first stages of bone damage, dislocation of the hip is carried out first and the stem is removed before elevation of the main femoral flap [5, 6]. In very difficult cases, the hip is left in place, the operated limb lying on the other. Dislocation and removal of the implant is performed after elevation of the femoral flap [2, 3].

Removal of the failed implant and pathological tissues

INCISION OF SKIN, SUBCUTANEOUS TISSUE AND APONEUROSIS

The length of the incision depends on many features: the level of the tip of the stem, the possible distal wedging of a cementless stem, a bone defect or a femoral deviation.

The exposure of the greater trochanter, of the anterior and posterior edges of the glutei muscles and of the different aspects of the capsule is made by sharp dissection and release of the fibrous tissue lying between the muscles. The entire mass of this fibrous tissue located between the pelvis and the femur will be henceforth referred to as "the capsule".

ELEVATION OF THE VASTUS LATERALIS MUSCLE FROM THE INTERMUSCULAR FASCIA; LOCATION OF THE LINEA ASPERA
(fig 2)

The linea aspera is located posteriorly and the muscle attachments are gently separated from the femur. The vastus lateralis muscle is cut 3 or 5 millimetres from the aponeurosis, following a cranial to caudal progression, and from the posterior to the anterior aspect. One by one, the perforating vessels emerging through the intermuscular fascia are very carefully individualised, dissected and ligatured. If this stage is neglected, there is a real risk of difficulty in controlling bleeding which may occur behind the fascia. The smooth dissection of the vastus lateralis muscle progressively reaches the femur, avoiding any elevation of the periosteum. It is still possible to begin the elevation of the femoral flap, but, especially in cases with significant bone stock loss, pseudarthrosis of the greater trochanter or notable femur deformities, we recommend the elevation of a bone strut from the linea aspera.

ELEVATION OF A BONE STRUT FROM THE LINEA ASPERA *(fig 3)*

The linea aspera is a strong anatomical structure made of cortical bone which remains present despite bone damage. The

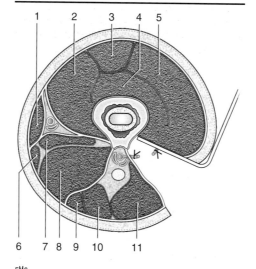

2   *Mid level, distal part of anatomical horizontal cut of right thigh. Lateral approach. Dissection of the vastus lateralis from the intermuscular aponeurosis. Careful ligature of the perforating vessels. 1. Sartorius muscle; 2. vastus medialis muscle; 3. rectus femoris muscle; 4 vastus intermedius muscle; 5. vastus lateralis muscle; 6. rectus medialis muscle; 7. medial adductor muscle; 8. great adductor muscle; 9. semimembranous muscle; 10. semitendinous muscle; 11. long head of biceps femoris.*

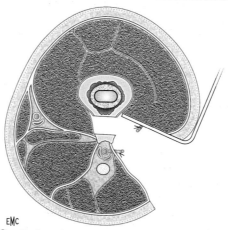

3   *Horizontal cut. Elevation of a stick of bone from the linea aspera (respecting aponeurotic attachments) gives a safe enlargement of the exposure and an additional zone of consolidation thanks to a final osteosynthesis with the same metallic wiring as that of the main femoral flap.*

elevation of a bone strut graft is suggested for two main reasons: first, to enlarge the exposure safely, and second, to create an additional zone of consolidation, with a significant callus of new living bone. It is possible to lift a thick cortical strut with total preservation of its own strong aponeurotic attachments. After lifting, the fragment spontaneously moves backwards and the posterior vessels and sciatic nerve slack off. Depending on the thickness and solidity of the bone, this section is performed either with a saw or by hammering with a thin narrow chisel (never use a thick bevelled chisel). This strut includes the gluteus maximus tendon, respecting its femoral attachment. At the end of the operation, this pedicled bone strut will be fixed by wiring to the femur diaphysis, in situ, or with

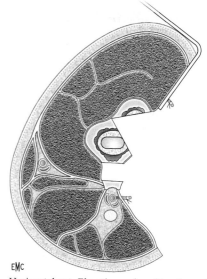

4   *Horizontal cut. Elevation and pushing forward of the main femoral flap. Preservation of all the muscle and aponeurotic attachments. No neurological or vascular risks.*

translation to fill the bone defect. This fixation allows control of the tension of the gluteus maximus muscle.

CUTTING AND LIFTING THE MAIN ANTEROLATERAL FEMORAL PEDICLED FLAP *(fig 4)*

This classical flap must include the totality of the greater trochanter. The cutting of the distal limit of the flap (according to the calculated level) is carefully carried out with a saw and, if necessary, with multiple drillings especially at the corners. Sometimes the risk of spiroid fracture can be prevented by temporary metallic wiring of the distal diaphysis. The flap must represent at least a third of the circumference of the femur. The saw and the thin, narrow chisel pass between the bone and the back of the stem. If the removal of the femoral prosthesis is impossible, it is usually easy to cut the anterior cortex from the back to the front cortex. If necessary, its section is facilitated by drilling performed anteriorly through the vastus lateralis muscle. To cut the trochanteric area, a large flat (not bevelled) chisel is used from the posterior to the anterior intertrochanteric line, passing trough the fossa digitalis, exactly at the limit between the capsule and the medial trochanter tip aspect.

DISSECTION OF THE CAPSULE

This stage will open the virtual and avascular space on the deeper side of the gluteus muscles and release their tension. The femoral flap is then gently pushed forward, completely preserving the attachments of the muscles, and remains so during the operation. A sharp dissection of the fibrous tissue all around the acetabular cavity naturally reaches the lateral wall of the pelvis. The circumference of the capsule

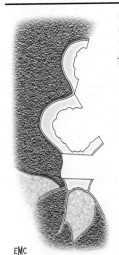

6 *Femur and flap cleaned safely and totally with sharp curettage. Fracture and perforation of the femur are eliminated for implantation of the new stem. Time- and blood-saving.*

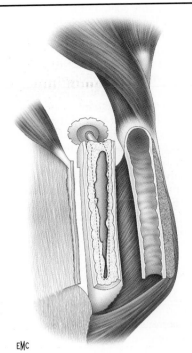

5 *Main femoral flap pushed forward, complete exposure of the damaged endocanal. Removal of any type of stem with preservation of the remaining bone stock.*

plug, bone console or egg cup) is removed with a chisel and progressive reaming. For distal locking, the final diameter of the canal must be slightly bigger than that of the stem.

Implantation of the new stem: osteosynthesis of the femur

The exposure is very satisfactory and without danger to vessels or nerves.

INSERTING THE STEM INTO THE FEMUR

The length of the stem allows it to be safely locked into the canal and to check that the length of the lower limb has been calculated exactly. The implant is firmly fixed onto the prosthesis holder and progressively introduced into the canal, without any hammering. Respecting the preoperative planning ensures a perfect and rapid positioning of the stem in length and size. The correct anteversion is checked in relation to knee flexion and to the orientation of the acetabular cup.

The recommended distal diameter of the stem must be smaller than the diameter of the canal. The stem must bridge any distal defect (cortex weakness, fracture, pseudarthrosis, surgical window). To ensure a level of locking without risk of overloading at the tip of the implant (*fig 1*), no more than 60 mm of the stem must be introduced in the canal.

DISTAL LOCKING OF THE STEM (fig 6)

The distal locking is calculated to be carried out with screws in the healthy diaphysis. Different ancillary devices are available to ensure safe insertion of the screws passing successively through the lateral cortex, the holes of the stem and the medial cortex. The procedure of locking is simple, reliable and fast thanks to the guides adapted to the stem-holder. The screws are tightened; their number depends on the type of stem, the quality of the diaphyseal cortex and the concept of the surgeon: at least two screws, and possibly up to four or five, are necessary. The prosthesis holder is then removed and impaction of the prosthetic head on the cone is carried out with reduction of the head into the cavity of the cup.

OSTEOSYNTHESIS OF THE FEMORAL FLAP AROUND THE STEM AND THE FEMUR (fig 7)

After the reduction has been performed, the operated limb is sustained in abduction. This stage of the osteosynthesis is of the greatest importance. The osteosynthesis must be as exact as possible to achieve the following goals: rebuild the femoral shape, facilitate

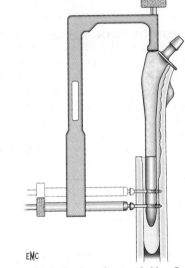

7 *Stem firmly fixed on the stem-holder. Guides for drilling and screwing for the stem locking.*

bone consolidation and ensure proximal stability of the stem. It is performed with metallic wiring which must be firmly tightened.

Restitution of an anatomical shape to the femur can be fully controlled. Simple repositioning in situ or translation of the femoral flap allows filling of any possible bone defects (for example, pseudarthrosis of the greater trochanter with lateral cortical defect) and a close contact between bone fragments which will trigger off the callus fusion and produce a very active and plastic new, living bone.

If there is a very large tulip-shaped deformity of the upper femur, either the lips of the flap overlap reciprocally or an additional longitudinal femorotomy is performed to reduce the volume of the cavity and obtain a close contact between bone and stem (hydroxyapatite coated or not). In some types of stem, two holes in its back allow two metallic wires to be passed (do not use strand cables because of the risks of acute wear and subsequent breakage). Each wire penetrates the flap from inside out. They will be firmly tightened on the superficial side of the greater trochanter so

is always fully and exactly delimited, even if a migration of the cup has occurred.

RESECTION OF THE CAPSULE, REMOVAL OF THE IMPLANT

The capsule must be opened only when its complete dissection has been performed. It seems better to keep it closed until the end of its complete release because it is easier to follow when the tissue is retained tightly by the prosthesis in situ.

First, the resection removes the previously dissected posterior, superior and anterior parts of the capsule. The implant is retrieved, tip first, head last. Second, after the inferior cul-de-sac of the capsule and the large granulomatous area with debris have been dissected around their outside aspect, resection of the inferior part of the capsule begins at the contact of the inferior part of the calcar region.

REPLACEMENT OF THE ACETABULAR COMPONENT

At this stage, if necessary, the treatment of the acetabulum is carried out, before that of the femoral part, so that any unnecessary bleeding of opened up bone surfaces can be avoided.

CLEANING THE FEMORAL CAVITY AND THE DEEP SIDE OF THE FEMORAL FLAP (fig 5)

Any pathological tissue (granulomatous tissues with debris, necrotic bone, interface membrane) is easily removed in totality from the widely exposed femoral cavity. The diaphyseal canal is verified along its length as well as its diameter: any obstacle (cement,

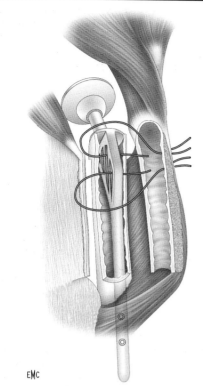

8 *Preparation of osteosynthesis of the flap(s). Control of the positioning of the greater trochanter with metallic wiring passing through holes in the stem back. The distal part of the flap is fixed with simple circumferential wiring.*

that its position can be controlled in height as well as laterally. The actual descent of the greater trochanter, performed to obtain satisfactory tension of the gluteus muscles, sometimes leads to a 1 or 2 cm resection at the distal end of the flap (*fig 8*).

Great care must be taken when driving the wire-passer through the strong aponeurotic attachments on the linea aspera: it must pass close to the femur to avoid tearing a vessel, artery or more frequently an inflated vein.

Special cases

PSEUDARTHROSIS OF THE GREATER TROCHANTER

Pseudarthrosis of the greater trochanter is a very worrying problem, which is worsened by the weakness of the bone tuberosity: demineralisation, fragmentation, fibrosis, etc. For these reasons, in our opinion a transversal cut of the fibrous tissue characterising non-union or signalling absence of bone must be strictly avoided at any level. To lift the main flap, the cut must always remain exactly the same: longitudinal. The one difference is the obvious weakness or the flexibility of the flap after its lifting. As previously described, the periprosthetic tissue must be resected in totality. It will be decided later if it is reasonable to resect the fibrous zone of pseudarthrosis and to attempt an osteosynthesis. If not, two solutions are possible:

– either the fibrous tissue is not resected and a close contact between the trochanteric fragment and the anterior or posterior edge of the main flap is obtained thanks to its translation;

– or if a thick pedicled bone strut has been elevated from the linea aspera, it may be moved and with translation will arrive in close contact with the trochanteric fragment.

EXTREMELY SEVERE BONE STOCK LOSS: THE "THREE-THIRDS" TECHNIQUE

A transfemoral approach with lifting of two pedicled flaps, the so-called "three-thirds" technique, can be suggested in cases of great difficulty in removing a stem. If a cemented or cementless stem is completely loose and mobile in the canal, lifting the anterolateral flap previously described is sufficient. In such a case, the transfemoral approach is chosen in order to clean the canal completely, to rebuilt the architectural shape of the upper femur safely and to restore a large bone stock loss thanks to flap consolidation. However, if the stem is gripped in a narrow canal and surrounded by dense bone, we suggest lifting two pedicled femoral flaps. The beginning of the approach is the same, but instead of cutting a simple stick of bone from the linea aspera, we recommend preparing and elevating a large pedicled flap from this region. In this way, the saw enters the canal directly in close contact with the implant, and cuts longitudinally going from distal to proximal. Finally, this additional flap is lifted and spontaneously goes backward. The last third of the diaphysis remains in continuity with the distal femur.

ADDITIONAL TRANSVERSAL OSTEOTOMY OF THE FEMORAL DIAPHYSIS

In extremely severe cases after successive failures, femur deformities can be impressive, producing pellucid cortex or deviations of the shaft. A tulip-shaped metaphysis makes it difficult to adapt the endocortical bone to the stem: it becomes necessary to perform longitudinal splits of the thin cortex and to adapt the endocortical bone to the stem, fastening the fragments with the final wiring. The presence of deviations of the femur is also very common, more frequently in varus and/or retroflexion. A transversal osteotomy performed exactly at the apex of the curved diaphysis will correct the deformity: the medial cortex must be firmly fastened to the stem by final wiring [5].

Implants

STEMS

Different stems, all cementless, are available. They are straight or curved, modular or not, with different types and numbers of screws,

hydroxyapatite coated or not. The concept is that of a long stem which bridges femoral lesions of varying extent without any voluntary distal wedging. The implant is stabilised by locking in the distal and healthy femur. A modularity of the neck allows for length adjustment, anteversion and offset of the stem. The presence or absence of a collar is disputable. A reliable prosthesis holder safely ensures the passage of the screws. These are either of a common or peg type with a proximal thread pitch that only fits in the first cortex (the lateral one is probably better). The required number of screws depends on both the stage of bone stock loss at the metaphyseal level and the possible weakness of the diaphyseal cortex.

Peroperative complications

With the transfemoral approach, the number of peroperative complications dramatically decreases. The wide exposure and the cautious lifting of the femoral flap(s) slack off the neighbouring vessels and nerves and allow the canal direction and diameter to be checked and femoral fractures to be treated.

Performed precisely, a regular transfemoral approach with distal locking incontestably saves time and bleeding.

Postoperative complications

No specific postoperative complications have been registered after a transfemoral approach. Thanks to preoperative planning and the excellent control of muscular tension, only 7 (3.8%) dislocations were found in 183 severe cases.

Postoperative care

Under the imperative condition of a solid osteosynthesis, getting out of bed and walking with partial weight-bearing with two crutches are possible a few days postoperatively. Full weight-bearing is progressively allowed according to the radiological appearance of consolidation.

Clinical and radiological results

We present below the clinical and radiological results of a multicentre study of 183 cases of revision performed using this technique, with a 1 to 11 year follow-up [6]:

First, it is necessary to insist on the severity of the bone stock loss in these cases: 75% of the patients' bone status was over Paprosky's stage 2A and stage 2 of the SOFCOT scores; the number of previous

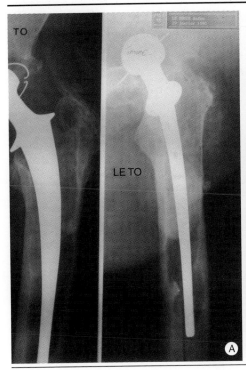

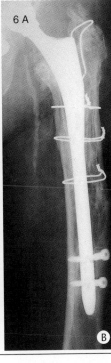

9 *A. Third failed cementation. Subsidence, pellucid cortex and femur deviation, invasive granuloma.*
B. Six year follow-up. Spontaneous rebuilding of the bone stock (neither bone graft nor bone substitute). Restoration of normal biomechanical sollicitations ensuring satisfactory bone restructuration.

allows perfect cleaning of lesions as well as for safe reimplantation of the new stem; the new living bone of the callus and the intense revascularisation of the femur are excellent ways to fight septic complications [5].

Indications

The combination of an anatomical transfemoral approach with a cementless, distally locked stem is routinely used for cases after a second revision. Independently of the classical scoring systems in current use, the indications for this technique seem to be cases of great bone stock loss, and periprosthetic or distal femur deviations, defects and/or discontinuities, as well as in pseudarthrosis of the greater trochanter. Possible and sometimes unpredictable peroperative risks of increased bone loss, an obviously difficult implant removal, a really invasive granulomatosis with pellucid cortex will also justify this indication. Complete cleaning of the bone cavities and the revascularisation of the entire femur increase the safety and duration of the results in septic cases. Carefully carried out according to precise preoperative planning, this technique saves time and bleeding and is recommended for difficult cases and in fragile and elderly patients.

revisions was more than two in 50% of these patients, reaching eight for one of them.

With regard to pain (10% painful), range of movement (85% with flexion over 100°) and walking (40% stable), the clinical results are really satisfactory. Globally, 60% of the patients are very satisfied, 30% have a good result and 10% have a poor score in relation to their preoperative status. A complete bone fusion was obtained in cases of distal fractures or pseudarthrosis, and definitive bone union was achieved in 7 out of 11 pseudarthroses of the greater trochanter. According to Brooker's classification, there were no cases in grade IV and a total absence of periprosthetic ossifications in 50% of patients. In five cases of failure of osseo-integration in the metaphyseal area, the stem was removed without any problem and a standard-sized stem was reimplanted in a rebuilt femur.

The specific target of the transfemoral approach with distal locking is the restoration of bone stock and stability of the stem *(fig 9)*. A complete preservation of the remaining bone is ensured peroperatively. In all cases, the consolidation of the femoral

flaps was obtained within the first six months. According to biomechanical laws, both reinforcement and restructuration of the cortex are faster on the medial than on the lateral side [1].

Concerning implant failures: the breakage of one stem and of thirteen screws was registered in 8 out of 183 patients.

Overloading at the distal locking level, represented by a cortical thickening, was present but painless in 36% of cases. Unlocking was required in 12 patients suffering from pain at the screw level: after simple removal of the screws, there was no more pain but a subsequent 5 to 12 mm subsidence.

In three patients suffering from persistent pain and presenting an evident absence of metaphyseal osteo-integration, the stem was easily unlocked and removed. In two patients a new standard-sized cemented stem and in one patient a cementless stem was re-implanted in a completely rebuilt femur.

In septic cases, with one or two stages, the transfemoral approach very effectively

References

[1] Picault C. Upper femoral intramedullary replacement in femoral failure of THR. In : Speciality day proceedings. Fourth EFORT Congress. Hip International, 1993 : 163-171

[2] Picault C. Consolidation and modelling of the femur with a cementless distally locked stem placed with transfemoral approach technique. In : Transfemoral approach and distally locked stem in femoral failures of total hip prosthesis. Montpellier : Sauramps Medical, 1999 : 53-63

[3] Picault C et al. Transfemoral approach: X-rays results in 120 consecutive cases of failed total hip replacement in humans compared with X-rays and histological results in animals. *J Jpn Orthop Assoc* 1995 ; 69 : 2-3

[4] Vielpeau C, Locker B, Van Neverbelde T, Heuguet V. Le risque infectieux en chirurgie orthopédique. *Encycl Méd Chir* (Éditions Scientifiques et Médicales Elsevier SAS, Paris), Techniques Chirurgicales-Orthopédie-traumatologie, 44-005, 1986 : 1-18

[5] Vives P, Picault C. Surgical technique. In : Transfemoral approach and distally locked stem in femoral failures of total hip prosthesis. Montpellier : Sauramps Medical, 1999 : 35-71

[6] Vives P, Plaquet JL, Leclair A, Blejwas B, Filloux JF. Tige de reprise verrouillée pour descellement des prothèses totales de hanche. Conception. Résultats préliminaires. *Acta Orthop Belg* 1992 ; 59 : 28-35

[7] Wagner H. Revisionsprothese für Hüftgelenk. *Orthopäde* 1989 ; 18 : 438-453

The infected hip prosthesis

A Lortat-Jacob

Abstract. – Infection of a total hip replacement poses one of the most difficult problems in orthopaedics. It may be difficult to make a definite microbiological diagnosis, although joint aspiration is of value. Treatment involves both medical and surgical management. Heavy antibiotic therapy is essential, but often there are multi-resistant microbes involved. For such microbes, a month of parenteral administration of two appropriate antibiotics is essential, followed by a further month with the two drugs given orally, and one of these should be continued orally for a third month. The surgery involves removal of the prosthesis and as much infected tissue as possible, thorough cleaning, and replacement of the prosthesis at an appropriate moment. Currently, this is usually performed as a two-stage procedure with an interval of about one month between removal and re-insertion. Femorotomy at the time of the prosthesis removal also allows complete removal of the femoral cement and curettage of the bone surfaces. Antibiotic-loaded cement is not essential, but is used with organisms which are sensitive to gentamycin. We often use interlocked stems for the femoral component when this is inserted at a second stage; this allows good "bridging" of the femorotomy. With these techniques, about 80% of patients will have a favourable result. However, the severity of the treatment and a failure rate of 20% emphasise the need to strive to prevent infection in major hip replacement surgery.

Keywords: hip, infected total hip replacement, infected prosthesis, hip revision, antibiotic cement, revision exchange of prosthesis.

Introduction

Infection around a hip prosthesis currently remains a significant problem, as the considerable decrease in the number of post-operative infections which occur has been counterbalanced by the steady increase in the number of prostheses implanted. In France, some 85,000 hip prostheses will be inserted during the year 2000, and this means that with a 1% infection rate, there will be some 850 new infections during that year.

Clinical presentations

ACUTE POSTOPERATIVE ABSCESS

This type of infection has become rare, with fever persisting after the operation, and the wound becoming red and hot. Blood should be taken for culture, as well as wound swabs if pus appears. Joint aspiration through healthy skin is wise, but antibiotherapy should await the result of cultures, except in the presence of septic shock.

Alain Lortat-Jacob, M.D., Professeur Faculté de médecine Paris-Ouest, Service Chirurgie Orthopédique et Traumatologique, Hôpital Ambroise-Paré, 9, avenue Charles de Gaulle, 92104 Boulogne cedex, France.

SUBACUTE INFECTION

The immediate post-operative course has been satisfactory, with the temperature having settled by the 5th day (considered the normal period), and the patient appears to be making reasonable progress. There may be some blood-stained or even clear discharge, which usually stops during a reasonably short time. Pain appears during the next few months, but there may be few worrying local signs. However, this symptom should always suggest the possibility of a deep infection which will require further investigation.

EARLY LOOSENING

This can suggest deep infection, and should always be considered even though the post-operative course had seemed to be relatively straight-forward. The mechanical symptoms which result may occur before the end of the first year, and radiography will reveal a progressive loosening of one or both elements of the prosthesis, which helps to confirm the diagnosis.

ACUTE SECONDARY ABSCESS

All seems to be going well. The prosthesis will have been forgotten by the patient, and the surgeon will be content with progress, until a febrile episode associated with acute pain in the joint rapidly develops. This can be associated with a bacteraemia resulting from medical procedures such as dental treatment, endoscopic examinations of the digestive tract or urinary system, or from a skin infection. Early diagnosis of a haematogenous infection allows early joint lavage combined with synovectomy.

INFECTION FOUND AT REVISION

Previously unsuspected infection is found in about 11% of hip prosthesis revisions [7, 23]. It is important to take wound swabs for culture during all hip revision operations performed for loosening.

Surgical techniques

SIMPLE LAVAGE WITH SYNOVECTOMY

Simple lavage with synovectomy is only indicated with acute postoperative infections, or during the first few days of an acute haematogenous infection.

■ *Approach*

The operation should be performed before antibiotic therapy is started. The original incision is re-opened and all infected granulation tissue is excised. Aponeuroses are cleaned with a rasp, and the newly formed capsule is opened (after changing gloves). Several wound swabs should be taken, and the whole area disinfected. The prosthesis is then dislocated to allow synovectomy.

■ *Cemented femoral component*

A cemented femoral component must be removed from its cement sheath, but the accetabular component can be left undisturbed. Portions of the excised synovium should be sent for histological and microbiological examination. The femoral component is then replaced into its cement sheath without any mechanical damage.

■ *Uncemented prostheses*

These cause greater problems, as although removal is often easy, their re-insertion is compromised by the necessary intramedullary curettage, which results in a loss of stability.

If an uncemented femoral component sits firmly in the femoral canal, it can be left in situ, and the synovectomy performed piecemeal. If it does have to be removed, either a larger size can be inserted after thorough cleaning of the medullary canal, or the femoral stem can be cemented in place.

■ *Irrigation fluids*

The use of skin disinfectants is not recommended for deep lavage, and povidone-iodine (Betadine®) loses its antiseptic properties in the presence of protein. Chlorhexidine is unsuitable as it only works in an alcoholic solution, and thus cannot be used in open wounds. Sterile water has only a mechanical cleaning action. Dakin's solution has similar mechanical advantages as well as a good antiseptic action, but it does necrose soft tissues. It is important to remember that antiseptics take time to work, and therefore they need to be left in the wound for the appropriate period.

■ *Instability after reduction*

Unfortunately, in a certain number of patients, instability can be produced by excision of soft tissues, and there is a serious risk of secondary dislocation. A prosthetic posterior offset anchored by screws may be required. This can also help to control any instability which may develop during the following few months as a result of exuberant scar tissue formation around the prosthesis. The infection itself can also result in dense scar tissue which may predispose to instability.

■ *Wound closure*

Suction drains are used, but continuous irrigation is not advised owing to the risk of contamination. If the organism is sensitive to gentamicin, appropriate "beads" (Septotal®) can be placed around the prosthesis, and also subcutaneously.

Exchange revisions

MEDICAL PREPARATION

As the revision of an infected hip prosthesis is a major and time-consuming surgical procedure, usually accompanied by considerable bleeding, it should only be undertaken after a careful assessment of the patient's general condition. The often-associated inflammatory anaemia must be corrected. Blood transfusion is almost certain to be required, but infection prevents the use of auto-transfusion, as well as the use of blood collected either at operation or in the early postoperative days.

A nutritional assessment, paying particular attention to the level of albumin, is important. It may be wise to delay surgery until any nutritional deficiencies have been corrected. It is unusual to have to resort to drip feeding.

The type of anaesthesia to be used should be decided by the anaesthetist. Unless there is an acute infection, antibiotics should be withheld until the results of intra-operative wound cultures are available.

REMOVAL OF THE PROSTHESIS AND PREPARATION OF THE BONE-PROSTHESIS INTERFACE

It is suggested in the literature that removal of a prosthesis should be performed by re-opening the original incision. The skin and subcutaneous tissues can be opened through the original incision, but it may be necessary to enlarge the deeper portions in order to allow the excision necessary to encourage healing of the infection. Cement is removed from the femoral neck, and an anterior window is performed to allow extraction of the distal portion. In fact, it is essential to have adequate exposure to allow thorough cleaning. Whether the prosthesis was inserted anteriorly (Hueter, Roy-Camille anterolateral approach or Watson-Jones approach), laterally (with trochanterotomy or by Hardinge's technique), or posteriorly, we recommend "opening" (femorotomy) the proximal part of the femur (fig 1).

■ *Femorotomy for cleaning* (fig 1)

With the patient in a lateral position, it is usually possible to re-open the original incision. The vastus lateralis is elevated carefully in order to preserve the blood supply to the femur. Trochanterotomy is performed and elevated with a strong forceps. It is then held in place by retracting pins.

Cemented femoral component

After dislocation of the joint, the femoral stem is removed from its cement sheath. An anterior femorotomy is then performed using an oscillating saw, cutting longitudinally down the lateral margin of the upper part of the femoral shaft. Care must be taken not to produce a distal spiral fracture. The saw cut then extends through both layers of cement and into the medial cortex, and must pass sufficiently far distally to allow removal of all the cement. A distal transverse saw cut allows the upper part of the femoral shaft to be opened out, with the mobile section remaining attached to the gluteus maximus (fig 1). The cavity is curetted and thoroughly cleaned after all the cement has been removed, and the femur is closed by double cerclarge.

Uncemented femoral component

Rarely, after mobilisation of the greater trochanter, the stem of the femoral prosthesis may be removed easily, but more often this is very difficult to do. Femorotomy can then be very useful. An oscillating saw cuts longitudinally down the lateral aspect of the femur just distal to the end of the stem. A transverse cut is made in the same way as used in the removal of a cemented prosthesis. A drill is then inserted through the lateral longitudinal cut in order to make postage stamp sized perforations of the medial cortex. These are then connected by cutting with a chisel, which will then allow opening of the proximal part of the femoral shaft. Even so, the prosthesis may still defy attempts at removal, and it may be necessary to use a curved chisel to divide any bone bridges which are holding it in place.

■ *Removal of the acetabular component*

This is done by using a hammer and chisel and usually presents no problems. Curettage is usually easy, but may be more difficult when there is a pelvic penetration perforation. In this case, removing the granulation is to be performed very cautiously.

■ *Closure*

The trochanter is replaced and anchored by cerclage. If the infecting organism is sensitive to gentamycin, we use beads; when it is insensitive, only suction drains are inserted.

■ *Postoperative care of the femorotomy*

Weight-bearing is allowed on the 45th day. This delay is to allow union of the trochanter as well as of the femorotomy. Any discomfort resulting from the transverse cut disappears by the 90th day. Weight-bearing will depend on the extent of the reconstruction, whether the revision has been completed in one or two stages, and if cement has been used.

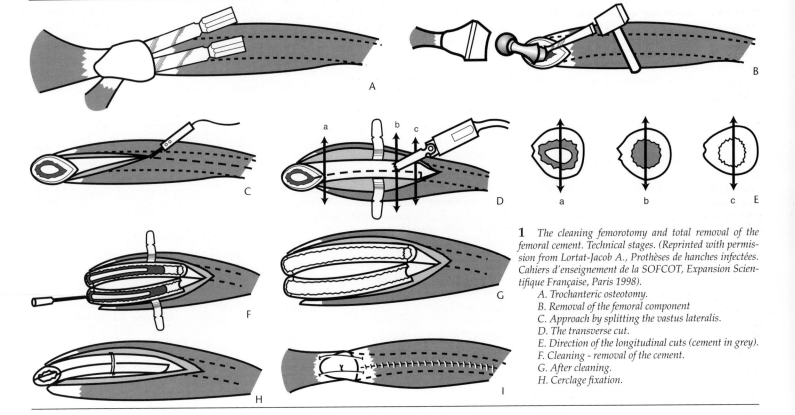

1 *The cleaning femorotomy and total removal of the femoral cement. Technical stages. (Reprinted with permission from Lortat-Jacob A., Prothèses de hanches infectées. Cahiers d'enseignement de la SOFCOT, Expansion Scientifique Française, Paris 1998).*
A. Trochanteric osteotomy.
B. Removal of the femoral component
C. Approach by splitting the vastus lateralis.
D. The transverse cut.
E. Direction of the longitudinal cuts (cement in grey).
F. Cleaning - removal of the cement.
G. After cleaning.
H. Cerclage fixation.

REVISION EXCHANGE OF THE PROSTHESIS *(fig 2)*

Insertion of the new prosthesis can either be done at the same time as the removal of the infected material (one-stage) or later on (two-stage). Whenever it is performed, reimplantating a prosthesis after infection raises difficult questions.

When reimplantation has been decided, it is important to use a prosthesis having the most appropriate mechanical qualities, as if the problem of infectious recurrence did not exist. "Therapeutic escalation" (use of a longer prosthesis, more cement) due to the possible recurrence of infection would be a double mistake, risking mechanical failure without limiting the risk of infection at a subsequent mechanical revision.

However, the possibility of recurrence of infection must never be forgotten. It is therefore very important to use a technique which will produce the least catastrophic result in case of infectious relapse.

These two principles are often incompatible, but both must guide the surgeon in selecting the best possible prosthesis, while avoiding "therapeutic escalation".

■ *The acetabular component*

The same considerations apply to replacement of the acetabular component, whether or not there has been local infection. Replacement combines the use of a cemented cup together with a reconstruction, using bank bone and a metallic sustaining plate

After thorough cleaning, and when there is only a small amount of bone loss, we use a classical cemented cup. It is not possible to use a non-cemented cup after infection as thorough debridement and cleaning makes the acetabular surface irregular, which interferes with primary stability of the component if no cement is used. In addition, the bone which has been infected does not have normal osteogenic powers.

When there is major loss of bone, support must be provided by a bone graft (from the bank) and a metallic device such as the sustaining plate. This device has a "claw" inferiorly which provides stability by passing under the transverse ligament of the acetabulum. The size selected depends on the width of the acetabular cavity. The superior portion is then screwed to the root of the socket, ensuring a position of neutral anteversion. The spaces between the device and the acetabular wall are filled with bone fragments. When there is a really large loss of bone substance, the roof is reconstructed, followed by the socket, before the metallic device is inserted. The new acetabular component is then cemented in place. If there is any significant likelihood of dislocation, then a retentive acetabular component should be used.

■ *The femoral component*

Three techniques are possible *(fig 2)*.

Standard prosthesis and insertion *(fig 2A)*

This can be used when there is no great loss of femoral bone stock, and when there will be no difficulties between the tip of the stem and the transverse part of the femorotomy. When the transverse cut is very distal, the prosthesis is entirely cemented in the zone

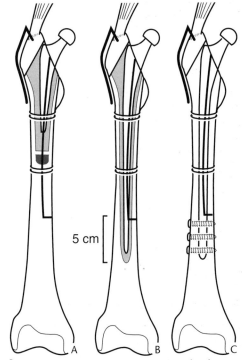

2 *The three options for reconstruction after femorotomy. (Reprinted with permission from Lortat-Jacob A., Prothèses de hanches infectées. Cahiers d'enseignement de la SOFCOT, Expansion Scientifique Française, Paris 1998).*
A. Standard prosthesis cemented only in the area which had been femorotomised.
B. A long stem prosthesis cemented in place, with the stem passing at least 5 cm distal to the femorotomy.
C. A long stem prosthesis fixed distally with screws and with no cement. The screws in certain cases can be inserted in the area of the femorotomy.

of the femorotomy. This is really the same as using a normal prosthesis, after a mechanical failure or an infection. However, it is important that the tip of the stem be well away from the transverse cut.

Cemented long-stem prosthesis

This is used when the transverse cut has been made more proximally and the stem should pass at least 5 cm distal to this area (rarely necessary) (fig 2B).

Cementless interlocked prosthesis (fig 2C)

This is another way to replace a loose prosthesis, pioneered by Vives [25] as being of use in major non-infected femoral reconstructions. The use of an associated bone allograft allows restoration of the proximal end of the femur and will bridge any weak areas resulting from previous operations. However, there are three technical problems which can be difficult to overcome:

1) The relative "height" of the prosthesis. The trochanterotomy allows relative lengthening or shortening, but it is difficult to assess this before the distal screws have been inserted. The degree of anteversion can be controlled by metaphyseal pieces of variable angles.

2) The screw fixation. The screws are inserted in the sagittal plane. This means that they pass through the longitudinal cut of the femorotomy. Sometimes, this will help to fix the femorotomy.

3) Allografts can help to replace loss of the femoral diaphysis, and their use does not seem to lead to a significant risk of infection [1, 26]. Very large defects require the use of bone bank femurs. Smaller defects can be filled with bone taken from bone bank femoral heads.

■ *Fixation of the trochanteric osteotomy (trochanterotomy)*

This is rarely simple, and problems may occur. In two-stage operations, the contact may be reduced by excision and by retraction. Cerclage alone is often insufficient, and specific hooks may be necessary. The size of the prosthesis may disturb the diaphyseal screw fixation of these hooks, and the reduction of the trochanter is often imperfect. This problem can be helped either by using Wagner's technique (approach through the gluteus medius) without trochanterotomy, or by opening the femorotomy posteriorly, thus preserving the trochanter intact. However, in practice neither of these two methods allows really good clearance and cleaning of the acetabulum. Wagner's technique may damage the nerve to the gluteus medius, and the modified femorotomy risks being fractured when being opened. However, in spite of these potential problems, trochanteric osteotomy has a definite place during revision of septic total hip replacements.

■ *Antibiotic cement*

The debate between the value of cemented and screwed prostheses is based only on mechanical properties, and does not really take account of the possible value of using antibiotic-loaded cement. Bucholtz [3] believes that local antibiotic prophylaxis assures control of infection, but in fact had only 77% of success, some only after several attempts. In addition, it is frequent to encounter persistent infections due to gentamycin-sensitive organisms, despite the previous use of gentamycin-loaded cement.

Clinical value

Clinical trials appear to confirm the value of antibiotic-loaded cement. A metastudy of 1414 revisions using antibiotic cement reported an 82.7% success rate, as opposed to 56.0% with cement alone.

Revision with cement alone

Published series using cement alone tend to be rather out of date and did not employ rigorous standards of medical and surgical management, and therefore are not comparable. Lai et al [13] report 26 cases of total revision for infection using plain cement with 24 successes; this was the same proportion they achieved when using antibiotic cement. Wilson [27] had a 91% success rate in 22 revisions for infection using antibiotic-loaded cement. However, there is always the possibility of producing ecological problems by using this material. While this risk is probably acceptable with gentamycin, it is greater with vancomycin. The appearance of *Staphylococci* resistant to the glycopeptides (vancomycin and teicoplanin) is causing considerable concern in the United States of America. It is likely that the use of sub-minimal doses of the glycopeptides may well be blamed, if major problems do develop. Therefore, at the present time we believe that mixing an antibiotic in the cement is to be avoided because:

– the mechanical effects are as yet unknown;

– the diffusion of the antibiotic is not certain;

– the clinical value has not been demonstrated;

– there may well be an ecological risk.

However, the use of aminoside-loaded cement prepared by reputable drug companies has a risk which can both be calculated and controlled. This is not so with the use of vancomycin.

Medical treatment, current theories

The medical management is just as important as the surgery, but unfortunately, at present there is no evidence to support an ideal antibiotic protocol. It is only possible to consider the treatment of infections in other areas, and the results of experimental bone infections in animals, of which the best

Table I. – Percentage of antibiotic found in the bone in relation to the serum level [8].

Betalactamines	10-30 %
Glycopeptides	10-30 % (100 % with continuous perfusion)
Aminosides	30 %
Fucidic acid	50 %
Quinolones	50-100 %
Rifampicin	40 %

It is thus obvious that if the microbes are sensitive to fusidic acid or quinolone, one can use the oral route at an early stage. Very favourable animal studies suggest that rifampicin should be used whenever possible, and intravenous administration (600 mg) gives twice the concentration shown by using the oral route (300 mg), although the latter can be used once the infection has been controlled.

known are those of Norden [19]. He suggests that the use of two antibiotics is better than one, and that prolonged treatment is essential to sterilise infected bones.

However, we consider that there are problems related to this medical therapy [16]:

– The molecules (therapy) should be chosen in relation to the antibiogram, but the antibiogram is only one factor which may influence the choice; another is the diffusion of the drug in bone.

– Large doses should be used. The level of the drug within bone depends on the serum levels. For example, methicillin and oxacillin, when used for bone infections, rapidly produce a high serum level, but they are also rapidly excreted by the kidneys. The serum levels are therefore not stable, and heavy daily doses (12gr/24hr) must be administered in smaller doses several times each day; this is difficult to do with tablets of 500 mg.

– The route of administration must depend on the quality of the bone (table I). Some antibiotic molecules are more useful in bone infections that others. When starting administration, we recommend the intravenous route in order to have a steady serum level during the first 24 hours (rifampicin).

– The duration of antibiotic therapy is not defined in the literature, and surgical articles are often imprecise on medical treatment. No prospective randomised study on this dilemma has been published, but we suggest that massive antibiotic therapy should be continued for at least a month.

– Heavy antibiotic therapy at the start of treatment can later be replaced by oral administration, particularly when the infection appears to be subsiding.

THERAPEUTIC PLAN

– Initial period: 0-30 days after revision, two-drug therapy using large doses parenterally.

– Period of consolidation: 30-60 days after revision, two oral drugs.

– Secondary phase: 60-90 days, a single oral drug.

This protocol is based on practical reasoning, and may require modification when used in certain situations.

Infections with methicillin-resistant staphylococci

The most popular antibiotics are the glycopeptides (vancomycin and teicoplanin). We like to use a permanent venous catheter in order to give these drugs intravenously for three months. This perfusion using an electrically driven syringe produces stable serum drug levels, and also a high level in bone [6].

Microbes sensitive to rifampicin

This drug is often vital as it is very efficient in bone infection, but there are potential if not real dangers: monotherapy, delay in commencing administration 24 hours after the start of another antibiotic, and because its rapid penetration into bone may produce a risk of the development of rifampicin-resistant organisms.

Early reduction of antibiotic administration

When the microbe is sensitive to antibiotics which act well within bone, it is possible to change to oral therapy after 21 days.

Indications and suggested management

We consider that lavage with synovectomy, one-stage reimplantation and two-stage reimplantation are now indicated in specific situations.

SIMPLE LAVAGE WITH SYNOVECTOMY

This is only indicated in two specific clinical situations.

Acute post-operative infection (0-21 days)

When an early acute infection develops, it is wise to perform an urgent lavage and synovectomy, followed by antibiotic therapy until the CRP has returned to normal. However, this problem is relatively rare, and more often the diagnosis is made only after the stage when lavage can be effective. In the literature, it seems that it is relatively effective (50% of success) when undertaken within 3 days, but it is worth trying until the 21st day.

Acute haematogenous infection

Haematogenous infection must be considered when:

– there has been a period during which the patient had no problem;

– there is a septic localisation with or without documented bacteriology;

– there is pain in the operated hip and fever.

The haematogenous infection begins in the articular cavity, the prosthesis being contaminated secondarily. The interface between bone and cement, or bone and prosthesis, is attacked by the infection in later on.

Urgent lavage and synovectomy can lead to healing, but there are two limits:

– Diagnosis of a haematogenous infection is not always easy, and late infections can result from intra-operative contamination with microbes of low virulence. In these cases, lavage is not effective. However, this lesser procedure is worth trying before considering the extremely serious step of removing the implant.

– Unfortunately, febrile syndromes in patients with prostheses are often managed in medical wards. The orthopaedic surgeon may only be consulted when severe septic arthritis has become apparent and major surgery may then be necessary.

REVISION IN ONE STAGE

One-stage revision is often indicated when there are relatively simple mechanical or infectious problems.

Mechanical problems

One-stage revision is possible when only minor reconstruction is necessary. A small graft to reinforce the acetabulum does not pose any great difficulty, but reconstruction of the femur is usually best combined with a two-stage revision, as much because of infection as because of mechanical indications. This also allows preparation of the necessary material: the size of the prosthesis and the size of the graft. One-stage revision is unwise when associated with a femorotomy, as the cement can leak out and imperil the fixation. It is best performed under better conditions, as explained by Laffargue et al [12] who found a high risk of complications in this situation. After one month, the femorotomy, although not yet well-united, will not allow any leakage of cement. Fixation can then be performed under better mechanical conditions. One-stage revision after femorotomy necessitates the use of an interlocked prosthesis (without cement), which is not necessarily directed in exactly the same direction as the original. For mechanical reasons, a two-stage procedure is much easier.

Infectious problems

When a one-stage revision is planned, it is essential to be absolutely certain of the character of the infecting microbe, and the excision of all the infected material must be assured. If the original cement has passed into the pelvis, a one-stage procedure is contraindicated, as total excision is impossible.

One-stage revision

This is less aggressive for the patient. When dealing with those who are frail, or when the excision has been difficult and extensive, one hesitates to expose such patients to a second operation. The technique of "all or nothing" can perhaps be considered an indication for a one-stage operation.

Results of one-stage revisions

Results are difficult to analyse, as no series limited to one-stage revisions is available, a selection always having been made by the surgeons. The Cochin Hospital team [21], reporting 90 cases of one-stage revision, found 17 failures due to recurrence of infection (80% success). This seems to be about the generally published figure, but it is difficult to compare different series. The follow-up is never the same, surgical techniques differ, and the antibiotic protocol is often rather vague. A meta-analysis found a 82.7% success rate with one-stage revision performed for infection and treated with antibiotic cement. Wroblewsky reported 91% of success with one-stage revision [28]. At the present time, it seems that with careful selection one can hope to cure three out of four patients with a one-stage revision, and to produce a functional result similar to that of an uninfected prosthesis. When the hip infection has been eradicated, the joint should be as good as one that has never had this problem. The functional results are certainly better after one-stage revisions, but this technique does not allow the surgeon to prepare the solution to difficult mechanical problems, or to make sure that the necessary bone grafts will be available. It is important never to forget that any operation may become infected, and this can happen even with two-stage revision. James et al [9] report 12% of infections after revisions of uninfected hips.

TWO-STAGE REVISIONS

Delaying replacement of an infected hip after removal of all infected material gives the best chance that antibiotics will control the infection. A meta-analysis of 191 cases reports a 93.4% success rate with cure of infection, using a two-stage procedure.

What is the ideal period between excision and replacement?

There is little published on this subject. Theoretically, the longer the delay, the greater the security. On the other hand, too long a delay can make the operation technically difficult. The Cochin Hospital team [21] found that for the functional results, a delay between the two stages was less satisfactory in 12 cases than in their other series of one-stage revisions. However, surgeons are all trying to shorten the period between the two stages.

Two-stage revisions with a short interval

At present, no one knows the ideal period between total removal of all infected material and the implantation of a new prosthesis. In this situation, we prefer a short period [5, 15], with the second stage performed when the CRP has returned to normal. Colyer [5] had the same rate of success with 28 cases re-operated upon before six months as he had after a delay of a year. The second stage is performed during the same admission, when the CRP is normal even though the ESR may remain raised.

After the primary removal of infected material, one must assess the biology (the ESR and the CRP) and the microbiology (cultures are taken from the drains about every five days).

If the drain fluid continues to contain microbes, a second excision and cleaning is indicated; this may also be indicated by the persistence of a raised CRP after a month.

The second stage is generally carried out at about the 30th day, and consists of a re-insertion if the infection appears to be biologically and clinically controlled, or of a further excision and cleaning when there is any possibility that infection is still present. We try to profit from the advantages of two stages (microbiological confirmation, efficacy of antibiotics, and time to solve mechanical problems) without having the inconveniences (more difficult surgery, more haemorrhage, and less good functional results). A short interval between two stages also avoids the functional problems associated with the absence of a prosthesis

and the patient's remaining in traction. However, there has been no statistical confirmation that this approach is correct, and indeed this would be difficult to prove.

THE USE OF SPACERS WITH ACRYLIC CEMENT

Although commonly used with knee prosthesis surgery, cement spacers impregnated with antibiotics have recently also been used in the hip [15, 20]. Younger [29] describes 61 cases, and of the 48 reviewed after re-implantation, there were only three failures. Migaud [17] reported three cases with one infected failure. The block of cement acts as a temporary prosthesis and makes life easier between the two stages. Re-implantation should also be easier.

To us, this method runs the risk of prolonging the infection. In fact, a block of cement delivers 17 times less antibiotic than a chain of beads [22]. However, the block is mechanically more satisfactory than a string of beads. Kendall [10] has shown that even if the liquid around the spacers was sterile, one could often find microbes adherent to the methacrylate. The success rate in controlling infection is little different to that following one-stage revision, and the benefit of spacers has not yet been demonstrated.

On mechanical grounds, the spacer's being in contact with the acetabulum would not appear to be compatible with the femorotomy. On functional grounds, we believe that a short interval between the two

stages makes it possible to avoid the functional invalidity which may occur after too long an interval.

With an interval of one month, retraction of the soft tissues is not difficult, and the re-implantation is relatively easy. It is important to remember that placing gentamycin beads in the cavity between stages is wise, especially when the microbes are sensitive to this antibiotic.

Conclusion

Infection of a hip prosthesis is a much-feared complication which demands rigorous multi-disciplinary medical and surgical management, in which the surgeon has the most thankless task. He or she was probably responsible for the infection, and then has to seek the patient's agreement to an often lengthy plan of management after consultation with the microbiologist and anaesthesiologist. Success demands close co-operation with the above team, and this must be fostered and nurtured by the surgeon. It is important to realise that no one technique can guarantee success. The use of a combination of several procedures (femorotomy with two-stage replacement, plus local and general antibiotics) may be best, although the exact role of each of these has never been demonstrated, and probably never will be. The principles that we recommend seem to us to be logical, but it seems highly unlikely that they will ever respond to scientific assessment.

References

[1] Alexeef M, Mahomed N, Morsi E, Garbuz D, Gross A. Structural allograft in two stage revisions for failed septic arthroplasty. *J Bone Joint Surg Br* 1996 ; 78 : 213-216

[2] Argenson JN, Drancourt M, Aubaniac JM, Huiskes R. Ciment à la vancomycine dans les infections à staphylocoque sur prothèse de hanche. Étude in vitro et clinique. *Rev Chir Orthop* 1996 ; 82 (suppl II) : 66-67

[3] Buchholtz HW, Elson RA, Engelbrecht E, Lodenkamper H, Ottger J, Siegel A. Management of deep infection of total hip arthroplasty. *J Bone Joint Surg Br* 1981 ; 63 : 342-353

[4] Chofi M, Langlais F, Fourastier J, Minet J, Renaud B, Cormier M. La pharmacocinétique de la vancomycine associée au ciment orthopédique. *Rev Chir Orthop* 1997 ; 83 (suppl II) : 20

[5] Colyer RA, Capello WN. Surgical treatment of the infected hip implant. Two stage reimplantation with a one month interval. *Clin Orthop* 1994 ; 298 : 75-79

[6] Desplaces N. Sepsis osseux gravex. In : Pourriat JL, Martin C éd. Principes de réanimation chirurgicale. Paris : Arnette Blackwell, 1995

[7] Espehaug B, Engesaeter LB, Vollset SE, Havelin LI, Langeland N. Antibiotic prophylaxis in total hip arthroplasty. *J Bone Joint Surg Br* 1997 ; 79 : 590-595

[8] Helwig ULF, Bretschneider M, Klotz R. Femoral cortical sleeve in revision arthroplasty. *Acta Orthop Scand* 1996 ; 67 : 424-430

[9] James ET, Hunter GA, Cameron HV. Total hip revision arthroplasty : does sepsis influence the results ? *Clin Orthop* 1982 ; 170 : 88-94

[10] Kendall RW, Duncan CP, Smith JA, Ngui Yen JH. Persistance of bacteria of antibiotic loaded acrylic depots. A reason for caution. *Clin Orthop* 1996 ; 329 : 273-280

[11] Kraay MJ, Goldberg VM, Figgie HE. Use of an antibiotic impregnated polymethyl methacrylate intra medullary spacer for complicated revision total hip arthroplasty. *J Arthroplasty* 1992 ; 7 : 397-402

[12] Laffargue PH, Delalande JL, Meyer E, Decoulx J. Voie transfémorale versus endofémorale dans les reconstructions prothétiques des prothèses totales de hanche descellées. *Rev Chir Orthop* 1996 ; 82 (suppl II) : 91

[13] Lai KA, Shen WJ, Yang CY, Lin RM, Lin CS, Jou IM. Two stage cementless revision THR after infection. Five recurrences in 40 cases. *Acta Orthop Scand* 1996 ; 67 : 325-328

[14] Langlais F, Bunetel L, Segui A, Sassi N, Cormier M. Ciments orthopédiques aux antibiotiques; Pharmacocinétique et taux osseux *Rev Chir Orthop* 1988 ; 74 : 493-503

[15] Lieberman JR, Callaway GH, Salvati EA, Pellici PM, Brause BD. Treatment of the infected total hip arthroplasty with a two-stage reimplantation protocol. *Clin Orthop* 1994 ; 301 : 205-212

[16] Lortat-Jacob A. Technique de prescription des antibiotiques en chirurgie orthopédique. *Encycl Méd Chir* (Éditions Scientifiques et Médicales Elsevier SAS, Paris), Techniques Chirurgicales - Orthopédie-Traumatologie, 44-088, 1997 : 1-4

[17] Migaud H, Chantelot C, Besson A, Gougeon F, Dubois HH, Duquennoy A. Prothèse temporaire en ciment imprégné d'antibiotiques au cours des arthroplasties en deux temps sur hanche infectée. *Rev Chir Orthop* 1997 ; 83 : 466-468

[18] Nestor BJ, Hanssen AD, Ferrer-Gonzales R, Fitzgerald RH Jr. The use of porous protheses in delayed reconstruction of total hip replacement that have failed because of infection. *J Bone Joint Surg Am* 1994 ; 76 : 349-351

[19] Norden Carl W. Lessons learned from animal models of osteomyelitis. *Rev Infect Dis* 1988 ; 10 : 103-110

[20] Oxborrow NJ, Stamer J, Andrews M, Stone MH. New uses for gentamycin impregnated polymethyl methacrylate spacers in two stage revision hip arthroplasty. *J Arthroplasty* 1997 ; 12 : 709-710

[21] Postel M. Infection des prothèses totales de hanche. Journées de Cochin, Paris, Mars 1991

[22] Salvati EA, Callaghan JJ, Brause BD, Klein RF, Small RD. Reimplantation in infection, elution of gentamycin from cement and beads. *Clin Orthop* 1986 ; 207 : 83-93

[23] Tsukayama DT, Estrada R, Gustilo RB. Infection after total hip arthroplasty. A study of the treatment of one hundred and six infections. *J Bone Joint Surg Am* 1996 ; 78 : 512-523

[24] Vielpeau C. Sauvetage des prothèses totales de hanche infectées. In : Cahier d'enseignement de la SOFCOT. Conférences d'enseignement. Paris : Expansion scientifique française, 1986 : 161-184

[25] Vives P, Mertl P, Marczuk Y, TranVan F. Possibilités d'une tige verrouillée dans les descellements fémoraux. *Rev Chir Orthop* 1997 ; 83 (suppl II) : 51

[26] Wang JW, Chen CE. Reimplantation of infected hip arthroplasties using bone allografts. *Clin Orthop* 1997 ; 335 : 202-210

[27] Wilson MG, Dorr LD. Reimplantation of infected total hip arthroplasties in the absence of antibiotic cement. *J Arthroplasty* 1989 ; 4 : 263-269

[28] Wroblewsky BN. One stage revision of cemented total hip arthroplasty. *Clin Orthop* 1986 ; 211 : 103-107

[29] Younger AS, Duncan CP, Masri BA, McGraw RW. The outcome of two-stage arthroplasty using a custom-made interval spacer to treat the infected hip. *J Arthroplasty* 1997 ; 12 : 615-623

Hip joint resection

A Lortat-Jacob

Abstract. – *Hip resection is a major procedure with significant effects on joint function. It should be considered only after conservative treatment has failed to control persistent and recalcitrant joint infection. The trochanteric-iliac coaptation described by R. Judet is now rarely indicated, as it cannot be followed easily by total replacement. In paraplegic patients, hip resection is used for inveterate sepsis often associated with major skin problems. Even if it does not produce a significant functional improvement, it can help to resolve some of the problems in achieving skin cover.*

Keywords: hip, resection, infection, infected hip prosthesis, trochanteric-iliac coaptation, cement removal, arthroplasty, trochanteric pressure sore.

Introduction

Girdlestone developed his technique of hip resection in order to overcome chronic septic arthritis of the hip joint. It involves removal of the femoral head and neck at the level of the trochanters. Although this specific technique is no longer employed, resection of the hip is still useful when dealing with infected prostheses, or with otherwise uncontrollable septic arthritis of the hip joint.

Hip resection for septic arthritis

This procedure is performed under appropriate antibiotic cover. The approach may be either that of Moore, Watson-Jones, or Hueter. The original incision may be re-opened when dealing with a postoperative infection (e.g. following repair of a fracture of the acetabulum or of the femoral neck). If the approach is difficult, it may be wise to enlarge the incision in order to allow really adequate exposure. Moore's approach can be extended by trochanterotomy, and an anterolateral approach can be converted to the more extensive Smith-Petersen approach by exposing the outer surface of the wing of the ilium.

Alain Lortat-Jacob, M.D., Professor, Service Chirurgie Orthopédique et Traumatologique, Hôpital Ambroise-Paré, 9, avenue Charles de Gaulle, 92104 Boulogne cedex, France.

The femoral neck is divided at its base with an oscillating saw. The acetabular cartilage is removed by curettage and the use of a dental burr, and the wound is closed over a drain.

It is wise to use an external fixator for 45 days, as this will allow early walking, while the immobilisation it produces will encourage healing and also reduce postoperative instability. During this period, knee mobilisation is started and weight-bearing is allowed after about three months.

Hip resection for infected prosthesis [2, 3]

The approach (*fig 1A*) should be made by re-opening the incision originally used to insert the prosthesis. The prosthesis is exposed by excising all the septic tissues, a total capsulectomy is performed, and bacteriological swabs are taken from different parts of the wound.

The prosthesis is dislocated; occasionally this can be helped by a trochanterotomy, which will also allow better exposure of the joint.

CEMENTED PROSTHESIS

■ **Removal of femoral component and cement**

Removal of the femoral part of the prosthesis is not difficult, as it usually slides easily out of its sheath of cement (*fig 1B*). However, removal of the cement itself can

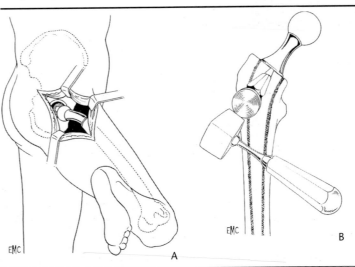

1 *Removal of a cemented prosthesis.*
A. Dislocation using a posterior approach and internal rotation.
B. The prosthesis is easily removed from the cement.

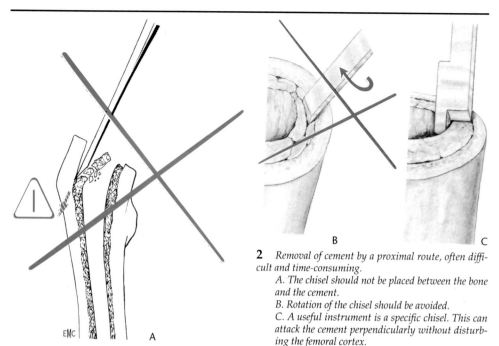

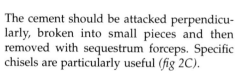

2 *Removal of cement by a proximal route, often difficult and time-consuming.*
A. The chisel should not be placed between the bone and the cement.
B. Rotation of the chisel should be avoided.
C. A useful instrument is a specific chisel. This can attack the cement perpendicularly without disturbing the femoral cortex.

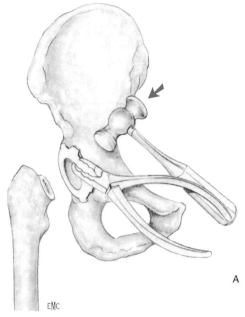

A

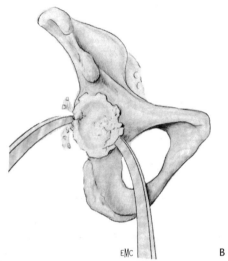

B

3 *Cleaning femorotomy (Reprinted with permission from Lortat-Jacob A, Prothèses de hanches infectées, Cahiers d'enseignement de la SOFCOT, Conférences d'Enseignement, Expansion Scientifique Française, Paris 1998).*
A. Opening the femur with a posterior flap.
B. Aspect of the femur after clearing.
C. Closing the femur with cerclage.

4 *A. Removal of the acetabular cup is usually easy.*
B. Removal of the acetabular cement is done under direct vision using a chisel.

be very tedious. It can take a long time, but must be done meticulously and carefully, avoiding in particular any major damage to the femoral shaft. Several special instruments have been devised, including long chisels of various designs, long gynaecological curettes of different shapes, sequestrum forceps, and appropriate "cold" illumination systems. Sometimes the cement can be removed fairly easily, but more often it has to be removed piecemeal using a hammer and a selection of chisels. Three important principles must be followed (fig 2) [2].

a) The chisels should never be used between the cement and the surrounding bone, as the bone may be more fragile than the cement and can easily be perforated (fig 2A).

The cement should be attacked perpendicularly, broken into small pieces and then removed with sequestrum forceps. Specific chisels are particularly useful (fig 2C).

b) Chisels should never be rotated when in the cement, as this can produce sufficient force to shatter the femoral cortex (fig 2B).

c) When it is virtually impossible to remove the cement by this means, it is wise to attack it from the distal aspect by using an anterior femorotomy (fig 3). This is best performed with the patient on his side, using an oscillating saw perpendicular to the cortex. The preliminary saw cut should extend to the distal cone of the cement; this can be detected by a change of resistance to the saw blade. The saw cut is then continued

proximally, dividing both the femoral cortex and the cement, and an anteriorly-based flap of cortex is raised. The cement can then be removed without great difficulty. The bone-cement interface is thoroughly curetted onto living bone; this helps to ensure adequate eradication of the sites of sepsis.

The femoral flap is closed with two loops of wire.

After femorotomy, the leg must be immobilised with traction for a month. If a new prosthesis is inserted, the stem must pass at least 5 cm distal to the cortical window. We no longer use a "femoral window", as these may not heal well and can considerably weaken the femoral shaft.

■ **Removal of the acetabular cup and its cement** (fig 4)

This is usually much easier. When the cup is loose, it can easily be removed by traction using an appropriate instrument

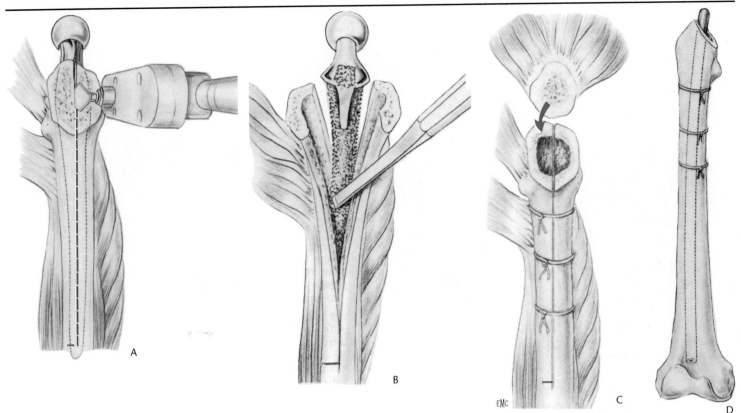

5 *Removal of an uncemented prosthesis.*
A. The trochanter is removed with its attached muscles, and the femur is split longitudinally on its lateral surface, but muscle attachments must be preserved.
B. When necessary, an anterior longitudinal split is also made. A chisel is used to separate the prosthesis from the bone.

C. After removal, the femur is restored with metallic cerclage, and the trochanter is reattached.
D. When the diaphysis is comminuted, a small medullary nail can be introduced before cerclage, in order to preserve an intramedullary canal and to allow a subsequent hip replacement.

(a "Farabeuf clamp"). When it is still attached firmly, a curved chisel (Smith-Petersen or Cauchoix) should be used gently to prise it free. The cement can usually be removed piecemeal and without great difficulty. The wound is closed over a drain, and immobilisation with traction is used for three weeks. Weight-bearing commences after three months.

■ *Uncemented prostheses* (fig 5)

Removal of uncemented prostheses can pose almost insoluble problems. It is often necessary to open the femur longitudinally, and then to use curved chisels if it has not been possible to remove the prosthesis by firm hammering.

It is important to open two flaps of femoral cortex, taking care to safeguard the vascularising attachments of muscles. The decision to do this should be made early, and before the vascular supply to the cortex has been destroyed by periosteal stripping. Cerclage wiring is used to close the defects, and the limb is supported in traction for six to seven weeks. If the sepsis can be adequately controlled, an intramedullary nail can inserted in order to preserve a medullary cavity into which another prosthesis can eventually be inserted.

■ *The use of an external fixator*

The use of an external fixator allows the formation of peri-articular fibrosis and healing of the infected cavity. It will also help to support body weight without actually creating a true joint between the greater trochanter and the acetabulum. After seven weeks when the fixator is removed, the proximal end of the femur is certainly free to move, but it does not pass into the buttock region, and the fibrous ankylosis is able to provide enough support for walking and standing. There is about 4 cm of shortening, and enough stability for reasonable activities. The insertion of another prosthesis is relatively easy. The use of an external fixator after this surgery also allows the immediate use of crutches and a wheel chair.

Specific problems and their solutions

SEPTIC ARTHRITIS OF THE HIP IN ASSOCIATION WITH A TROCHANTERIC PRESSURE SORE IN PARAPLEGICS *(fig 6)*

The necessary procedure involves resection of the hip, closure with an island flap raised from the buttock, and the application of an external fixator. Our technique [9, 10] is as follows.
1) The sore is excised including granulation tissue. It is often helpful to stain the wound with methylene blue. Bacteriological swabs are taken after the sore and scar tissue have been excised.

2) The incision is extended laterally from the distal margin of the excision wound, and should reach the inferior border of the tendon of gluteus maximus. It then passes transversely and posteriorly toward the posterosuperior iliac spine.

3) The tendon of gluteus maximus is mobilised from its distal insertion making sure to ligate the first perforating artery. The block of skin and muscle is raised, leaving the sciatic nerve in a deeper plane, thus creating the necessary musculocutaneous flap.

The femur is resected with an oscillating saw at the subtrochanteric level, thus allowing removal of the head and neck of the femur, together with all infected material. There is often a very free issue of blood at this stage. Closure is performed by using the buttock flap which resulted from resection of the original pressure sore and which should be of sufficient size to fill the defect.

4) Application of an external fixator: Three short but strong pins (of at least 5 mm diameter) are placed posterolaterally in the femoral shaft and must be well spread out. Two connected groups of pins are inserted into the ilium: one group of three above the acetabulum, and another, also of three (or more), into the iliac crest.

The reduction is made by allowing the upper end of the femoral shaft to move proximally and thus to fill the area from which the musculocutaneous flap was raised.

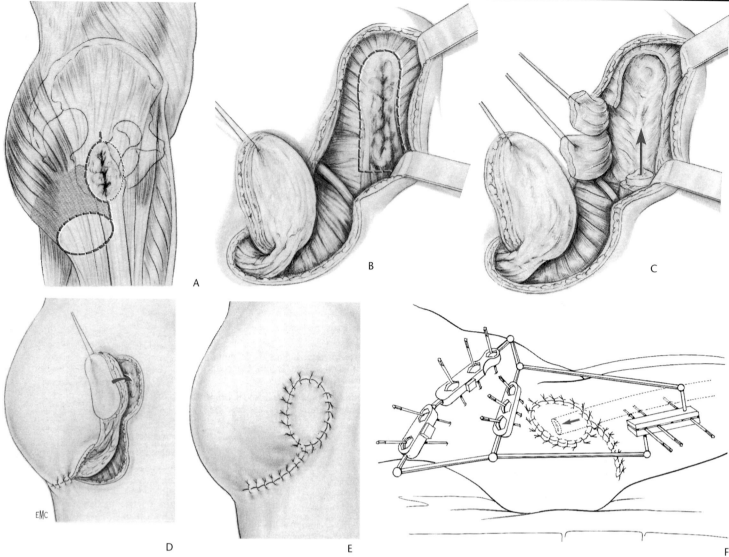

6 *Excision of the hip for arthritis associated with a trochanteric pressure sore in a paraplegic patient.*

A. Lateral approach to excise the scar prolonged to below the insertion of gluteus maximus. A skin island of sufficient size to replace the excised scar is mobilised.

B. After division of the tendon of gluteus maximus, the distal part of this muscle is raised in continuity with the skin island. The peri-trochanteric muscles are divided.

C. The femur is divided distal to the trochanteric crest with an oscillating saw, and its "stump" moves proximally toward the acetabulum.

D. The hip muscles are repaired as well as possible, and the gluteus maximus island flap is used to fill the trochanteric defect.

E. The donor area can be primarily closed as the femur has been proximally displaced.

F. An iliofemoral external fixator is applied for a month.

5) The flap covers the resected area, and the wound is closed in two layers with drainage.

6) Antibiotics are continued until the patient is apyrexial. They are prescribed according to the results of both the peroperative bacterological swabs and then by the cultures taken twice weekly from the wound drainage.

7) The drains remain in place until the wound is well-healed and there is no further discharge. A very considerable volume of fluid drains from the cavity created by removal of the prosthesis; it is usual to leave the drains in situ for at least 15 days. This also helps to prescribe the appropriate antibiotics, but it can become difficult to decide when the drains should be removed. This will depend on the volume of drainage and the extent of wound healing. If the wound is entirely water-tight, the drains can be removed and any fluid which continues to collect can then be evacuated by repeated aspirations.

Septic discharge after hip resection [8]

THE VASTUS LATERALIS MUSCULOCUTANEOUS FLAP *(fig 7)*

The acetabular cavity is an important space which is likely to become infected. When this occurs after debridement and repeated excisions, obliteration by a muscle flap may be helpful. The vastus lateralis muscle flap is the simplest to use.

A lateral incision is made to the femoral condyle. The anterior skin margin is elevated.

The rectus femoris and vastus lateralis are separated, followed by mobilisation of the vastus lateralis from the inter-muscular septum and the rectus femoris. The dissection should continue 12 cm distal to the intertrochanteric crest. The muscle is turned to fill the acetabular cavity, and the wound is closed with drainage.

An external fixator is applied for about seven weeks.

Sterile fistula after hip resection

Sterile discharge from a sinus after hip resection does not always arise from a recurrence of infection. It can often be the result of excess fluid being produced due to lack of adequate healing. Apyrexia, lack of positive cultures and normal blood tests support this diagnosis. The principle of treatment is to ensure a water-tight closure after having adequately filled the cavity. This can only be done by using the tissues which are locally available, a musculo-cutaneous gluteus maximus flap, a V-Y advancement of this muscle, or a flap from the tensor fascia lata. It is essential to use an external fixator to allow good tissue healing, and thus to reduce the size of the cavity.

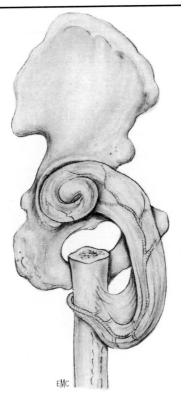

7 *A vastus lateralis flap. This is useful when there is continual hip sinus drainage. It is essential to fill the post-excision cavity by "rotating" the distal portion of the vastus lateralis which has been raised through a long lateral incision. It may be stripped from the femur up to 10 cm distal to the inter-trochanteric crest.*

The result of resection of the head and neck [1, 2, 12]

Girdlestone's operation gives mediocre results, and stability is poor, necessitating the use of two crutches or sticks. The shortening is significant, often more than 5 cm, which can lead to shoe problems. However, it does relieve pain and often restores useful mobility. The overall result is more favourable in relatively thin people and in those with strong arms. The results seem to be much better when a contact between the femur and the actebabulum ("linked resection") is created. This is the principal aim of the external fixator. In paraplegic patients, paradoxically the operation improves the sitting position, but it may lead to skin pressure problems and the risk of recurrence of pressure sores.

Trochanteric-iliac coaptation

This operation was described in 1964 by R. Judet, who had been surprised by the good clinical results which could be associated with a failed hip arthrodesis. Thus, it appeared that bone fusion was not absolutely necessary to produce a satisfactory situation, in which a certain mobility improved the functional result. The principle was to place the greater trochanter under the acetabulum. This medial

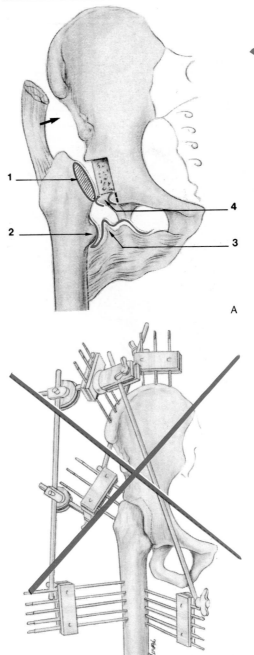

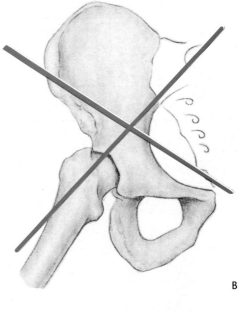

8 *The trochanteric-iliac coaptation of R. Judet. The idea is to stabilise the greater trochanter under the acetabulum.*
A. Several technical points are important: 1. Wide excision of the femoral neck ; 2. resection of the lesser trochanter ; 3. resection of the distal soft tissues ; 4. resection of the posterior lip of the acetabulum.
B. It is essential to avoid forcing the neck into abduction, as this can lead to stiffness in this position.
C. External fixation is advised only when the femoral pins can be applied in only one plane, otherwise there is a risk of producing a stiff knee.

displacement reduced both the dead space and the likelihood of a recurrence of the infection [6, 7].

TECHNIQUE *(fig 8)*

Adequate medical preparation is essential, as this procedure is larger than a simple resection, and there is often considerable bleeding.

The hip is resected in the manner already described. The coaptation is obtained after a rather more extensive resection of the neck, proceeding distally to the inter-trochanteric crest. The trochanter is then trimmed, and the medial displacement is achieved by excision of the medial soft tissues, the capsule and the adductors. The trochanter should remain without restraint within the acetabular cavity. It is essential to avoid an abduction position as this is incompatible with a useful functional result.

An ilio-femoral external fixator is applied. R. Judet originally advised the use of screws to keep the trochanter in the acetabulum, but it soon became apparent that an external fixator gives better fixation without leaving metal in the hip region. Modern fixators do not produce knee stiffness, and transverse iliac pins are usually used. The apparatus is removed after seven weeks, and weight-bearing commences three months after the surgery.

RESULTS

Trochanteric-iliac copatation is designed to produce stability with moderate mobility. However, reports in the literature suggest that:

– There was an improvement in stability, but that only one in four patients were eventually able to walk without using a walking stick.

Table I. – Three types of intervention feasible after serious hip infection.

	Technical difficulty	Relief of pain	Mobility	Stability	Effort on knee and spine	Later THR
Arthrodesis	+++	Very good	0	+++	++	+
Resection of head and neck	0	Very good	Very good	0	0	+++
Trochantericiliac coaptation	++	Average	Poor	Variable	+++	±

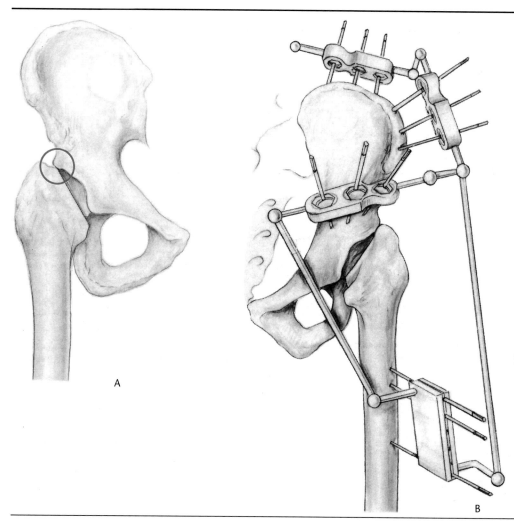

A

B

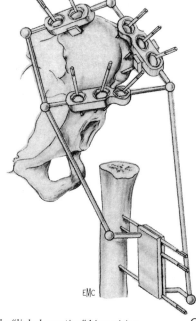

9 *The "linked resection" hip excision.*
A. Rather than creating a true trochanteric-iliac coaptation, which may have dire consequences for the knee and is difficult to follow with a total replacement, it is better to produce contact between the proximal end of the femur and the acetabulum.
B. This contact is obtained by the use of an ilio-femoral external fixator with reduction of the ilio-femoral space. Only moderate medial displacement is used.
C. The stability sometimes subsequently decreases, but often remains sufficient to reduce the leg length discrepancy, and to allow useful weight-bearing.

C

– This improvement in stability is obtained at the expense of mobility. Very few patients regained more than 50° of flexion. Those with the least mobility were more stable.

– The degree of pain relief obtained was very variable; rarely was there an improvement to more than "4" on the scale of Merle d'Aubigné.

Criteria for selecting hip resection or trochanteric-iliac coaptation [4, 5, 11] *(table I)*

The possibility of secondary arthroplasty and the publication of very mediocre results after coaptation have necessitated a review of the indications for this operation. Nowadays, it seems that it is rarely indicated, as it is very difficult to insert a total replacement at a later date, and also because the necessary medial displacement of the head has a deleterious effect on the associated knee. Simple excision should normally be the first choice, particularly as we now use external fixation to produce better weight-bearing *(fig 9)*. The rare indications for a copatation seem to be after postoperative infections and avascular necrosis of the femoral head following a trans-cervical fracture. When recommending this salvage operation, it is always important to remember the possibility of total replacement at a future date, and therefore to conserve the appropriate bone stock and anatomy.

References

[1] Ahlgren SA, Gudmundsson G, Bartholdsson E. Function after removal of a septic hip prosthesis: a survey of 27 Girdlestone hips. *Acta Orthop Scand* 1980 ; 51 : 541-545

[2] Bourne RB, Hunter GA, Rorabeck, CH, Macnab JJ. A six-year follow-up of infected total hip replacements managed by Girdlestone's arthroplasty. *J Bone Joint Surg Br* 1984 ; 66 : 340-343

[3] Campbell A, Fitzgerald B, Fischer WD, Hamlblen DL. Girdlestone pseudarthrosis for failed total hip replacement. *J Bone Joint Surg Br* 1978 ; 60 : 441-442

[4] Courtois B, Delarue P, Le Saout J, LeNen G. Cinquante neuf ablations de prothèses de hanche. Comparaison entre l'ablation simple et le coaptation. *Rev Chir Orthop* 1982 ; 68 : 523-529

[5] Frank A. Coaptation ou résection de hanche. [thèse], Paris-Ouest, 1979

[6] Letournel E. La coaptation trochantéro-iliaque. In : Actualités de chirurgie orthopédique. Paris : Masson, 1973

[7] Letournel E. La coaptation trochantéro-iliaque. *Rev Chir Orthop* 1975 ; 61 (suppl II) : 115-119

[8] Lortat-Jacob A. Tratement chirurgical de l'infection articulaire. *Encycl Méd Chir* (Éditions Scientifiques et Médicales Elsevier SAS, Paris), Techniques Chirurgicales-Orthopédie-traumatologie, 1990, 44-085, : 1-18

[9] Lortat-Jacob A. Traitement chirurgical des escarres. *Encycl Méd Chir* (Éditions Scientifiques et Médicales Elsevier SAS, Paris), Techniques Chirurgicales-Orthopédie-traumatologie, 44-072, 1992 : 1-14

[10] Lortat-Jacob A, Lortat-Jacob S, Jouanin TH, Beaufils PH. L'arthrite de hanche chez le paraplégique. *Rev Chir Orthop* 1984 ; 70 : 383-388

[11] Marotte JH, Cohen E, Lord G, Blanchard JP, Guillamon JL. Résultats comparés des résections et coaptation de hanche pour arthrite septique. *Rev Chir Orthop* 1982 ; 68 : 517-522

[12] Petty W, Goldsmith S. Resection arthroplasty following infected total hip arthroplasty. *J Bone Joint Surg Am* 1980 ; 62 : 889-896

Arthrodesis of the hip

A Lortat-Jacob

Abstract. — *Arthrodesis of the hip is not an easy operation and the long term results are poor. Internal screw fixation together with external fixation should avoid knee stiffness (the femoral part of the fixator must be in a single plane, and postoperative knee physiotherapy should start as early as possible). Difficulty in achieving fusion often necessitates bone grafting, which should be done before the external fixator has to be removed. The possibility of later converting an arthrodesis to a total hip replacement must always be borne in mind and local anatomy respected. In view of the problems which are often associated with a successful hip fusion, this operation is nowadays rarely indicated.*

© 2000, Editions Scientifiques et Médicales Elsevier SAS. All rights reserved.

Keywords: hip, arthrodesis of the hip, intra-articular arthrodesis, extra-articular arthrodesis, iliofemoral external fixation.

Introduction

Since the world-wide acceptance of total hip replacement (THR) for very many hip problems, the indications for arthrodesis of this joint are now rare, and it is a procedure which has practically disappeared from our repertoire. In addition, several arthrodesis techniques are now contraindicated as they do not allow insertion of a THR at a later date [4].

Arthrodesis may be extra-articular or intra-articular [6]. In pre-antibiotic days, extra-articular procedures were developed to avoid the risks of spreading infection or major surgical blood-letting. These techniques should be abandoned, as a very long period of postoperative immobilisation is required. They have been superseded by intra-articular procedures.

Three criteria for hip arthrodesis

Position: Fusion of a hip has severe repercussions for both static and dynamic function of the knee and of the spine. The ideal position for a stiff hip does not exist (fig 1, 2, 3).

Alain Lortat-Jacob, M.D., Professor, Service Chirurgie Orthopédique et Traumatologique, Hôpital Ambroise Paré, 9, avenue Charles de Gaulle, 92104 Boulogne cedex, France.

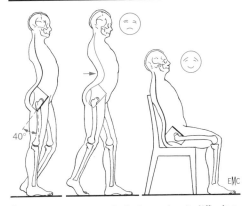

1 *Fusion in too much flexion makes it difficult to stand.*

In the sagittal plane, adequate flexion is important to allow sitting, while extension is better for standing. The position in this plane must be decided individually for each patient, who should be involved in this discussion. A young active person who works standing up would be better with a hip fixed in nearly full extension. An older and more sedentary individual will prefer rather more flexion. In practice, the acceptable range is between 20 to 40 degrees of flexion.

An ideal position for all of life's daily activities simply does not exist, and the best compromise seems to be:

– flexion, 20 degrees in young people, who prefer to be relatively "upright", and 40 degrees for older people, who prefer to sit;

– adduction, 10 degrees, which is approximately the position of the hip during walking;

– rotation: neutral or very slight external rotation.

IMMOBILISATION OF THE ARTHRODESIS

This is difficult in view of the very considerable forces involved, which produce considerable leverage on the arthrodesis. A long hip-spica extending from nipples to toes, and often also including the opposite leg down to the lower part of the thigh, should no longer be used. In addition to being difficult to tolerate, it is very likely to make the knee irretrievably stiff, a potential problem which always haunts the surgeon. A stiff hip with a stiff knee is a major disability, as it renders the foot inaccessible (for putting on shoes, washing, etc.). The classical iliofemoral plate may also cause problems, and this is one of the reasons why R. Schneider [7] (fig 4, 5) combined this procedure with an osteotomy and with medial displacement of the diaphysis of the femur. However, this produces genu valgum, which itself will give long-term difficulties. This procedure should be abandoned as it is difficult to convert to a THR. The best fixation is "mixed": screws which maintain contact between the femoral head and the acetabulum, and an iliofemoral external fixator to reduce stresses on the arthrodesis.

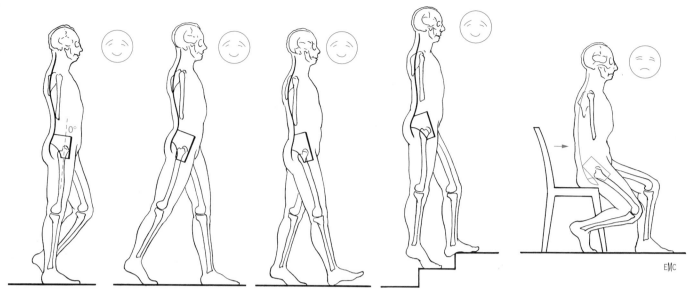

2 *Fusion in extension allows walking and stair climbing, but produces a lumbar kyphosis when sitting, which can partly be disguised by sitting on the edge of the seat.*

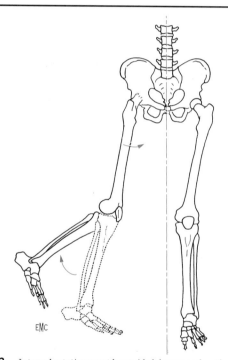

3 *Internal rotation must be avoided, because when the knee is flexed the foot moves away from the body.*

FUSION

As the bone surfaces between the head and the acetabulum are relatively small, it is often difficult to achieve bone fusion. This may be helped considerably by using a complementary bone graft.

The technique of intra-articular arthrodesis of the hip *(fig 6A, B, C, D, E)*

Correct positioning in strict lateral decubitus is very important and special supports are useful. It is very important to examine the mobility and position of the spine to make certain that the hip is fused in the desired degree of flexion *(fig 7).*

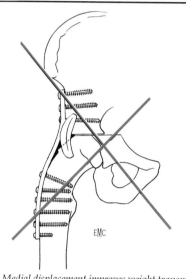

4 *Medial displacement improves weight transmission and allows the use of a plate. However, this medialisation should be abandoned as it has a very deleterious effect on the knee.*

SURGICAL APPROACH *(fig 6A)*

It is very important to respect the muscles, as they may be essential if a THR is to be inserted at a later date. It is often possible to retract posteriorly the glutei and to use a modified Moore's approach. However, if there is the least difficulty, it is wise to perform a trochanterotomy *(fig 8).*

PREPARATION OF THE BONE SURFACES *(fig 6B)*

Posterior dislocation. Because the femoral head prevents a clear view of the acetabulum, it is wise to deal with this first. It is ideal to produce two flat surfaces, one horizontal at the superior part of the head, and one vertical at the level of the fossa of the ligamentus capitis femoris. However, the destruction of the head, which is one of the indications for the arthrodesis, may make this impossible to achieve, and a simple "freshening" of the remaining femoral head is all that can be done.

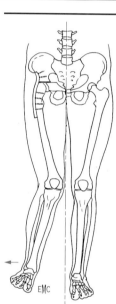

5 *Medialisation of the femoral shaft produces genu valgus.*

Adequate exposure of the acetabulum is often difficult *(fig 6C)*, and it is often necessary to mobilise the proximal end of the femur by dividing the soft tissues at the base of the femoral neck. The anterior capsule is exposed by traction through a hook passed under the base of the neck, and then excised. A retractor can then be put under the transverse ligament of the acetabulum.

Exposure of the acetabulum is then completed by widely dividing the peripheral capsule and using retracting pins inserted into the superior margin.

"Freshening" and preparation of the acetabulum should be designed "to match" that of the femoral head *(fig 6D)*. The ideal is to make two perpendicular cuts, but this is rarely possible and simple "freshening" is all that can be achieved. The bone tissue removed should be carefully saved and can be packed into the acetabulum after reduction of the joint.

After the head has been returned to the acetabulum, the position is maintained by

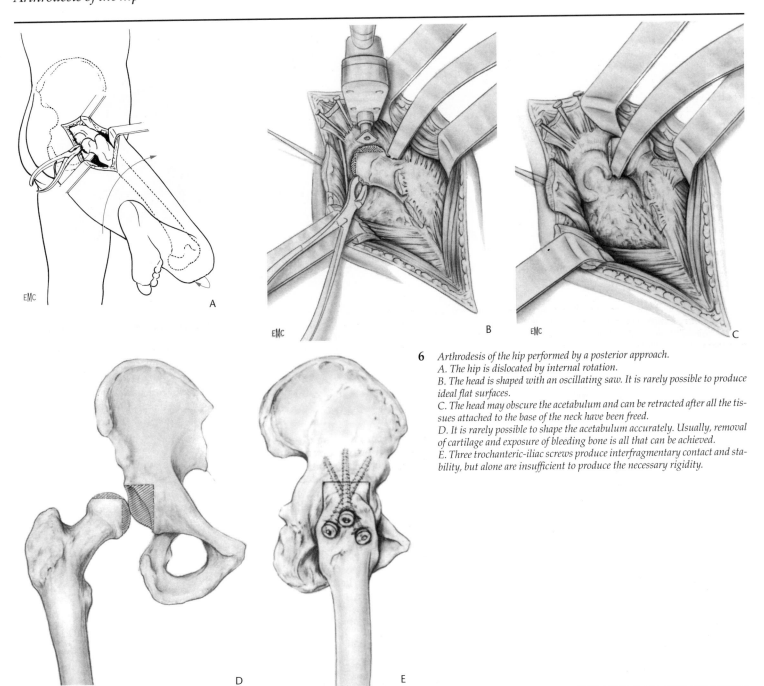

6 *Arthrodesis of the hip performed by a posterior approach.*
A. The hip is dislocated by internal rotation.
B. The head is shaped with an oscillating saw. It is rarely possible to produce ideal flat surfaces.
C. The head may obscure the acetabulum and can be retracted after all the tissues attached to the base of the neck have been freed.
D. It is rarely possible to shape the acetabulum accurately. Usually, removal of cartilage and exposure of bleeding bone is all that can be achieved.
E. Three trochanteric-iliac screws produce interfragmentary contact and stability, but alone are insufficient to produce the necessary rigidity.

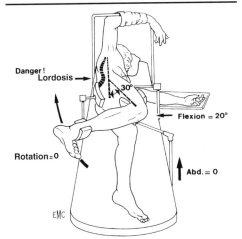

7 *The chosen position for the arthrodesis is maintained on the table by the use of special supports. It is always important to consider the degree of lumbar lordosis, as this can often cause problems.*

resting the leg in a special support. It is important to have as much bone contact as possible, and the position is maintained by two pins.

Two or three femoroiliac screws are then inserted *(fig 6E)* with the aim of restricting micro-movements. These screws are either Maconer 50 or Venable (diameter 70 mm). The previously inserted pins can be used as direction indicators and are removed as the screws are inserted. This fixation is often difficult. As the superior portion of the acetabulum contains the best quality bone, the first screw should be vertical and pass through the superior part of the head. The next two screws should be directed posterosuperiorly and anterosuperiorly. Their insertion should be controlled by radiography.

The wound is closed with drainage, using a deep strong resorbable suture and then interrupted sutures for the subcutaneous tissues and for the skin.

Application of an iliofemoral external fixator

External fixation is now an integral part of hip arthrodesis, as screw fixation alone cannot allow walking. Plaster spica immobilisation should no longer be used. There are two requirements for whatever fixation is used; it must not produce knee stiffness and it must be adjustable. This means that only fixators which allow osteotaxis should be used, as fixators composed of two elements do not allow any necessary adjustment.

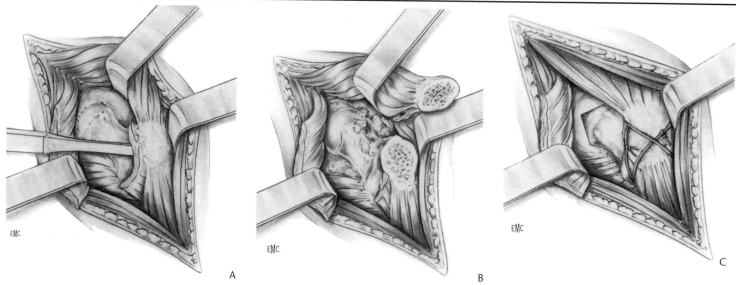

8 *Trochanterotomy may improve the exposure. It may be performed routinely, or only when there are difficulties.*
A. When a Moore's approach is inadequate, the trochanter can be elevated with a chisel.

B. After trochanterotomy, the hip can be both anteriorly and posteriorly dislocated.
C. The trochanter must be re-attached at the end of the operation. Double cerclage with steel wire is used.

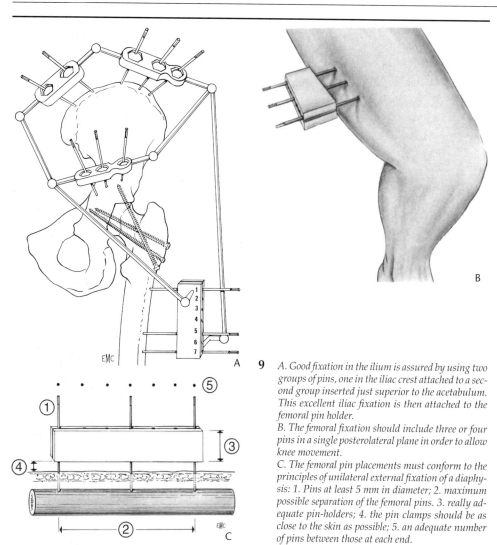

9 *A. Good fixation in the ilium is assured by using two groups of pins, one in the iliac crest attached to a second group inserted just superior to the acetabulum. This excellent iliac fixation is then attached to the femoral pin holder.*
B. The femoral fixation should include three or four pins in a single posterolateral plane in order to allow knee movement.
C. The femoral pin placements must conform to the principles of unilateral external fixation of a diaphysis: 1. Pins at least 5 mm in diameter; 2. maximum possible separation of the femoral pins. 3. really adequate pin-holders; 4. the pin clamps should be as close to the skin as possible; 5. an adequate number of pins between those at each end.

connected to whatever fixator is being used. A group of two or three pins is then inserted just proximal to the superior aspect of the acetabulum, and no preliminary tapping should be done. A finger passed into the acetabulum can ensure that the pins have not been placed too low. These pins always have a very good grip and when "joined together" produce a very solid group. Connection of these two groups of iliac pins produces excellent fixation.

The femoral pins (*fig 9B, C*) are inserted in the usual fashion [5]:

– they should be at least 5 mm in diameter;

– the pin holder should be as long as possible, thus giving control in the femoral diaphysis as far distal as possible;

– the pin holder should have a good "grip" of the pins, and should be as close to the skin as possible;

– enough pins should be used, at least four.

These femoral pins should be positioned to prevent stiffness of the knee. They should be posterolateral, thus allowing early knee movement and exercise.

The external fixator can be used in two ways: as an accessory to internal screw fixation, or by itself, when internal fixation has been technically impossible.

POSTOPERATIVE CARE

Patients are allowed to stand up early, but weight-bearing is rarely possible before four months. It can be difficult to be sure that good bone union has occurred, as radiography can be misleading. Early bone grafting can often be helpful, and active knee physiotherapy should continue for at least as long as the external fixator is in place.

Two groups of pins should be used for the ilium (*fig 9A*). One group of four pins is inserted into the iliac crest, although this can be difficult with the patient in a lateral position. The left hand should identify the wing of the ilium, and the pins can then be inserted between the thumb and the index finger. The tortuous shape of the bone means that the pins have to pass in different directions. If the patient is very obese, it may be wise to make a small incision to ensure correct pin placement. The pins are

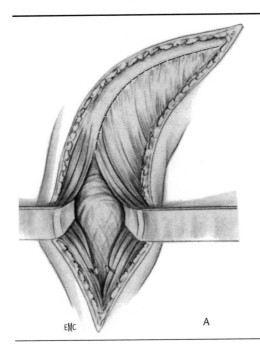

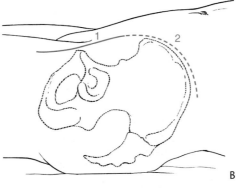

10 A. *The Watson-Jones anterior approach. This can easily be extended to become a Smith-Petersen approach by elevating the muscles from the outer wing of the ilium.*
B. *An arthrodesis by an anterior approach. 1. Watson-Jones incision; 2. For difficult cases, this can be extended to the iliac crest (Smith-Petersen).*

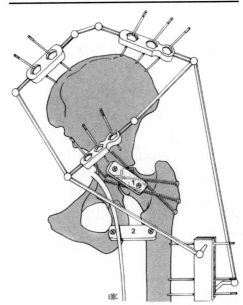

12 *A secondary graft is often necessary. 1. A direct local graft which can be used when local conditions allow. 2. A Brittain-Trumble ischio-trochanteric graft.*

Specific cases

OTHER SURGICAL APPROACHES

An anterior approach may be used, such as the Watson-Jones approach *(fig 10)*.

With a large cushion or pad under the abnormal hip, the incision starts at the anterosuperior iliac spine and passes to the greater trochanter. The gluteus medius is separated from the tensor fascia lata, and three retractors help to expose the joint, one below and one above the femoral neck. The third is placed anterior to the acetabulum. The capsule is excised and the head dislocated anteriorly by adduction and external rotation.

LACK OF BONE CONTACT *(fig 11)*

After the necessary wide excision of all diseased and abnormal tissue, there may be very little surface left to produce adequate bone contact between the remains of the femoral head and the acetabulum. This situation can be improved by packing a cancellous bone graft taken from the trochanter into this gap. It is wise to avoid using cortical bone, as this is more liable to become infected and may act as a foreign body. The plasticity of cancellous bone allows better packing into the defect and also leads to better resistance to infection. Among the most difficult arthrodesis situtions is the case of hips from which a total replacement has been removed. Very little remains of the femur, and in fact it is often necessary to place the proximal end of the femoral diaphysis within the acetabulum. However, this may result in considerable knee problems, and it is probably wiser to convert the situation to a complete hip excision.

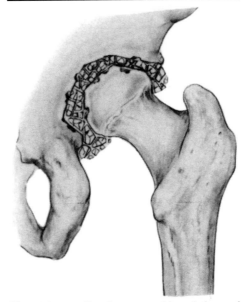

11 *All the cancellous bone removed is packed around the arthrodesis. If necessary, this can be supplemented by bone taken from within the greater trochanter.*

SECONDARY BONE GRAFTING [10]
(fig 12)

This is often essential when there is very poor bone contact, chronic sclerotic osteomyelitis, or difficulty in stabilising a real or potential nonunion. In addition, it is most unwise to leave an external fixator in place for more than five months, and this is another indication for relatively early bone grafting. It should be performed as soon as there is any doubt as to the progress of bone fusion (before the third month). The Brittain-Trumble technique is useful and uses a large cortical graft placed between the femur and the ischium.

It is probably wise to screw the graft to the trochanter, taking great care of the sciatic

nerve. If the graft is "high", the nerve passes anterior, but more often it is left lying posterior.

Results of hip arthrodesis [1, 2, 8, 9]

When the hip is fused in a good position, it can provide good short-term functional results. Pain-free stability allows walking without aids. However, in the longer term, problems arise from the spine and the knee and often cause considerable concern.

Indications for hip arthrodesis [3]

Nowadays, hip fusion is rarely indicated, as the fairly favourable short-term result usually deteriorates. Low back pain and degeneration of the knee, which may affect both left and right, can be difficult to treat. Thus, the indication for a possible THR rather than an arthrodesis must always be considered in the light of the expected longevity of the patient. By contrast, after twenty years, a THR is likely to be worn out, but the spine and hip will have been preserved. Currently, the main indications for hip arthrodesis are the sequelae of infection of this joint: haematogenous osteomyelitis, infections after acetabular surgery and haematogenous septic arthritis. However, even these indications are becoming rare, and it is always important not to forget the possibility of a secondary THR.

References ➤

References

[1] Barnhardt T, Stiehl JB. Hip fusion in young adults. *Orthopedics* 1996 ; 19 : 303-306

[2] Demigneux F, Rainaut JJ, Cedart CL. Étude de la hanche opposée aux arthrodèses. *Rev Chir Orthop* 1968 ; 54 : 649-656

[3] Evrard J, Hourtoulle P, Roure JL, Merle d'Aubigné R. Les arthrodèses de hanche pour arthrite septique. Étude critique. *Rev Chir Orthop* 1985 ; 71 : 87-93

[4] Kostuik J, Alexander D. Arthrodesis for failed arthroplasty of the hip. *Clin Orthop* 1984 ; 188 ; 173-182

[5] Lortat-Jacob A. Traitement chirurgical de l'infection articulaire. *Encycl Méd Chir* (Elsevier, Paris), Techniques chirurgicales - Orthopédie-Traumatologie, 44-085, 1990 : 1-18

[6] Merle d'Aubigné R, Ramadier JO. L'arthrodèse de hanche. In : Traumatismes anciens. Rachis membres inférieurs. Paris : Masson, 1959

[7] Müller ME, Allgöwer M, Schneider R, Willennegger H. Manual of internal fixation; techniques recommended by the AO-group. New York : Springer-Verlag, 1980 : 388-389

[8] Roberts CS, Fetto JF. Functional outcome of hip fusion in the young patient. *J Arthroplasty* 1990 ; 5 : 89-96

[9] Romness DW, Morrey BF. Total knee arthroplasty in patients with prior ipsilateral hip fusion. *J Arthroplasty* 1992 ; 7 : 63-70

[10] Teinturier P. Arthrodèse de la hanche. Lambeau pédiculé avec vissage ischio-fémoral. *Rev Chir Orthop* 1966 ; 52 : 645-649

Osteotomies of the upper femur: varisation, valgisation, derotation

| ME Müller

Abstract. – *Despite the overwhelming success of total hip replacement, the intertrochanteric osteotomy still remains a valuable alternative.*
This chapter outlines the principles of the healing process induced by a varus or valgus osteotomy in a diseased hip joint, as described by Pauwels [11]. *The most important aspect is the relationship between the change of the femoral neck angle, the medial or lateral displacement of the femoral shaft and the stresses developed in both compartments of the knee joint. AO angled blade plates allow the impaction of both surfaces of the osteotomy and early weight-bearing. Preoperative graphic planning is mandatory for intertrochanteric osteotomy; the details of such planning are provided. The techniques of the six essential types of osteotomy for the treatment of dysplastic hips, post-traumatic malunion or nonunion, or the early signs of arthritic hip are also described, as well as the shortening procedure (1-3 cm) at the level of the lesser trochanter.*

© 2002, Editions Scientifiques et Médicales Elsevier SAS. All rights reserved.

Keywords: hip, femoral osteotomies, intertrochanteric osteotomy, dysplastic hip, varus osteotomy, valgus osteotomy, subtrochanteric shortening osteotomy.

Introduction

An intertrochanteric osteotomy is a transverse osteotomy of the femur between the greater and lesser trochanters. If the resected bone wedge is medial, the osteotomy is called an adduction or varus osteotomy. If it is localised laterally, it is an abduction or valgus osteotomy. If in addition the femoral shaft is partially resected, we speak of a shortening osteotomy. If necessary, varus and valgus osteotomies are combined with an internal or external rotation, or performed simultaneously with a pelvic osteotomy.

With an intertrochanteric osteotomy, the angle between the axis of the neck and the axis of the femur can be altered in three planes: frontal (abduction/adduction), sagittal (flexion/extension), and transverse (external/internal rotation).

Three types of displacement are possible: medial or lateral, anterior or posterior, lengthening or shortening.

In Europe, for the 20 year period between 1950 and 1970, the intertrochanteric osteotomy was the treatment of choice for osteoarthritic hips. Is this treatment only of great historical significance today? This may be the case for advanced osteoarthritis, but intertrochanteric osteotomies are still performed in young adults after slipped femoral epiphysis, for dysplastic hips, for post-traumatic arthritic changes, etc., as well as in leg length discrepancies of 2 to 2.5 cm following a total hip replacement.

In addition, the more than 65 year old simple transverse displacement osteotomy of McMurray [3] has gained new disciples. This procedure seems to change the direction of only the stresses, but in suitable cases, the remodelling of the direction of the bone trabeculae can have a long-lasting effect in relieving pain.

Aims and interrelated phenomena

AIMS

For an intertrochanteric osteotomy, Pauwels [10] demonstrated that knowledge of the distribution of the load (external forces) and the stress (effect of forces inside bone and cartilage) in the proximal femur are primordial. If the direction of the stresses in the proximal femur changes, the orientation of the bone trabeculae in the femoral head and neck is remodelled. If the weight-bearing surface of the joint is reduced and/or the length of the lever arm of the abductor muscles is shortened, the load becomes higher and the stresses increase. Osteoarthritic changes begin and the development of an arthritic hip is pre-programmed.

Pauwels [9, 10] wanted to reverse this process by using the varus osteotomy. He tried to increase the weight-bearing joint surface and to lengthen the lever arm of the abductor muscles. He calculated that after the osteotomy the load would be reduced 3 to 6 times. This is the biomechanical principle of the healing effect of a varus intertrochanteric osteotomy described by Pauwels in 1950 (*fig 1*). Pauwels, and later R. Bombelli [1], F. Langlais [2], M.E. Müller [6] and R. Schneider [12, 13], demonstrated astonishing results, with restoration of a quite normal hip joint space lasting 10, 20 or more years after the operation.

INTERRELATED PHENOMENA BETWEEN VARUS/VALGUS OSTEOTOMIES AND MEDIAL/LATERAL DISPLACEMENT OF THE FEMORAL SHAFT (*fig 2*)

Under normal conditions, the axis of the knee joint is at right angles to the axis of the body, or vertical line, and parallel to the floor. The mechanical axis links the centres of the femoral head, and of the knee and ankle joints, and is parallel to the tibia. The

Maurice E Müller, Prof. Dr. med., Maurice E. Müller Foundation for Continuing Education, Research and Documentation in Orthopedic Surgery, Murtenstrasse 35 / P.O. Box 8354, CH-3001 Bern, Switzerland.

All references to this article must include: Müller ME. Osteotomies of the upper femur: varisation, valgisation, derotation. Editions Scientifiques et Médicales Elsevier SAS (Paris). All rights reserved. Surgical Techniques in Orthopaedics and Traumatology, 55-470-A-10, 2002, 9 p.

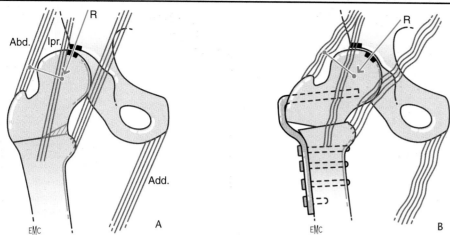

1 *A. Biomechanical background of the varus osteotomy in a painful dysplastic hip.*
B. After a varus osteotomy, the weight-bearing area and the lever arm of the muscle forces (that is, the distance be-tween the centre of the femoral head and the abductors) are increased and the abductor muscles are released (Pau-wels [9]).

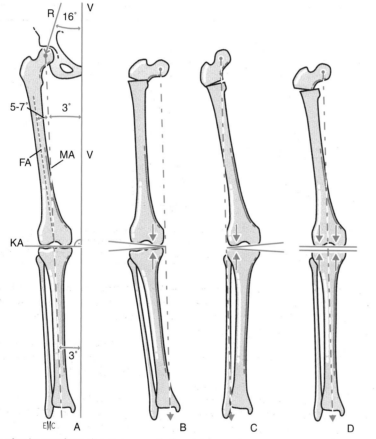

2 *Influence of an intertrochanteric osteotomy on the knee joint.*
A. Physiological axial and angular correlation of the lower extremity. The mechanical axis (MA) goes through the centre of the femoral head, the centre of the knee, and the centre of the ankle. It subtends an angle of 3° with the vertical (V) and 5°-7°, depending on the sex of the patient, with the anatomical axis of the femoral shaft (FA). The axis of the knee joint (KA) is perpendicular to the vertical, and the angle which the resultant (R) of the compres-sive forces on the hip subtends with the vertical is 16°.
B. A simple varus osteotomy without medial displacement induces a varus knee joint with overloading of the me-dial compartment and a shortening of the femur.
C. A simple valgus osteotomy without lateral displacement induces a lengthening of the femur and a valgus knee joint with overloading of the lateral compartment.
D. Physiological loading conditions of the knee joint are realised with a medial displacement in a varus osteotomy or a lateralisation of the femoral shaft in a valgus osteotomy (see Fig. 6).

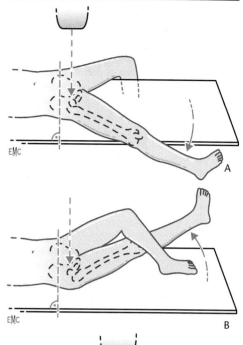

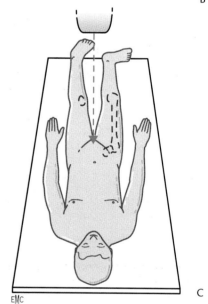

3 *A. Functional a-p X-ray in maximal abduction of both legs. The foot of the opposite leg hangs over the table.*
B. Functional a-p X-ray in maximal adduction, the opposite leg crossed over the involved leg.
C. In unilateral malunion, the normal hip should be internally rotated when the a-p X-ray of the pelvis is taken.

angles between the mechanical and the vertical lines measure 3°; between the vertical line and the femoral axis the angle is 5-7° (usually 5° for a man and 7° for a woman) *(fig 2A)*. The compressive force R evokes stresses in the hip joint during the support period of gait. The angle of the R line (resulting from the forces of the body weight and the abductor muscles) to that of the vertical axis measures 16°. In order to obtain symmetrical weight-bearing of both compartments of the knee joint after a varus osteotomy, a medial displacement is needed. On the contrary, with a valgus osteotomy, a lateralisation of the femoral shaft is indicated.

Prerequisites for inter-trochanteric osteotomy

PREOPERATIVE X-RAYS

A pelvic X-ray is essential for diagnosis. It is centred 2 cm above the symphysis of the pelvis, the patient being in the prone

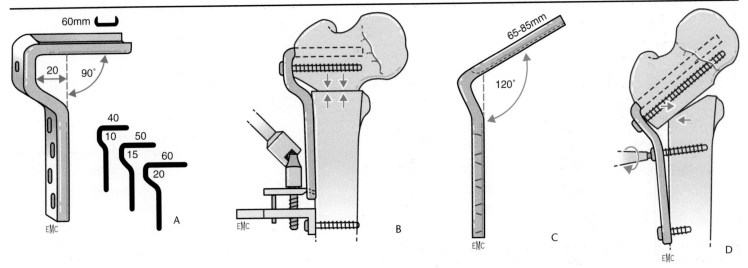

4   *The two angled blade plates with U-profile and the technique of impaction of both osteotomy surfaces.*
A. The right-angled blade plate with its 3 possible medial displacements (offsets) of 10, 15 and 20 mm and 3 different blade lengths (40, 50, 60 mm).

B. Impaction of the osteotomised bone surfaces with the tension device.
C. The 120° double-angled blade plate.
D. Distal fixation of the 120° plate with a short screw, impaction with the second screw.

position. The knees must touch each other. To determine the best position of the femoral head in the acetabulum, the situation of the hip joint in maximal abduction and adduction must be checked on a functional X-ray. To test the abduction on the right side, the left leg must be maximally abducted and if possible hang outside the table (*fig 3A*). To measure the possible adduction, the opposite leg is crossed over the involved leg in order to fix the pelvis (*fig 3B*). If it is necessary to correct a malunion of a trochanteric fracture, the normal hip should be internally rotated (*fig 3C*). Of course, for the preoperative planning it is necessary to determine the contours of the normal hip on the opposite side.

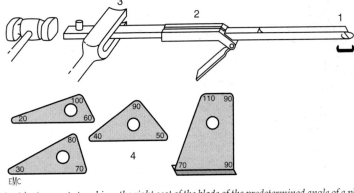

5   *The important instruments to achieve the right seat of the blade of the predetermined angle of a plate. The seating chisel with U-profile (1), the chisel guide (2) and the slotted hammer (3), the three triangular positioning plates and the quadrangular positioning plate (4). Other instruments needed: inserter-extractor, impactor, Kirschner wires.*

PLATES FOR IMPACTION OF THE OSTEOTOMISED BONE SURFACES

Impaction is possible with the standard right-angle blade plate (*fig 4A*) and the 120° double-angled blade plate with a U-profiled blade (*fig 4C*) developed in 1960 by M.E. Müller specifically for intertrochanteric osteotomies. These allow the surgeon to deeply impact both osteotomised surfaces. The removable tension device allows a compression of more than 50 kg for the 90° standard plate (*fig 4B*) or for the 120° plate by using a special technique (*fig 4D*). With such a plate, the patient can move his leg actively the day after surgery and get up a few days later. The standard plate is available with 3 different offsets of 10, 15 or 20 mm.

SPECIAL INSTRUMENTS (*fig 5*)

Preoperative graphic planning is necessary before each intertrochanteric osteotomy. Without such planning, the use of the most important instruments – the seating chisel together with its aiming device, the triangular and quadrangular plates and the Kirschner wires – is quite impossible. An image intensifier is no substitute for a three-dimensional concept. The AO angled blade plates for osteotomy in the proximal femur have a U-profile and a fixed angle. Before the blade of the plate can be inserted into the femoral neck, a window has to be made with a large drill or a chisel, and a channel has to be prepared with the seating chisel having a U-profile. The fixed angle between blade and plate may cause initial difficulties; these will soon be overcome by the preoperative planning and the aiming devices. The slotted hammer controls the rotation of the seating chisel.

Surgical procedures [4, 5, 6, 8]

THE 6 STANDARD TYPES OF OSTEOTOMY (*fig 6*)

The six standard types of intertrochanteric osteotomy require wedge excision, displacement (offset) and fixation.

– Standard varus osteotomy of 20°; right angled hip plate, offset of 15 mm, medial wedge of 20° (*fig 6A*).

– Varus osteotomy of 30° with translation of the lesser trochanter; right-angled hip plate with offset of 20 mm (*fig 6B*).

– Simple valgus osteotomy of 20° with a proximal wedge; right-angled hip plate with offset of 10 mm (*fig 6C*).

– Valgus osteotomy of 30° with physiological knee joint; 120° double-angled hip plate and bone graft to lateralise the femoral shaft (*fig 6D*).

– Repositioning valgus osteotomy: for nonunion of the femoral neck, the nonunion line has to be placed at nearly a right angle to the resulting compressive forces acting on the femoral neck. This requires resection of two bone wedges laterally. Therefore, often the wedge should have an angle of 50° (*fig 6E*).

– Shortening osteotomy: resection of a quadrilateral wedge for shortening of 2 to 2.5 cm (*fig 6F*).

Most of the angle corrections in the frontal plane are combined with a lateral or medial

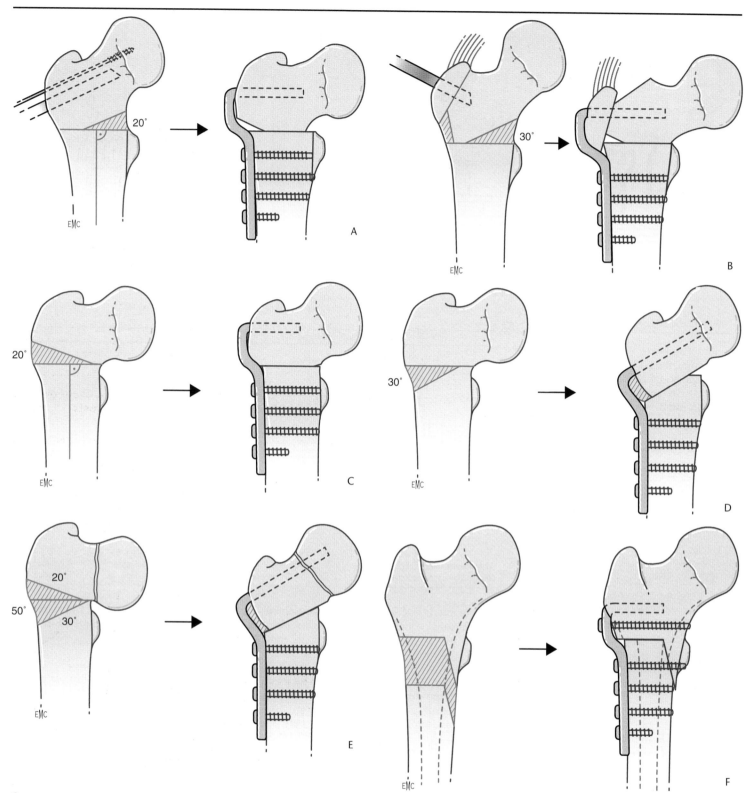

6   *The 6 essential types of intertrochanteric osteotomy: wedge excision, displacement (offset) and fixation.*

A. Standard varus osteotomy of 20°; right angled hip plate, offset of 15 mm, medial wedge of 20° (similar preoperative planning see Fig. 9, technique see Fig. 10).

B. Varus osteotomy of 30° with translation of the greater trochanter: right-angled hip plate with offset of 20 mm (technique see Fig. 11).

C. Simple valgus osteotomy of 20° with proximal wedge: right-angled hip plate with offset of 10 mm.

D. Valgus osteotomy of 30° with physiological knee joint: 120° double-angled hip plate and bone graft to lateralise the femoral shaft (technique of compression see Fig. 4D).

E. For nonunion of the femoral neck, the nonunion line has to be placed nearly at a right angle to the resulting compressive forces acting on the femoral neck. Resection of two bone wedges laterally. Therefore, often the wedge should have an angle of 50° (technique see Figs. 12 and 13).

F. Resection of a quadrilateral wedge for shortening of 2 to 2.5 cm (technique see Fig. 14).

displacement, the so-called offset. In 60% of the examples, the standard angled plate is used, and in praxis, more than 90% of these osteotomies are fixed with the standard blade plate. The first step in an intertrochanteric osteotomy is the transverse osteotomy of the

femur just above the lesser trochanter in order to correct the rotational deformity.

Each excised bone wedge will be reintroduced or pushed between the bone fragments at the end of the procedure.

CORRECTION OF A ROTATION AND A FLEXION DEFORMITY

These corrections must be incorporated in the planning of the procedure. The amount of rotation to be corrected is marked by 2 Kirschner wires before the osteotomy *(fig 7)*.

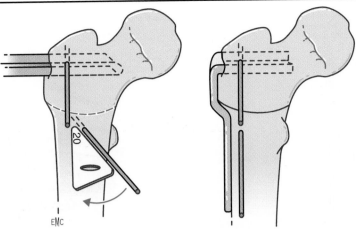

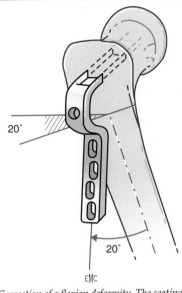

7   *Correction of a rotational deformity. Before the intertrochanteric osteotomy, two Kirschner wires are placed perpendicular to the shaft above and below the foreseen osteotomy line. After the osteotomy and the derotation, the two Kirschner wires must be parallel to one another.*

8   *Correction of a flexion deformity. The seating chisel must be introduced into the femoral neck at an angle of 20° extension. A flexion contraction is corrected by removing a wedge with a dorsal base. At the end of the procedure, the wedge is inserted ventrally into the osteotomy.*

A flexion deformity has to be corrected with a slight rotation of the seating chisel when making the track for the blade of the plate (fig 8).

PREOPERATIVE GRAPHIC PLANNING (fig 9)

A sketch of the desired final result using two transparent tracing papers is mandatory for intertrochanteric osteotomies. The sketch must be drawn the day before surgery and often takes more time than the surgery itself. After the operation, the sketch must match the final result. Figure 9 describes the details of the different steps in planning a varus intertrochanteric osteotomy of 30°. This same type of graphic planning can be used for all types of varus osteotomy.

■ **Step-by-step graphic planning for a simple varus (adduction) osteotomy of 30°**

1) Diagram of the a-p X-ray of a dysplastic hip.

2) Trace the contours of the proximal femur on a transparent tracing paper (A). Mark the axis of the femoral shaft (FA) with a dotted line and trace a line that is perpendicular to FA and crosses the femoral shaft just at the upper level of the lesser trochanter. This is the intertrochanteric osteotomy line (IO).

3) Trace the contours of the acetabulum on a second transparent sheet (B) and draw in the femoral shaft axis (FA) as a dotted line.

4) Superimpose drawing B on drawing A, and turn drawing A to determine the ideal position of the head in the acetabulum (30° of adduction). Once the best joint congruity has been found, trace the proximal femur and the osteotomy line (IO) from sheet A onto sheet B. Also draw the femoral shaft axis (FA) from sheet A onto sheet B. Sheet B now has the outline of the acetabulum and the proximal femur in the correct position. The angle subtended by the original femoral axis and the femoral axis in the corrected position corresponds to the desired angle of adduction of 30°.

5) Keep sheet B over sheet A and move sheet A until the femoral axes (FA) on both drawings overlie one another. Move sheet B up or down until the distal tip of the proximal fragment overlaps the osteotomy line (IO) on the distal fragments of sheet A by 5 to 8 mm (d). This represents the impaction of the proximal fragment into the cancellous surface of the distal fragment. In this example, the knee joint is normal. (If the femoral axes (FA) are superimposed, then the knee joint alignment will remain unchanged. To compensate for a valgus knee, the femoral shaft has to be lateralised, and to compensate for a varus knee, it must

be medialised.) In this case, the shortening resulting from the osteotomy measures 16 mm.

6) Sheet B now has an outline of the acetabulum and the osteotomy fragments are in their correct relationship to one another. Place the blade plate template under sheet B and bring the plate into the

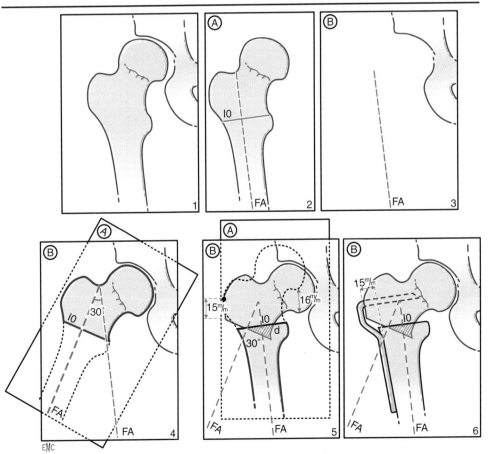

9   *Preoperative graphic planning of a simple varus (adduction) osteotomy of 30° (described in detail in the text).*

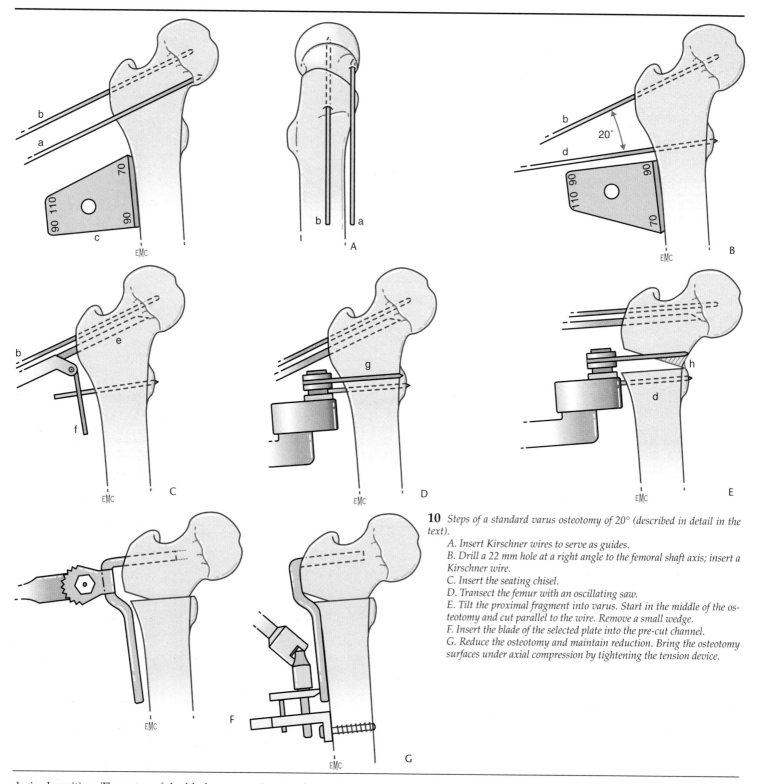

10 *Steps of a standard varus osteotomy of 20° (described in detail in the text).*
A. Insert Kirschner wires to serve as guides.
B. Drill a 22 mm hole at a right angle to the femoral shaft axis; insert a Kirschner wire.
C. Insert the seating chisel.
D. Transect the femur with an oscillating saw.
E. Tilt the proximal fragment into varus. Start in the middle of the osteotomy and cut parallel to the wire. Remove a small wedge.
F. Insert the blade of the selected plate into the pre-cut channel.
G. Reduce the osteotomy and maintain reduction. Bring the osteotomy surfaces under axial compression by tightening the tension device.

desired position. The entry of the blade must be at least 12-15 mm above the osteotomy line. The medial displacement of the distal fragment can be measured, and the right angled blade plate with a displacement of 10, 15 or 20 mm is chosen accordingly (here 15 mm). The plate is traced onto the drawing. We now know the offset (15 mm) and the length of the blade (50-60 mm).

STANDARD STEPS OF A VARUS INTERTROCHANTERIC OSTEOTOMY OF 20° (fig 10)

This type of procedure, described below, has given satisfaction in more than a hundred intertrochanteric osteotomies performed in our department.

– Incision: start at the tip of the greater trochanter and make a straight lateral incision of 20 cm. Open the fascia in line with the skin incision. Reflect the vastus lateralis forwards and medially. Insert one bone retractor medially around the calcar and one laterally above the neck just medial to the tip of the greater trochanter. Open the joint capsule in line with the neck axis and examine the joint. Put a Kirschner wire (a) on and along the neck and insert the tip into the border of the femoral head. This Kirschner wire serves as the guide to the direction of the neck axis. The second Kirschner wire (b) is inserted into the greater trochanter parallel to Kirschner wire a and parallel to the upper edge of the 70° quadrangular plate (c). The Kirschner wire b is the guide wire for the insertion of the seating chisel with its aiming devise. Kirschner wire a can now be removed (fig 10A).

– Drill a 2 mm hole at a right angle to the femoral shaft axis 0.5 cm distal to the site of the planned osteotomy, approximately in the middle of the lesser trochanter. Insert a

Kirschner wire of 2 mm ø into this hole *(fig 10B)*.

– About 2 cm above the site of the planned osteotomy, open the cortex of the femur with an osteotome in preparation for insertion of the seating chisel (e). The seating chisel is then inserted parallel in both planes, frontal and sagittal, to the second Kirschner wire (b). The seating chisel is aimed at the centre of the femoral neck and is inserted to a depth of 4.5 cm. The angle which the flap of the seating chisel (f) subtends either above or below with the shaft will represent the amount of flexion or extension through the osteotomy (here 0) *(fig 10C)*.

– Protect the soft tissues posterior to the osteotomy with a broad bone retractor. With an oscillating saw (g), transect the femur at a right angle to its long axis *(fig 10D)*.

– Using the seating chisel as a handle, tilt the proximal fragment into varus. Start in the middle of the osteotomy and cut parallel to the Kirschner wire (d). Remove a small wedge (h) *(fig 10E)*.

– Remove the seating chisel and insert the blade of the selected right-angled osteotomy plate carefully into the pre-cut channel *(fig 10F)*.

– Reduce the osteotomy and maintain reduction by clamping the plate to the shaft. Check the rotational alignment of the leg in extension and in flexion. Fix the tension device to the femur and bring the surfaces of the osteotomy under axial compression by tightening the tension device *(fig 10G)*.

VARUS INTERTROCHANTERIC OSTEOTOMY OF 30° OR MORE WITH DISTAL TRANSFER OF GREATER TROCHANTER AND SHORTENING OF FEMORAL NECK

A varus osteotomy of 30° or more usually involves a distal transfer of the greater trochanter and shortening of the femoral neck *(fig 11)*.

– Before the greater trochanter is osteotomised, cut a hole in the middle of the trochanter by means of a chisel and then drive the seating chisel 15 mm deep through this hole in the greater trochanter into the femoral neck. Remove the seating chisel and osteotomise the greater trochanter. Insert a Kirschner wire (d) at a right angle to the shaft *(fig 11A)*.

– Introduce the seating chisel into the femoral neck in the usual fashion. Perform the intertrochanteric osteotomy parallel to the Kirschner wire and excise the medial wedge of 30° from the proximal fragment. Remove the seating chisel and shorten the femoral neck 5 to 10 mm. Tilt the neck/head fragment into varus *(fig 11B)*.

– Pass the blade of the right angled blade plate through the previously U-shaped cut in the greater trochanter and then insert the blade into the previously cut channel in the femoral neck *(fig 11C)*.

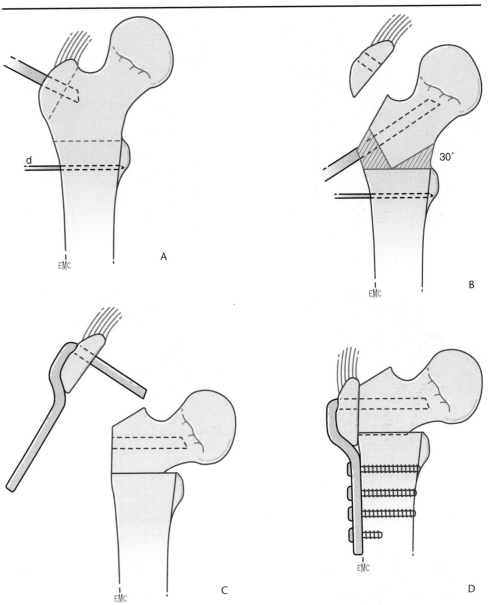

11 *Technique of distal transfer of the greater trochanter and of shortening of the femoral neck at the time of a varus osteotomy of 30° (described in the text).*
A. Osteotomy of the greater trochanter.
B. Intertrochanteric osteotomy and excision of medial wedge from the proximal fragment. Shortening the femoral neck.
C. Insertion of the blade into the pre-cut channel in the femoral neck.
D. Compression of the osteotomy and fixation of the plate.

– Compress the osteotomy with the tension device and fix the plate to the femur *(fig 11D)*.

VALGUS INTERTROCHANTERIC OSTEOTOMY (REPOSITIONING OSTEOTOMY) *(fig 12, 13)*

The aetiology is usually a malunion after a pertrochanteric fracture or nonunion of a neck fracture. These can be fixed with the standard compression blade plate only if the angle of the resected wedge is 20° or less. If a wedge of 50° has to be excised, we resect two wedges: one of 30° from the distal fragment and one of 20° from the proximal fragment. For a nonunion, we must be sure that the femoral head is still alive. Figures 12 and 13 show the principles and the tactical steps of a repositioning osteotomy.

■ *Principles of a repositioning osteotomy* *(fig 12)*

Note that the tip of the blade is inserted into the inferior segment of the head. After the transverse osteotomy, a 20° wedge is cut from the proximal fragment. The external rotation is corrected. A 30° wedge is then cut from the distal fragment adjacent to the intertrochanteric osteotomy (IO) line. Note that the angle between the seating chisel and the shaft is 110° and the angle between the plate and shaft is 50° *(fig 12A)*.

In lateralising the shaft, one must remember that the minimal permissible contact area between the osteotomy surfaces is one-third of the diameter of the shaft. Sometimes a bone graft (a) is inserted between the neck and the plate *(fig 12B)*.

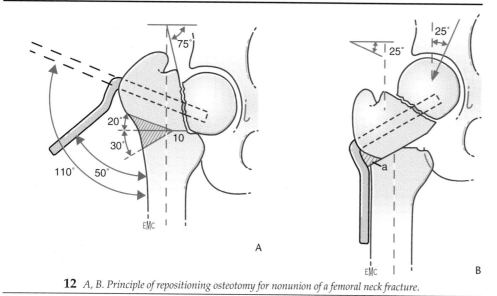

12 *A, B. Principle of repositioning osteotomy for nonunion of a femoral neck fracture.*

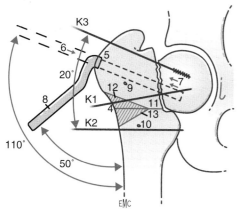

13 *Tactical steps of a repositioning osteotomy of 50° with a 120° angle blade plate (described in detail in the text).*

■ Step-by-step repositioning osteotomy *(fig 13)*

1) A 2-mm Kirschner wire (K1) is placed over the femoral neck.

2) A second 2 mm Kirschner wire (K2) is inserted at right angles to the shaft axis at the level of the lesser trochanter.

3) A 2.5 mm threaded Kirschner wire (K3) is inserted through the tip of the greater trochanter at a 20° angle to K2 in the frontal plane and parallel to K1 in the transverse plane. K1 is removed.

4) Two-thirds of the planned osteotomy are marked with the saw.

5) The portal of entry for the seating chisel is prepared.

6) The seating chisel is inserted parallel to K3. Its guide is tilted 10° dorsally in order to subsequently carry out a 10° extension osteotomy. Note that the seating chisel is inserted into the inferior half of the femoral head.

7) The seating chisel is removed.

8) The chosen blade of the 120° angled plate is inserted.

9/10) Two parallel Kirschner wires are inserted, one on each side of the osteotomy, for rotational control.

11) The transverse osteotomy is completed. Then, any rotational deformity is corrected.

12) Resection of a 20° cranial wedge parallel to the seating chisel in both planes.

13) Resection of the distal wedge of 30°. Once this wedge is resected, the shaft is abducted and the plate is fixed to the shaft with a short screw. The osteotomy is then placed under compression by insertion of the remaining screws, which pull the shaft towards the plate *(fig 4D).*

SHORTENING OPERATION *(fig 14)*

This procedure is used mostly in leg length discrepancies of 1-3 cm following a THR. The big advantage here is that the patient can usually walk after one week with the help of only one stick.

■ *Technique*

The following technique is used for an inter- and subtrochanteric shortening osteotomy of 2.5 cm and fixation with a right-angled blade plate having an offset of 10 mm.

– Expose the intertrochanteric area and insert three Kirschner wires perpendicular to the femoral shaft. The Kirschner wire a is inserted in the tip of the greater trochanter and serves as a guide to the femoral neck axis. The Kirschner wires b and c are inserted more anteriorly at about a 45° angle to the frontal plane. Measure the distance between b and c. Note the quadrangular positional plate (d) which assists the insertion of the most proximal Kirschner wire at 90° to the shaft axis *(fig 14A).*

– Insert the seating chisel at right angles to the shaft. Use the oscillating saw to resect whatever length of bone you wish between 1-3 cm. If possible, preserve the attachment of the lesser trochanter to the proximal fragment and shape the distal fragment into a slight cone *(fig 14B).*

– Remove the seating chisel, insert the right-angled blade plate and a proximal long screw in the hole in the bend of the plate. Reduce the osteotomy and rotate the distal fragment until Kirschner wires b and c are parallel. Measure the distance between Kirschner wires b and c. Fix the plate to the femur with a bone-holding clamp and insert the tension device. As soon as the fragments are impacted and the desired shortening is achieved, fix the plate to the shaft *(fig 14C).*

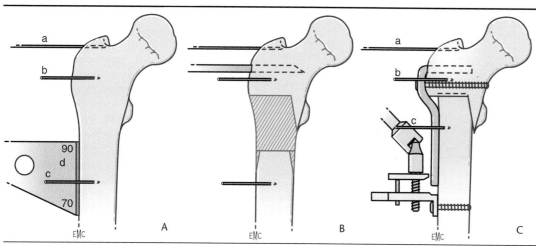

14 *Technique of an inter- and subtrochanteric shortening osteotomy of 2.5 cm and fixation with a right-angled blade plate with an offset of 10 mm.*
A. Insertion of Kirschner wires (a, b, c).
B. Resection of bone.
C. Reduction of osteotomy and fixation of the plate to the shaft.

References

[1] Bombelli R. Osteoarthritis of the hip. Classification and pathogenesis. The role of osteotomy as a consequent therapy. Berlin : Springer-Verlag, 1983

[2] Langlais F, Bombelli R, Maquet P, Jacomy LP. Ostéotomies de l'extrémité supérieure du fémur. *Encycl Méd Chir* (Éditions Scientifiques et Médicales Elsevier SAS, Paris), Techniques chirurgicales - Orthopédie-Traumatologie, 44-654, 1989

[3] McMurray TP. Osteoarthritis of the hip. *J Bone Joint Surg Br* 1940 ; 22 : 716

[4] Müller ME. Intertrochanteric osteotomy in the treatment of the arthritic hip joint. In : Tronzo RG ed. Surgery of the hip joint. Philadelphia : Lea and Febiger, 1973 : 627-643

[5] Müller ME. Intertrochanteric osteotomies in adults: planning and operating technique. In: Cruess RL, Mitchell NS eds. Surgical management of degenerative arthritis of the lower limb. Philadelphia : Lea and Febiger, 1973 : 53-64

[6] Müller ME. Intertrochanteric osteotomy: Indication, preoperative planning, technique. In : Schatzker J ed, The intertrochanteric osteotomy. Berlin : Springer-Verlag, 1984 : 25-66

[7] Müller ME, Allgöwer M, Schneider R, Willenegger H. Manual of internal fixation. Berlin : Springer-Verlag, 1979 : 85-93, 357-371

[8] Müller ME, Krushell R. Intertrochanteric osteotomies. *Surg Musculoskelet Syst* 1990 ; 3 : 2833-2858

[9] Pauwels F. Atlas zur Biomechanik der gesunden und kranken Hüfte. Prinzipien, Technik und Resultate einer kausalen Therapie. Berlin : Springer-Verlag, 1973

[10] Pauwels F. Biomechanics of the normal and diseased hip. Theoretical foundation, technique and results of treatment. Berlin : Springer-Verlag, 1976

[11] Pauwels F. Biomechanical principles of varus/valgus intertrochanteric osteotomy (Pauwels I and II) in the treatment of osteoarthritis of the hip. In : Schatzker J ed, The intertrochanteric osteotomy. Berlin : Springer-Verlag, 1984 : 3-23

[12] Schneider R. Die intertrochantere Osteotomie bei Coxarthrose. Berlin : Springer-Verlag, 1979

[13] Schneider R. Intertrochanteric osteotomy of the hip joint. In : Schatzker J ed, The intertrochanteric osteotomy. Berlin : Springer-Verlag, 1984 : 135-168

Osteonecrosis of the femoral head

P Gallinaro
A Massè

Abstract. – Since the natural history of untreated non-traumatic avascular necrosis (AN) of the femoral head results in a very poor outcome, several surgical procedures have been proposed to treat this disease:
– Procedures aimed at reducing intramedullary pressure: the core decompression, proposed by Ficat, is widely used as it gives excellent results in Stage I and some Stage II patients, while it is unacceptable for later stages.
– Procedures aimed at moving the necrotic area out of the weight-bearing zone: the anterior wedge flexion osteotomy proposed by Schneider is best indicated for young, well-motivated patients with a diagnosis of Stage II or III "idiopathic" avascular necrosis.
– Procedures aimed at restoring the bone supply inthe necrotic area: vascularised fibular grafting is a technically-demanding procedure, indicated in symptomatic AN developed to Ficat Stage II or III in relatively young and well-motivated patients.
The majority of the surgical procedures described in this chapter are more technically-demanding than a hip replacement, result in a lengthy period of disability and do not provide totally predictable results. Nonetheless, conservative surgery still has an important place in carefully-selected patients and in the early stages of this crippling disease.

© 2000, Editions Scientifiques et Médicales Elsevier SAS. All rights reserved.

Keywords: hip, avascular necrosis, core decompression, osteotomy, vascularised bone graft.

Introduction

Untreated non-traumatic avascular necrosis (AN) of the femoral head results in a very poor outcome, due to the high percentage of collapse of the head, ranging from 70% to 100% of cases, depending on the stage of the disease [7, 20, 22, 29, 33].

Ficat and Arlet described a classification system based on standard radiographs, consisting of four stages (I to IV) to be applied to symptomatic patients [8, 9]; to this staging system, Hungerford added a stage "0", pre-clinical and pre-radiographical. The classification of Ficat was later modified by several authors, based on magnetic resonance imaging. In 1992, the Association Internationale de Recherche sur la Circulation Osseuse (ARCO) proposed a classification based on the staging system of Ficat and Arlet and including both the quantification and the location of the involvement (*table I*). Mont and Hungerford, in a recent overview of non-traumatic

Table I. – *The Ficat-Arlet staging system modified according to the Association Internationale de Recherche sur la Circulation Osseuse.*

Stage	Characteristics
0	Bone-biopsy results consistent with avascular necrosis; normal findings on all other tests
I	Positive scintiscan or magnetic resonance image, or both; lesions subdivided into medial, central, or lateral depending on location of involvement of femoral head
I-A	< 15 % involvement of femoral head*
I-B	15-30 % involvement of femoral head*
I-C	> 30 % involvement of femoral head*
II	Radiographic abnormalities (mottled appearance of femoral head, osteosclerosis, cyst formation, and osteopenia); no signs of collapse of femoral head on radiographs or computerised tomography scan; positive scintiscan and magnetic resonance image; no changes in acetabulum; lesions subdivided into medial, central or lateral
II-A	< 15 % involvement of femoral head*
II-B	15-30 % involvement of femoral head*
II-C	> 30 % involvement of femoral head*
III	Crescent sign; lesions subdivided into medial, central, or lateral depending on location of involvement of femoral head
III-A	< 15 % crescent sign or < 2 mm depression of femoral head**
III-B	15-30 % crescent sign or 2 to 4 mm depression of femoral head**
III-C	> 30 % crescent sign or 4 mm depression of femoral head**
IV	Articular surface flattened radiographically and joint space shows narrowing; changes in acetabulum with evidence of osteosclerosis, cyst formation and marginal osteophytes

* as determined on magnetic resonance imaging
** as determined on anteroposterior and lateral radiographs.
(rewritten from Mont, 1995 [20])

Paolo Gallinaro, M.D., Professor.
Alessandro Massè, M.D.
Centro Traumatologico Ortopedico, Via Zuretti 29, I-10126 Torino, Italy.

All references to this article must include: Gallinaro P and Massè A. Osteonecrosis of the femoral head. Editions Scientifiques et Médicales Elsevier SAS (Paris). All rights reserved. Surgical Techniques in Orthopaedics and Traumatology, 55-470-B-10, 2000, 6 p.

avascular necrosis of the femoral head, suggested that this staging system be adopted as the international standard classification of this disease [20].

In an effort to improve the prognosis of avascular necrosis, several surgical procedures have been proposed, aimed at preventing the collapse of the subchondral bone and at slowing the progress of degenerative changes.

These procedures can be grouped, depending on the desired goal, as follows:

– procedures aimed at reducing intramedullary pressure;

– procedures aimed at moving the necrotic area out of the weight-bearing zone;

– procedures aimed at restoring the bone supply in the necrotic area.

Procedures aimed at reducing intramedullary pressure

Arlet and Ficat first recognised the therapeutic effect of core decompression on AN of the femoral head and described its rationale. Observing the raised intramedullary pressures and retarded venous sinusoidal drainage in the proximal femur, they developed the hypothesis that vascular stasis and prolonged ischaemia were factors involved in the pathogenesis of AN [1, 8, 9]. According to Ficat, "the effect of a core biopsy is similar to that of a decompression operation for a nerve tunnel syndrome or a fascial release for a muscle compartment syndrome".

SURGICAL TECHNIQUE

With the patient supine on the fracture table, the hip is placed in a neutral position. A 5° to 10° internal rotation is helpful, as it places the femoral neck parallel to the floor. A 8 to 10 cm skin incision is made, starting proximal to the vastus lateralis tubercle of the greater trochanter, and extending distally along the posterior edge of the vastus lateralis itself.

The fascia lata is therefore split in correspondence to the skin incision. The vastus lateralis is stripped anteriorly with a periosteal elevator in order to expose the lateral aspect of the greater trochanter. A cortical window is made just below the trochanteric ridge, wide enough to allow the introduction of the trephine (fig 1).

A hollow trephine, 8 or 6 mm in diameter, is then introduced into the neck of the femur through this window. The coring device is directed into the anterosuperior portion of the femoral head until the tip arrives within 5 mm of the subchondral plate (fig 2); its manipulation is controlled, both in the anteroposterior and lateral planes, with an

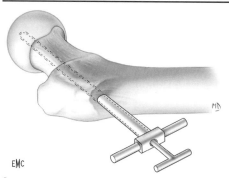

1 *A cortical window is made just below the trochanteric ridge, wide enough to allow for the introduction of the trephine.*

2 *A hollow trephine, 8 or 6 mm in diameter, is introduced into the neck of the femur through this window: the coring device is directed into the anterosuperior portion of the femoral head.*

image intensifier. A second channel is made with a smaller trephine in a different direction. As hyperpressure exists in the bone marrow around the necrotic area, some authors recommend to drill up to, but not through, the border of the necrosis.

The core specimens thus obtained are then sent for histological examination. The forage channels are left open.

AFTERCARE

Aftercare is strongly dependent on the patient's age, weight and collaboration.

Usually, partial weight-bearing is not indicated before 40 days. Full weight-bearing is permitted at three months.

DISCUSSION

The efficacy of core decompression is controversial, and the orthopaedic literature has not clearly defined the role for this procedure, considered as the only treatment [14, 17].

Ficat reports good clinical results in 94% of Stage I and 82% of Stage II of his classification. Fairbank recently reported the long-term results of core decompression, with a 15 year survival rate of 90% in Stage I, 66% in Stage II, 23% in Stage III [7].

These results are similar to those reported by other authors: Smith, in an average 3 year follow-up, reports the failure of the core

decompression (defined as performance of a subsequent operation) in 16% of Stage I, 80% of Stage II, and 10% of Stage III hips [28].

It seems reasonable to conclude that the rate of success of the core decompression is largely dependent on:

– the accuracy of the diagnosis: excluding transient osteoporosis, reflex sympathetic dystrophy;

– the correct timing: core decompression gives excellent results in Stage I and some Stage II patients, while it is unacceptable for later stages [10];

– the correct surgical procedure: neck fracture has been described as a frequent complication of core decompression [13]; a simple means to eliminate this complication is to avoid an approach which is too distal.

Procedures aimed at moving the necrotic area out of the weight-bearing zone

Many different osteotomy techniques have been proposed to move the necrotic area, which is usually located in the anterosuperior part of the femoral head, out of the weight-bearing zone. The type of osteotomy to be performed is controversial, as osteotomies have been proposed on every plane, each with its own rationale.

Merle d'Aubigné first introduced varus osteotomy to load the intact far lateral part of the femoral head [19]; Saito gave as an indication for varus osteotomy the presence of more than one-third of the head intact, laterally [24].

A valgus-extension osteotomy has been proposed by Pauwels and Bombelli, in order to move the necrotic area laterally and posteriorly, and to enlarge the weight-bearing surface by loading the so-called capital drop osteophyte [2, 18, 23]. In opposition to this technique, it has been remarked that this osteophyte is poorly developed in Stage III, contrary to Stage IV necrosis, in the presence of osteoarthritic modifications that make this indication debatable for a salvage procedure [6, 25].

As the anterosuperior part of the femoral head is usually involved in the necrosis, an osteotomy aimed at moving the necrotic area anteriorly seems to be the most logical solution. This may be achieved either by rotating the head and neck anteriorly, as proposed by Sugioka, or by performing an anterior wedge flexion osteotomy, as proposed by Schneider [10, 11, 30].

Sugioka, by using the Japanese roengtenographic staging system of idiopathic femoral head necrosis (comparable to the Ficat classification) reported a 73% success rate of his procedure in Stage III and a 70% rate in Stage IV, after a follow-up from 3 to 16 years [31]. However, the rotational osteotomy did not give the same good results outside Japan: Tooke had a 41% rate of revision to hip replacement at 39 months [32]. Dean, reporting a 83% rate of early failure, concluded that the "Sugioka anterior rotational osteotomy...should not be performed in Caucasian patients. It does give satisfactory early pain relief, perhaps through joint denervation produced by the capsulotomy, but the procedure appears to compromise further the blood supply of the femoral head..." [5]; he gives as an explanation for these results the fact that the anterior rotation of the femoral head stretches the quadratus femoris, therefore flattening and obstructing the posterior branch of the medial circumflex artery. This author hypothesises that the posterior capsule of the hip may be more lax in Japanese patients, allowing for anterior rotation of the neck without compromising the flow through this artery.

Schneider, in 1969, at the Congress of the Orthopaedic Swiss Society, proposed a flexion intertrochanteric osteotomy aimed at rotating the intact posterior portion of the femoral head into the weight-bearing portion of the acetabulum; this osteotomy became popular in Europe due to its efficacy when carefully planned and performed on well-selected patients [26].

TECHNIQUE OF THE FLEXION OSTEOTOMY

■ *Planning the osteotomy*

Pre-operative planning of the osteotomy is based on evaluation of the following parameters:

Radiological: an A.P. view to evaluate the angle of the neck (valgus or varus), the morphology of the trochanteric area, the condition of the opposite hip and the likelihood of its future deterioration. These criteria enable the surgeon to select the right point to introduce the osteotome, the level of the osteotomy, and the amount of displacement. Two craniocaudal views at 15° and 30° to assess the amount of flexion necessary. An axial view to evaluate the extent of the healthy posterior sector of the head and any anteversion of the neck. MRI, even if absolutely mandatory in the diagnosis of the osteonecrosis, gives no

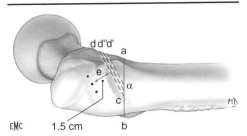

3 α= flexion angle; a-b= first osteotomy; c-d= second osteotomy; e= distance between the second osteotomy and the entry point of the blade.

supplementary information useful for the osteotomy planning. A CT scan allows a precise evaluation of the location and the extent of the lesion.

Amount of flexion: it is necessary to put the necrotic area out of load when the hip is flexed about 20°, as occurs during walking. Therefore, it is necessary to add a further 20° to the flexion which makes the necrotic area disappear in the craniocaudal x-ray. The necessary angle of flexion (α) is calculated. In recent years, we have tended to increase the limit, because it is not always possible to achieve the exact pre-operative calculation of correction. However, we suggest that the limit should be 50° of flexion.

Fixation device: the osteotomy site is stabilised with an AO right-angle or 95° blade-plate; usually, the blade does not exceed 50 mm in length.

■ *Surgical procedure* [10, 11, 26]

With the patient supine on the fracture table, the leg is draped to allow free movement during the operation.

The anterolateral approach is used as a rule: the anterior portion of the medius gluteus and the tendon of the minimus gluteus are cut, and longitudinal capsulotomy is performed to allow inspection of the femoral head, eliminating the need for intraoperative radiography. Some surgeons do not perform the arthrotomy, in which case each step of the operation requires fluoroscopic control. Guide wires are inserted to achieve the planned flexion. The first osteotomy "a-b" is performed at a right angle to the diaphysis and just proximal to the lesser trochanter, and is not completed (*fig 3*). The second osteotomy is performed on the "c-d" plane according to the α angle calculated preoperatively. In order to achieve a complete congruence of the osteotomy surfaces, "a-b" should be equal to "c-d". This can be achieved either directly or by subsequent trial osteotomy (d', d").

The seating chisel for the blade-plate has to be inserted parallel to the plane of the second osteotomy "c-d", inferiorly in the femoral head and posteriorly in the neck. Its entry point is 1.5 to 2 cm proximal to the "c-d", and should correspond to the middle portion of the "c-d" length (*fig 4*).

The blade is inserted almost completely, the first osteotomy is completed and the bone

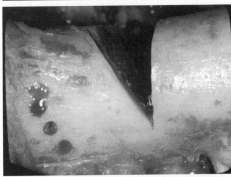

4 *The operative field: the seating chisel for the blade-plate has to be inserted parallel to the plane of the second osteotomy "c-d"; its entry point has to be 1.5 to 2 cm proximal to the "c-d", and should correspond to the middle portion of the "c-d" length.*

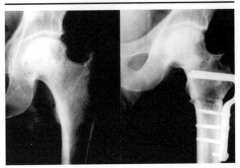

5 *Pre-operative and post-operative X-rays of a flexion osteotomy performed on a 43 year old male; the osteotomy site is stabilised with an AO right-angle or 95° blade-plate. The blade usually does not exceed 50 mm in length.*

wedge removed to allow contact between the osteotomy planes. Before removing the wedge, the osteotomy surfaces are marked to avoid rotational errors. The plate is positioned on the femoral shaft, the osteotomy site is compressed and the plate secured with a single screw. Rotation is checked, and, if satisfactory, the plate is fully secured: if not, the holding screw is released and the necessary rotational adjustment made before securing the plate (*fig 5*).

If the α angle, i.e. the flexion to be reached, exceeds 30°, psoas release is mandatory to avoid flexion deformity.

Some authors have combined the osteotomy with curettage of the necrotic bone and packing of the remaining cavity with autogenous bone graft from the iliac crest [25].

■ *Errors and pitfalls* [11]

– placing the blade too anteriorly, thus jeopardising the congruence of the osteotomised surfaces;

– inserting the blade too distally: the amount of bone between the blade and the osteotomy is reduced and consequently the stability of the fixation is threatened;

– placing the blade correctly from the point of view of the osteotomy, but not in the axis of the femoral neck. The main risk is that the blade may penetrate the posterior cortex, particularly in anteverted hips, with possible damage to the blood supply of the head.

– omitting to tenotomise the ileo psoas tendon and Bertin's ligament when high degree flexion osteotomies are performed; the risk in such circumstances is a fixed flexion deformity.

AFTERCARE

A regime of passive mobilisation of the hip is begun in the first few days: active abduction and flexion are usually contraindicated before 40 days. If there is a tendency to hip flexion, patients are told to lie prone for a short period every day during the first few months; weight-bearing is not allowed before 3 to 6 months.

DISCUSSION

The results of the series reported in the literature are difficult to compare, due to the differences in the indications for this operation. Most authors agree that intertrochanteric osteotomy for the treatment of AN of the hip does not give totally predictable results, and that patient characteristics, pathogenesis of the AN, stage and extent of the lesion, as well as pre-operative range of motion, all play an important role in the final outcome [10, 12, 18, 25].

Patient characteristics: young patients are the best candidates for intertrochanteric osteotomy. The upper age limit is generally around 45 years; however, in our experience, good results can be achieved even in patients up to 60 years. Furthermore, the operation must be avoided if there is poor patient compliance or if he/she is not highly motivated to accept a lengthy period of disability.

Pathogenesis: "idiopathic" AN represents the best indication, while intertrochanteric osteotomy should be avoided in cases of underlying metabolic disease or in the presence of a systemic condition that has been treated with chemotherapy or corticosteroids.

Stage and extent of the lesion: the Ficat Stage III lesions or late Stage II can be successfully treated with intertrochanteric osteotomy, while Stage IV is a contraindication. As to the extent of the necrotic area, the best results can be obtained in those patients who have a necrosis angle of less than 200°, calculated according to Kerboull as the sum of the arc of the surface involved measured in A-P and lateral radiographs [4, 12, 16]; we give a more limited indication, avoiding osteotomy if the lesion has reached the surface in the craniocaudal views at 30°, or if the lesion exceeds the fovea shape in the A-P view.

Range of motion: all authors agree that the passive range of motion has to be normal or slightly reduced: flexion should be to at least 110°, and adduction to 20° [12].

Recently, Scher reported 87% satisfactory outcomes at 10 years after intertrochanteric flexion osteotomy [25]. This result is in agreement with our findings and has led us to justify this operation with these very limited indications, as well as on the basis of the absence of serious technical problems in case of a subsequent total hip prosthesis.

Procedures aimed at restoring bone supply in the necrotic area

Judet [15] first introduced the muscle-bone pedicle graft of the greater trochanter on fractures of the femoral neck. Meyers and Palazzi used a similar procedure in treating Ficat's Stages I-II AN, reporting good results. Implantation of a vascular pedicle into the femoral head was attempted by Hori, who reported new bone formation around the vascular pedicle [38]. None of these procedures could provide a mechanical support to the subcondral bone. Rrecently, an increasing number of papers report good results with the use of free vascularised fibular grafting in treating AN of the femoral head: vascularised fibular grafting introduces not only a source of mesenchymal stem cells and a vascular supply, but also a structural bone graft able to provide articular support [27, 35, 37].

TECHNIQUE OF VASCULARISED FIBULAR GRAFTING

■ *Pre-operative planning*

Besides the standard pre-operative imaging, some authors suggest the need for arteriography to confirm that the patient's vascular pattern, distal to the trifurcation of the femoral artery, is intact.

■ *Surgical procedure* [3, 34, 35]

The operation can be performed either with the patient supine or in lateral decubitus on the fracture table. The hip and the lower limb are prepared and draped as a single sterile field; a tourniquet is placed on the thigh. Usually, the femur and the fibula are approached simultaneously by two separate teams to lower operative times.

Operative procedure on the femur

The femur is approached through an anterolateral incision: the lateral aspect of the proximal part of the femur is exposed through the interval between the tensor fasciae latae and the gluteus medius (*fig 6*). The vastus lateralis is then reflected from the vastus ridge for approximately 5 cm to expose the bone (*fig 7*).

Anteriorly, the origin of the vastus intermedialis is carefully released to create a gap that provides a shorter route for the ascending vessels. To avoid damaging the vessels and the femoral nerve, the dissection must not exceed the fat layer medial to the

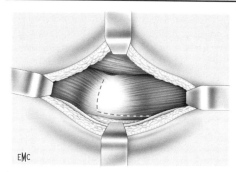

6   *The femur is approached through an anterolateral incision: the lateral aspect of the proximal part of the femur is exposed through the interval between the tensor fasciae latae and the gluteus medius.*

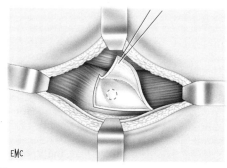

7   *The vastus lateralis is then reflected from the vastus ridge for approximately 5 cm to expose the bone.*

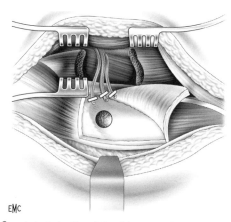

8   *Anteriorly, the origin of the vastus intermedialis is carefully released to create a gap that provides a shorter route for the ascending vessels. The ascending branch of the lateral circumflex artery is identified and carefully mobilised with two veins for a length of about 4 cm: haemostatic clips are placed on the end of each of the three vessels.*

vastus intermedialis. The donor vessel is usually the ascending branch of the lateral circumflex artery, which can be identified as it runs laterally between the vastus intermedialis and the rectus femoris. The artery and two veins are carefully mobilised for a length of about 4 cm; haemostatic clips are placed on the end of each of the three vessels (*fig 8*).

Under fluoroscopic control, a guide wire is inserted into the femoral neck and directed into the centre of the necrotic area. Cannulated reamers are progressively used over the guide pin; the maximum size of the reamer depends on the largest diameter of the fibular graft, being usually 16 mm in females and 19 mm in males. The reaming extends to within 3-5 mm from the articular surface of the femoral head. Cancellous bone graft is then harvested from the greater trochanter and packed into the cavity.

Operative procedure on the fibula

The tourniquet is inflated to an appropriate pressure.

The fibula is approached through a lateral incision. The muscles are reflected off the fibula. The deep fascial layer is incised anteriorly and posteriorly. Anteriorly, the interosseous membrane is incised along its length. The pedicle lies posteriorly, directly under the flexor hallucis longus.

The distal cut is performed at least 10 cm from the tip of the lateral malleolus, while the second cut is usually 15 cm proximal to the first. In the distal wound, the pedicle is dissected free from the muscle for a length of 5 cm: two haemostatic clips are placed across the pedicle. After the pedicle has been transected, the fibular graft is freed from the leg.

Forty mL of heparinised lactate Ringer's solution are injected into the artery and both veins. A 3-0 absorbable suture is passed circumferentially around the distal part of the periosteum and vascular pedicle, to avoid stripping of the periosteum and the pedicle at the insertion of the graft into the core.

Placement of the graft

The fibular graft is inserted into the femoral head beneath the subchondral bone, within the cancellous bone graft: the pedicle is located superiorly and anteriorly. The fibular graft is then secured to the femur with a Kirschner wire (*fig 9*). With the help of an operating microscope, the arterial and venous anastomoses are performed with 8-0 or 9-0 interrupted nylon sutures. Both incisions are closed over drains.

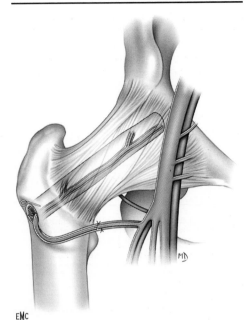

9 *The fibular graft is inserted into the femoral head beneath the subchondral bone, within the cancellous bone graft: the pedicle is located superiorly and anteriorly. The fibular graft is then secured to the femur with a Kirschner wire.*

AFTERCARE

Non-weight-bearing ambulation is begun with a walker or crutches as of the first postoperative days, and continued for 6 weeks, after which partial weight-bearing is started, progressing to full weight-bearing within 6 months after surgery.

DISCUSSION

According to Brunelli and Urbaniak, this technique is indicated in symptomatic AN developed to Ficat Stage II or III in relatively young patients (under 40 years according to Urbaniak, under 55 according to Brunelli) and who are well-motivated. These indications appear to be very close to those given for the rotational osteotomy; however, we did not find any study which compared the outcome of these two techniques.

Recently, Scully published a comparison of the outcome of core decompression and vascularised fibular grafting. By using total hip arthroplasty as the end point, the survival rate was significantly higher at fifty months for vascularised fibular grafting, both for Ficat Stage II (89%) and Stage III (81%) lesions [27]. Even in the presence of such promising results, it has been pointed out that vascularised fibular grafting requires a great deal of technical expertise, implies a prolonged period of restricted weight-bearing and is affected by considerable morbidity associated with the graft donor site [20, 36].

Conclusions

The place remaining for conservative surgery of avascular necrosis is becoming more and more reduced, due to progress in the field of total hip replacement and to the increasing demand from patients for an immediate and optimal result. The majority of the surgical procedures described here are more technically-demanding than a hip replacement, result in a lengthy period of disability and do not give totally predictable results. Nonetheless, conservative surgery still has an important place in carefully-selected patients and in the early stages of the disease.

Researchers in many orthopaedic fields have recently focused their attention on the effects of growth and differentiating factors on the bone healing process: cytokines, bone morphogenetic proteins and angiogenic factors have been used successfully in animal experimental models of AN. Their use in human therapy, in combination with conservative surgical techniques, as suggested by Mont, may represent the next, fundamental step in the treatment of this crippling disease [21].

Acknowledgements. – The authors would like to thank Dr. Vincenzo Lancione for his help in the preparation of the illustrations.

References ➤

References

[1] Arlet J. Nontraumatic avascular necrosis of the femoral head. Past, present and future. *Clin Orthop* 1992 ; 277 : 12-20

[2] Bombelli R. Osteoarthritis of the hip. Berlin : Springer-Verlag, 1976

[3] Brunelli G, Brunelli F. Free fibular bone grafts in the treatment of idiopathic necrosis of the femoral head. In : Brunelli G ed. Textbook of microsurgery. Paris : Masson, 1988 : 409-411

[4] Canadell J, Aguilella L, Azcarate R, Valenti JR. The place of intertrochanteric osteotomy in the treatment of idiopathic necrosis of the head of the femur. *Int Orthop* 1986 ; 10 : 41-46

[5] Dean M, Cabanela ME. Transtrochanteric anterior rotational osteotomy for avascular necrosis of the femoral head: long term results. *J Bone Joint Surg Br* 1993 ; 75 : 597-601

[6] D'Souza SR, Sadiq S, Northermore-Ball MD. Proximal femoral osteotomy as the primary operation for young adults who have osteoarthritis of the hip. *J Bone Joint Surg Am* 1998 ; 80 : 1428-1438

[7] Fairbank AC, Bhatia D, Jinnah RH, Hungerford DS. Long-term results of core decompression for ischaemic necrosis of the femoral head. *J Bone Joint Surg Br* 1995 ; 77 : 42-49

[8] Ficat P, Arlet J. Ischémie at nécrose osseuses. Paris : Masson, 1977

[9] Ficat RP. Idiopathic bone necrosis of the femoral head: early diagnosis and treatment. *J Bone Joint Surg Br* 1985 ; 67 : 3-9

[10] Gallinaro P. Chirurgie conservatrice des nécroses de la tête fémorale. In : Cahier d'enseignement de la SOFCOT. Conférences d'enseignement. Paris : Expansion scientifique française, 1992 : 99-110

[11] Gallinaro P, Rossi P, Giacometti R, Massè G. Idiopathic osteonecrosis of the femoral head. Treatment by flexion osteotomy. *Italian J Orthop Trauma* 1982 ; VIII : 131-134

[12] Gottschalk F. Indications and results of intertrochanteric osteotomy in osteonecrosis of the femoral head. *Clin Orthop* 1989 ; 249 : 219-222

[13] Hopson CN, Siverhus SW. Ischemic necrosis of the femoral head. *J Bone Joint Surg Am* 1988 ; 70 : 1048-1051

[14] Iorio R, Healy WL, Abramowiz AJ, Pfeifer BA. Clinical outcome and survivorship analysis of core decompression for early osteonecrosis of the femoral head. *J Arthroplasty* 1998 ; 13 : 34-41

[15] Judet H, Judet J, Gilbert A, Garcia R. Traitement des nécroses idiopathiques de la tête fémorale par greffon Péroniere vascularisé. *Rev Chir Orthop* 1987 ; 73 : 209-210

[16] Kerboull M, Thomine J, Postel M, Merle d'Aubigné R. The conservative surgical treatment of idiopathic aseptic necrosis of the femoral head. *J Bone Joint Surg Br* 1974 ; 56 : 291-295

[17] Koo K, Kim R, Ko G, Song H, Jeong S, Cho S. Preventing collapse in early osteonecrosis of the femoral head. *J Bone Joint Surg Br* 1995 ; 77 : 870-874

[18] Maistrelli G, Fusco U, Avai A, Bombelli R. Osteonecrosis of the hip treated by intertrochanteric osteotomy. A 4 to 15 years follow-up. *J Bone Joint Surg Br* 1988 ; 70 : 761-766

[19] Merle d'Aubigné R, Postel M, Mazabraud A, Massias P, Gueguen J. Idiopathic necrosis of the femoral head in adults. *J Bone Joint Surg Br* 1965 ; 47 : 612-633

[20] Mont MA, Hungerford DS. Non-traumatic avascular necrosis of the femoral head. *J Bone Joint Surg Am* 1995 ; 77 : 459-474

[21] Mont MA, Jones LC, Einhorn TA, Hungerford DS, Reddi AH. Osteonecrosis of the femoral head. Potential treatment with growth and differentiation factors. *Clin Orthop* 1998 ; 355 : 314-335

[22] Ohzono K, Saito M, Takaoka K, Ono K, Saito S, Nishina T, Kadowaki T. Natural history of nontraumatic avascular necrosis of the femoral head. *J Bone Joint Surg Br* 1991 ; 73 : 68-72

[23] Pauwels F. Biomechanics of the normal and diseased hip. Berlin : Springer-Verlag, 1976

[24] Saito S, Ohzono K, Ono K. Joint-preserving operations for idiopathic avascular necrosis of the femoral head. Results of core decompression, grafting and osteotomy. *J Bone Joint Surg Br* 1988 ; 70 : 78-84

[25] Scher MA, Jakim I. Intertrochanteric osteotomy and autogenous bone-grafting for avascular necrosis of the femoral head. *J Bone Joint Surg Am* 1993 ; 75 : 1119-1133

[26] Schneider R. Die intertrochantere osteotomie bei coxarthrose. Berlin : Springer-Verlag, 1979

[27] Scully SP, Aaron RK, Urbaniak JR. Survival analysis of hips treated with core decompression or vascularized fibular grafting because of avascular necrosis. *J Bone Joint Surg Am* 1998 ; 80 : 1270-1275

[28] Smith SW, Fehring TK, Griffin WL, Beaver WB. Core decompression of the osteonecrotic femoral head. *J Bone Joint Surg Am* 1995 ; 77 : 674-680

[29] Stulberg BN, Davis AW, Bauer TW, Livine M, Easley K. Osteonecrosis of the femoral head: a prospective randomized treatment protocol. *Clin Orthop* 1991 ; 268 : 140-151

[30] Sugioka Y. Transtrochanteric rotational osteotomy in the treatment of idiopathic and steroid-induced femoral head necrosis, Perthes' disease, slipped capital femoral epiphysis, and osteoarthritis of the hip: indications and results. *Clin Orthop* 1984 ; 184 : 12-23

[31] Sugioka Y, Hotochebuchi T, Tsutsui H. Transtrochanteric anterior rotational osteotomy for idiopathic and steroid-induced necrosis of the femoral head: indications and long-term results. *Clin Orthop* 1992 ; 277 : 111-120

[32] Tooke SM, Amstuz HC, Hedley AK. Results of transtrochanteric rotational osteotomy for femoral head osteonecrosis. *Clin Orthop* 1987 ; 224 : 150-157

[33] Tooke SM, Nugent PJ, Bassett LW, Nottingham P, Mirra J, Jinnah R. Results of core decompression for femoral head osteonecrosis. *Clin Orthop* 1988 ; 228 : 99-104

[34] Urbaniak JR, Coogan PG, Gunneson EB, Nunley JA. Treatment of osteonecrosis of the femoral head with free vascularized fibular grafting. *J Bone Joint Surg Am* 1995 ; 77 : 681-694

[35] Urbaniak JR, Harvey EJ. Revascularization of the femoral head in osteonecrosis. *J Am Acad Orthop Surg* 1998 ; 6 : 44-54

[36] Vail PT, Urbaniak JR. Donor-site morbidity with use of vascularized autogenous fibular grafts. *J Bone Joint Surg Am* 1996 ; 78 : 204-211

[37] Wood MB, Gilbert A. Femoral head osteonecrosis. In : Microvascular bone reconstruction. London : Martin Dunitz, 1997 : 161-169

[38] Yoo MC, Chung DW, Hahn CS. Free vascularized fibula grafting for the treatment of osteonecrosis of the femoral head. *Clin Orthop* 1992 ; 277 : 128-138

Resection of periacetabular tumours (Segment II) and reconstruction

R Kotz
R Windhager

Abstract. – *Periacetabular wide resection for malignant bone tumours is technically-demanding because of the vicinity of major vessels and nerves, and reconstruction is difficult because the acetabulum is the weight-bearing part of the pelvis. Different approaches to the tumour region are possible and partly determined by the extent of the tumours. Three-dimensional models of the pelvis are necessary to design a custom-made tumour prostheses and allow for better preoperative planning of the osteotomies, and thus safe surgical margins. The different methods of reconstruction include saddle prostheses, custom-made and modular tumour prostheses and allografts. In the case of a small tumour, a flail hip with shortening of the affected leg can be a sufficient solution.*

Keywords: pelvic ring, pelvic region, malignant bone tumour, periacetabular resection, wide resection, pelvic prosthesis, saddle prosthesis.

Introduction

Resection of iliac segment II – the periacetabular region – requires surgery in one of the most challenging pelvic regions, due to the fact that the femoral neurovascular bundle passes it ventrally and the ischiatic nerve passes it dorsally. Furthermore, the hip joint is also involved and, in most cases, resection of the femoral head or the proximal femur is also necessary. Curative surgery aimed at avoiding local recurrences requires resection of the tumour with wide margins [2]. If this can be achieved, the life expectancy of the patient equals that of persons undergoing amputation of the leg with wide resection margins within the pelvic region. When hemipelvectomy is replaced by pelvic resection with limb salvage, this surgery requires considerably greater efforts, because wide resection margins must be observed proximally as well as distally of the tumour; at the same time, the vital structures for the leg must be maintained. Because the prognosis is better with neoadjuvant chemotherapy, especially in patients suffering from highly-malignant tumours such as osteosarcoma and Ewing's sarcoma, but also due to the tumour-shrinking effect, amputations within the

Rainer Kotz, M.D., Professor and Chairman, Department of Orthopaedics, Medical Faculty of the University of Vienna, Währinger Gürtel 18-20, A-1090 Wien, Austria.
Reinhard Windhager, M.D., Professor and Chairman, Department of Orthopaedics, Medical Faculty of the University of Graz, Austria.

pelvic region are necessary only in rare cases. Hemipelvectomy is indicated when extensive bone and soft tissue resection is necessary, in addition to nerve resection, which renders reconstruction difficult; a poor functional outcome has to be expected.

Reconstruction of the acetabular region is much more difficult as compared to mere ilium type I, ischium type III reconstruction, or reconstruction of the os pubis, because the acetabulum is the weight-bearing part of the pelvis. Possible reconstruction methods are the "flail leg" with shortening and fixing of the residual thigh at the iliac wing (iliofemoral coaptation). Of course, the necessary shortening of the leg (of 8 cm or more) by this type of surgery does not allow a sufficient gait afterwards, and these patients require at least a stick for support and compensation of the leg length discrepancy by an appropriate shoe. Reconstruction by allografts or endoprostheses might preserve the adequate leg length. In the case of endoprostheses, we may choose between a saddle prosthesis [5], a custom-made pelvic prosthesis [6] or a modular pelvic prosthesis [3].

Surgical technique

Exact preoperative staging using imaging procedures such as CT and MRI is mandatory. The manufacture of a three-dimensional model can be advisable to investigate the methods of resection and reconstruction. In singular cases, depicting the vascular system is also a precondition. Preoperative bowel preparation, urological and rectal clinical investigations are recommended. A rapid infusion system during operation and postoperative intensive care is mandatory.

For periacetabular resection, a skin incision is made along the ilium [4] (*fig 1*). In the case of huge tumours and those that are difficult to operate, an additional dorsal approach along the sciatic nerve might facilitate resection and guarantee oncological safety (wide resection margins). Via the anterior approach, the iliac artery and vein and the femoral nerve are prepared, and the hypogastric artery and vein are clamped, cut and ligated. During retroperitoneal preparation of the vessels, the ureter is transferred medially and the sciatic notch is prepared. After ventral and dorsal exposition of the tumour, at a safety distance of some centimetres from the tumour, the upper part of the femur is exposed. Thereafter, the gluteal muscles and the fasciae latae tensors must be prepared from the lateral tumour. If the tumour is huge and positioned dorsally, a dorsal exposition of the sciatic nerve is favourable. For this purpose, the patient is turned in a prone position, and by a dorsal incision (*fig 1*), the sciatic nerve is prepared from the incisura ischiadica towards the proximal thigh. Whereas the gluteus maximus muscle and the respective neurovascular bundle are separated medially as far as possible, the

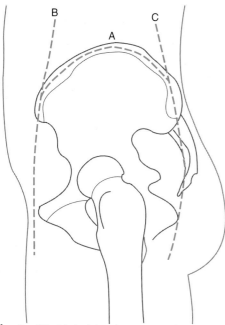

1   *Possible skin incisions for resection of periacetabular tumours. The skin incision (A) along the iliac crest can be extended anteriorly or posteriorly along the dotted lines B and C. B and C represent a combined anterior and posterior approach with skin incisions along the femoral neurovascular bundle and the sciatic nerve respectively. This combined approach is suitable for periacetabular tumours with a large extent of soft tissue.*

gluteus medius and minimus muscles remain attached to the tumour in order to achieve wide resection margins. For performance of the osteotomies, it has proved favourable to make a model of the pelvis based on the data gained from the CT, as mentioned earlier, and to simulate surgery on this model to ensure wide resection. Four osteotomies must be performed: the ischium and the pubis from a ventral approach, the femur, and finally

the ilium from a ventral and dorsal access. The second incision permits a good view on the ischium and ilium without touching the n. ischiadicus. Only after cutting the sacrotuberal and the sacrospinal ligaments can the resected part be moved. After dissection of the iliac and gluteus medius muscles, both covering the tumour, it can be removed.

Methods of reconstruction

The method of construction depends on the extension of the tumour and the size of the resected part. If the size of the remaining os ilium is sufficient, good bridging of the defect can be achieved with a saddle prosthesis (*fig 2*). If the femoral head can be maintained, a good result with a shortened leg can be achieved without reconstruction by repositioning the femoral head in the resection hole (*fig 3*). In the case of a huge defect, other reconstruction methods such as implantation of allografts (*fig 4*) into the pelvis and/or the femur, or modular or custom-made pelvic prostheses, have to be applied (*fig 5*). A custom-made prosthesis can be ordered by the surgeon, based on the pelvic model and produced by a company specialised in this field. The advantage of such a pelvic model with an integrated prosthesis is the possibility to subsequently perform adequate surgery with wide resection margins, as well as to obtain advance information on the mode of fixation of the prosthesis to the residual bones. Implantation of a pelvic prosthesis is indicated not only when type II resection is necessary, but also when type I and type IV resections have to be performed (inner hemipelvectomy); otherwise, support of the

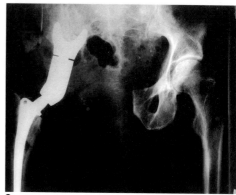

2   *Reconstruction with a saddle prostheses: The saddle acts as a spacer between the remaining part of the ilium and the femur and allows for flexion and rotation.*

leg can hardly be achieved. The functional outcome depends on the method of reconstruction and the size of the tumour. In any case, long-term immobilisation with a plaster cast for 6 to 12 weeks is necessary, and subsequently, the patient must be provided with a brace for at least half a year in order to prevent dislocation.

Complications

A high rate of complications has to be expected, including neural lesions (25%), haematomas (5-10%) and infections (15-50%). Furthermore, the time-consuming surgery accompanied by high blood loss is often associated with acute complications in the operation room and during the first postoperative days, such as lung embolism and respiratory difficulties (10%) due to massive transfusions.

Postoperative complications should be treated surgically as early as possible,

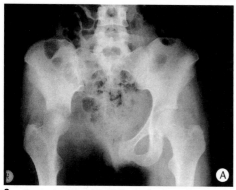

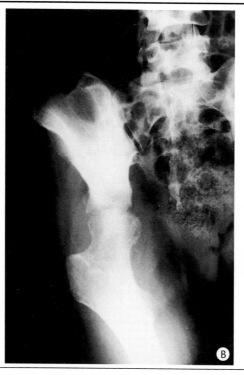

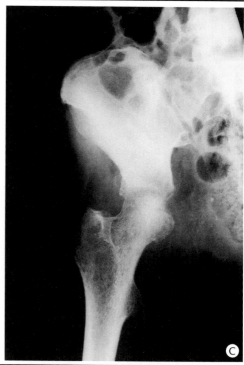

3   *Reconstruction by iliofemoral coaptation (A). In cases of small periacetabular resection and salvage of the femoral head, an iliofemoral pseudarthrosis can be attempted. In this case, the cartilage of the femoral head and the remaining one-third of the acetabulum had been removed, already giving fibrous stability 11 weeks postoperatively both in adduction and abduction (B, C).*

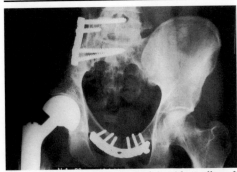

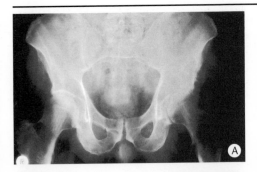

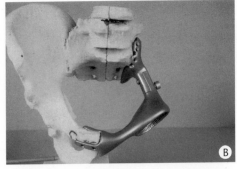

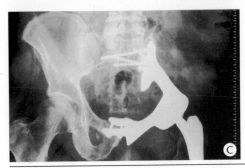

4   *Reconstruction of the hemipelvis with an allograft fixed to the contralateral pubis and the sacrum by osteosynthesis plates. The femoral head had been replaced by a bipolar prosthetic head.*

5   *A. Chondrosarcoma of the left periacetabular region involving the hip joint.*
B. Construction of a three-dimensional individual model with the help of CT scan data. For reconstruction of the removed hemipelvis, a custom-made prosthesis has been manufactured.
C. X-ray control two years after implantation of the custom-made prosthesis, fixed without cement to the sacrum and the contralateral pubic rim.

because a large quantity of haematoma may accumulate in the huge wound hole, which in turn may cause infections. Some authors propose the use of a suction system to avoid formation of huge holes.

In the literature, there has been great variation regarding the functional results achieved. Following pelvic resection and reconstruction, a mean value of 20 out of 30 possible points [1] is achieved, mainly due to poor values for stability, force and complications.

To date, there is no agreement on the surgical treatment of periacetabular tumours, which ranges from external to internal hemipelvectomy without or with reconstruction using allografts, saddle prostheses, custom-made and modular pelvic prostheses. The difficulty in establishing exact guidelines for the treatment often results in a delay in the management of these patients, which sometimes leads to an inoperable situation. Consequently, for this particular group of patients, early admission to a specialised tumour centre is absolutely mandatory.

References

[1] Enneking WF, Dunham W, Gebhardt MC, Malavar M, Pritchard DJ. A system for the functional evaluation of reconstructive procedures after surgical treatment of tumours of the musculoskeletal system. *Clin Orthop* 1993 ; 286 : 241-246

[2] Enneking WF, Spanier SS, Goodman MA. A system for the surgical staging of musculoskeletal sarcoma. *Clin Orthop* 1980 ; 153 : 106-120

[3] Gradinger R, Rechl H, Hipp E. Pelvic osteosarcoma. Resection, reconstruction, local control, and survival statistics. *Clin Orthop* 1991 ; 270 : 149-158

[4] Letournel E. The treatment of acetabular fractures through the ilioinguinal approach. *Clin Orthop* 1993 ; 292 : 62-76

[5] Nieder E, Elson RA, Engelbrecht E, Kasselt MR, Keller A, Steinbrink K. The saddle prosthesis for salvage of the destroyed acetabulum. *J Bone Joint Surg Br* 1990 ; 72 : 1014-1022

[6] Windhager R, Karner J, Kutschera HP, Polterauer P, Salzer Kuntschik M,, Kotz R. Limb salvage in periacetabular sarcomas: review of 21 consecutive cases. *Clin Orthop* 1996 ; 331 : 265-276

Resection of ischiopubic tumours (pelvic region 3)

N Fabbri
M Mercuri
M Campanacci†

Abstract. – The obturator ring (region 3) is not a common site for pelvic tumours. Surgical margins are crucial for tumour control. Limb salvage surgery with a wide margin is usually possible and in most circumstances reconstruction is not needed. The proximity of important neurovascular structures and viscera, and potentially severe complications require careful staging, planning, and a multidisciplinary approach. An ilio-inguinal incision with a perpendicular vertical branch in the genitofemoral region is routinely used. Extension of this standard incision may be required in order to improve exposure. Care must be taken to avoid injuries to the femoral neurovascular bundle, urethra, and bladder. Reconstruction of the abdominal wall should be carried out to prevent herniations. The perioperative complication rate is high and ranges from 30% to 40%. Disease free survival (DFS) is more than 80% for low grade tumours and 35% to 40% for high grade tumours. Functional results are satisfactory in more than 80% of cases.

Keywords: pelvis, malignant bone tumour, ischiopubic tumour, obturator ring resection.

Introduction

Limb salvage surgery for malignant pelvic tumours is a valuable option and a reliable alternative to hemipelvectomy. Tumour control remains the most important issue and correlates with the achievement of an adequate surgical margin [3, 7, 12, 15, 16, 21]. The minimum surgical margin required for tumour control is a wide margin which implies the en bloc removal of the tumour, completely surrounded by normal tissue [9]. A pelvic resection is therefore a reasonable option when an adequate surgical margin can be obtained or when an amputation does not offer a better margin; if chances of tumour control are the same, the restoration of a functional result superior to hemipelvectomy becomes the rationale for a limb-sparing procedure.

Pelvis and sacrum are divided into four anatomical regions and pelvic resections are classified according to Enneking et al [8]. Obturator ring (region 3) resections are less commonly performed than either iliosacral (regions 1 and 4) and periacetabular

Nicola Fabbri, M.D.
Mario Mercuri, M.D.
Mario Campanacci†, M.D.
Department of Musculoskeletal Oncology, Istituto Ortopedico Rizzoli,
Via Pupilli 1, 40136 Bologna, Italy.

(region 2) resections, comprising about 20% in large series [3, 7, 12, 15, 16]. The malignant tumours most frequently located in region 3 are chondrosarcomas (primary and secondary) and Ewing's sarcoma [2, 20]. The resection of pelvic tumours located in region 3 (ischium and pubis) is in general a less complex and demanding procedure for both the surgeon and the patient when compared to iliosacral and periacetabular resections. Indeed, tumour expansion and consequent surgical dissection is frequently less extensive; furthermore, a stable femorosacral continuity and an essentially normal weight-bearing capability are usually maintained with no need for reconstruction. However, the necessity of adequate surgical margins, the proximity to relevant neurovascular structures and viscera, and potentially severe intra and postoperative complications are key factors to be kept in mind for successful management of these lesions. The value of an appropriately placed and performed biopsy cannot be overemphasised [5]. A poorly performed biopsy complicates future surgical management, makes the achievement of an adequate margin without (or even with) amputation sometimes impossible and compromises disease control [13, 14].

Because of the need to excise the biopsy track en bloc with the tumour [7], the biopsy should be placed along the line of the incision required for definitive surgery.

A thorough review of the regional anatomy and careful preoperative planning based on tumour staging studies are essential steps. A multidisciplinary team approach including urologists, plastic, general and vascular surgeons is recommended. Even when no visceral nor neurovascular involvement is suspected on preoperative staging studies, team members should be available because of the risk of intraoperative complications and the subsequent need for repair.

Surgical technique

PATIENT PREPARATION

Lower bowel preparation and urinary catheter insertion should be carried out routinely. A urinary catheter maintains the bladder deflated and allows easier identification of the urethra during surgery; the latter is especially valuable in males because of its anatomical relationship with the pubic symphysis.

Moreover, intraoperative methylene blue injection through the catheter may be very helpful in revealing bladder lacerations. According to preoperative multidisciplinary evaluation and planning, ureteral stent placement should be considered when

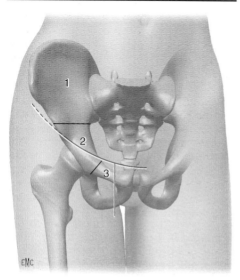

1 *The standard ilioinguinal incision with a descending vertical branch. Its relationship to pelvic regions 1, 2, and 3 is shown.*

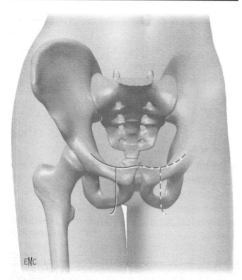

2 *Bilateral incision for bilateral obturator ring resection.*

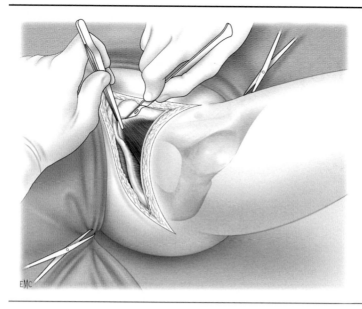

3 *Dissection through the vertical incision. The hip is abducted and externally rotated, the external surface of the ring is exposed. The external obturator muscle is released from the foramen at an appropriate distance from the tumour.*

tumour involvement is at least suspected, or ureteral dissection anticipated. Perioperative antibiotics are definitely recommended; due to potential contamination from urinary and/or gastrointestinal tracts, gram-negative bacteria coverage should be considered along with routine prophylaxis.

OPERATIVE TECHNIQUE

The patient is placed supine; the abdomen, pelvis and ipsilateral lower limb are prepared and draped in the surgical field that extends from the posterior to the anterior midline including the pubic symphysis and from the rib cage to the ipsilateral toes. When a bilateral obturator ring resection is planned, the entire abdomen, pelvis and both lower extremities are included in the operative field.

Different incisions and techniques have been reported in the literature [4, 7, 10, 11, 18]. The biopsy track (full thickness from the skin to

the tumour) must be included in the incision line and planes of dissection, and removed en bloc with the tumour. In order to incorporate the biopsy, the incision frequently needs to be adjusted.

We routinely use an ilioinguinal incision: from the anterior superior iliac spine extending to the symphysis following the superior border of the pubis. A descending vertical incision approximately perpendicular to the ilioinguinal incision is usually performed to improve exposure of the obturator ring [4]. This vertical incision begins in proximity to the symphysis (usually 3-6 cm) and spans over the genitofemoral region *(fig 1)*. When a bilateral obturator ring resection is planned, a bilateral ilioinguinal incision with a descending vertical branch is required *(fig 2)*.

In specific circumstances dictated by tumour location and extension, the exposure can be further improved by:

– extending the ilioinguinal incision laterally and/or across the symphysis;

– starting the vertical incision more laterally;

– extending the vertical incision to the ischial tuberosity and eventually to the subnatal crease.

The ilioinguinal fascia is exposed and incised, the spermatic cord (males) or round ligament (females) identified and retracted. While care must be taken to protect the spermatic cord, the round ligament can actually be sacrificed without consequences. The inguinal ligament, rectus abdominal and pyramidal muscles are released from the pubis exposing the superior aspect of the symphysis. By blunt finger dissection the retropubic space (space of Retzius) is entered and developed exposing the posterior wall of the symphysis. The bladder is gently retracted backwards, the urethra identified and the inferior pubic arch can then be palpated. During this phase, attention should be paid to the retropubic venous plexus, a potential source of significant

bleeding. Laterally, with the ipsilateral hip and knee flexed and externally rotated, the femoral sheath containing the femoral vessels is identified, dissected and elevated from the osteomuscular plane after ligation and division of a few branches to the abdominal wall, including the deep circumflex iliac and inferior epigastric vessels. With the hip fully abducted and externally rotated, dissection through the vertical incision is carried out. The pectineal, adductor and gracilis muscles are divided at an appropriate distance from the tumour; the iliopsoas muscle is laterally retracted and the outer surface of the obturator ring is exposed *(fig 3)*. The external obturator and quadratus muscles are divided exposing the inferior portion of the hip joint capsule and the ischium just distal to the acetabulum. Elevation of the femoral vessels and lateral retraction of the iliopsoas muscle and femoral nerve allow adequate exposure of the entire superior pubic ramus up to the iliopubic eminence. The obturator vessels and nerve are sacrificed and the pubic region is prepared for the medial osteotomy which is performed through the symphysis, or the contralateral pubis, as dictated by tumour extension, using either an osteotome or a Gigli saw. In both circumstances, attention should be paid to protect the urethra and the retropubic venous plexus. The lateral osteotomies through the superior pubic ramus and ischium are then performed at the chosen level *(fig 4)*. Sometimes, tumour extension requires a lateral osteotomy through the acetabulum. Applying gentle traction, the residual external rotators (internal obturator, superior and inferior gemellus muscles) are divided from the femur, and hamstrings from the ischial tuberosity, carefully avoiding the sciatic nerve. By externally rotating the specimen, the pelvic floor musculature is divided from the inner aspect of the ischium. The sacrospinous and sacrotuberous ligaments are then cut and the specimen removed; because of its proximity to the

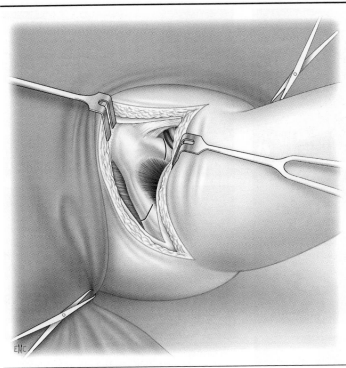

4 *Lateral retraction of the femoral vessels allows adequate exposure of pubis and ischium. Osteotomies can then be performed at the chosen level.*

symphysis will allow adequate exposure. Lateral tumour expansion and the need to resect part of the acetabulum require lateral extension of the incision up to the anterior superior iliac spine and along the anterior portion of the iliac crest. In these circumstances, more lateral placement of the vertical incision will also improve the exposure, reducing the lateral flap length. Hip dislocation is usually required to remove a significant portion of the acetabulum. Tumour extension in the ischium, a difficult region to expose adequately, may be addressed by extending the vertical incision to the ischial tuberosity, and eventually in the subnatal crease.

Given the need to remove the biopsy site en bloc with the tumour, an inappropriately placed biopsy may require an atypical incision, either for a resection or an amputation. Plastic surgery counselling as well as assistance for evaluation of skin flap viability and potential need for soft tissue reconstruction, with regional or free flaps, are mandatory for these patients.

Tumour involvement of the femoral vessels requires en bloc removal of the vessels with the specimen and appropriate replacement by vascular surgeons.

ischial spine, care must be taken to avoid injuries to the pudendal nerve during this phase. Careful haemostasis and frequent irrigation is recommended throughout the procedure. Accurate soft tissue reconstruction of the abdominal wall should then be performed augmenting the repair with either synthetic (Marlex® mesh) or biological (fascial allograft) material in order to prevent herniations. Routine wound closure over suction drains is then undertaken (*fig 5*).

POSTOPERATIVE CARE

Given the extent of surgery, postoperative intensive care monitoring is frequently needed. Drains should not be removed until drainage is minimal. Perioperative antibiotics should be continued for a few days and discontinued only after drain removal.

Special circumstances

Specific tumour location in the obturator ring may require a modified standard incision. When the tumour is located close to the symphysis, extension of the ilioinguinal incision well across the

Results

COMPLICATIONS

A number of reports on limb salvage surgery for pelvic tumours are currently available in the literature; they uniformly emphasise a high complication rate ranging from 30% to 50% [1, 3, 7, 12, 15, 16, 19, 21]. This includes wound healing problems (20%-40%), infection

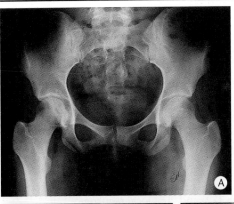

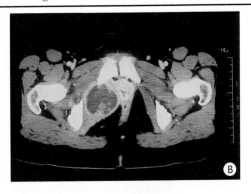

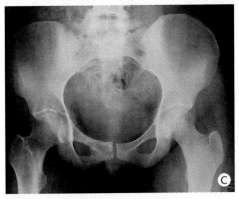

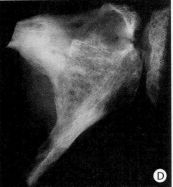

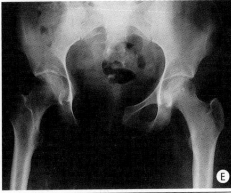

5 *Twenty-one year-old female with Ewing's sarcoma of the right pubis.*
A. Standard AP view at presentation.
B. CT scan at presentation.
C. Standard AP view obtained one year later, after adjuvant chemotherapy and radiation therapy. No evidence of tumour on CT scan for the same period. Resection was then performed to improve local control.
D. Radiograph of the resected specimen. The medial osteotomy was performed through the contralateral pubis.
E. Standard AP view obtained 6 months after surgery. Two years later the patient is disease free with an excellent result.

(20%-30%), nerve palsies (5%-15%), visceral injuries (5%-10%), vascular injuries (3%-5%), deep venous thrombosis and pulmonary embolism (10%-30%), perioperative mortality (0-10%). A recent review has combined data from all reports since 1989, obtaining an overall complication rate of 33% (23% wound related) and a perioperative mortality close to zero [6].

Although data on the specific risk for each type of procedure are scant, type 3 resections seem to be more commonly associated with urological complications, mostly involving the bladder and urethra (30%-40%), such as intraoperative lacerations and/or postoperative urinary incontinence [3, 7, 15]. In males, postoperative impotence, usually of organic origin, is a specific risk for type 3 resections.

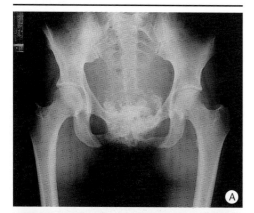

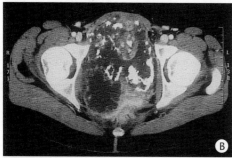

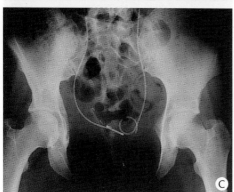

6 *Thirty-three year old female with large secondary chondrosarcoma arising from the pubic symphysis. A bilateral obturator ring resection was performed. Ureteral stents were placed before surgery and the tumour was removed en bloc with part of the bladder.*
A. Standard AP view at presentation.
B. CT scan of the pelvis at presentation showing tumour expansion in the lower pelvis.
C. Postoperative AP view; note ureteral stents still in place.

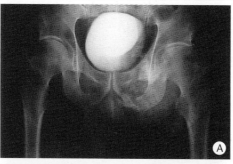

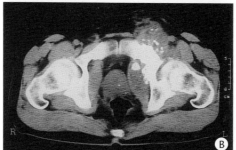

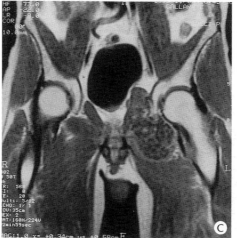

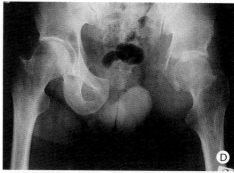

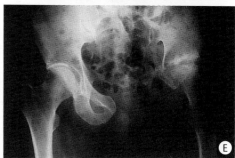

7 *A forty-two year old male with secondary chondrosarcoma of the obturator ring involving the acetabulum, left side. A resection including the inferomedial portion of the acetabular wall was performed; the femoral head was dislocated to allow the acetabular osteotomy.*
A. Standard AP view at presentation.
B. CT scan of the pelvis at presentation showing involvement of the left acetabulum.
C. Coronal MRI scan at presentation confirming acetabular involvement.
D. Standard AP view 3 months after surgery.
E. AP view 5 years after surgery. The patient developed progressive left hip pain and instability, requiring the use of a crutch. The radiograph shows avascular necrosis of the femoral head with collapse and advanced degenerative changes. The patient remains continuously disease free from chondrosarcoma.

Both urinary problems and impotence are more common in bilateral obturator ring resections [3] because of the more extensive dissection connected with this procedure (fig 6). Type 3 resections including part of the acetabulum have also been associated with hip instability and avascular necrosis of the femoral head [3, 15]. Residual stability of the hip joint should always be carefully assessed intraoperatively before closure, and acetabular autograft or allograft reconstruction undertaken if necessary. An effort should always be made to avoid femoral head dislocation whenever possible, thus reducing the risk of avascular necrosis. If this is unavoidable, care should be taken to reduce dislocation time, preserve the ligamentum teres if possible and minimise soft tissue stripping from the proximal femur (fig 7).

ONCOLOGICAL OUTCOME

There is solidly based evidence that tumour stage, surgical margin and local recurrence correlate with prognosis of pelvic sarcomas, regardless of location. Large series show a 5 year disease free survival ranging from 77% to 95% for low-grade and 25% to 55% for high-grade lesions [1, 3, 12, 15, 16, 17, 21]. Combining all the data published after 1989, an overall survival rate of 37% and a local recurrence rate of 17% have been reported [6]. Wide margin achievement is reported in 50% to 70% of cases. Overall local recurrence rates range from 15% to 30% and increase to more than 50% when associated with inadequate margins (contaminated, marginal or intralesional).

Few data are available for the subgroup of type 3 resections; two large studies reported a 17% and 20% local recurrence rate [3, 15, 16].

FUNCTIONAL RESULTS

Functional outcome is satisfactory (excellent or good using either MSTS or ISOLS scores) in 81%-100% according to different experiences [3, 15, 16].

In most circumstances, femorosacral continuity can be maintained through a stable hip joint preserving an essentially normal function. If part of the acetabulum is resected with the obturator ring, the hip joint may become unstable if not appropriately reconstructed, compromising the functional result with pain and sometimes necessitating a cane or crutch (*fig 7*).

Conclusions

Surgical management of pelvic tumours remains one of the most challenging problems in orthopaedic oncology. When the likelihood of tumour control (i.e. type of surgical margin) is the same as for hemipelvectomy, and the functional result can reasonably be expected to be superior to that offered by amputation and prosthetic fitting, a pelvic resection should be

considered. This is frequently the case for tumours located in region 3 because in most instances they can be adequately resected with no significant impact on function.

Hemipelvectomy is seldom required; however, patients presenting local recurrence after a previous limb-sparing procedure should be regarded as candidates for amputation unless a wide margin can be achieved with certainty or the amputation will not provide a better margin. In these cases, tumour grade, absence or presence of metastases, and life expectancy of the patient should be taken into appropriate account while deciding between ablative and conservative options. Careful staging and

preoperative planning, a multidisciplinary approach, achievement of adequate surgical margins and awareness of the high risk of severe complications are crucial issues. Advances in diagnostic and staging modalities, the application in most high-grade tumours of adjuvant chemotherapy and sometimes radiation therapy, as well as surgical experience accumulated over the past 30 years have definitely improved the outcome of patients affected by primary malignant bone tumours of the pelvis. If local tumour control can be achieved, an overall 5 year survival of more than 80% for low grade lesions and of 35% to 40% for high grade lesions can reasonably be expected.

References

[1] Apffelstaedt JP, Driscoll DL, Karakousis CP. Partial and complete internal hemipelvectomy: complications and long term follow-up. *J Am Coll Surg* 1995 ; 181 : 43-48

[2] Campanacci M. Bone and soft tissue tumors. Wien : Springer-Verlag, 1999

[3] Campanacci M, Capanna R. Pelvic resections: the Rizzoli Institute experience. *Orthop Clin North Am* 1991 ; 22 : 65-86

[4] Campanacci M, Langlais F. Les resections du bassin pour tumeurs. *Encycl Méd Chir* (Éditions Scientifiques et Médicales Elsevier SAS, Paris), Techniques chirurgicales - Orthopédie-Traumatologie, 44-505, 1992 : 1-7

[5] Campanacci M, Mercuri M, Gamberini G. Biopsy. *Chir Organi Mov* 1995 ; LXXX : 113-123

[6] Conrad EU 3rd, Springfield D, Peabody TD. Pelvis. In : Simon MA, Springfield D eds. Surgery for bone and soft-tissue tumors. Philadelphia : Lippincott-Raven Publishers, 1998

[7] Enneking WF, Dunham WK. Resection and reconstruction for primary neoplasms involving the innominate bone. *J Bone Joint Surg Am* 1978 ; 60 : 731-746

[8] Enneking WF, Dunham WK, Gebhardt MC, Malawer MM, Pritchard DJ. A system for the classification of skeletal resections. *Chir Organi Mov* 1990 ; LXXV (suppl 1) : 217-240

[9] Enneking WF, Spanier SS, Goodman MA. A system for the surgical staging of musculoskeletal sarcoma. *Clin Orthop* 1980 ; 153 : 106-120

[10] Karaharju EO, Korkala OL. Resection of large tumors of the anterior pelvic ring while preserving functional stability of the hip. *Clin Orthop* 1985 ; 195 : 270-274

[11] Karakousis CP. Abdominoinguinal incision in resection of pelvic tumors with lateral fixation. *Am J Surg* 1992 ; 164 : 366-371

[12] Kawai A, Huvos AG, Meyers PA, Healey JH. Osteosarcoma of the pelvis. *Clin Orthop* 1998 ; 348 : 196-207

[13] Mankin HJ, Lange TA, Spanier SS. The hazards of biopsy in patients with malignant primary bone and soft-tissue tumors. *J Bone Joint Surg Am* 1982 ; 64 : 1121-1127

[14] Mankin HJ, Mankin CJ, Simon MA. The hazards of the biopsy, revisited. *J Bone Joint Surg Am* 1996 ; 78 : 656-662

[15] O'Connor MI, Sim FH. Salvage of the limb in the treatment of malignant pelvic tumors. *J Bone Joint Surg Am* 1989 ; 71 : 481-494

[16] Ozaki T, Hillmann A, Lindner N, Blasius S, Winkelmann W. Chondrosarcoma of the pelvis. *Clin Orthop* 1997 ; 337 : 226-239

[17] Shin K, Rougraff BT, Simon MA. Oncologic outcomes of primary bone sarcomas of the pelvis. *Clin Orthop* 1994 ; 304 : 207-217

[18] Steel HH. Partial or complete resection of the hemipelvis. An alternative to hindquarter amputation for periacetabular chondrosarcoma of the pelvis. *J Bone Joint Surg Am* 1978 ; 60 : 719-730

[19] Stephenson RB, Kaufer H, Hankin FM. Partial pelvic resection as an alternative to hindquarter amputation for skeletal neoplasms. *Clin Orthop* 1989 ; 242 : 201-211

[20] Unni KK. Dahlin's bone tumors. Philadelphia : Lippincott-Raven Publishers, 1996

[21] Windhager R, Karner J, Kutschera HP, Polterauer P, Salzer-Kuntschik M, Kotz R. Limb salvage in periacetabular sarcomas. Review of 21 consecutive cases. *Clin Orthop* 1996 ; 331 : 265-276

Hip rotationplasty

W Winkelmann

Abstract. –   *For the adequate surgical control of malignant tumours of the lower pelvis or the proximal part of the femur with involvement of the hip joint, hip rotationplasty is a surgical alternative to disarticulation of the hip and hemipelvectomy, especially in patients who are still growing. After en bloc resection of the tumour-bearing part of the proximal thigh, the hip joint and the lower pelvis, the distal part of the femur with the knee joint and leg is rotated 180 degrees and fixed to the lateral side of the pelvis. Patients with a rotationplasty retain the feeling of having a complete leg because they retain intact proprioception, as well as superficial and deep sensitivity of the foot. Prosthetic fitting is considerably better than after hip disarticulation or hemipelvectomy. Not only is the prosthesis smaller but it can be actively used with the knee joint functioning as the hip joint and with the ankle joint functioning as the knee joint. From the oncological point of view, rotationplasty is completely comparable to ablative surgery. Rotationplasty has the lowest rate of postoperative complications when compared with all other operative forms of limb salvage.*

Keywords: hip, rotationplasty, hip disarticulation, hemipelvectomy, pelvic tumour.

Introduction

The idea of replacing the knee joint by rotating the foot 180 degrees was conceived by Borggreve [2]. Salzer introduced rotationplasty to the surgical treatment of malignant tumours of the distal femur [3]. Development of this technique was further advanced by the author, by performing a rotationplasty of the hip joint in the treatment of malignant tumours of the proximal femur, either with or without involvement of the hip joint, or malignant tumours of the lower pelvis.

In addition to rotating the foot 180 degrees so that it functions as a knee joint, we rotated the knee joint 180 degrees to function as a hip joint [4, 5].

We classify rotationplasty procedures as belonging in two main groups – type A and type B – which are further divided into subgroups (*fig 1*) [1, 6]:

Type A1 rotationplasty is for malignant tumours of the distal femur and type AII for malignant tumours of the proximal tibia.

Type B includes all forms of hip rotationplasty and is subdivided into type

BI hip rotationplasty for malignant tumours of the proximal femur with no involvement of the hip joint, type BII hip rotationplasty for malignant tumours of the proximal femur with involvement of the hip joint, and type BIII hip rotationplasty for tumours that require complete resection of the femur, with further subdivision into BIIIa for children and BIIIb for adults.

Indications

– Malignant tumours of the proximal femoral bone with an extensive extra-osseous soft tissue component and hip joint involvement.

– Malignant tumours of the pubic and or ischial bone with an extensive extra-osseous soft tissue component and hip joint involvement.

Positioning and skin incisions

The patient must be positioned in the mobile lateral position on the non-affected side. The proximal skin incision is oval-shaped. It begins 3 cm distal to the inguinal ligament, crosses the anterior superior iliac spine,

continues laterally, courses behind the greater trochanter into the anal cleft, and finally, must be extended medially to its starting point. The distal skin incision, again oval-shaped, begins medially 8 cm above the knee joint space, courses to lateral, crosses the head of the fibular bone, and must be continued to dorsal below the popliteal fossa and medial to its starting point.

The proximal skin incision should match up with the distal incision after partial resection of the thigh and a 180° rotation of the distal femur. A third skin incision on the dorsal thigh combines the proximal and distal incisions (*fig 2*).

Surgical technique

After performing the incision on the dorsal thigh, the preparation of the sciatic nerve should ensure that there is no contact between the nerve and the tumour. The gluteus maximus muscle must be detached crosswise from the femoral tuberosity and the fascia lata. The sciatic nerve and its branches (common peroneal nerve and tibial nerve) are visible after crosswise cutting off the biceps femoris muscle. The branches innervating the thigh muscle must be cut, and the sciatic, peroneal and tibial nerves should be mobilised down to the popliteal fossa (*fig 3*).

Winfried Winkelmann, M.D., Professor, department of Orthopaedic Surgery, Westfälische Wilhelms-University, Münster, Germany.

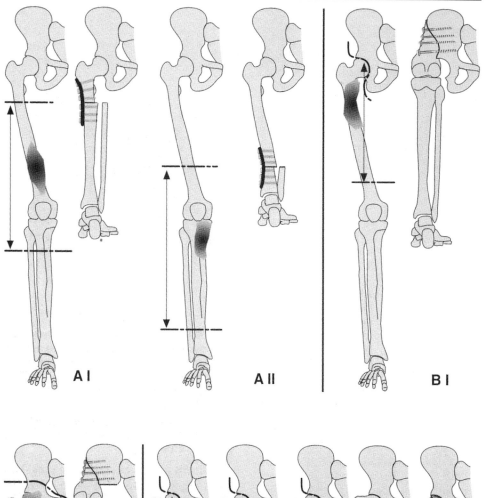

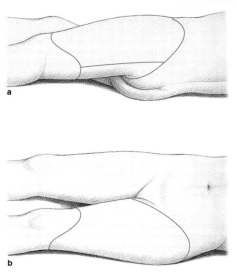

2 *Positioning of the patient and skin incisions. (Reproduced with permission from Bauer R, Kerschbaumer F, Poisel S, eds. Orthopädische Operationslehre, Becken und untere Extremität 1995 © Georg Thieme Verlag.)*

Depending on the localisation and size of the tumour, as much as possible of the iliopsoas muscle should be preserved. In case of a proximal femoral tumour, the surgeon should proceed with caution because a soft tissue component often involves the origin of the iliopsoas tendon.

The proximal parts of the adductor muscles near the symphysis should be spared. After periosteal incision, osteotomy of the iliac bone is performed cranially to the acetabulum.

Distally, the tendon of the quadriceps muscle and the distal parts of the medial and lateral vastus muscles must be retained to allow construction of a soft tissue flap. Dorsally, the tendons and the distal parts of the biceps femoris and semimembranosus muscles must be spared. The length of the distal femoral bone should be sufficient to allow its attachment to the outside of the iliac bone after 180° rotation of the femur and adjusting the shape of the bone *(fig 5)*.

An osteotomy has already been performed cranially to the acetabulum; after an osteotomy of the symphysis or the adjacent pubic bone, the detached pelvic bone can be pulled down and laterally. In the inner part of the pelvis, the piriformis muscle, the sacrospinal and sacrotuberal ligaments and the obturator nerve and vessels must be cut. Taking great care with the pudendal nerve and the internal pudendal vessels to the pelvic floor, the muscles are disinserted.

The great vessels proximally and distally must be clamped and cut, and finally, the thigh and the lower part of the pelvis can be removed *(fig 6)*.

The remaining lower leg should be rotated 180° and the distal femoral bone shaped and adjusted to match with the outside of the

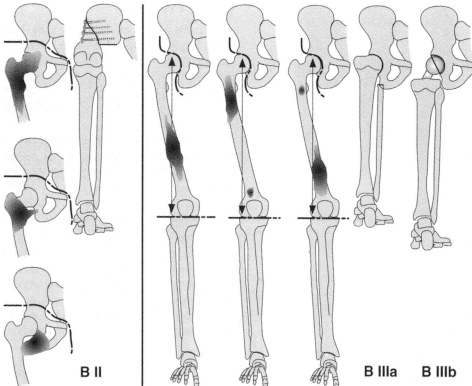

1 *Classification of rotationplasties according to Winkelmann. (Reproduced with permission from Bauer R, Kerschbaumer F, Poisel S, eds. Orthopädische Operationslehre, Becken und untere Extremität 1995 © Georg Thieme Verlag.)*

The proximal skin incision should be followed by the preparation of the femoral artery, vein and nerve. The femoral nerve must be cut distal to the inguinal ligament. Among all the branches of the femoral vessels, only those to the proximal adductor muscles should be spared.

The pelvic origins of the sartorius, gracilis and rectus femoris muscles must be detached *(fig 4)*. The tendons of the gluteus medius and minimus muscles should be detached from the greater trochanter to allow visualisation of the greater sciatic foramen.

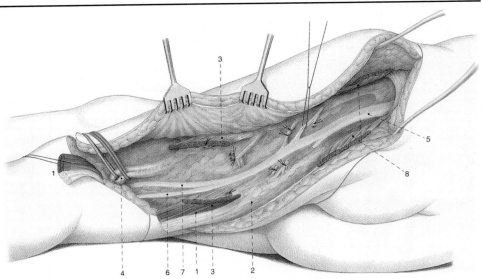

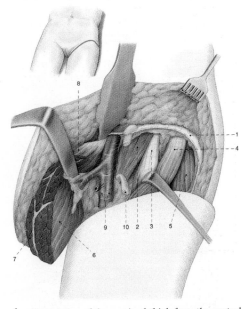

3 *Preparation of the thigh from the dorsal skin incision. 1. Biceps femoris m.; 2. biceps femoris m., long head; 3. biceps femoris m., short head; 4. popliteal vessels; 5. sciatic nerve; 6. common peroneal nerve; 7. tibial nerve; 8. gluteus maximus m. (Reproduced with permission from Bauer R, Kerschbaumer F, Poisel S, eds. Orthopädische Operationslehre, Becken und untere Extremität 1995 © Georg Thieme Verlag.)*

4 *Preparation of the proximal thigh from the ventral incision. 1. Fascia lata; 2. ilopsoas m.; 3. pectus femoris m.; 4. sartorius m.; 5. tensor fasciae latae m.; 6. adductor mm.; 7. gracilis m.; 8. pectineus m.; 9. femoral vessels; 10. femoral nerve. (Reproduced with permission from Bauer R, Kerschbaumer F, Poisel S, eds. Orthopädische Operationslehre, Becken und untere Extremität 1995 © Georg Thieme Verlag.)*

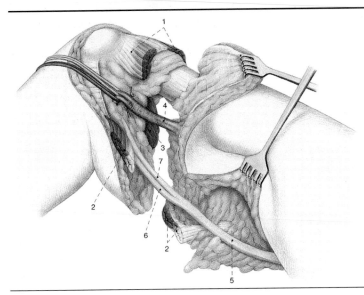

5 *Preparation of the distal thigh 1. Vastus medialis and vastus lateralis muscles; 2. biceps femoris muscle; 3. semimembranosus muscle; 4. femoral vessels; 5. sciatic nerve; 6. common peroneal nerve; 7. tibial nerve. (Reproduced with permission from Bauer R, Kerschbaumer F, Poisel S, eds. Orthopädische Operationslehre, Becken und untere Extremität 1995 © Georg Thieme Verlag.)*

iliac bone. After freshening the cortical iliac bone, the femur is attached to the iliac bone with lag screws *(fig 7)*.

In hip rotationplasty type B I and type B III, the distal femur should be screwed to the ilium in 5 – 10 degrees of abduction *(fig 8A)*. The weight (vector of force) on the rotated knee joint is least when the knee is placed as far medial as possible in the longitudinal axis *(fig 8B)* [7].

Reconstruction of the soft tissues includes connection of the tendons of the biceps femoris and the semimembranosus muscles with the iliopsoas tendon. This increases the

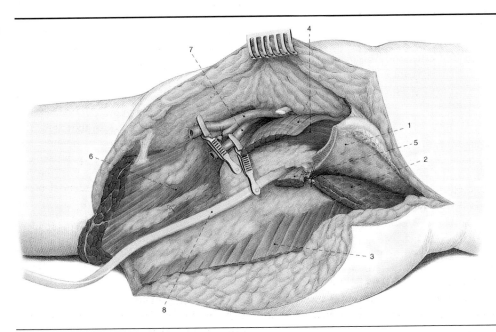

6 *Situs after resection of the thigh and the lower pelvis. The remaining part of the iliac bone is prepared subperiostally. 1. Iliac bone (osteotomised); 2. gluteus medius and gluteus minimus muscles; 3. gluteus maximus muscle; 4. iliopsoas muscle; 5. piriformis muscle; 6. adductor muscles; 7. femoral vessels (clamped and cut); 8. sciatic nerve. (Reproduced with permission from Bauer R, Kerschbaumer F, Poisel S, eds. Orthopädische Operationslehre, Becken und untere Extremität 1995 © Georg Thieme Verlag.)*

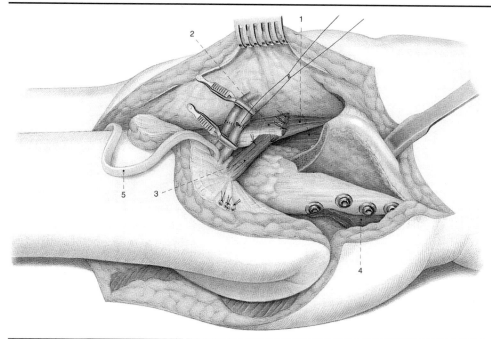

7 *After 180 degrees rotation, the distal femoral bone is attached to the iliac bone with lag screws. The iliopsas muscle (1) is connected with the tendons of the biceps femoris muscle (2) and the semimembranosus muscle (3); 4. gluteus medius and minimus muscles; 5. sciatic nerve. (Reproduced with permission from Bauer R, Kerschbaumer F, Poisel S, eds. Orthopädische Operationslehre, Becken und untere Extremität 1995 © Georg Thieme Verlag.)*

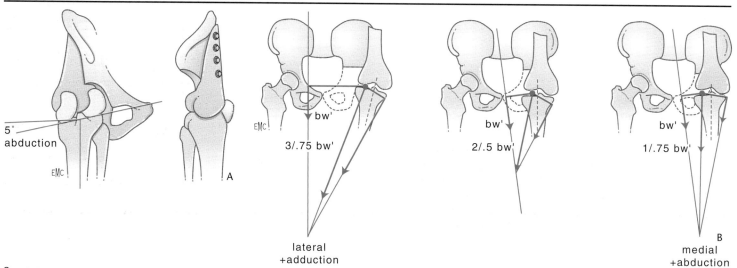

8 A. In type BI and type BII hip rotationplasty the distal femur should be screwed to the ilium in 5-10 degrees of abduction.

B. The weight (vector of force) on the rotated knee joint is least when the knee is placed as far as possible medially and the longitudinal axis is placed in slight abduction.

flexion of the (hip-)knee joint, which will later be performed mainly by the gastrocnemius muscle. Then, an end-to-end anastomosis of the great vessels is performed.

In (hip-)knee flexion of 70°, the tendons of the gluteus medius and minimus muscles and the remaining part of the gluteus maximus muscle must be connected to the soft tissue flap and around the knee cap with the fascia of the lower leg (fig 9). The remaining parts of the adductor muscles again have to be attached to the fascia of the lower leg. The only function of the adductor is to fill the wound. The function of the gluteal muscles is (hip-)knee extension. The sciatic nerve has to be placed subcutaneously and medially. The skin suture must ensure connection of the proximal and distal skin incisions which often are very incongruent (fig 10).

Complications

To prevent circulatory disorders caused by an arterial or venous thrombus, the greater vessels have to be flushed with heparin-NaCl after their incision. Post-operative treatment with heparin is obligatory.

If the adjustment of the proximal femur to the outside of the iliac bone has not been performed properly, the outcome could be a mechanical malrotation of the axis of the remaining leg. Later, this would make prosthesis fitting more difficult.

Should the remainder of the adductor muscles be too great, a compartment syndrome may result. Temporal lymphostasis of the rotated lower leg for about four weeks nearly always follows surgery.

Treatment after surgery

A plaster cast must be applied to the pelvis and the leg post-operatively until complete fusion of the distal femur with the pelvic bone has occurred. After four weeks, the plaster is incised to allow passive motion exercises of the former knee joint which is now a hip hinge. Active and passive motion exercises of the foot are always possible.

■ *Prosthesis*

A standard prosthesis has a leather cuff. The shape is best adapted to that of the contralateral leg and the leather cuff adjusted accordingly. The foot is embedded in synthetic leather shaped to form a lower leg and the prosthesis is cushioned further around the foot with thermoplastic soft foam (fig 11). Full weight-bearing with the prosthesis depends on the fusion of the

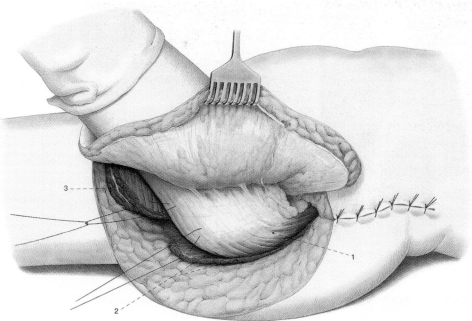

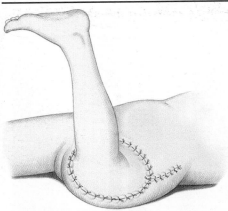

10 *The different sizes of the skin flaps are matched together and the wound is closed in the usual manner. (Reproduced with permission from Bauer R, Kerschbaumer F, Poisel S, eds. Orthopädische Operationslehre, Becken und untere Extremität 1995 © Georg Thieme Verlag.)*

9 *In 70 degrees (hip) knee flexion the gluteus maximus muscle (2) as well as the remaining part of the adductor muscles (3) are attached as well to the distal femoral tendon-muscle flap as to the fascia of the lower leg (1). (Reproduced with permission from Bauer R, Kerschbaumer F, Poisel S, eds. Orthopädische Operationslehre, Becken und untere Extremität 1995 © Georg Thieme Verlag.)*

References

[1] Baumgartner R, Botta P. Amputation und Prothesenversorgung der unteren Extremität. Stuttgart : Enke, 1995

[2] Borggreve J. Kniegelenkersatz durch das in der Beinlängsachse um 180° gedrehte Fußgelenk. *Arch Orthop Trauma Surg* 1930 : 28 : 175-178

[3] Salzer M, Knahr K, Kotz R. Treatment of osteosarcoma of the distal femur by rotationplasty. *Arch Orthop Trauma Surg* 1981 : 99 : 131-139

[4] Winkelmann W. Umdrehplastiken. In : Bauer R, Kerschbaumer F, Poisel S, eds. Orthopädische Operationslehre 2/II; Becken und untere Extremität. Stuttgart : Thieme-Verlag, 1995 : 314-340

[5] Winkelmann W. Hip rotationplasty for malignant tumors of the proximal part of the femur. *J Bone Joint Surg Am* 1986 ; 68 : 362-369

[6] Winkelmann W. Classification of rotationplasty. *Campells Oper Orthop* 1992 ; 8 : 208

[7] Winkelmann W. Rotationplasty. *Orthop Clin North Am* 1996 ; 27 : 503-523

distal femur to the ilium. Walking with the prosthesis should be learned with the help of a physiotherapist and, if possible, under gait analysis control.

In addition, patients should be fitted with a swimming prosthesis that will allow them to move around freely in public swimming pools and to swim. The swimming prosthesis has a special hollow system which fills up with water and therefore does not float *(fig 11E, F, G, H)*.

To protect the Achilles tendon, knee flexion (foot extension) is blocked at 110 degrees. In patients with type BI or type BII hip rotationplasty, a rotation adaptor is fitted into the lower leg portion of the prosthesis to minimise the weight of rotation on the fixed knee joint.

Figure 11 ➤

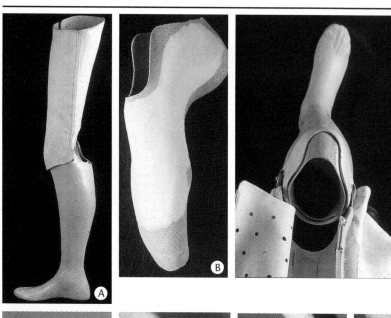

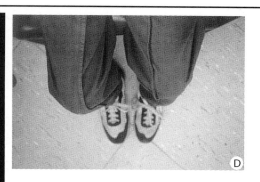

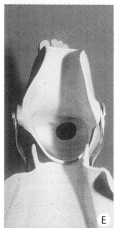

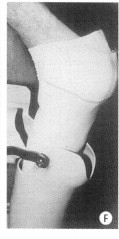

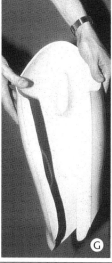

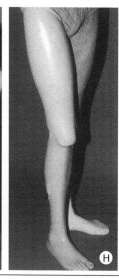

11 *Prosthetic care after rotationplasty.*
A. Standard prosthesis.
B, C. The foot is embedded in a special inner shoe.
D. The upper shaft of the prosthesis should have the same length as the contralateral thigh.
E, F, G, H. Swimming prosthesis.

Hip disarticulation

R Baumgartner

Abstract. – The main reasons for amputations in the area of the hip joint are tumours and trauma. Peripheral vascular occlusive diseases, which are responsible for the great majority of lower extremity amputations, only exceptionally lead to hip disarticulation or even hemipelvectomy.

In trauma, hip disarticulation is often associated with open pelvic fractures and avulsion of the urethra and the rectum.

It is recommended to preserve an ultra-short femoral stump. This makes prosthetic fitting more difficult, although not impossible, but contributes to a larger and more symmetrical loading area in sitting as well as in standing with the prosthesis.

The posterior flap technique with the gluteus maximus muscle covering the end of the stump is described in detail. Full end bearing requires a shortening of the ischial nerve proximal to the acetabulum.

Depending on the localisation and the malignancy of a tumour, or the extent of tissue lesions in trauma, the wound may also be closed by means of anteriorly or medially based musculocutaneous flaps.

With the Canadian-type hip disarticulation prosthesis, ambulation is possible in unilateral amputations.

Keywords: hip, hip disarticulation, Canadian-type prosthesis.

Introduction

Only 1 to 2% of all lower extremity amputations and disarticulations are performed at the hip joint. In addition, these are quite different in many respects from more peripheral amputation levels. Although peripheral vascular diseases are the major cause for lower extremity amputations (80 to 90% of such amputations), this is not valid in the hip and pelvic area. For about 50% of hip disarticulations, **malignant tumours** are the most important cause. The localisation of the tumour and its pattern of spread dictate the operative technique. In about 25%, **trauma** is the cause. Except for avulsion injuries, polytrauma caused by compression by a truck tyre may even result in bilateral hip disarticulation and, in addition to it, open infected pelvic fractures, ruptures of the urethra, the rectum and the spleen. **Peripheral vascular diseases** lead to hip disarticulation mostly in the case of infections of obliterated arterial grafts or of arterial occlusion at the bifurcation of the

René Baumgartner, M.D., Orthopaedic Surgeon, Emeritus Professor, Department of Prosthetics, Orthotics & Rehabilitation, University of Münster, Klinik und Poliklinik für Technische Orthopädie und Rehabilitation, Westfälische Wilhelms-Universität, Münster, Germany. Langwisstr. 14, Zumikon, Switzerland.

aorta. In the case of infection, the complete removal of the graft is imperative. **Gas gangrene** and **failures of total hip replacement** are less frequent causes of hip disarticulation. Finally, **congenital limb deficiencies** might include the absence of an entire limb with pelvic deformities and a coxa vara at the opposite side.

Selection of the amputation level

Hip disarticulation is indicated only if there is no way to preserve part of the femur. In case of malignancy, rotationplasty according to Borggreve-van Nes is the better solution with regard to quality of life. The ultra-short femoral stump is another important alternative. Due to severe muscle imbalance, this stump goes into a flexion and abduction position and cannot be fitted with a regular above-knee prosthesis. Also, it makes prosthetic fitting with a Canadian-type hip prosthesis more difficult than in hip disarticulation. This is why Persson [5] supports the point of view of many prosthetists that it is better to remove a remaining femoral neck. However, the ultra-short femoral stump contributes to enlarging the weight-bearing surface in sitting, which

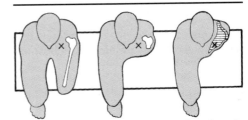

1 *The weight-bearing surface in sitting depends on the level of amputation. X = ischial tuberosity. (Reproduced with permission from Baumgartner R, Botta P. Amputation und Prothesenversorgung an der unteren Extremität. Stuttgart : Enke, 1995 © Georg Thieme Verlag.)*

is particularly important in bilateral amputation at the level of the hip *(fig 1)*. On the other hand, hemipelvectomy is indicated only if it is impossible to perform a hip disarticulation; hemipelvectomy causes even more severe problems in sitting and prosthetic fitting.

Whatever the level of amputation selected, the aim is to achieve a stump which is as peripheral as possible, free from pain, and permitting total weight-bearing at the bottom. In order to preserve length, skin grafts might become necessary to cover soft tissue defects outside the weight-bearing areas.

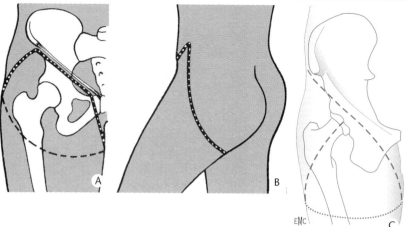

2 *Different flap techniques.*
A, B. Long posterior flap. (Reproduced with permission from Baumgart-ner R, Botta P. Amputation und Prothesenversorgung an der unteren Extremität. Stuttgart : Enke, 1995 © Georg Thieme Verlag.)
C. Maurer's anterior raquet-type technique.

Operative techniques

From an anatomical and functional point of view, a long posterior musculocutaneous flap consisting of full skin with the gluteus maximus and the hamstring muscles presents the ideal coverage of the stump. However, it is also possible to close a stump by means of an anterior or anteromedial musculocutaenous flap, depending on the local conditions provided by the lesion.

POSTERIOR FLAP TECHNIQUE
(fig 2A, B)

The incision begins parallel to the full length of the inguinal ligament. The posterior flap follows the contours of the gluteus medium muscle. Maurer [3] recommended a racquet type incision. This makes soft tissue closure easier, but has the disadvantage of being a triangular skin closure with the risk of wound healing problems.

The patient is in a supine position with the entire pelvis elevated by at least 5 cm. A urinary catheter is recommended, especially for female patients, and is left in place for the first postoperative days.

Even if it is impossible to apply a tourniquet, blood loss will not exceed that of an average orthopaedic operation if gentle tissue handling and careful haemostasis are strictly observed.

Before performing the skin incision and subcutaneous incision down to the muscular fascia, it is advisable to use a skin marker.

With the retractor dividing the wound only in the distal direction, the femoral vessels are isolated and ligated first. Maurer [3] suggested to ligate first the artery, then the vein only after the extremity has been held for 2 - 3 minutes in an elevated position. The femoral nerve is severed by means of a clean cut, well proximal to the inguinal ligament *(fig 3A)*.

Then, the anterior muscles originating from the inguinal ligament are dissected transversally one by one at about 1 cm distance from the inguinal ligament. This

will facilitate tissue closure. In order to minimise blood loss, the use of the electric knife is recommended. The same procedure applies for the adductors (the obturator vessels being ligated) and the pelvi-trochanteric muscles. Once they are all divided except for the dorsal group consisting of the hamstrings and the gluteus maximus muscle, the hip joint is opened by a T-shaped incision *(fig 3B)*. Now, the hip is dislocated anteriorly with the extremity held in hyperextension and external rotation, in order to put tension on the tissues of the posterior flap which will be made. The long amputation knife first separates these remaining soft tissues from the posterior part of the femur, following the skin incision previously made *(fig 3C, D)*. This procedure causes minimal blood loss if it lasts only a few seconds and is immediately followed by compression of the flap for about one minute. Then, the deep femoral vessels are identified and ligated. The sciatic nerve with its artery has to be clamped first, then prepared without any traction up to the level of dissection just proximal to the acetabulum *(fig 3E)*. The artery of the sciatic nerve must be ligated before the nerve is dissected by means of a clean cut. This shortening of the sciatic nerve is necessary to avoid the amputee's sitting on the nerve stump which might be a cause of stump and phantom pain.

As for the acetabulum, the cartilage should not be removed, as it represents a natural barrier. However, in cases of osteoarthritis or malnutrition, it is recommended to resect the prominent part of the acetabular angle.

Now, the posterior musculocutaneous flap must be bevelled to obtain a soft tissue closure without tension *(fig 3F)*. After insertion of 2 suction drains, the fascia of the dorsal flap is sutured to the inguinal ligament. The posterior skin flap usually needs further adaptation to the short anterior flap and is sutured by using the moccasin technique *(fig 3F)*. Dog-ears should

be strictly avoided as they may cause hygiene problems and interfere with the prosthetic requirements.

WOUND DRESSING

Adhesive tapes, bandages or plaster casts tend to reduce further traction to the sutures and to compress the large cavity between the soft tissue flaps. One must be aware of the risk of pressure sores at the sacrum and the anterior iliac spine.

Postoperative management and prosthetic fitting

With the posterior flap technique, the patient can be mobilised in a vertical position with increasing weight-bearing at the stump end within the first postoperative days.

The Canadian-type hip prosthesis developed by McLaurin and Foort [4] in 1953 permits prosthetic fitting with surprisingly good results in terms of function and cosmesis *(fig 4)*. The patient stands or sits on a pelvic bucket. Lateral displacement of the pelvic bucket during the stance phase is avoided by means of a medial rim comparable to the ischial containment socket for transfemoral stumps. The prosthetic hip joint is displaced anteriorly; its knee is recurvated which offers full stability in the stance phase. In the swing phase, a pelvic tilt causes flexion of the hip and the knee joint [6].

For bilateral hip disarticulations, the same principle is applied – with limited success, however, as locomotion by means of a wheelchair is less energy consuming and more comfortable.

The wheelchair has to be adapted to the elevated centre of gravity due to the absence of the extremities. The amputee's body has to be secured with sitting shells and safety belts.

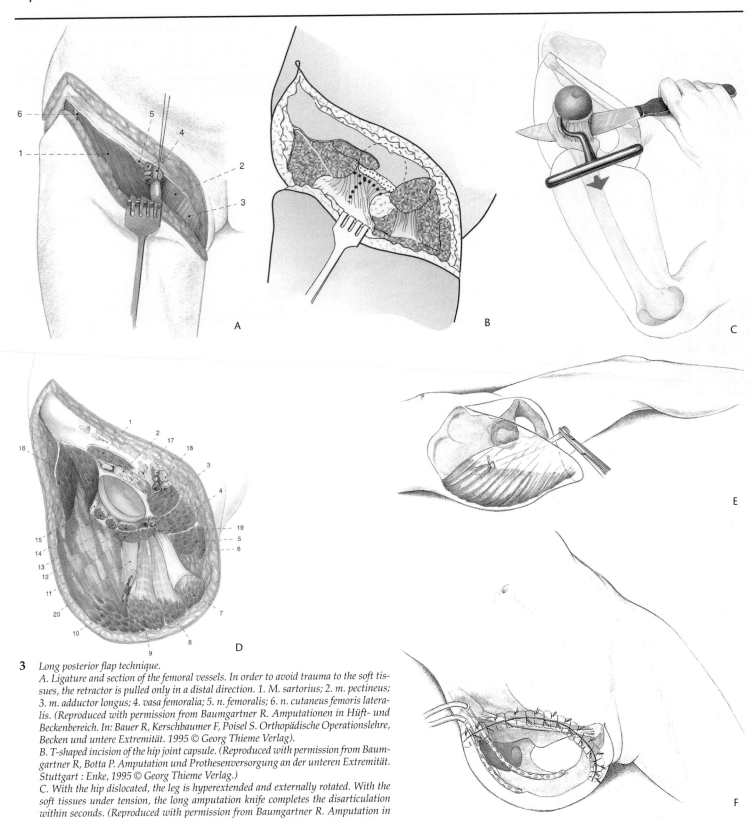

3   Long posterior flap technique.

A. Ligature and section of the femoral vessels. In order to avoid trauma to the soft tissues, the retractor is pulled only in a distal direction. 1. M. sartorius; 2. m. pectineus; 3. m. adductor longus; 4. vasa femoralia; 5. n. femoralis; 6. n. cutaneus femoris lateralis. (Reproduced with permission from Baumgartner R. Amputationen in Hüft- und Beckenbereich. In: Bauer R, Kerschbaumer F, Poisel S. Orthopädische Operationslehre, Becken und untere Extremität. 1995 © Georg Thieme Verlag).

B. T-shaped incision of the hip joint capsule. (Reproduced with permission from Baumgartner R, Botta P. Amputation und Prothesenversorgung an der unteren Extremität. Stuttgart : Enke, 1995 © Georg Thieme Verlag.)

C. With the hip dislocated, the leg is hyperextended and externally rotated. With the soft tissues under tension, the long amputation knife completes the disarticulation within seconds. (Reproduced with permission from Baumgartner R. Amputation in Hüft- und Beckenbereich. In: Bauer R, Kerschbaumer F, Poisel S. Orthopädische Operationslehre, Becken und untere Extremität. 1995 © Georg Thieme Verlag).

D. The long posterior flap. Note the sciatic nerve with its artery. 1. M. satorius; 2. m. iliopsoas; 3. m. pectineus; 4. m. adductor longus; 5. m. adductor magnus; 6. m. gracilis; 7. m. semimembranosus; 8. m. semitendinosus; 9. m. biceps femoris. Caput longum; 10. m. gluteus maximus; 11. m. quadratus femoris; 12. m. gemellus inferior; 13. m. obturator internus; 14. m. gemellus superior; 15. m. piriformis; 16. m. tensor fasciae latae; 17. n. femoralis; 18. vasa femoralia; 19. vasa obturatoria; 20. n. ischiadicus. (Reproduced with permission from Baumgartner R. Amputation in Hüft- und Beckenbereich. In: Bauer R, Kerschbaumer F, Poisel S. Orthopädische Operationslehre, Becken und untere Extremität. 1995 © Georg Thieme Verlag).

E. Shortening of the sciatic nerve proximally to the acetabulum. (Reproduced with permission from Baumgartner R. Amputation in Hüft- und Beckenbereich. In: Bauer R, Kerschbaumer F, Poisel S. Orthopädische Operationslehre, Becken und untere Extremität. 1995 © Georg Thieme Verlag).

F. Double suction drainage; final closure with interrupted sutures avoiding dog-ears. (Reproduced with permission from Baumgartner R. Amputation in Hüft- und Beckenbereich. In: Bauer R, Kerschbaumer F, Poisel S. Orthopädische Operationslehre, Becken und untere Extremität. 1995 © Georg Thieme Verlag).

Figure 4 and references ➤

3

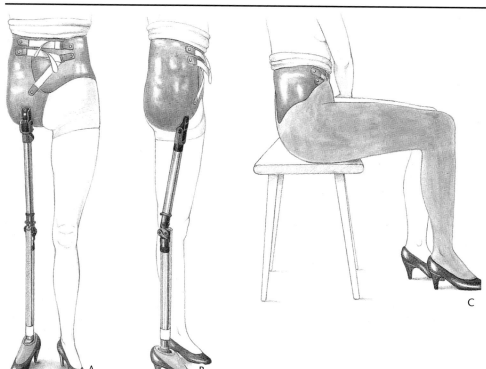

4 *A modern version of Colin McLaurin's Canadian-type hip disarticulation prosthesis. (Reproduced with permission from Baumgartner R. Amputation in Hüft- und Beckenbereich. In: Bauer R, Kerschbaumer F, Poisel S. Orthopädische Operationslehre, Becken und untere Extremität. 1995 © Georg Thieme Verlag).*

References

[1] Baumgartner R, Botta P. Amputation und Prothesenversorgung an der unteren Extremität. Stuttgart : Enke, 1995 : 182-191, 327-333

[2] Baumgartner R. Amputation in Hüft- und Beckenbereich. In: Bauer R, Kerschbaumer F, Poisel S eds. Orthopädische Operationslehre, Becken und untere Extremität. 1995 : 411-417 © Georg Thieme Verlag.

[3] Maurer P. Désarticulation de la hanche. *Encycl Méd Chir* (Éditions Scientifiques et Médicales Elsevier SAS, Paris), Techniques chirurgicales - Orthopédie-traumatologie, 44-106, 1960 : 7-8

[4] McLaurin CA. Hip disarticulation prosthesis, report n° 15, Toronto : Prosthetic Services Center, Department of Veterans Affairs, 1954

[5] Persson BM. Hip disarticulation, transiliac and sacroiliac amputations. In: Murdoch G, Wilson AB eds. Amputation: Surgical practice and patient management. London : Butterworth-Heinemann, 1995 : 141-144

[6] Radcliffe CW. The biomechanics of the Canadian-type hip disarticulation prosthesis. *Artif Limbs* 1957 ; 4 : 29-38

Hemipelvectomy (hindquarter amputation)

W Winkelmann

Abstract. – *A hemipelvectomy is required for primary malignant tumours or bone metastases of the bony pelvic girdle, and soft tissue sarcomas which cannot be resected with adequate surgical margins and without sacrificing too much of the pelvis and the neurovascular supply to the lower limb. Depending on the size and location of the tumour and the soft tissue extension, different levels of amputation and soft tissue removal are necessary. Therefore, we can distinguish the lower, total or extended hemipelvectomy. The morbidity from hemipelvectomy is high; wound problems from infection and flap necrosis are the most common problems. To avoid a flap necrosis, the preservation of the internal iliac vessels is very important. In the extended hemipelvectomy, the rate of wound problems is higher if the blood supply to the posterior flap is further diminished by the osteotomy and resection of the lateral part of the sacrum. The Canadian hip disarticulation prosthesis or its modifications are the standard prosthetic fitting.*

Keywords: hip, pelvis, hemipelvectolmy, hindquarter amputation, pelvic tumours.

Indication

Hemipelvectomy is indicated for malignant tumours of the pelvis involving the hip joint and the sciatic nerve.

Types of hemipelvectomy
(fig 1)

– Lower hemipelvectomy: for malignant tumours of the lower pelvis (fig 1A).

– Total hemipelvectomy: for malignant tumours involving the entire hip bone (fig 1B).

– Extended hemipelvectomy: for malignant tumours involving the whole hip bone, sacroiliac joint and parts of the sacrum (fig 1C).

Positioning and skin incisions

The patient lies in a lateral position on his unaffected side. The skin incision runs underneath the groin from medial to lateral,

Winfried Winkelmann, Professor Dr. med., Department of Orthopaedic Surgery, Westfälische Wilhelms-University, Münster, Germany.

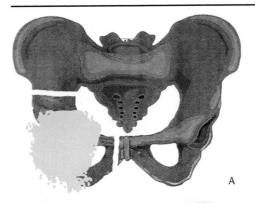

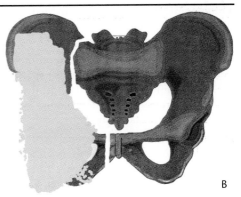

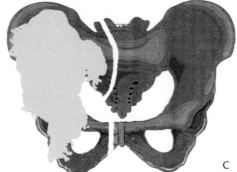

1 *Types of hemipelvectomy.*
A. Lower hemipelvectomy.
B. Total hemipelvectomy.
C. Extended hemipelvectomy.

and then along the iliac crest to the posterior iliac spine. It then bends distally behind the greater trochanter into the gluteal fold up to the adductors. Medially, it meets the beginning of the anterior incision (fig 2).

Surgical technique

After dividing the inguinal ligament and separating the abdominal wall muscles from the iliac crest, the inferior epigastric vessels

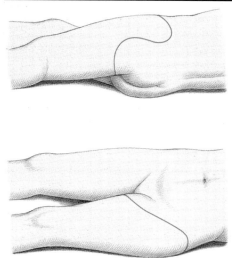

2 *Positioning of the patient and skin incisions. (Reproduced with permission from Winkelmann W. Beckenamputationen. In : Bauer R, Kerschbaumer F, Posiel S eds. Orthopädische Operationslehre 2/II; Becken und untere Extremität. Stuttgart : Thieme, 1995 © Georg Thieme Verlag.)*

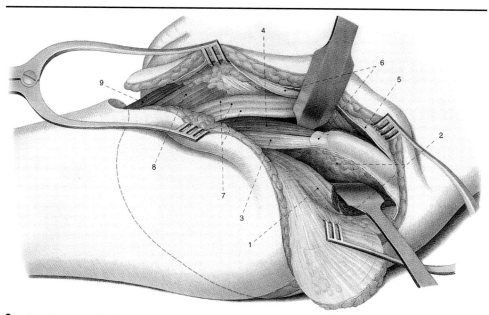

3 *Anterior approach to the pelvis. 1. Tensor fascia lata m.; 2. gluteus medius m.; 3. sartorius m.; 4. iliopsoas m.; 5. oblique externus et internus mm.; 6. inguinal ligament; 7. femoral vessels and nerve; 8. pectineus m.; 9. gracilis m. (Reproduced with permission from Winkelmann W. Beckenamputationen. In : Bauer R, Kerschbaumer F, Posiel S eds. Orthopädische Operationslehre 2/II; Becken und untere Extremität. Stuttgart : Thieme, 1995 © Georg Thieme Verlag.)*

are exposed, ligated and divided. Deep within the retroperitoneal space, the external iliac vessels and femoral nerve are identified and prepared (*fig 3*). The external iliac artery and vein are separated, individually clamped, doubly ligated (proximally with an additional needle suture), and divided. The femoral nerve is ligated and divided as far proximally as possible.

In type I hemipelvectomy, the tumour extension in almost all cases allows sparing the internal iliac vessels. The iliopsoas muscle is transected and the iliac bone exposed subperiostally (*fig 3*).

In type II and type III hemipelvectomies, depending on the extra-osseous extension of the tumour, the ilopsoas muscle must be divided at the level of L5/S1 or even higher. Of the internal iliac vessels, at least the superior gluteal vessels and nerves should be spared, if possible. In type II hemipelvectomy, the anterior sacro-iliac ligaments are exposed and divided stepwise. Severe bleeding from the presacral venous plexus is common at this stage of the operation.

Distally, the rectus abdominis and adductor muscles are detached from the pubic bone, which is subperiostally prepared medially up to the symphysis pubis. Depending on the intra-osseous extension of the tumour, the osteotomy of the pubic bone is planned, normally 1 cm lateral to the symphysis pubis. Injury to the bladder or urethra should be avoided during preparation and osteotomy of the pubic bone with a Gigli saw.

Dorso-laterally, in type I hemipelvectomy, the tensor fascia lata muscle and the gluteus medius muscle are dissected from the iliac crest. The gluteus maximus muscle is

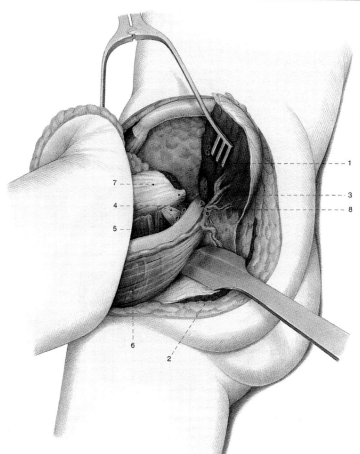

4 *Postero-lateral approach to the pelvis in type I hemipelvectomy 1. Gluteus medius and minimus mm.; 2. gluteus maximus m.; 3. piriformis m.; 4. gemellus superior m., obturator internus m., gemellus inferior m.; 5. quadratus femoris m.; 6. semitendinosus m.; 7. vastus lateralis m.; 8. glutealis inferior vessels, gluteus inferior nerve. (Reproduced with permission from Winkelmann W. Beckenamputationen. In : Bauer R, Kerschbaumer F, Posiel S eds. Orthopädische Operationslehre 2/II; Becken und untere Extremität. Stuttgart : Thieme, 1995 © Georg Thieme Verlag.)*

separated from the gluteus medius muscle, transected at its insertion at the greater trochanter and proximal femur, and retracted posteriorly. Vessels and nerves to the gluteus maximus muscle are preserved. The preservation of the gluteus maximus muscle is possible in almost all cases of hemipelvectomy type II or type III. The

greater sciatic foramen is prepared. The sciatic nerve is ligated and sharply divided; the pirifomis, gemelli and obturator internus muscles are dissected. The inferior gluteal vessels and nerves are clamped, ligated and dissected as well (*fig 4, 5*). From the inner and outer sides, retractors are brought into the sciatic foramen and, in type I

Hemipelvectomy (hindquarter amputation)

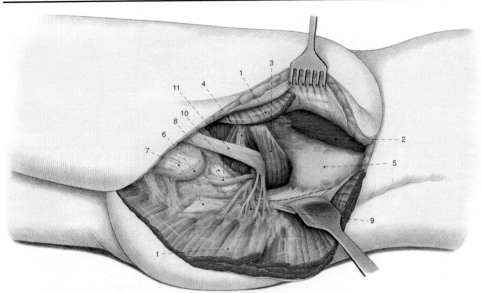

5 *Postero-lateral approach to the pelvis in type III hemipelvectomy. 1. Gluteus maximus m.; 2. gluteus minimus m.; 3. piriformis m.; 4. gemelli mm. and obturator internus m.; 5. iliac bone, posterior part; 6. ischial bone; 7. sacro-tuberal ligament; 8. sacro-spinal ligament; 9. gluteus inferior nerves and vessels; 10. pudendus nerve; 11. sciatic nerve. (Reproduced with permission from Winkelmann W. Beckenamputationen. In : Bauer R, Kerschbaumer F, Posiel S eds. Orthopädische Operationslehre 2/II; Becken und untere Extremität. Stuttgart : Thieme, 1995 © Georg Thieme Verlag.)*

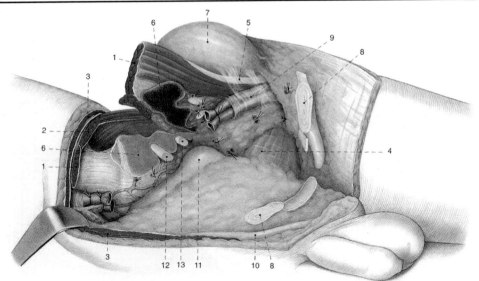

6 *View into the pelvis after osteotomy of the sacrum in type III hemipelvectomy. 1. Psoas major m.; 2. quadratus lumborum m.; 3. oblique externus and internus mm; 4. obturator internus m.; 5. femoral nerve; 6. sacrum (osteotomised); 7. tumour; 8. symphysis pubis; 9. iliaca communis vessels; 10. spermatic cord; 11. rectum; 12. sacralis I nerve root; 13. sacralis II nerve root. (Reproduced with permission from Winkelmann W. Beckenamputationen. In : Bauer R, Kerschbaumer F, Posiel S eds. Orthopädische Operationslehre 2/II; Becken und untere Extremität. Stuttgart : Thieme, 1995 © Georg Thieme Verlag.)*

hemipelvectomy, the iliac bone is osteotomised with a Gigli saw just above the hip joint. The hip is manipulated into maximal abduction and external rotation to open the inner pelvic area. The obturator nerve and vessels are clamped, ligated and dissected. After retraction of the bladder, the levator ani muscle and the coccygeus muscles are dissected.

After bringing the patient into a more prone position in type II and type III hemipelvectomy, the posterior iliac crest is exposed by detachment of the obliquus abdominis externus, obliquus abdominis internus and latissimus dorsi muscles. After dissection of the lumbo-dorsal fascia, the iliocostalis, quadratus lumborum and sacrospinal muscles and the iliolumbar ligaments are detached as well.

In type II hemipelvectomy, the posterior sacro-iliac ligaments are divided and the iliac bone is dislocated in the sacro-iliac joint.

In type III hemipelvectomy, depending on the intrasacral extension of the tumour, more or less of the sacrum will have to be resected. Kirschner wires are drilled in an exactly anterior-posterior direction from the inner to the outer side of the sacrum. With broad chisels, the osteotomy of the sacrum is performed along these Kirschner wires. Because the sacral nerve roots S3 to S5 are very important for the innervation of the bladder and the rectum, it is important to avoid damaging them. During this part of the operation, severe bleeding is unavoidable. This can only be controlled after the osteotomy of the sacrum, and therefore after the amputation has been completed *(fig 6)*. The anaesthetists and surgeons should be prepared for this specific phase of the operation which can be highly dangerous for the patient.

After a careful check of the ligated vessels and insertion of two large Redon drains, the gluteus maximus muscle is sutured to the divided margins of the inguinal ligament and the medial and lateral abdominal wall muscles.

The fascia and subcutaneous tissues are closed *(fig 7)*. In most cases, the overlying skin is resected so that the closure is free of tension and creases. Wide compression dressings are applied over the wound to prevent deep haematoma.

Prosthesis [1, 2]

The Canadian type prosthesis designed by C. A. McLurin in 1953 [3] permits good results in hip disarticulation. In hemipelvectomy, however, the same quality result is more difficult to achieve when a larger amount of the pelvis has been removed. The ischial tuberosity and the iliac crest are the most important landmarks.

The amputee sits rather than stands on the prosthetic socket *(fig 8)*. Therefore, amputation techniques should avoid operative scars in the weight-bearing area as well as "dog-ears".

During the stance phase, the pelvis will tend to tilt medially. This tendency is controlled by a rim at the inner side of the ramus ossis publis (the same principle applies for the ischial containment socket in transfemoral stumps). Lateral displacement of the prosthesis is also controlled by a precise fit over the iliac crests. In hemipelvectomy, the telescoping of the pelvis is reduced by means of a socket design which stimulates the iliac crest at the amputed side and which covers the lower part of the rib cage.

Stability is achieved by positioning the hip joint on the anterior part of the socket. This alignment permits stability during the stance phase. In the swing phase, the prosthetic hip and knee joints are activated by tilting the pelvis in the frontal plane.

Results are best in unilateral hip disarticulation. As a rule, a cane is used for walking on uneven ground. In hemipel-

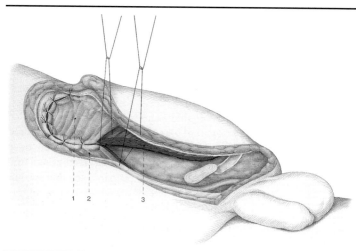

7 *Wound closure. 1. Gluteus medius m.; 2. obliqus abdominis externus m.; 3. gluteus maximus m. (Reproduced with permission from Winkelmann W. Beckenamputationen. In : Bauer R, Kerschbaumer F, Posiel S eds. Orthopädische Operationslehre 2/II; Becken und untere Extremität. Stuttgart : Thieme, 1995 © Georg Thieme Verlag.)*

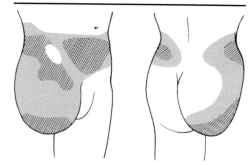

8 *The amputee sits rather than stands on the prosthetic socket. Amputation techniques should therefore avoid scars in the weight-bearing area. (Reproduced with permission from Baumgartner R, Botta P. Amputation und Prosthesenversorgung der unteren Extremiät. Enke 1995 © Georg Thieme Verlag.)*

vectomy, the distance the patient can walk is limited. In bilateral amputations, it is still possible for the patient to walk, but most prefer a wheelchair with an extended wheelbase, a seat bucket and a safety belt.

References

[1] Baumgartner R, Botta P. Amputation und Prosthesenversorgung der unteren Extremität. Stuttgart : Thieme, 1995 : 327-333

[2] Lyquist E. Biomechanics of the hip disarticulation prosthesis. In : Murdoch G, Wilson AB Jr eds. Amputation. Oxford : Butterworth-Heinemann, 1996

[3] McLaurin CA. The Candian hip disarticulation prosthesis. *Artif Limbs* 1957 ; 22-28

[4] Winkelmann W. Beckenamputationen. In : Bauer R, Kerschbaumer F, Posiel S eds. Orthopädische Operationslehre 2/II; Becken und untere Extremität. Stuttgart : Thieme, 1995 : 3345-3353

Resection and reconstruction in proximal femoral malignancies

F Langlais

Abstract. – For primary tumours of the proximal femur which do not involve the hip joint, a wide margin, favoured by precise per-operative planning, is the most important factor in the oncologic prognosis. Significant functional improvement is obtained by reconstructing the proximal femur by a composite allograft total hip prosthesis: the tendons of the patient's gluteal muscles are sutured to the tendons of the allograft, achieving good control of active abduction and stability.

When the primary tumour has extended to the hip joint, en bloc resection of the proximal femur, of the articulation, and of the acetabular zone is necessary, followed by reconstruction by a composite femoral total hip replacement (THR) and a bulk acetabular allograft.

In metastases, the palliative tumour excision is treated by a standard reconstruction THR without allograft. The aim of this more simple operation is to achieve a stable hip (if possible by a transtrochantereric slide-digastric approach) with early and painless full weight-bearing.

Keywords: hip, femur, primary malignant tumour, metastasis at the proximal femur, wide excision, composite THR, reconstruction prosthesis, acetabular reconstruction.

The proximal femur is a common target for malignant tumours.

The proximal femur is the second most common site of primary bone tumours, after the knee (distal femur and proximal tibia). Reconstruction usually involves total hip arthroplasty, which is now generally performed using the allograft-prosthesis composite technique. The allograft is composed primarily of bone, often with a tendon component. When used in combination with chemotherapy, femoral reconstruction allows to salvage the limb in nine-tenths of the cases and to cure the tumour permanently in two-thirds of the cases.

The femoral metaphysis is the main site of development of limb bone metastases. When internal fixation is not feasible, palliative excision of the tumour, followed by implantation of a total reconstruction prosthesis, is performed. This technique allows early ambulation and provides significant improvements in self-sufficiency.

Introduction

We will discuss three surgical techniques for proximal femoral malignancies.

Frantz Langlais, M.D., Professor and Chairman, Department of Orthopaedic and Reconstructive Surgery (S.C.O.R.), University Hospital Sud, 16, boulevard de Bulgarie, 35056 Rennes, France.

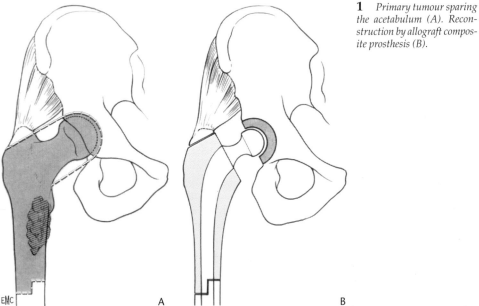

1 *Primary tumour sparing the acetabulum (A). Reconstruction by allograft composite prosthesis (B).*

Radical treatment of primary tumours (sparing the acetabulum) by the allograft-prosthesis composite technique (fig 1). This is the preferred technique in primary tumours (osteosarcoma, chondrosarcoma, Ewing's tumour, malignant fibrous histiocytoma, etc.) requiring extensive excision [4, 11]. In a very small number of cases, it can be used for the curative treatment of an apparently solitary metastasis from a primary tumour that appears to be cured; in this situation, it sometimes allows complete eradication of the malignant disease (e.g. in patients with thyroid cancer).

Palliative treatment in proximal femoral metastases (fig 2). Surgeons resort to this method only when internal fixation is not feasible because of extensive osteolysis or if it has failed because of tumour progression. In the latter situation, the internal fixation usually consisted of a screw-plate or reconstruction nail. The palliative technique

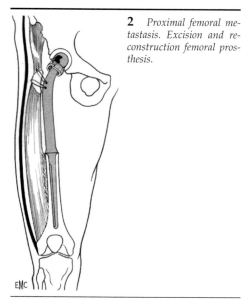

2 *Proximal femoral metastasis. Excision and reconstruction femoral prosthesis.*

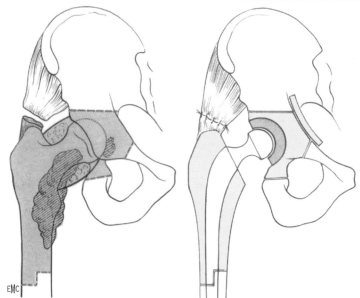

3 *Primary tumour extended to the acetabulum: reconstruction by an acetabular and femoral allograft composite total hip prosthesis.*

consists of resection followed by arthroplasty. Its goal is not to achieve mandatory complete tumour excision, but rather to reduce the tumour burden and to allow early painless weight-bearing and, if appropriate, early adjuvant treatment, for instance by radiation. In most cases, a reconstruction prosthesis without an allograft is implanted, ensuring excellent stability and ambulation within the first few postoperative days [9, 17].

Treatment of primary tumours of the proximal femur extended to the acetabulum (fig 3). The method used varies with the extent of the tumour and the general health status of the patient. In young patients who can be treated by extensive excision, we reconstruct the femur using the allograft-prosthesis composite technique, and the acetabulum using a massive acetabular allograft. In patients whose general condition is less satisfactory, the acetabulum is not reconstructed, and a saddle prosthesis, articulating with the lower edge of the iliac wing, is implanted [1].

Resection-reconstruction of primary tumours sparing the acetabulum

PRINCIPLES OF RESECTION AND RECONSTRUCTION

■ *Planning the resection*

The bone lesion is removed by cutting at least 3 cm under the edge of the tumour identified by MRI. The soft tumour tissue is excised with a 1 to 2 cm margin around the areas of suspected involvement on imaging studies. The joint is considered to be spared by the tumour if the proximal pole of the lesion is at a distance from the attachment of the synovial membrane on the femoral neck, and if there is no MRI evidence of a joint effusion. When an effusion is seen, it is

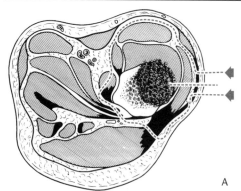

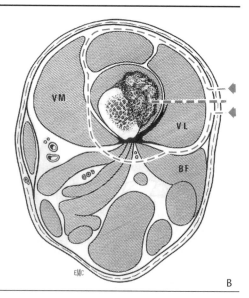

4 *Primary tumour of the proximal femur: resection margins at the level of the lesser trochanter (A) and of the diaphysis (B).*
VM: Vastus medialis; VL: vastus lateralis; BF: biceps femoris.

aspirated to look for malignant cells. If any are found, single-block removal of the acetabulum is performed.

In tumours confined to the proximal femur, the following structures are removed as a single block with the bone (fig 4A, B):

– the capsular sheath, attached to the trochanteric line; a 2 cm-wide capsular flange can be left adjacent to the acetabulum and used to stabilise the prosthesis;

– the greater trochanter and a flange of the gluteus medius and gluteus minimus tendons attached to it;

– the distal tendon of the ilio-psoas muscle and the distal part of this muscle contiguous to the capsule;

– the quadriceps overlying the bone defect, i.e. the entire rectus femoris, the vastus lateralis with the lateral intermuscular septum to which it is attached, and the vastus medialis;

– the trochanteric attachments of the gemelli, obturator, and quadratus femoris muscles, as well as the femoral attachments of the adductors and the gluteus maximus.

■ *Planning the reconstruction*

A total hip prosthesis is generally used in adults. In young patients with an open acetabular growth plate, the preferred method is implantation of a bipolar femoral prosthesis [18] without acetabular resurfacing. The stem is cemented into the diaphysis and allograft. Use of antibiotic-loaded bone cement provides immediate stabilisation of the allograft and, at the same time, produces high levels of antibiotics around the operative site, thus protecting the prosthesis and allograft from infection during the bacteremic episodes common during chemotherapy. Furthermore, chemotherapy slows bone ingrowth, giving added importance to the immediate stable fixation provided by cementing. Ten-year outcomes in patients with cemented prostheses are encouraging. However, the acetabular cup and the part of the stem located within the remaining femur can be implanted without cement, but cement should be used to secure the stem to the allograft.

The size of the stem should be selected so that the stem lodges firmly within the femoral shaft at the resection site, after removal of the cancellous bone but without reaming of the endocortex. The length of the stem located within the patient's femur should be about 120 to 150 mm. We generally use a Charnley Kerboull type prosthesis, whose 22-mm head causes very little wear of the polyethylene cup. The cup can be either standard or equipped with a posterosuperior wall that passively limits the risk of posterosuperior dislocation.

■ *Planning the allograft*

We use a cryopreserved, non-irradiated [8, 13] allograft including 2 to 3 cm of the tendons attaching the gluteus medius and minimus muscles to the greater trochanter. The allograft should be wide enough to accommodate the previously-selected prosthesis [6]. The allograft-prosthesis composite technique is the method that provides the best active abduction, because it allows reimplantation of the medius and minimus gluteus muscles. To date, there is no failproof method for directly reimplanting tendons onto a metallic prosthesis. Thus, reimplantation on an allograft is the only means of obtaining a satisfactory functional outcome (with a 4/5 or 5/5 active abduction score in over two-thirds of cases). Furthermore, reimplantation of the soft tissues onto the allograft provides good passive stability and, in our experience, reduces the risk of prosthetic dislocation despite the extensive muscular resection. The allograft is interfaced with the patient's femoral shaft by a step-cut junction, which provides excellent control of rotations. This may contribute to reducing shear rotation strains on the femur-prosthesis interface, thus increasing the life-span of prosthetic bonding.

THE STEPS OF THE RESECTION

■ *Positioning the patient and making the incision*

The patient is lying on one side. A folding field is placed at the anterior aspect of the table to receive the limb during reconstruction.

The total length of the incision is about 30 cm: a 20 to 25 cm incision along the lateral aspect of the shaft, following the axis of the femur, is carried 8 to 10 cm into the buttock by slightly angling the direction of the incision backwards. The incision circumscribes the biopsy track, at a distance of about 10 to 15 mm from it. The subcutaneous tissue and fascia lata are incised using the same pattern, but are removed in a single block with the tumour. On either side of the biopsy site, the fascia lata is opened longitudinally. The aponeurosis of the gluteus maximus is incised, and the muscle is dissociated.

■ *Posterior then anterior dissection*

With the limb in extension and internal rotation (*fig 5A, B*), the piriformis, the

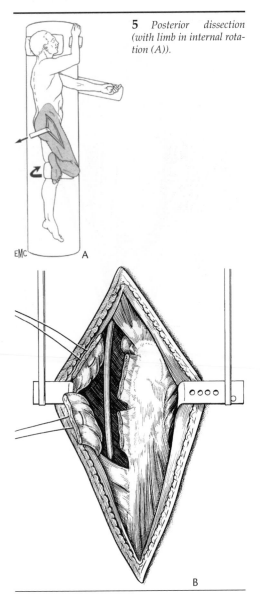

5 *Posterior dissection (with limb in internal rotation (A)).*

curtain formed by the gemelli, the obturator internus, and the quadratus femoris are identified and severed 2 to 3 cm from the posterior intertrochanteric line. A traction suture is inserted into their proximal ends. The ischiadic nerve is protected by pulling the cut muscles over to the back. The vastus lateralis is separated from the fascia femoralis, and the intermuscular septum is cut at the line of attachment of the vastus lateralis. The ischiadic nerve is identified at the upper edge of the diaphyseal gluteus maximus tendon and is displaced medially. The attachment of the deep portion of the gluteus maximus is severed 2 cm from the linea aspera. The dissection is carried downward to the site of the planned bony resection.

The thigh is then placed in slight flexion and external rotation (*fig 6A, B*). The quadriceps is separated from the femoral aponeurosis, all the way to the dihedral angle formed by the medial edge of the vastus medialis and the anterior aspect of the adductor muscles, travelling posterior to the tensor fasciae latae and the sartorius. The ilio-psoas muscle is cut above the lesser trochanter, and the body of the muscle is

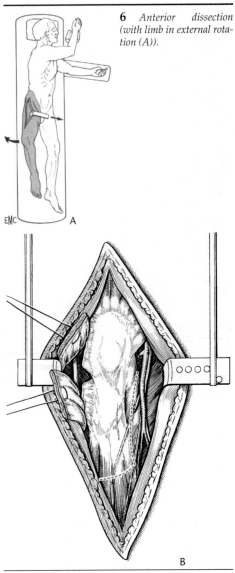

6 *Anterior dissection (with limb in external rotation (A)).*

retracted medially, sometimes in its entirety, but often after dissociation of the muscle, leaving a few fibres adherent to the capsule. Medially, several branches of the deep femoral artery are ligated, most notably the medial circumflex artery and the trunk of the quadricipital and lateral circumflex arteries. Some branches of the femoral nerve for the rectus femoris and vastus lateralis are severed.

■ *Proximal and distal sections*

The anterior and posterior edges of the gluteal muscles are isolated, and the muscles are cut using a diathermic scalpel, leaving a 1 to 2 cm ruff on the trochanter. The tumour is approached by passing between the deep aspect of the gluteal muscles and the superficial aspect of the capsule. The muscles are lifted using two or three Steinmann pin retractors. The top of the greater trochanter is marked by a needle and the distal cut is made 150 mm below (*fig 7A*).

The quadriceps is cut using a diathermic scalpel, above the bony section. The distance between the supra-acetabular pin and the level of the resection is measured (here, 180 mm). At completion of the reconstruction stage, the distance between the

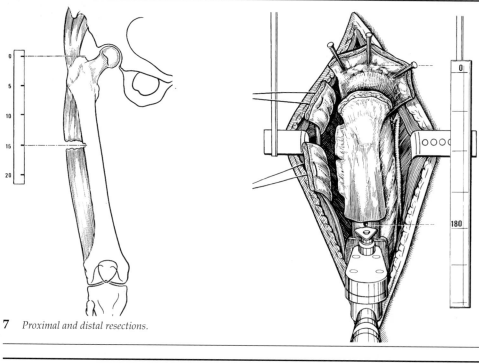

7 *Proximal and distal resections.*

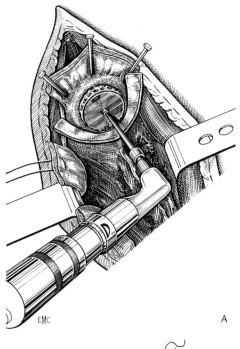

A

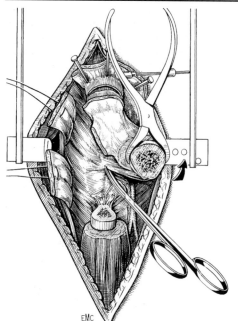

A

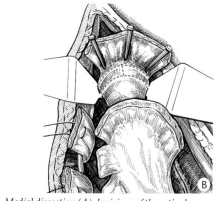

B

8 *Medial dissection (A). Incisions of the articular capsule (B).*

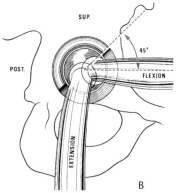

B

9 *Preparing the patient's acetabulum (A) and cup positioning (B).*

level of the bony section and the pin should be kept unchanged to ensure that the two lower limbs remain of equal length (*fig 7B*).

■ ***Medial dissection*** (*fig 8A, B*)

During this last step of the dissection, the distal end of the metaphyseal fragment is grasped using forceps and gradually lifted in abduction. This places tension on the muscles attached to the linea aspera: the gluteus maximus posteriorly and the adductor muscles medially. Clips are placed on the perforating arteries, which travel within the attachments of the adductor muscles. The muscles are severed one by one, working from the bony resection site to the femoral head, as the proximal femur is increasingly abducted. The external obturator muscle is cut at the lower edge of

the capsule. At this point, the only remaining connection between the femoral epiphysis and the acetabulum is the capsular sheath, which is cut circumferentially 2 cm from the acetabular rim. The head is removed through a superior longitudinal incision through the capsular flange.

THE RECONSTRUCTION STAGE

■ ***Preparing the acetabulum*** (*fig 9A, B*)

The limb is placed in the folding field, the capsule is cut into two flaps attached inferiorly, and the pulvinar is resected. The acetabulum is prepared as usual for THR. While this is being done, the acetabular cup is cemented at 10° of anteversion and 35° of horizontal tilt.

■ ***Preparing the femur***

Rotary broaches are used to remove the cancellous bone. Care should be taken to check that the stem of the prosthesis enters the shaft only with considerable friction and lodges securely at the desired level.

■ ***Preparing the allograft*** (*fig 10A*)

A proximal femur allograft is used. It is a "combined" allograft, as it associates bone (proximal femur) and tendons (trochanteric attachments of the terminal gluteal tendons). The shaft is cut 2 to 3 cm further down than necessary. The allograft is reamed until its diameter equals at least that of the distal femoral preparation. The epiphysis is cut at the intertrochanteric line. A rotary broach is used to remove the metaphyseal cancellous bone. The match between the prosthesis and allograft is checked.

A step-cut junction (5 to 8 mm high) is fashioned to ensure rotational stability of the allograft [14].

■ ***Cementing the prosthesis***

The prosthesis is cemented after distal obturation. A low-viscosity, antibiotic-loaded cement is injected using a syringe,

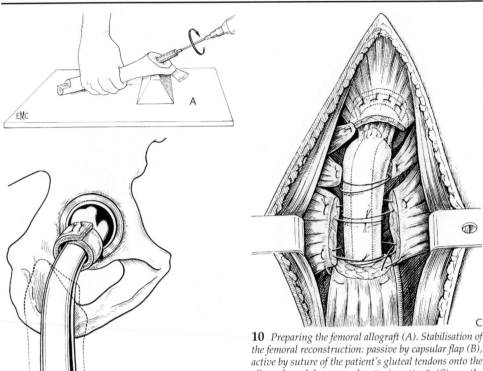

10 *Preparing the femoral allograft (A). Stabilisation of the femoral reconstruction: passive by capsular flap (B), active by suture of the patient's gluteal tendons onto the allograft and by muscular "reinsertion" (C) on the allograft.*

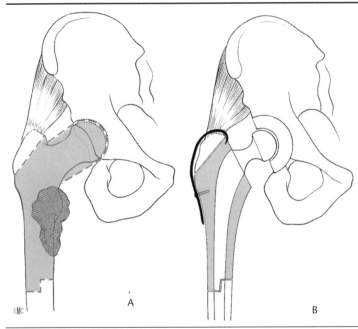

11 *Primary tumour sparing the major trochanter: approach through a trochanteric osteotomy (A). Reconstruction by a femoral allograft on which the patient's trochanter is fixed by a hookplate (B).*

from distal to proximal. The recipient femur is injected first. The prosthesis is then introduced into the cement-filled allograft. Lastly, the stem of the prosthesis is pushed into the recipient femur.

■ *Stabilising the prosthesis* (fig 10B, C)

Three means are used to achieve stabilisation.

– Passive stabilisation of the head is obtained by performing an overlapping suture of the two capsular flaps to the upper edge of the neck. The flaps left attached to the area of the acetabular horns constitute a powerful anti-dislocation sling that does not limit prosthesis motion [16].

– Active stabilisation by the gluteus medius and minimus muscles plays a key role [11, 15]. Strong reattachment is achieved by securing the intramuscular tendinous lamina of the patient's gluteus muscles to the allograft tendons, using a overlapping suture. The other muscles are moved closer to the prosthesis. A few autografts (collected, for instance, from the acetabular anchoring sites) can be added to the junction, as well as chips from the medial part of the resected femoral head, if this structure is clearly free of cancer.

– The superficial planes are painstakingly reconstructed, taking special care to suture the fascia lata and the gluteus maximum aponeurosis. Several suction drains are inserted.

■ *After-care*

The patient is left in bed for about one week. Isometric contractions of the quadriceps and passive extension-flexion movements of the knee are started early, with the patient lying on the side. Walking with two crutches and no weight-bearing is allowed during the first 20 days, then with slight weight-bearing until the sixth week. Only then are abductor exercises started. Use of a crutch on the contralateral side is recommended during the first three months, until attachment of the gluteal muscles to the allograft is complete. Chemotherapy can be restarted on the tenth postoperative day.

■ *Special case: other abductor reconstructions* (fig 11A, B)

In most patients, there is extensive spread of the tumour to the greater trochanter, requiring its resection and that of the gluteus medius and maximus tendons. This is the technique described above. In some moderately aggressive tumors, however (e.g. chondrosarcoma), MRI findings convincingly demonstrate that the tumour is at a distance from the greater trochanter. In this situation, a transtrochanteric osteotomy can be performed, starting from the attachment ridge of the vastus lateralis and removing a 4-cm high and 10-mm thick fragment from the greater trochanter. At the end of the procedure, this fragment is placed on the trochanteric area of the recut allograft and secured using a hook plate. After-care is the same as above.

OUTCOMES AND COMPLICATIONS

After extensive excision, the oncologic outcome is favourable in three-quarters of patients whose post-chemotherapy tumour necrosis studies indicate a good response.

Postoperative dislocation is the main mechanical complication [3]. It is extremely rare if a capsular sling is fashioned and care is taken to ensure that the two lower limbs are of equal length. To obtain satisfactory abductor muscle function, abduction exercises should not be started until the healing process is well advanced. This is true whether the reconstruction technique involved suturing the patient's tendons to the allograft tendon, or internal fixation of the greater trochanter.

Data from the literature show far better functional outcomes with the allograft-prosthesis composite technique [5, 10, 21] than with reconstruction prostheses [19]. Reconstruction prostheses do not allow satisfactory reattachment of the abductor muscles and result in a significant limp in one-third of cases; in addition, 4/5 or 5/5 abduction strength is achieved in only one-third of cases [9]. The risk of dislocation is almost completely eliminated with the allograft-prosthesis composite technique, which provides 4/5 or 5/5 abduction strength in two-thirds of cases.

Resection-reconstruction for palliative excision of a metastasis

PRINCIPLES OF THE RESECTION AND RECONSTRUCTION *(fig 2)*

Whereas in the radical resections described above, top priority is given to achieving complete excision, which is the key to a full recovery, here complete excision is not feasible. The main goal of the procedure is to provide short-term functional gains to a patient with a limited life expectancy. To achieve this, the tumour burden must be reduced in a way that allows rapid resumption of function with minimal morbidity. Adjuvant treatments can then be used to further reduce the tumour. The challenge is therefore to strike the best compromise between the extent of the excision, and the stability of the joint during active and passive motion. At the femur, most of the tumour is removed, and a mechanically satisfactory prosthesis implantation site is identified, based on the appearance of the cortices on plain radiographs since the reconstruction prosthesis rests on the cut bone surface. Either a single-block prosthesis (from a range including several resection lengths) or a modular prosthesis can be used. Modular prostheses are more versatile, and the risk of junction corrosion, which is their main disadvantage, is irrelevant in patients with a limited life expectancy. Sagittal orifices in the trochanteric region are useful for securing the abductor muscles. A 32-mm head provides good passive stability, and its shorter life span is of no consequence in these patients. For the acetabular reconstruction, if the bone is not involved, a cup with a posterosuperior wall limiting the risk of dislocation should be used. If the texture of the bony acetabulum is altered by the tumour or by osteoporosis, augmentation by acetabular rings is used. If needed, long screws anchored in healthy bone in the iliac wing or obturator ring are used to increase the stability of the cemented cup. If the acetabulum is known to be uninvolved by the tumour, a bipolar prosthesis can be used since it offers very good stability. The allograft-prosthesis composite technique is not recommended in the palliative treatment of metastases because its main advantage is to allow reattachment of the muscles, which is not a priority in palliative procedures, since these require only moderate muscle resection. In addition, the allograft-prosthesis composite technique is a burdensome procedure that is justified only for curative therapy.

Stabilisation of the prosthesis is an essential goal since early weight-bearing to improve

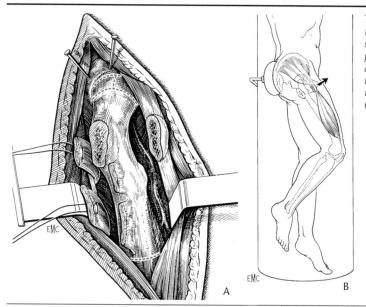

12 *Palliative resection of a metastasis, and femoral reconstruction prosthesis. Approach through a trochanteric digastric osteotomy (A). The trochanter anterior displacement is obtained by hip flexion (B).*

quality of life is the main reason for the procedure. To achieve this goal, a digastric muscle is fashioned from the gluteus medius, greater trochanter and vastus lateralis. The capsule is left in place so that an overlapping suture can be made above the prosthetic neck. At the end of the procedure, the trochanter is secured to the lateral part of the prosthesis to improve stability. If resection of the trochanter or vastus lateralis is required, the hip is stabilised by suturing the tendons of the gluteus medius and minimus muscles to the deep aspect of the fascia lata.

EXCISION *(fig 12A, B)*

The patient is placed on the side as for the radical procedure. The skin incision is the same. After incision of the fascia lata, a digastric muscle is prepared by identifying the anterior and posterior edges of the gluteus medius and minimus muscles, and distally the vastus lateralis, which is separated from the lateral intermuscular septum. Marginal resection is performed to provide access to the deep aspect of the quadriceps muscle. The tumour is often confined to the bone, and in this case is dissected in the subperiosteal or extraperiosteal plane, whichever is associated with less bleeding. If the tumour has spread to the muscle, it is dissected at the junction with healthy tissue. The trochanter is then cut from back to front, and left attached to the glutei and vastus. The hip is placed in flexion. This displaces the trochanteric fragment anteriorly. The joint capsule can then be opened, leaving two capsular flaps as in the radical procedure. The hip is dislocated. The level of the femoral resection is determined in relation to the upper edge of the greater trochanter. The proximal femur is resected.

RECONSTRUCTION *(fig 13)*

The preparation and acetabular cementing phases are as described above. Cementing of the femoral component is done by injecting a low-viscosity antibiotic-loaded cement through a syringe. Stability is provided by a cup with a posterosuperior wall, a large diameter femoral head, and a capsular sling tightened at the upper edge of the neck. The trochanter is put back in place with the limb in extension and wired on the prosthesis. Ambulation with weight-bearing is allowed as early as the first week if it is painless, with two crutches, then with an ordinary cane.

No effort should be made to obtain marked flexion of the hip during the first six weeks, which is the time needed for the periarticular soft tissues to heal. Radiation therapy (and, if appropriate, chemotherapy) can be restarted on the tenth postoperative day.

The outcomes and complications seen with reconstruction prostheses have been discussed above (comparison of the allograft-prosthesis composite technique and the reconstruction prosthesis technique).

Primary femoral tumour with spread to the acetabulum

We will describe single-block excision of the proximal femur, hip joint, and acetabulum *(fig 3)*. Reconstruction is achieved using the allograft-prosthesis composite technique at the femur and an allograft at the acetabulum [2, 7, 12]. The saddle prosthesis technique will be described in the section on pelvic tumours.

A tumour of the proximal femur with spread to the acetabulum requires single-block excision of the proximal femur, entire intracapsular part of the joint, and acetabular part of the coxal bone. The boundaries of the resected acetabular area consist of a horizontal line at the upper edge of the capsule, and two lines on the ischiopubic and iliopubic rami.

The approach is a "Y" whose vertical segment allows dissection of the femur and

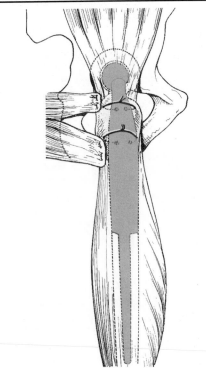

13 *Reconstruction prosthesis stabilisation. The trochanter is fixed by metal wires into the prosthesis. The piriformis and gluteus maximus tendons are reinserted.*

whose two other segments are carried anteriorly and posteriorly to allow lifting of the gluteal muscles and exposure of the anterior and posterior columns of the acetabulum. The steps of the resection phase are the same as above: preparation of the anterior and posterior aspects of the femur, section of the gluteal tendons, and preparation of the anterior and posterior edges of the acetabulum. The femur is cut and the medial aspect of the femur dissected. After performing the three acetabular osteotomies, the femur and acetabulum can be removed. Femoral reconstruction is achieved using the allograft-prosthesis composite technique. At the acetabulum, an allograft is secured to the ilium by two large screws and to the iliopubic and ilioischiatic rami by additional screws. Two autografts 6 to 7 cm in length and 1 to 2 cm in width, harvested from the contralateral iliac wing, are placed at the deep aspect of the allograft.

EXCISION

The first step is to harvest any allografts that may be needed from the contralateral iliac wing.

■ *Approach* (fig 14)

The Y-shaped approach is derived from the Ollier approach. The vertical segment is an incision about 15 cm long made along the lateral aspect of the femur, through the biopsy site. The proximal end of this incision is 4 to 5 cm under the ridge of the vastus lateralis, on the greater trochanter. Posteriorly, the incision is carried toward the

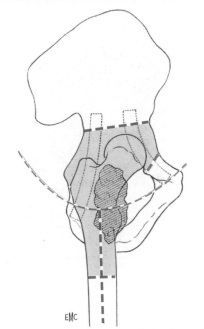

14 *Primary femoral tumour extended to the acetabulum. A triradiated Y-shaped Ollier's approach is used.*

posterosuperior iliac spine along the axis of the fibres of the gluteus maximus, as in the Kocher-Langenbeck approach. Anteriorly, the incision extends more horizontally through the tensor fasciae latae and sartorius, all the way to the medial edge of the iliopsoas muscle. The anterior and posterior edges of the gluteus minimus and medius muscles are isolated, and the tendons are cut 1 to 2 cm from the greater trochanter. The iliac bone is exposed 2 to 3 cm above the upper attachment of the capsule by lifting the gluteus muscles from the joint capsule using Steinmann pin retractors.

■ *Preparing the femoral excision*

This step is carried out as described above.

■ *Preparing the acetabulum*
(fig 15A, B, C)

The anterior edge of the capsule is dissected to allow access to the anterior edge of the iliac bone, which is exposed to the emergence of the superior pubic ramus. Hohmann retractors are placed on either side of this area, taking care to avoid the obturator bundle. The bone is cut using a saw. The quadratus femoris and gemelli muscles are detached from the posterior intertrochanteric line and reclined posteriorly to protect the ischiadic nerve. The upper third of the ilioischiatic ramus is exposed and cut using a saw protected by Hohmann retractors.

Using a rasp and under control of the surgeon's finger, the deep medial aspect of the acetabulum is exposed, working from its anterior and posterior edges toward its superior edge. A protective gauze pad is put in place.

■ *Section of the femoral shaft and periacetabular area*

The femoral shaft is cut, then pulled gradually in abduction and severed from its medial connections all the way to the inferior edge of the joint, where the external obturator muscle is cut. The pelvis is cut using a saw, horizontally, at the upper edge of the capsular attachment. The femur, joint and acetabulum are then removed as a single block, after section of a few extensions of the sacrosciatic ligaments.

RECONSTRUCTION

■ *Acetabular reconstruction*

An allograft is used to reconstruct the acetabulum (fig 16).

When the adjustment is satisfactory, fixation is achieved using four large screws. Two screws go from the roof of the allograft acetabulum toward the iliac wing of the recipient and two are used for fixation of the pubis and ischium. These cannulated screws are introduced on pins inserted through the pubic and ischiatic anchoring holes of the cup; the pubic pin is centred in the medullary cavity of the pubis and the ischiatic pin passes through the ischial tuberosity. The cup can then be cemented in place, tilted at the desired angle. Finally, the two autografts are placed at the deep aspect of the acetabulum, along the anterior and posterior columns.

■ *Femoral reconstruction*

Femoral reconstruction, stabilisation, and soft tissue closure are performed as described above. Full weight-bearing is not allowed until the third month.

This complex reconstruction technique provides similar functional outcomes to those seen with an allograft-prosthesis composite. However, the long term outcomes [20] are not well known, since our earliest cases now have follow-ups of only ten years.

Conclusion

In primary malignant tumours of the proximal femur, modern techniques using a composite hip prothesis, associating a prosthesis and an allograft (composed of bone and, whenever possible, of tendon) have provided significant functional gains, most notably with respect to stability and abductor muscle reattachment, without increasing morbidity rates. When reconstruction of the pelvis is also needed, the acetabular allograft technique can be useful and has yielded extremely encouraging medium-term results. In the palliative treatment of metastases, the simpler reconstruction prosthesis technique significantly improves quality of life and causes little morbidity.

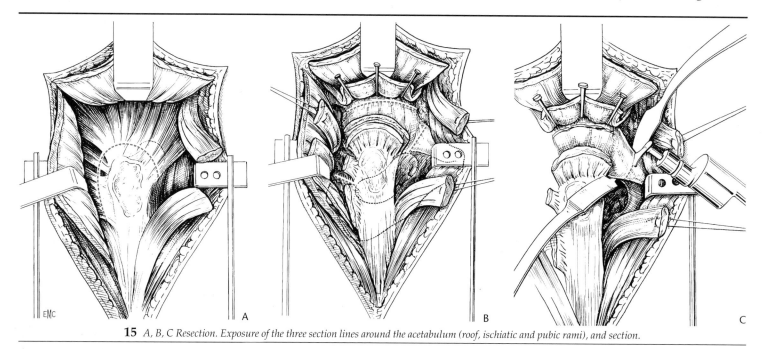

15 *A, B, C Resection. Exposure of the three section lines around the acetabulum (roof, ischiatic and pubic rami), and section.*

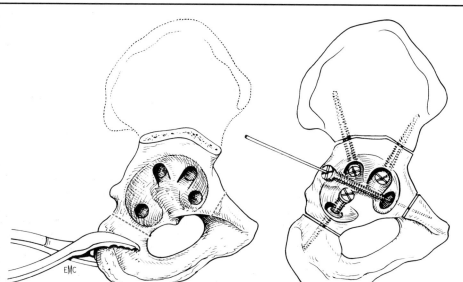

16 *Reconstruction. Fixation of the acetabular allograft to the patient's remaining pelvic bone.*

References

[1] Aboulafia AJ, Buch R, Mathews J, Li W, Malawer M. Reconstruction using the Saddle prosthesis following excision of primary and metastatic periacetabular tumors. *Clin Orthop* 1995 ; 314 : 203-213

[2] Abudu A, Grimer RJ, Cannon SR, Carter SR, Sneath RS. Reconstruction of the hemipelvis after excision of malignant tumours. *J Bone Joint Surg Br* 1997 ; 79 : 773-779

[3] Anract P, Coste J, Vastel L, Jeanrot C, Mascard E, Tomeno B. Proximal femoral reconstruction with mega prosthesis versus allograft prosthesis composite (41 cases). *Rev Chir Orthop* 2000 ; 86 : 278-288

[4] Clarke H, Berry D, Sim F. Salvage of failed femoral megaprostheses with allograft prosthesis composites. *Clin Orthop* 1998 ; 356 : 222-229

[5] Gitelis S, Heligman Quill G, Piasecki. The use of large allografts for tumor reconstruction and salvage of the failed total hip arthroplasty. *Clin Orthop* 1988 ; 231 : 62-70

[6] Giurea A, Paternostro M, Heinz-Peer G, Kaider A, Gottsauner-Wolf F. Function of reinserted abductor muscles after femoral replacement. *J Bone Joint Surg Br* 1998 ; 80 : 284-287

[7] Harrington KD. The use of hemipelvic allograft or autoclaved graft for reconstruction after wide resections of malignant tumors of the pelvis. *J Bone Joint Surg Am* 1992 ; 74 : 331-341

[8] Hernigou P, Delepine G, Goutallier D, Julieron A. Massive allografts-sterilized by irradiation. Clinical results. *J Bone Joint Surg Br* 1993 ; 75 : 904-913

[9] Langlais F, Aubriot JH, Postel M, Tomeno B, Vielpeau C. Prothèse de reconstruction de hanches pour tumeur. *Rev Chir Orthop* 1986 ; 72 : 415-425

[10] Langlais F, Delepine G, Dubousset JF, Missenard G. Composite prostheses in malignant tumors : rationale and preliminary results of 42 cases. In : Langlais F, Tomeno B eds. Limb salvage. Berlin : Springer Verlag, 1991 : 1-826

[11] Langlais F, Thomazeau H, Attali JY, Haykal G, Dréano T. Functionnal improvement of proximal femoral reconstructions by allografts composite prostheses (22 cases). 9th Symposium International Society of Limb Salvage (ISOLS), New York, 1997 : [abstract] : 60

[12] Langlais F, Vielpeau C. Allograft of hemipelvis after tumor resection. Technical aspects of 4 cases. *J Bone Joint Surg Br* 1989 ; 70 : 58-62

[13] Loty B, Courpied JP, Tomeno B, Postel M, Forest M, Abelanet R. Bone allografts sterilised by irradiation. Biological properties, procurement and results of 150 massive allografts. *Int Orthop* 1990 ; 14 : 237-242

[14] Markel M, Wood S, Bogdanske J, Rapoff A, Kalscheur V, Bouvy B et al. Comparison of allograft/endoprosthetic composites with a stepcut or transverse osteotomy configuration. *J Orthop Res* 1995 ; 13 : 639-641

[15] Markel M, Wood S, Bogdanske J, Rapoff A, Kalscheur V, Bouvy B et al. Comparison of healing of allograft/ endoprosthetic composites with three types of gluteus medius attachment. *J Orthop Res* 1995 ; 13 : 105-114

[16] Masterson E, Ferracini R, Griffin A, Wunder J, Bell R. Capsular replacement with synthetic mesh : effectiveness in preventing postoperative dislocation after wide resection of proximal tumors ansd prosthetic reconstruction. *J Arthroplasty* 1998 ; 13 : 860-866

[17] Postel M, Langlais F. Prosthesis for reconstruction after upper epiphyseal-diaphyseal resection for tumor. Chicago : Year book of orthopaedic and traumatic surgery, 1978 : 102-105

[18] Rock M. The use of Bateman bipolar proximal femoral replacement in the management of proximal femoral metastatic disease. In : Yamamuro T ed. New developments for limb salvage in musculoskeletal oncology. Tokyo : Springer-Verlag, 1989 : 1385-1417

[19] Unwin P, Cannon S, Grimer R, Kemp H, Sneath R, Walker P. Aseptic loosening in cemented custom-made prosthetic replacements for bone tumors of the lower limb. *J Bone Joint Surg Br* 1996 ; 78 : 5-13

[20] Windhager R, Karnert J, Kutschera HP, Polterauer P, Salzer-Kuntschik M, Kotz R. Limb salvage in periacetabular sarcomas. *Clin Orthop* 1996 ; 331 : 265-276

[21] Zehr R, Enneking W, Scarborough M. Allografts-prosthesis composite versus megaprosthesis in proximal femoral reconstruction. *Clin Orthop* 1996 ; 322 : 207-223

Hip arthroscopy

R Villar
A Arora

Abstract. – Hip arthroscopy has gradually evolved over the past two decades. In the 1980s, the procedure was restricted to very few centres in the world, and pursued by few experts. Since then, there has been considerable technological and methodological advance, but the procedure is still limited to specialist centres. The anatomical location and the strong ligaments surrounding the hip joint make access difficult as compared to other joints.

Lately, there has been increased acceptance of hip arthroscopy, but although it is a well-established procedure, it is by no means the cure for everything. There are increasing indications for the procedure, but controlled studies are still lacking. This chapter describes the technique and indications developed at a large specialist hip practice, and reviews the results and complications of hip arthroscopy. Anatomy and specialist instrumentation have been described with an emphasis on the technique – the key to the success of this procedure. Pathologies such as chondral defects, labral lesions, loose bodies, septic arthritis, synovitis and osteoarthritis are discussed, being appropriate indications for hip arthroscopy. Complications can occur, but can largely be avoided with care and experience.

Keywords: hip, arthroscopy, acetabular labral lesions, osteochondral defects, osteoarthritis, loose bodies.

Introduction

Hip arthroscopy has gradually evolved over 20 years of considerable technical and methodological advance. The evolution of this procedure is still limited to specialist centres, due to its demanding nature and the technical difficulty in accessing this joint. In 1977, Gross [19] reported the use of arthroscopy in the adolescent hip affected by a slipped femoral epiphysis. Subsequently, there were two reports of arthroscopy following total hip replacement [28, 29]. In 1986, Eriksson [11] described the forces necessary to distract the hip for arthroscopy.

During the last decade, this technique has become increasingly accepted as indications have expanded, and the number of trained professionals has increased. There have been many publications concerning the usefulness of hip arthroscopy for various intra-articular lesions [7, 12, 20].

Richard Villar, BSc MA MS FRCS, Consultant Orthopaedic Surgeon, Addenbrooke's Hospital Cambridge, United Kingdom, Clinical Director, Cambridge Hip and Knee Unit, Cambridge Lea Hospital, Cambridge, United Kingdom.
Arvind Arora, MS MMSc Mphil, Research Fellow, Hip & Knee Unit, Cambridge Lea Hospital, Cambridge, United Kingdom.

Anatomy of the hip joint

The hip joint is a deep-seated, ball and socket synovial joint which does not at first sight lend itself to arthroscopic access. The important extra-articular structures that lie anteriorly are the lateral femoral cutaneous nerve, femoral nerve, femoral artery and vein. Posteriorly lies the sciatic nerve, and laterally, the superior gluteal nerve. These structures can be injured while using the anterior and posterior portals for hip arthroscopy. Byrd et al [4] described the lateral safe zone over the top of the entire breadth of the greater trochanter which makes a lateral portal the safest option.

Dvorak et al [9] have shown that 80% of the femoral head can be seen using the lateral and anterior portals. The fovea and inferior part of the femoral head were best identified from the anterior approach. Robinson and Villar [26] reported that 90% of the acetabulum can be seen using the lateral portal.

The transverse ligament is seen inferiorly; below it lies the inferior recess. This is a common place to see loose bodies, but they are often inaccessible for retrieval. However, certain centres advocate hip arthroscopy without traction, in which case loose body retrieval from the inferior recess is said to be easier. The acetabular labrum is clearly seen anteriorly and posteriorly, only the superior portion being difficult to identify because of its proximity to the site of arthroscopic entry through the capsule. This portion can be seen using the anterior or anterolateral portal. The labrum overlies the hyaline cartilage of the acetabulum, except for an area at the margins of the acetabulum, where it is separated by a distinct labral groove. Surrounding the labrum is the perilabral sulcus, where the synovial membrane blends with the base of the labrum.

Instrumentation

Many instruments used in hip arthroscopy are of similar design to those used in knee arthroscopy. Extended arthroscopes (22.5 cm) are available, as are extended operating instruments. Many manual and powered instruments are available with curved handles and ends to facilitate access to more remote areas of the joint around the femoral head. For the majority of hip arthroscopies, our centre will use a standard length arthroscope, and extended operating instruments for any therapeutic manoeuvres required.

Mainly a 70°, 4.5-mm arthroscope is used in hip arthroscopy to provide a wide field of view. A high flow rate mechanical pump is useful, though not essential, for a good fluid flow. Sterile normal saline solution is used for irrigation through a 15-gauge 6" cardiac needle. The pressure generated by these pumps also helps in controlling the bleeding which otherwise can obscure the field of view. It is important to avoid high pressures and to continually check the needle position, as these can lead to considerable fluid extravasation.

A variety of convex full radius chondroplasty blades is available. They can be used for trimming chondral flaps and labral tears without damaging the femoral head. Wide ranges of cannulae are available for instrumentation or retrieval of loose bodies.

Technique

The equipment required for hip arthroscopies are: the distraction apparatus, video unit, mechanical water pump unit and image intensifier. The operating theatre must be large enough to accommodate all this equipment along with the surgical and anaesthetic teams. Arthroscopy without distraction has been described [8, 23], but it is not widely used in this practice. Some do advocate it widely and some suggest a combination of hip arthroscopy with and without traction at different stages of the operation. There is clearly a place for both techniques. At many centres, a distraction system is popular, as it provides good access and visualisation. It was noted by Dorfmann and Boyer [7] that the hip is divided into two regions. The peripheral region, which can be visualised without traction, consists of the peripheral femoral head, femoral neck, labrum and synovium. The second is the articular region, comprising the head of the femur and the acetabular surface. This requires a distraction system for proper visualisation. The distraction of this joint can be easily achieved atraumatically and without the use of excessive force. The force required to distract the hip by 10 mm can be reduced from 900 N to 300 N with the use of anaesthetic muscular relaxants [11].

The hip joint is firmly held by surface tension forces produced by the synovial fluid. This can be easily overcome by inserting a 22-gauge spinal needle, which allows the air to flow in and equalise the pressure inside the joint. This further reduces the forces required to distract the hip.

There are two methods for distracting the hip joint. A standard orthopaedic traction table can be used, on which the patient is placed supine and the affected hip is extended and abducted 25° [3]. The central perineal pole is placed to provide a lateral force as well as counter-traction to the longitudinal pull *(fig 1)*. This results in a vector that is aligned in the direction of the femoral neck. The other leg is positioned to

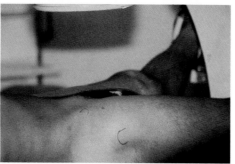

1 *Supine position with markings for the greater trochanter, anterior superior iliac spine and the point of entry when using an anterior approach. (Photograph © R. Villar).*

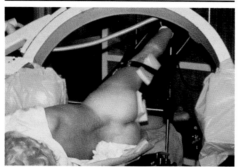

2 *Lateral position using a specialised hip distractor. The leg is abducted by 30° and the C-arm is in position. (Photograph © R. Villar).*

permit easy access to the image intensifier and also provides a counter force to balance the traction.

The other method is by using a specialised hip distractor. Here, the patient is placed in a lateral position as seen in figure 2. We prefer using this position [30]. When the patient is in a lateral position, the foot is firmly secured in a traction boot. This is then fixed to a leg rest frame that is connected to the distractor. A perineal bar is carefully positioned between the legs and placed against the perineum. The leg should be abducted 30° and the hip joint lateralised using the perineal bar. This relaxes the superolateral capsule and allows an optimal vector force for distraction along the neck of femur. Following this, the image intensifier should be positioned to take an oblique anteroposterior view. The C-arm of the image intensifier should be tilted towards the feet to allow good access to the operative site, whilst an image of the hip is taken to ascertain the position. At this stage, a trial distraction is performed. The image intensifier can be repositioned as required. A force of 25 kg is usually enough to allow sufficient distraction, but sometimes as much as 50 kg may be needed. The aim here is to see a slight increase in joint space, as full distraction may not be possible due to the vacuum present inside the joint. After distractibility has been established, traction is released. This minimises traction time and is called the "Trial of Traction" [30]. After release of the traction, the skin is prepared and the area is draped by a sterile, adhesive isolation drape.

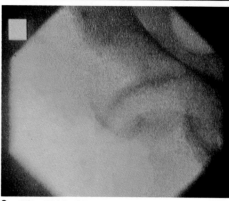

3 *The "Trial of Traction". Typically, no more than 2-3 mm of distraction will be seen at this stage. (Photograph © R. Villar).*

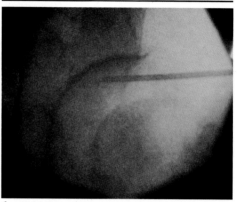

4 *The joint space increases dramatically the moment a needle enters the joint. (Photograph © R. Villar).*

There are various portals used for hip arthroscopy. We prefer using a lateral portal at our centre for this procedure. The other portals used are anterior, posterior, and a medial portal, which has more recently been used by Hasan and Al-Sabiti [20] in congenital dislocation of the hip.

The lateral portal is chosen approximately 2 cm above the greater trochanter. The position of the skin incision is a vital part of gaining accurate access to the hip joint proper, as the angle of "attack" to the lateral part of the joint is critical. In the obese patient, the positioning of the skin incision is harder – such individuals also tend to bleed more. Traction is reapplied and a 22-gauge spinal needle is introduced into the joint under image intensifier control. This releases negative intra-articular pressure and helps the joint to open up *(fig 3, 4)*. The joint is next distended with 10 to 30 ml of normal saline. After this, the spinal needle is removed and two 15 gauge cardiac needles are introduced under image intensifier control, one lateral and one slightly anterior. A flexible Nitinol® guide wire is passed through the posterior of the two needles. This ideally ends in the cotyloid fossa without touching the head of the femur. Now, a 1 cm incision is made around this needle and the needle is then withdrawn, leaving the guide wire in position. An arthroscope sheath with a cannulated sharp trochar is passed over this guide wire, until it is felt to penetrate the joint capsule. This sharp trochar is exchanged for a blunt cannulated trochar and the arthroscope sheath is then advanced towards the cotyloid fossa. The blunt trochar and guide wire are then removed and a standard length (4.5 mm) 70° arthroscope is inserted down the sheath into the hip joint. The more anterior needle is used for inflow of irrigation fluid, while the arthroscopic sheath functions as an outflow.

The anterior portal is used with the patient supine on a traction table. The foot is firmly secured in the traction boot and the hip is abducted 25°. A "Trial of Traction" is performed under image intensifier control. The portal of entry is about 6.5 cm distal to the anterior superior iliac spine. This is roughly where a vertical line dropped from the anterior superior iliac spine intersects a horizontal line extended forwards from the tip of the greater trochanter. At this point, the instrument penetrates the muscle belly of the sartorius and rectus femoris, before entering through the anterior capsule of the hip joint. Care must be taken of neurovascular structures such as the lateral femoral cutaneous nerve, femoral nerve and the ascending branch of lateral circumflex femoral artery near this portal of entry.

A posterior portal was described by Goldman [16]. He performed hip arthroscopy through an open procedure. The sciatic nerve is in very close proximity and thus has to be protected by direct visualisation. This approach was used for removal of a bullet embedded in the posterior part of the femoral head.

Additional portals are established according to need and depending on the pathology present. A 15-gauge needle and a guide wire are introduced under arthroscopic visualisation. Placing the needle near to the pathology makes the procedure much easier. Usually a 5.7 mm plastic cannula is introduced using the sharp and blunt trochars over the guide wire. The arthroscopic hook, and other instruments, can be introduced through this cannula.

Indications and results of hip arthroscopy

In the 1980s, hip arthroscopy was restricted to use by a few experts [8, 15]. Now, this procedure has gradually evolved into a widely-accepted technique, though it is still restricted to specialised centres. This is probably due to the demanding nature of this procedure and the lack of experienced personnel. The procedure itself is well-established and many limitations have been resolved. It is considered to be of value in assessing and treating the adult patient with pain in the hip of uncertain cause. The frequency of indication for hip arthroscopy in the authors' practice is shown in Table I.

Table I. – Indications for hip arthroscopy.

Indications	Patients %
Undiagnosed hip pain	35
Osteoarthritis	30
Labral pathology	10
Loose bodies	10
Osteochondral defects	5
Sepsis	
Ligamentum teres	10
Trauma	
Synovitis	

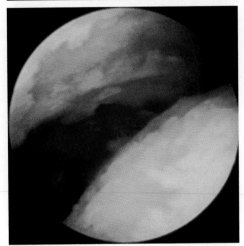

5 *Gross osteoarthritic destruction of the hip. It is unlikely hip arthroscopy will make a major difference here. (Photograph © R. Villar).*

OPERATIVE INDICATIONS AND RESULTS

■ *Undiagnosed hip pain*

Arthroscopy of the hip is considered to be of value in assessing and treating the adult patient with pain in the hip of uncertain cause. In a series of 328 patients, a preoperative diagnosis was reached in 174 patients (53%) by using arthrography, CT or MRI, while the remaining 154 were diagnosed as having "idiopathic hip pain". Arthroscopy altered the diagnosis in 176 hips (53%) [1].

■ *Osteoarthritis* (fig 5)

Hip arthroscopy is used for joint debridement and washout. It can also be used for removal of chondral flaps, a torn degenerate labrum and intra-articular impinging osteophytes. This may be useful for planning osteotomies around the hip joint, though this is as yet unproven. Arthroscopic debridement is a well-established procedure for many joints, and in some cases of hip debridement has been shown to provide symptomatic relief for up to two years [30]. The more severe the osteoarthritis, the less likely it is that arthroscopic debridement will be successful, either technically or clinically.

■ *Removal of loose bodies* (fig 6)

Loose bodies are frequent findings during hip arthroscopy. Their removal can usually

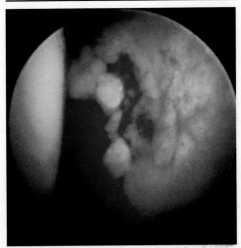

6 *Multiple loose bodies of synovial osteochondromatosis seen in the cotyloid fossa. (Photograph © R. Villar).*

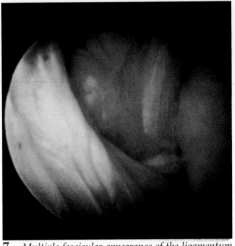

7 *Multiple fascicular appearance of the ligamentum teres with its insertion into the femoral head. (Photograph © R. Villar).*

be accomplished through a cannula, though occasionally larger loose bodies need to be broken down, using powered shavers or mechanical crushers before extraction. Removal is not always possible and patients should be warned of this beforehand.

In synovial osteochondromatosis, loose bodies can be removed arthroscopically [31]. This improves function, relieves pain and may reduce the chances of joint destruction. Keene and Villar reported the removal of intra-articular bony fragments after traumatic hip dislocation [22]. Foreign bodies can also be removed, either from the hip joint [6] or even a total hip arthroplasty [29].

■ *Ligamentum teres rupture*

The ligamentum teres is unmistakable when seen (fig 7). Its rupture has been reported and classified in 20 patients out of 472 consecutive hip arthroscopies [18]. The clinical presentation varied from groin pain, to thigh pain, to clicking of the hip.

■ *Acetabular labrum tears* (fig 8)

Labral tears are a common cause of hip pain associated with clicking or locking. MRI and

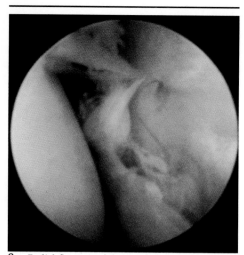

8 *Radial flap tear of the acetabular labrum. (Photograph © R. Villar).*

arthrography are not always helpful in diagnosing these lesions [10], though their success rate has improved in recent years. These tears can be seen and effectively treated by hip arthroscopy. Lage et al [25] reported that 62% of tears were located anteriorly in their series. Acetabular labrum tears associated with radiological signs of arthritis do poorly after hip arthroscopy, when compared to those without any signs of arthritis [12].

■ *Synovitis*

Synovectomy for both synovitis [17] and for treatment of pigmented villonodular synovitis [21] has been described. The results are uncertain, but it has been suggested that arthroscopy may help in making an early diagnosis, so that arthroscopic synovectomy might perhaps be more effective.

■ *Hip sepsis*

Hip arthroscopy is an effective way to wash out a septic hip. Chung et al [5] reported 9 cases of septic arthritis of the hip joint treated by arthroscopic lavage in children. Similar good results have been reported following this procedure in adults.

■ *Other uses*

As the popularity of hip arthroscopy increases, so do the indications. Drilling of osteochondral lesions, retrieval of post-traumatic bony fragments, foreign body removal, labral repair, the management of avascular necrosis [27], are all possibilities. Hip arthroscopy in children [24] is a very new field, currently with few protagonists.

Complications

The complications of hip arthroscopy are mostly of neural origin. Prolonged distraction of the joint can cause a varying degree of neurapraxia. Glick [14] reported 8 sciatic and pudendal transient nerve palsies and breakage of one instrument in the joint in a series of 60 patients. Eriksson [11] has reported paraesthesia following damage to the lateral cutaneous nerve of the thigh. Villar [30] reported transient femoral nerve palsy, albeit due to a misplaced local anaesthetic injection. Iatrogenic scuffing of articular cartilage during the insertion of either arthroscope or operating instrument can occur. Funke and Munzinger [13] reported complications early in the learning curve, but with care and experience the incidence can be reduced. Theoretically, hip arthroscopy without traction might reduce the chances of neural damage. The so-called "Trial of Traction" is important in this regard. Perineal tearing and bruising can be caused by the perineal bar. There have been no published reports of sepsis following the hip arthroscopy, though there is now one case in the Cambridge series. Bartlett reported a case of cardiac arrest as a result of intra-abdominal extravasation of fluid during arthroscopic removal of a loose body in a patient with an acetabular fracture [2].

The future

Hip arthroscopy has gradually evolved over the past two decades. Indications are constantly appearing and are being successfully applied. As minimally invasive surgery develops further, as it surely will, the future of hip arthroscopy is secure.

References

[1] Baber YF, Robinson AH, Villar RN. Is diagnostic arthroscopy of the hip worthwhile? *J Bone Joint Surg Br* 1999 ; 81 : 600-604

[2] Bartlett CS, Di Felice GS, Buly RL, Quinn TJ, Green DS, Helfet DL. Cardiac arrest as a result of intraabdominal extravasation of fluid during arthroscopic removal of a loose body from the hip joint of a patient with an acetabular fracture. *J Orthop Trauma* 1998 ; 12 : 294-299

[3] Byrd JW. Hip arthroscopy utilizing the supine position. *Arthroscopy* 1994 ; 10 : 275-280

[4] Byrd JW, Pappas JN, Pedley MJ. Hip arthroscopy: an anatomic study of portal placement and relationship to the extra-articular structures. *Arthroscopy* 1995 ; 11 : 418-423

[5] Chung WK, Slater GL, Bates EH. Treatment of septic arthritis of the hip by arthroscopic lavage. *J Pediatr Orthop* 1993 ; 30 : 444-446

[6] Cory JW, Ruch DS. Arthroscopic removal of a 44 caliber bullet from the hip. *Arthroscopy* 1998 ; 14 : 624-626

[7] Dorfmann H, Boyer T. Arthroscopy of the hip: 12 years of experience. *Arthroscopy* 1999 ; 15 : 67-72

[8] Dorfmann H, Boyer T, Henry P, Debie B. A simple approach to hip arthroscopy. *Arthroscopy* 1988 ; 4 : 141-142

[9] Dvorak M, Duncan C, Day B. Arthroscopic anatomy of the hip. *Arthroscopy* 1990 ; 6 : 264-273

[10] Edwards DJ, Lomas D, Villar RN. Diagnosis of the painful hip by magnetic resonance imaging and arthroscopy. *J Bone Joint Surg Br* 1995 ; 77 : 374-376

[11] Eriksson E, Arvidsson J, Arvidsson H. Diagnostic and operative arthroscopy of the hip. *Orthopedics* 1986 ; 9 : 169-176

[12] Farjo LA, Glick JM, Sampson TG. Hip arthroscopy for acetabular labral tears. *Arthroscopy* 1999 ; 15 : 132-137

[13] Funke EL, Munzinger U. Complications in hip arthroscopy. *Arthroscopy* 1996 ; 12 : 156-159

[14] Glick JM. Complications of hip arthroscopy by the lateral approach. In : Sherman OH, Minkoff J eds. Current management of complications in orthopaedics. Arthroscopic surgery. Baltimore : Williams and Wilkins, 1990 : 93-201

[15] Glick JM, Sampson TG, Gordon RB, Behr JT, Schmidt E. Hip arthroscopy by the lateral approach. *Arthroscopy* 1987 ; 3 : 4-12

[16] Goldman A, Minkoff J, Price A et al. A posterior arthroscopic approach to bullet extraction from the hip. *J Trauma* 1987 ; 27 : 1294-1300

[17] Gondolph-Zink B, Puhl W, Noack W. Semiarthroscopic synovectomy of the hip. *Int Orthop* 1998 ; 12 : 31-35

[18] Gray AJ, Villar RN. Rupture of the ligamentum teres of the hip. An arthroscopic classification. *J Bone Joint Surg Br* 1997 ; 79 (suppl 1) : 96

[19] Gross R. Arthroscopy in hip disorders in children. *Orthop Rev* 1977 ; 6 : 43-49

[20] Hasan AR, Al-Sabiti A. Arthroscopy of the hip in congenital dislocation [abstract]. *J Bone Joint Surg Br* 1995 ; 77 (suppl I) : 3

[21] Janssens X, Van Meirhaeghe J, Verdonk R et al. Diagnostic arthroscopy of the hip joint in pigmented villonodular synovitis. *Arthroscopy* 1987 ; 3 : 283-287

[22] Keene G, Villar RN. Arthroscopic loose body retrieval following traumatic hip dislocation. *Injury* 1994 ; 25 : 507-510

[23] Klapper R, Silver D. Hip arthroscopy without traction. *Contemp Orthop* 1989 ; 18 : 687-693

[24] Kuklo TR, MacKenzie WG, Keeler KA. Hip arthroscopy in Legg-Calve-Perthes disease. *Arthroscopy* 1999 ; 15 : 88-92

[25] Lage LA, Patel JV, Villar RN. The acetabular labral tear: an arthroscopic classification. *Arthroscopy* 1996 ; 12 : 269-272

[26] Robinson AH, Villar RN. State of the art hip arthroscopic techniques. In : Parisien JS ed. Current techniques in arthroscopy. Stuttgart : Thieme, 1998 : 149-160

[27] Ruch DS, Satterfield W. The use of arthroscopy to document accurate position of core decompression of the hip. *Arthroscopy* 1998 ; 14 : 617-619

[28] Shifrin L, Reis N. Arthroscopy of a dislocated hip replacement: a case report. *Clin Orthop* 1980 ; 146 : 213-214

[29] Vakili F, Salvati E, Warren R. Entrapped foreign body within the acetabular cup in total hip replacement. *Clin Orthop* 1980 ; 150 : 159-162

[30] Villar RN. Hip arthroscopy. Oxford : Butterworth-Heinemann, 1992 : 149-159

[31] Witwity T, Uhnmann RD, Fischer J. Arthroscopic management of chondromatosis of the hip joint. *Arthroscopy* 1988 ; 4 : 55-56

Soft tissue coverage of trochanteric and sacral sores

C Oberlin
C Touam
N Ameur
P Greant
A Bhatia

Abstract. –   The orthopaedic or plastic surgeon must differentiate the various types of decubitus ulcer. Pressure sores in debilitated patients affected by life-threatening disease or cachexy must be excluded from surgery. Sores must be surgically treated only in patients presenting a good general status or in patients who are permanently paralysed.

The decubitus ulceration corresponds to an ischaemic necrosis due to hyperpressure. The cutaneous defect is only part of a usually very large ischaemic area which includes subcutaneous tissue, muscle, deep infection of the bone, etc.

The first and major step of the surgical procedure is extensive debridement, with a systematic excision of all ischaemic or infected tissues. This part of the operation is the most difficult and requires an experienced surgeon.

The second step is to provide the defect with solid, thick and gliding tissue in order to prevent a recurrence of the ulceration.

Trochanteric ulcers are routinely treated with the tensor fascia lata flap, and sacral sores with the gluteal musculocutaneous rotation flap, while ischiatic ulcerations can generally be closed primarily, less often with a flap harvested from the posterior aspect of the thigh.

Keywords: pressure sores, sacral sores, trochanteric sores, ischiatic sores, cutaneous flap, musculocutaneous flap.

Introduction

Many different procedures are available to reconstruct trochanteric and sacral sores [1-4, 7, 8, 10, 16, 17].

The aim of this short chapter is to propose a few reliable technical tools to the orthopaedic surgeon faced with a pressure sore. However, the surgeon must be aware of the extreme difficulty in treating pressure sores if certain conditions are not present, such as good nutritional status of the patient, an excellent nursing team, possibly an air bed system, etc.

This chapter concerns only the surgical aspects and considers three locations of pressure sores: sacral, trochanteric and ischiatic.

Christophe Oberlin, *Professeur des Universités, Praticien Hospitalier.*
Chabane Touam, *Praticien Adjoint.*
Noreddine Ameur, *Orthopaedic Surgeon.*
Hopital Bichat, Service d'Orthopédie-Traumatologie, 46 rue Henri-Huchard, 75877 Paris cedex 18, France.
Philippe Greant, *Plastic Surgeon.*
Hôpital de Jolimont Haine Saint-Paul, Belgique.
Anil Bhatia, *Hand and Plastic Surgeon.*
L 3 Mantri Avenue II, Pashan Pune 411008, India.

Sacral sores

Although some new techniques are now available [2, 10, 17], the gluteus maximus flap is the most commonly used, in its musculocutaneous form, to cover a sacral defect [3, 5, 9, 11, 14]. This is usually a fairly bloody procedure and should only be performed in patients who are in a reasonable state of health.

DIFFICULTY

Using the basic technique, the gluteus maximus flap can be performed without the assistance of a flap specialist and without previous experience of this specific flap. Detailed close dissection of the vessels is not required. However, previous cadaveric surgical experience with this flap is advised.

ANATOMY

The gluteus maximus is a large muscle arising from the sacrum, the external surface of the wing of the ilium, and the thoracolumbar fascia. It passes distally to insert into the fascia lata and the greater trochanter of the femur.

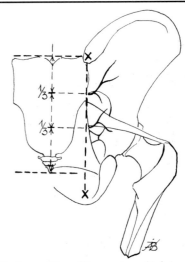

1 *Surface markings of the superior and inferior gluteal arteries.*

It has two main vascular pedicles, derived from the internal illiac artery *(fig 1)*. The superior gluteal artery, the most important branch of the internal iliac, passes over the piriformis muscle and supplies the superior part of the muscle. The inferior gluteal passes under the piriformis, accompanied by the sciatic nerve and the posterior nerve of the thigh.

The skin and subcutaneous portion of the flap are vascularised by perforating branches from the gluteal muscle. The gluteal muscle is innervated by the inferior gluteal nerve. It plays an important part in maintaining an upright position, and in nonparalysed patients, a portion of this muscle should be left in situ. The flap can survive on either one of the two possible vascular pedicles.

Although more than a dozen techniques have been described for raising a gluteal flap, we describe two, both of which preserve muscle function.

■ Gluteal rotation flap

In the treatment of sacral sores in paraplegics, it is wise to remember that recurrences are common, and to use a rotation flap, which if necessary can be further advanced at a later date. If the primary management is by one or more island flaps, further surgery can be very difficult indeed. However, the raising of a rotation flap of the gluteus muscle can be a very bloody procedure.

Basic design of a gluteal rotation flap

Whatever type of flap is planned, it is important to mark on the skin the site of the vascular pedicles of the gluteus maximus. A line joins the posterior iliac spine and the ischial tuberosity. The vertical axis of the sacrum is then divided into three equal parts. The superior pedicle is situated at the junction of the upper and middle thirds, and the inferior pedicle at the junction of the middle and lower thirds (*fig 1*).

The area of scar to be excised is then marked, and a distally-based flap is designed (*fig 2*). Superiorly, it should not pass over the iliac crest, and distally, it can extend to the trochanteric region.

• Technique

After incising the skin and subcutaneous tissue, the gluteal fascia is opened, and by blunt dissection the space between the gluteus maximus and medius is developed. This also allows mobilisation of the superior pedicle and separation of the muscle from the sacrum without risk to its blood supply.

The superior and medial part of the muscle is divided for 4-5 cm near its distal insertion, conserving the inferior fibres, and the flap is advanced with very light traction. It is then relatively easy to feel the structures which are preventing adequate movement of the flap, and these are released by separating the origin of the muscle from the sacrum.

The flap can then be advanced adequately to cover the defect, and this leaves the

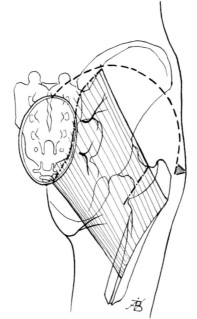

2   *The incisions for a rotation musculocutaneous gluteal flap. This passes distal and below the iliac crest, but should not expose the greater trochanter. The insertion is raised from the sacrum, leaving only the inferior fibres. The superior border is then divided a few centimetres proximal to its insertion, to allow the flap to be rotated.*

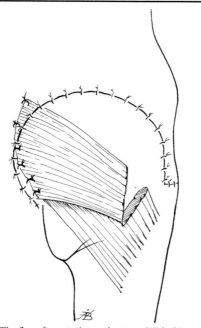

3   *The flap after rotation and suture. With this technique, the procedure can be repeated if there is a recurrence of ulceration.*

inferior part of the body of the muscle to continue to act normally. The donor site can usually be closed without difficulty, by using a small "back-cut" (*fig 3*).

This flap will cover defects as large as 15 cm x 12 cm.

■ Gluteus maximus musculocutaneous island flap

This is a relatively rapid technique which does not necessitate dissection near the vascular pedicles. It is useful for small and medium-sized defects [5, 11, 12].

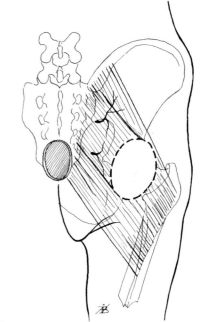

4   *The principle of the island muscular gluteal flap.*

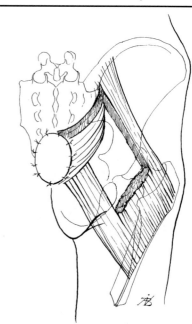

5   *The muscular pedicle remains attached to the sacrum, thus avoiding all risk of damage to the vessels.*

The principles are:

– to raise a flap of skin with an appropriate portion of underlying muscle (*fig 4*);

– to leave intact the muscular origin from the sacrum, so as to protect the vessels from any traction which may occur during transfer of the flap (*fig 5*).

Design of the gluteus maximus island flap (*fig 6*)

The direction of the fibres of the muscle, and the outlines of the flap, with a maximum of 6-7 cm of length and 4-5 cm of width, are marked on the skin. This should allow primary closure of the donor site.

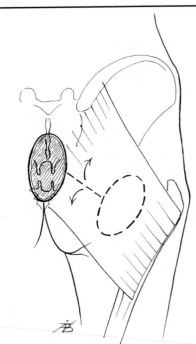

6   *The incisions for an island flap. A further incision joining the site of the flap and the lesion may be indicated if the graft cannot be transferred by tunnelling. However, this increases scarring.*

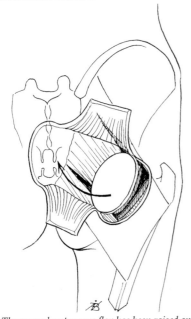

7   *The musculocutaneous flap has been raised and can now be rotated.*

Ideally, the flap is "tunnelled" to fill the defect. If this is impossible, the skin has to be incised, and then closed after transferring the flap *(fig 7)*.

At this site, the flap can often be slightly smaller than the defect, which can often be reduced by mobilising the local skin.

- *Technique*

The margins of the skin flap are incised, and the lateral portion of the underlying gluteus maximus is also divided to expose the gluteus medius. The fibres of the maximus are then separated on either side of the

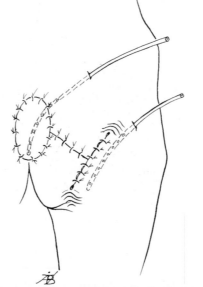

8   *The flap in place, and the donor site closed primarily over drainage.*

island, superficial to the gluteus medius, to allow the flap to be raised *(fig 7)*.

After the flap has been rotated to fill the defect, it should be sutured in place, but without excess tension. The donor site is closed with drainage *(fig 8)*, and a bandage spica is applied.

Postoperative management

Ideally, the patient should be nursed on a water bed for the first 4-6 weeks. Attention must be given to nutrition, hydration, oxygenation and to the correction of anaemia.

■ **Variations**

A pure gluteal muscle flap can be covered with a split-skin graft, thus reducing the chances of breakdown at the donor site.

A pure island flap will allow better rotation, but may limit advancement. Occasionally, it is wise to perform bilateral flaps in order to cover a midline defect, but this is unacceptable functionally in non-paralysed patients, as it considerably weakens the muscles of the buttocks [3].

■ **Indications**

The gluteus maximus musculocutaneous flap is the method of choice for covering large sacral defects, whether midline or near the midline.

■ **Advantages**

These flaps have a more reliable vascular supply than the classical cutaneous rotation flaps in this area.

■ **Disadvantages**

As a result of its constituents, this is a thick flap. However, any resulting "deformity" quickly disappears.

Theoretically, it is undesirable to use an important muscle in patients who are not paralysed, but in practice, very little if any functional disability results.

The magnitude of the operation, with a major concomitant blood loss in debilitated patients, can also be a problem, and therefore careful pre- and postoperative management are mandatory.

Trochanteric sores

This location is routinely covered by a tensor fascia lata musculocutaneous flap [4, 13, 15, 18].

DIFFICULTY

The tensor fascia lata musculocutaneous flap is easy to perform. Detailed close dissection of the vessels is not required.

For the basic technique, this flap can be performed without the assistance of a flap specialist, and without previous experience of this specific flap. In addition, it may be undertaken without previous experience of this flap in the laboratory.

ANATOMY

The tensor fascia lata arises from the anterosuperior iliac spine and the adjacent part of the iliac crest; it measures 10-15 cm. It inserts into the iliotibial tract. It receives its blood supply from the lateral circumflex femoral artery which enters the muscle about 8 cm distal to the anterosuperior iliac spine.

BASIC DESIGN

Classically, the anterior incision follows a line between the anterior spine and the external tubercle of the tibia *(fig 9)* and commences about 8 cm distal to the spine. This also marks the anterior border of the tensor fascia muscle. The flap can extend two-thirds of the way down the thigh, and may thus be 30 cm in length. It normally ends some 10 cm proximal to the knee joint. A width of about 6-7 cm will usually allow primary closure, and this can be tested by squeezing the lateral part of the thigh between two hands. Closure of the donor site rarely causes problems, due to the excellent blood supply of the neighbouring skin.

TECHNIQUE

The flap usually includes the skin, subcutaneous tissue and the fascia lata. It has a proximal base, and it is not necessary to mobilise the vascular pedicle. It is easy to raise this flap with a good plane of cleavage between the fascia lata and the vastus lateralis. The defect in the fascia lata is left

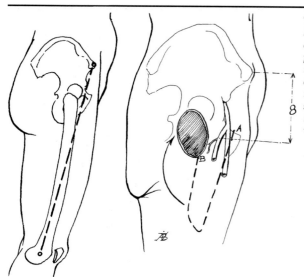

9 *The skin incisions of the tensor fascia lata musculocutaneous flap. The anterior incision follows a line joining the anterior superior iliac spine and the external condyle of the femur. The origin of the vascular pedicle, comprising the lateral circumflex femoral artery, is marked 8 cm distal to the anterior spine. The posterior incision descends from the anterior border of the defect. This design will allow primary closure of the donor site.*

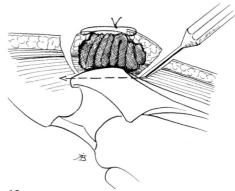

12 *The technique advised for excision of a deep fibrotic and infected trochanteric sore, often involving bone. The wound is "closed" by firm suture over an antiseptic pack, and is then removed in toto with any infected portions of the greater trochanter.*

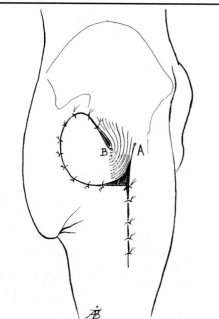

10 *The flap after rotation. There is usually an unsightly fold of skin which resolves spontaneously, leaving good mobile skin over the greater trochanter.*

open. The exact design of the flap will depend, of course, on the defect which is to be covered:

– simple rotation of the flap *(fig 10)*: the flap is turned 90 degrees posteriorly to cover an ulcer over the greater trochanter;

– advancement-rotation *(fig 11)*: the most fleshy part of the flap is advanced to fill the defect. This will temporarily produce a defect at the distal point of the flap, which can be closed by using the incisions illustrated.

POSTOPERATIVE MANAGEMENT

Suction drainage is left in place for 8 to 10 days, and the wound is supported with a bandage spica.

VARIATIONS

Normally, this is a long flap, which can cover even the largest trochanteric ulcers. It can also be used to cover an associated

11 *The musculocutaneous tensor fascia flap after simple advancement. Note that the posterior incision follows the posterior border of the defect, and this produces a wider flap. The distal portion of the donor site can be closed primarily by the use of the two incisions (A and B).*

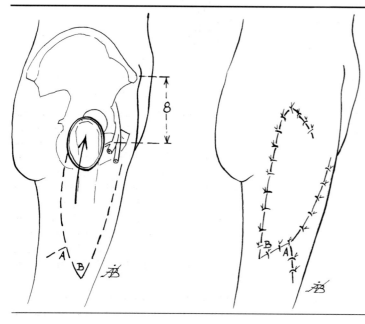

sacral sore; in this case, it may be necessary to excise the skin bridge separating these two lesions.

If the vastus lateralis is also included in this flap, very large defects can be closed. In addition, this provides a muscle base for the distal part of the flap, which is not so if only the fascia lata is raised. It may also allow an even longer skin flap to be used. There are several perforating cutaneous arteries which arise in the vastus lateralis, and these will improve the vascularisation of the distal end of long flaps when this muscle is incorporated. Thus, the use of both these muscles will considerably increase the size of the flap, and thus allow cover of relatively enormous defects.

INDICATIONS

This is the flap of choice to cover trochanteric sores in paraplegics. The results of the procedure depend not only on the general state of the patient, but also on the adequacy of the excision of dead tissue. This may necessitate removal of a portion of the greater trochanter.

These large ulcers may have to be excised in toto after an antiseptic pack has been sutured in the cavity *(fig 12)*. An osteotomy is usually required to remove infected portions of the trochanter.

A similar technique may help to avoid recurrence of a chronic ischial bursa which may underlie a skin ulcer at this site.

ADVANTAGES

No very fine dissection of vessels is required, and the donor site can normally be closed primarily.

The tensor fascia lata advancement rotation flap covers pressure sores with muscle.

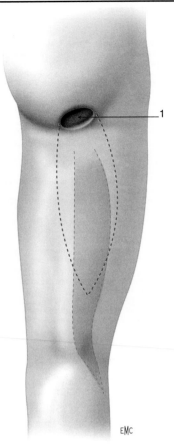

13 *Incision of a biceps musculocutaneous flap for ischiatic pressure sore. The axis of the skin paddle follows a line joining the ischiatic tuberosity to the head of the fibula. 1. pressure sore.*

DISADVANTAGES

This flap, when rotated, can produce an unsightly fold of skin, although this normally disappears spontaneously. Rotation advancement flaps do not have this problem.

Ischiatic sores

In the ischiatic area, the problem is that of a deep bone infection rather than a problem of a soft tissue defect.

Thus, a partial excision of the prominent ischiatic tuberosity and excision of adhesive tissues routinely permits primary closure after a simple soft tissue release. This can include a release and more proximal reattachment of the proximal insertion of the muscles inserted on the ischiatic process.

However, in some cases, the use of a coverage flap is still required [4, 6, 8, 12, 16, 19].

If both trochanteric and ischiatic sores have to be treated, a longer tensor fascia lata flap can cover both areas in the same procedure.

In other cases, a flap from the thigh is needed, such as a long biceps V-Y musculocutaneous advancement flap or a

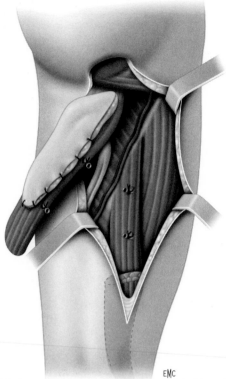

14 *Harvesting the flap. The long head of the biceps is sectioned at the level of the distal skin incision. The musculocutaneous flap is retracted proximally, while muscle and paddle are closely tied together. Some vascular pedicles to the biceps muscle are divided. The proximal pedicle is preserved.*

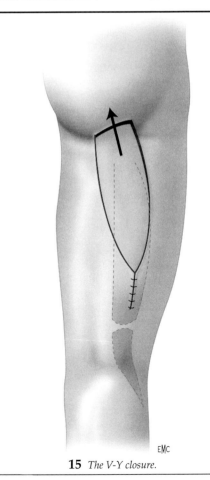

15 *The V-Y closure.*

vastus lateralis musculocutaneous flap [4, 13, 18].

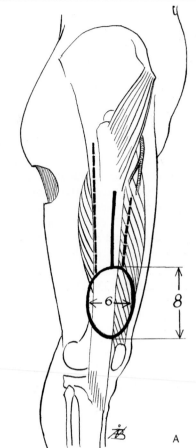

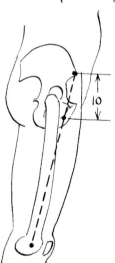

16 *The skin incisions for the vastus lateralis musculocutaneous flap (A) and for the pure muscular flap (B). The flap is based on a line joining the anterior superior iliac spine and the lateral femoral condyle. The skin flap is taken from the more distal part of the thigh, and should not be greater than 6 x 8 cm.*

BICEPS MUSCULOCUTANEOUS FLAP

A triangular paddle is outlined on the posterior aspect of the thigh, distal to the skin defect (*fig 13*). The general axis of the paddle follows the axis of the long head of the biceps muscle (along a line joining the ischiatic tuberosity to the head of the fibula). The muscle is identified distally and sectioned. Some distal muscular vascular pedicles are divided (*fig 14*), allowing proximal advancement. The donor site is then closed, using the "V-Y" procedure (*fig 15*).

Despite the apparent simplicity of this technique, one must be aware of the relative difficulty of preserving adequate vascularisation to the entire skin paddle [6].

In large defects, the semimembranosus and the biceps can be used in association.

VASTUS LATERALIS MUSCULOCUTANEOUS FLAP

■ *Basic design*

A line is drawn on the skin, joining the anterior superior iliac spine and the lateral femoral condyle (*fig 16A*). The incision starts 10 cm distal to the anterior spine and follows this line. The flap is designed according to the requirements and is usually anterior to the iliotibial band, in the region well-supplied by perforating branches from the lower portion of the vastus lateralis muscle (*fig 16B*).

Technique

The skin and subcutaneous tissues are divided to outline the skin flap on the lateral surface of the thigh, and this is deepened through the iliotibial tract. This exposes the vastus lateralis, which is mobilised from the distal end and is separated without difficulty from the rectus femoris. It may be more difficult to separate it from the vastus intermedius, and there may be some bleeding. Care must be taken in the more proximal part of the thigh to avoid damaging the vascular pedicle, but this need not be specifically isolated.

It is important during this dissection to avoid any damage to the tensor fascia lata, which might prevent the future use of this

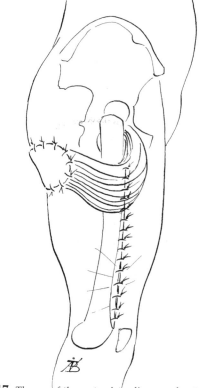

17 *The use of the vastus lateralis musculocutaneous flap to cover an ulcer in the ischial region.*

muscle as a graft to supplement the vastus lateralis flap.

The donor site is closed primarily with drainage (*fig 17*).

Acknowledgements – Figures 1-12, 16 and 17 were originally published in Oberlin C, Bastian D, Greant P. Les lambeaux pédiculés de couverture des membres. Expansion Scientifique Française, Paris, 1994.

References

[1] Akguner M, Karaca C, Atabey A, Menderes A, Top H. Surgical treatment for ischial pressure sores with gracilis myocutaneous flap. *J Wound Care* 1998 ; 7 : 276-278

[2] Ao M, Mae O, Namba Y, Asagoe K. Perforator-based flap for coverage of lumbosacral defects. *Plast Reconstr Surg* 1998 ; 101 : 987-991

[3] Baran CN, Celebioglu S, Civelek B, Sensoz O. Tangentially split gluteus maximus myocutaneous island flap based on perforator arteries for the reconstruction of pressure sores. *Plast Reconstr Surg* 1999 ; 103 : 2071-2076

[4] Bovet JL, Nassif T, Guimberteau JC, Baudet J. The vastus lateralis musculocutaneous flap in the repair of trochanteric pressure sores: technique and indications. *Plast Reconstr Surg* 1982 ; 69 : 830-834

[5] Chen TH. Bilateral gluteus maximus V-Y advancement musculocutaneous flaps for the coverage of large sacral pressure sores: revisit and refinement. *Ann Plast Surg* 1995 ; 35 : 492-497

[6] Foster RD, Anthony JP, Mathes SJ, Hoffmann WY. Ischial pressure sore coverage: a rationale for flap selection. *Br J Plast Surg* 1997 ; 50 : 374-379

[7] Ger R. The surgical management of decubitus ulcers by muscle transposition. *Surgery* 1971 ; 69 : 106

[8] Hayashi A, Maruyama Y, Saze M, Okada E. The lateral thigh V-Y flap for the repair of ischial defects. *Br J Plast Surg* 1998 ; 51 : 113-117

[9] Koshima I, Moriguchi T, Soeda S, Kaxata S, Ohta S, Ikeda A. The gluteal perforator-based flap for repair of sacral pressure sores. *Plast Reconstr Surg* 1993 ; 91 : 678-683

[10] Kroll SS, Rosenfield L. Perforator-based flaps for low posterior midline defects. *Plast Reconstr Surg* 1988 ; 81 : 561-566

[11] Maruyama Y. A gluteus maximus island flap for the repair of a sacral decubitus ulcer. *Br J Plast Surg*, 1980 ; 33 : 150-155

[12] Masquelet A, Gilbert A. An atlas of flaps in limb reconstruction. London : Martin Dunitz, 1995

[13] Minami RT, Hentz VP, Vistnes LM. Use of vastus lateralis muscle flap for coverage of trochanteric pressure sores. *Plast Reconstr Surg* 1977 ; 60 : 364

[14] Minami RT, Mills R, Pardoe R. Gluteus maximus musculocutaneous flaps for repair of pressure sores. *Plast Reconstr Surg* 1977 ; 60 : 242

[15] Nahai F, Hill L, Hester TR. Experiences with the tensor fascia lata flap. *Plast Reconstr Surg* 1979 ; 63 : 788

[16] Rajacic N, Gang RK, Behbehani A. Treatment of ischial pressure sores with an inferior gluteus maximus musculocutaneous flap: an analysis of 31 flaps. *Br J Plast Surg* 1994 ; 47 : 431-434

[17] Rawat SS, Mathur BS. Transverse lumbar flap for sacral bed sores. *Plast Reconstr Surg* 1991 ; 88 : 154-158

[18] Schmidt AB, Fromberg G, Ruidisch MH. Applications of the pedicled vastus lateralis flap for patients with complicated pressure sores. *Spinal Cord* 1997 ; 35 : 437-442

[19] Yamamoto Y, Tsutsumida A, Murazumi M, Sugihara T. Long-term outcome of pressure sores treated with flap coverage. *Plast Reconstr Surg* 1997 ; 100 : 1212-1217

Index
Volume 6 - Pelvic ring and hip
Surgical Techniques in Orthopaedics and Traumatology

A

Acetabuloplasty..................................... 55-420-A-10
55-440-E-10
– : lateral shelf...................................... 55-420-D-10
Amputation
– : Boyd's, for proximal femoral deficiency.. 55-430-B-10
– : hemipelvectomy............................... 55-480-B-10
– : hip disarticulation............................ 55-480-A-10
– : Syme's, for proximal femoral deficiency . 55-430-B-10
Ankylosis
– : hip 55-450-A-10
Armature, acetabular reconstruction............ 55-450-D-10
Arthritis
See: Septic arthritis
Arthrodesis, hip
– : ankylosed hips................................. 55-450-A-10
– : extra-articular.................................. 55-460-E-10
– : intra-articular................................... 55-460-E-10
Arthroplasty, complications
– : acetabular loosening........................ 55-450-B-10
– : acetabular reconstruction 55-450-D-10
– : acetabular revision........................... 55-450-E-10
– : dislocations of total hip.................... 55-440-A-10
– : infected total hip.............................. 55-460-C-10
– : revision after loosening, hip 55-460-E-10
– : revision, failed femoral prosthesis 55-460-B-20
– : revision, femoral side....................... 55-460-A-10
Arthroscopy, hip 55-480-D-10

B

Bone, graft
– : femoral revision, cancellous allografting 55-460-A-10
– : femoral revision, impaction grafting 55-460-A-10
– : femoral tumours, combined allograft...... 55-480-C-10
– : hip, acetabular deficiencies................ 55-450-B-10
– : hip arthrodesis 55-460-E-10
– : hip, morsellised allografts, acetabular
reconstruction................................... 55-450-D-10
55-450-E-10
– : hip, shelf operations 55-420-A-10
– : vascularised, avascular necrosis.............. 55-470-B-10

C

Casts
– : spica, hip 55-410-D-10
Cement
– : acetabular component....................... 55-450-D-10
– : allograft, femoral revision 55-460-A-10
– : antibiotic, infected prosthesis.................. 55-460-B-20
– : Exeter cementing technique, femur.......... 55-430-D-20
– : removal, femoral cavity, extended
trochanter... 55-440-C-10
– : removal, hip resection....................... 55-460-D-10
Cerebral palsy
– : hip 55-430-A-10
Charnley cup
– : hip instability................................... 55-440-A-10
– : long posterior wall............................ 55-440-A-10
Classification
– : acetabular deficiencies 55-450-B-10
– : acetabular fractures 55-400-F-10
– : avascular necrosis, femoral head.............. 55-470-B-10
– : Delbet-Colonna, femoral neck fractures.. 55-410-B-10
– : Gillespie, congenital femoral deficiency.. 55-430-B-10
– : pelvic ring fractures.......................... 55-410-A-10
– : pelvic ring fractures, children................. 55-410-B-10
– : Pipkin, femoral head fractures................ 55-400-B-10

– : rotationplasty................................... 55-470-E-10
– : total hip arthroplasty........................ 55-430-D-10
– : trochanteric and subtrochanteric
fractures.. 55-400-E-10
Coaptation, trochanteric-iliac................... 55-460-D-10
Congenital anomalies
– : femoral deficiency............................ 55-430-B-10
– : hip, developmental dysplasia 55-410-E-10
– : hip, dislocation................................ 55-410-E-10
– : hip, total replacement....................... 55-440-E-10
– : proximal femoral deficiency.................... 55-430-B-10

D

Dislocation
– : high, total hip arthroplasty 55-440-E-10
– : isolated hip...................................... 55-400-B-10
– : low, total hip arthroplasty................. 55-440-E-10
– : total hip prosthesis........................... 55-440-A-10
Dunn's operation.................................... 55-420-E-10
Dysplasia dislocation, hip
– : conservative treatment...................... 55-410-D-10
– : open reduction................................. 55-410-D-10

F

Femur
– : approach, transfemoral 55-400-A-10
– : approach, transfemoral, failed femoral
prosthesis.. 55-460-B-20
– : approach, transfemoral, revision total
hip arthroplasty................................. 55-460-B-10
– : approach, Watson-Jones................... 55-400-A-10
– : Dunn's operation.............................. 55-420-E-10
– : Exeter cementing technique................... 55-430-D-20
– : femoral cavity, cement removal.............. 55-440-C-10
– : femoral head, fractures...................... 55-400-B-10
– : femoral head, necrosis....................... 55-400-D-10
55-400-F-10
55-420-E-10
– : femoral head, osteonecrosis............... 55-470-B-10
– : femoral head, Perthes' disease 55-420-D-10
– : femoral head, shelf operations.................. 55-420-A-10
– : femoral malignancies........................ 55-480-C-10
– : femoral neck fracture........................ 55-400-C-10
– : femoral neck fracture, children................ 55-410-B-10
– : femoral neck, Kramer's osteotomy 55-420-E-10
– : femoral neck lengthening................... 55-430-C-10
– : femoral neck, non-union 55-400-D-10
– : femoral osteotomies in cerebral palsy...... 55-430-A-10
– : femoral revision............................... 55-440-A-10
– : femoral revision after loosening 55-460-B-10
– : femoral stem prosthesis, cementless 55-440-D-10
– : femorotomy in infected hips 55-460-B-20
– : osteotomies, upper femur 55-470-A-10
– : proximal femoral deficiency.................... 55-430-B-10
– : slipped capital femoral epiphysis.............. 55-420-E-10
– : tumour of the proximal femur,
rotationplasty.................................... 55-470-E-10
– : upper femoral fractures, children............. 55-410-B-10
Fixation, external
– : iliofemoral....................................... 55-460-E-10
Fixation, internal, hip
– : acetabular cup.................................. 55-450-B-10
– : cementless distally locked stem 55-460-B-20
– : cementless stem................................ 55-440-D-10
– : cementless implant 55-460-B-10
– : dynamic hip screw............................ 55-400-C-10
55-400-E-10
– : Ender nail.. 55-400-E-10

– : Gamma nail...................................... 55-400-E-10
– : pelvic ring injuries............................ 55-410-A-10
– : press-fit cup..................................... 55-440-D-10
55-450-B-10

Fixation, internal, lower extremities
See: Nailing
Flaps
– : hip, cutaneous.................................. 55-480-E-10
– : hip, musculocutaneous...................... 55-480-E-10
See also: Pressure sores
Fracture, acetabular
– : approaches....................................... 55-400-F-10
– : children 55-410-B-10
Fracture, children
– : acetabular 55-410-B-10
– : congenital dysplasia and femoral
reconstruction................................... 55-440-E-10
– : femoral osteosynthesis 55-460-B-20
– : femoral revision, allograft...................... 55-460-A-10
– : femoral revision, failed femoral
prosthesis.. 55-460-B-20
– : pelvic ring.. 55-410-B-10
– : upper femoral 55-410-B-10
Fracture, hip
– : femoral head 55-400-B-10
– : femoral neck..................................... 55-400-C-10
– : femoral neck, non-union 55-400-D-10
– : ipsilateral hip and shaft..................... 55-400-C-10
– : subtrochanteric 55-400-E-10
– : trochanteric 55-400-E-10
Fracture, leg
See: Femur
Fracture, pelvic ring
– : injury classification 55-410-A-10
– : stabilisation techniques...................... 55-410-A-10

H

Hip, adult
– : acetabular deficiencies....................... 55-450-B-10
55-450-E-10
– : acetabular reconstruction................... 55-450-D-10
– : acetabular reconstruction, femoral
malignancies 55-480-C-10
– : acetabular revision 55-450-E-10
– : ankylosed hips.................................. 55-450-A-10
– : approach, acetabulum 55-400-A-10
– : approach, in femoral malignancies.......... 55-480-C-10
– : approach, Kocher-Langenbeck................ 55-400-A-10
55-400-F-10
– : approach, Ludloff.............................. 55-400-A-10
– : approach, Smith-Petersen 55-400-A-10
55-420-C-10
– : approach, supra-acetabular region.......... 55-420-A-10
– : approach, transfemoral 55-400-A-10
– : approach, transgluteal....................... 55-400-A-10
– : approach, transtrochanteric............... 55-400-A-10
– : approach, Watson-Jones.................... 55-400-A-10
55-400-D-10
– : approaches, general 55-400-A-10
– : arthrodesis....................................... 55-460-E-10
– : arthroplasty, ankylosed hips 55-450-A-10
– : arthroplasty, artificial hip joint in total
hip.. 55-430-E-10
– : arthroplasty, cement removal, femoral
cavity.. 55-440-C-10
– : arthroplasty, cementless total hip 55-440-D-10
– : arthroplasty, constrained total hip 55-440-A-10
– : arthroplasty, dislocations of total hip 55-440-A-10
– : arthroplasty, dysplasia and total hip 55-440-E-10

– : arthroplasty, hemiarthroplasty............... 55-400-C-10
– : arthroplasty, revision total hip, femoral
    approach... 55-460-B-10
– : arthroplasty, total hip........................ 55-430-D-10
– : arthroplasty, tribology of total hip.......... 55-430-E-10
– : arthroscopy.................................... 55-480-D-10
– : Bernese periacetabular osteotomy........... 55-420-C-10
– : cement removal, femoral cavity 55-440-A-10
– : Charnley cup 55-440-A-10
– : Chiari osteotomy 55-420-B-10
– : congenital dislocation 55-420-B-10
– : disarticulation 55-480-A-10
– : dislocation 55-400-B-10
– : dislocations of total hip prostheses 55-440-A-10
– : dysplasia, congenital 55-420-A-10
                                                    55-430-C-10
– : dysplastic hip 55-470-A-10
– : hemipelvectomy 55-470-E-10
– : infected hip prosthesis 55-460-B-20
– : infected hip prosthesis, resection 55-460-D-10
– : intertrochanteric osteotomy 55-400-D-10
– : ischiopubic tumours 55-470-D-10
– : non-union, femoral neck 55-400-D-10
– : periacetabular tumours........................ 55-470-C-10
– : resection, hip joint............................ 55-460-D-10
– : revision, failed femoral prosthesis 55-460-B-20
– : rotationplasty 55-470-E-10
– : sacral, trochanteric, ischiatic sores 55-480-E-10
– : subtrochanteric and trochanteric
    fracture 55-400-E-10
– : triple pelvic osteotomy (Tönnis).............. 55-410-E-10
– : upper femur osteotomies...................... 55-470-A-10
See also: Femur. Pelvic ring

Hip, children
– : acetabular fracture............................ 55-410-B-10
– : cerebral palsy................................. 55-430-A-10
– : congenital dislocation 55-420-B-10
– : congenital femoral deficiency 55-430-B-10
– : dysplasia, congenital 55-420-A-10
                                                    55-430-C-10
– : dysplasia, developmental (DDH)............ 55-410-B-10
– : dysplasia dislocation 55-410-D-10
– : limb reconstruction........................... 55-430-B-10
– : Pavlik's harness............................... 55-410-D-10
– : pelvic fractures............................... 55-410-B-10
– : pelvic ring fracture 55-410-B-10
– : Perthes' disease 55-420-D-10
– : proximal femoral deficiency 55-430-B-10
– : rotationplasty 55-430-B-10
– : slipped capital femoral epiphysis 55-420-E-10
– : upper femoral fracture........................ 55-410-B-10

I

Infection, orthopaedic surgery
– : femoral revision 55-460-C-10
– : infected hip prosthesis 55-460-C-10
– : infected hip prosthesis, joint resection..... 55-460-D-10
Instability, hip
– : ankylosed hips 55-450-A-10
– : dislocations.................................. 55-440-A-10

J

Judet R
– : coaptation, trochanteric-iliac.................. 55-460-D-10

K

Kocher-Langenbeck procedure, hip.............. 55-400-F-10

L

Leg
– : proximal femoral deficiency...................... 55-430-B-10
Lengthening
– : femoral neck.................................... 55-430-C-10

N

Nailing
– : Ender nail 55-400-E-10
– : Gamma nail.................................... 55-400-E-10
Necrosis
– : avascular, hip dysplasia........................ 55-410-D-10
                                                    55-430-C-10
– : cartilage 55-420-E-10
– : femoral head, acetabular fractures 55-400-F-10
– : femoral head in neck fractures 55-400-D-10
– : femoral head, osteonecrosis.................. 55-470-B-10
– : slipped capital femoral epiphysis............. 55-420-E-10

O

Orthosis
– : hip 55-440-A-10
Osteoarthritis, hip
– : arthroscopy.................................... 55-480-D-10
Osteosynthesis
– : femoral, in cerebral palsy...................... 55-430-A-10
Osteotomy
– : Bernese periacetabular 55-420-C-10
– : Chiari 55-420-B-10
– : double, triple pelvic (Tönnis) 55-410-E-10
– : dysplastic hip................................. 55-470-A-10
– : extended trochanter for cement removal 55-440-C-10
– : femoral... 55-470-A-10
– : femoral neck lengthening 55-430-C-10
– : femoral osteotomy in cerebral palsy 55-430-A-10
– : innominate, Perthes' disease 55-420-D-10
– : intertrochanteric.............................. 55-400-D-10
                                                    55-470-A-10
– : Kramer's base of femoral neck 55-420-E-10
– : Pauwels 55-400-D-10
– : pelvic, in DDH................................ 55-410-E-10
– : pelvic, innominate (Salter).................... 55-410-E-10
– : pelvic, Pemberton, hip 55-410-E-10
– : pertrochanteric 55-420-E-10
– : Southwick's pertrochanteric.................. 55-420-E-10
– : subtrochanteric shortening.................... 55-470-A-10
– : valgisation 55-400-D-10
– : valgus, femur.................................. 55-470-A-10
– : varus, femur................................... 55-470-A-10

P

Palsy
– : hip, cerebral 55-430-A-10
Pelvic ring
– : approaches..................................... 55-410-A-10
– : Bernese periacetabular osteotomy............ 55-420-C-10
– : fractures, children 55-410-B-10
– : fractures, dislocations......................... 55-410-A-10
– : injury classification........................... 55-410-A-10
– : innominate osteotomy (Salter)................ 55-410-E-10
– : ischiopubic tumours........................... 55-470-D-10
– : osteotomy in DDH............................ 55-410-E-10
– : Pemberton osteotomy.......................... 55-410-E-10
– : periacetabular tumours 55-470-C-10
Perthes' disease............................... 55-420-B-10
                                                   55-420-D-10

Plate
– : acetabular fractures........................... 55-400-F-10
– : pelvic ring injuries 55-410-A-10
– : proximal femur fractures 55-400-E-10
Pressure sores
– : sacral, trochanteric, ischiatic................... 55-480-E-10
– : trochanteric, hip joint resection................ 55-460-D-10
Prosthesis for amputation
– : Canadian type................................. 55-480-A-10
                                                   55-480-B-10
Prosthesis, hip
– : acetabular reconstruction..................... 55-450-D-10
– : acetabular revision............................ 55-450-E-10
– : acetabular ring................................ 55-450-B-10
– : after rotationplasty........................... 55-470-E-10
– : ankylosed hips 55-450-A-10
– : cement removal 55-440-C-10
– : cementless THA............................... 55-440-D-10
– : constrained total hip 55-440-A-10
– : dislocations of total hip....................... 55-440-A-10
– : failed femoral................................. 55-460-B-20
– : femoral endoprosthesis 55-400-C-10
– : femoral revision............................... 55-460-A-10
– : infected 55-460-C-10
– : infected, resection............................ 55-460-D-10
– : material for.................................... 55-430-D-10
– : pelvic 55-470-C-10
– : saddle 55-470-C-10
– : THA, congenital hip disease.................. 55-440-A-10
– : THA revision.................................. 55-460-B-10
– : total hip arthroplasty......................... 55-430-D-10
– : tribology of THR 55-430-E-10
– : trochanteric and subtrochanteric
    fractures 55-400-E-10
Pseudarthrosis
– : femoral head fractures 55-400-B-10
– : femoral neck................................... 55-400-D-10
– : pelvic ring fractures 55-410-A-10
– : proximal femur fractures 55-400-E-10

R

Rotationplasty
– : proximal femoral deficiency.................... 55-430-B-10
– : tumour of the proximal femur 55-470-E-10
– : Van Nes 55-430-B-10

S

Screw
– : dynamic hip screw 55-400-C-10
                                                   55-400-E-10
Septic arthritis
– : hip, arthrodesis............................... 55-460-E-10
– : hip, joint resection............................ 55-460-D-10
Skin coverage, general
See: Pressure sores
Skin coverage, hip
– : sacral, trochanteric, ischiatic regions........ 55-480-E-10

T

Tumour
– : femoral malignancies.......................... 55-480-C-10
– : hemipelvectomy 55-480-B-10
– : hip disarticulation............................. 55-480-A-10
– : ischiopubic 55-470-D-10
– : periacetabular 55-470-C-10
– : proximal femur, rotationplasty................ 55-470-E-10